The Human Bone Marrow: Anatomy, Physiology, and Pathophysiology

Volume I

Editors

Sidney Trubowitz, M.D.
Veterans Administration Medical Center
East Orange, New Jersey
and
Professor of Medicine
CMDNJ-New Jersey Medical School
Newark, New Jersey

Stephen Davis, M.D.
Veterans Administration Medical Center
East Orange, New Jersey
and
Associate Professor of Medicine
CMDNJ-New Jersey Medical School
Newark, New Jersey

CRC Press, Inc.
Boca Raton, Florida

Library of Congress Cataloging in Publication Data
Main entry under title:

The Human bone marrow.

Bibliography: p.
Includes indexes.
1. Marrow—Diseases—Diagnosis. 2. Marrow—Biopsy, Needle. 3. Marrow—Examination. 4. Diagnosis, Cytologic. I. Trubowitz, Sidney, 1911– . II. Davis, Stephen, 1943– . [DNLM: 1. Bone marrow. WH 380 H918]
RC645.7.H85 616.4′1 81-18195
ISBN 0-8493-6105-2 (v. 1) AACR2
ISBN 0-8493-6106-0 (v. 2)

Direct all inquiries to CRC Press, Inc., 2000 Corporate Blvd., N.W., Boca Raton, Florida, 33431.

International Standard Book Number 0-8493-6105-2 (Volume I)
International Standard Book Number 0-8493-6106-0 (Volume II)

Library of Congress Card Number 81-18195
Printed in the United States

THE EDITORS

Sidney Trubowitz, M.D., is a graduate of Columbia College, Columbia University in New York City and received his medical degree from Rush Medical College (University of Chicago). On completion of his clinical training he was called to active duty and served in the Pacific Theatre during World War II for some 3 years. On his return to civilian life he spent a year at the National Transfusion Center in Paris and then joined the Veterans Administration Medical Center, East Orange, New Jersey where he served as Chief of the Hematology Section. He is Professor of Medicine, New Jersey College of Medicine, Newark New Jersey. His major research interests have centered on the alkaline phosphatase of granulocytes and on the structure and function of the bone marrow matrix. He is a member of the American College of Physicians, the American Society of Hematology, and the Royal Society of Tropical Medicine.

Stephen Davis, M.D., graduated magna cum laude from Brooklyn College of Pharmacy, Long Island University in Brooklyn, New York and obtained his doctorate in medicine at New York's Mount Sinai School of Medicine. His training in neoplastic and blood diseases was obtained at the National Cancer Institute (NIH), Bethesda, Maryland and the Tufts-New England Medical Center, Boston, Massachusetts. He served as Chief of the Oncology-Hematology Section at the Veterans Administration Medical Center, East Orange, New Jersey and Associate Professor of Medicine, New Jersey Medical School, Newark, New Jersey. His research interests are varied but have concentrated on normal and malignant lymphocyte biology, thymic hormones, and human and experimental lung carcinomas. He is also active in many scientific societies particularly the American Society of Clinical Oncologists, the American Society of Hematology, and the American Association for Cancer Research.

CONTRIBUTORS

Hal E. Broxmeyer, Ph.D.
Assistant Member
Sloan Kettering Institute for Cancer Research and
Assistant Professor
Cornell University
New York, New York

Professor Wenceslao Calvo, M.D.
Department of Clinical Physiology
University of Ulm
Federal Republic of Germany

Stephen Davis, M.D.
VA Medical Center
East Orange, New Jersey and
Health Research Institute
Fairleigh-Dickinson University
Madison, New Jersey and
Associate Professor of Medicine
CMDNJ-New Jersey Medical School
Newark, New Jersey

E. Kelemen, M.D., D.Sc.
Professor of Medicine
Semmelweis University Medical School
Budapest, Hungary

Alexander Nakeff, Ph.D.
Assistant Professor
Cancer Biology in Radiology
Mallinckrodt Institute of Radiology
Washington University School of Medicine
St. Louis, Missouri

Young K. Park, M.D.
Assistant Professor
CMDNJ-New Jersey Medical School
Attending Physician
VA Medical Center
East Orange, New Jersey

Pietro Rambotti, M.D.
Assistant Professor of Medicine
Instituto di Clinica Medica Generale e Terapia Medica del Universita di Perugia
Perugia, Italy

Nydia G. Testa, M.D., Ph.D.
Senior Research Scientist
Paterson Laboratories
Christie Hospital and
Holt Radium Institute
Manchester
Great Britain

Sidney Trubowitz, M.D.
VA Medical Center
East Orange, New Jersey and
Professor of Medicine
CMDNJ-New Jersey Medical School
Newark, New Jersey

TABLE OF CONTENTS
THE HUMAN BONE MARROW:
ANATOMY, PHYSIOLOGY, AND PATHOPHYSIOLOGY

Volume I

Volume II

TABLE OF CONTENTS

Volume I

Chapter 1

INTRODUCTION

Sidney Trubowitz and Stephen Davis

In all epochs and in all places blood assumed a place of special importance in human experience. Blood was thought to be inextricably tied to the life force itself, a concept expressed in countless ways in the recorded literature of all people. Aristotle,[1] on observing the rhythmic motion of the anlage of the heart of a bird's embryo, saw it as the origin, the source of life itself, and the very embodiment of the soul. Blood stirred the imagination of both the poet and the philosopher, and though the latter may have couched his thoughts in more prosaic phrases, his insights were no less poetic.

A major and significant advance in the comprehension of the composition of blood was made in 1673, when Leeuwenhoek described red blood cells and lymphocytes in a small drop of lymph he placed under the lens of his microscope. Hewson[2] later identified these forms in blood itself.

The origin of the blood cells remained obscure for some 200 years. As late as 1858, Virchow,[3] in his celebrated lectures on cellular pathology, described the whole history of the red cell as "still invested with a mysterious obscurity, inasmuch as no positive information has even at the present time been obtained with regard to the origin of these elements." Virchow knew that nucleated red blood cells exist in the blood during the first few months of fetal life, and since he postulated that the nonnucleated red corpuscles could not propagate, he rejected all theories which assumed red cell propagation by vesicle formation in the blood and argued that "everything points to a probability of a supply from without." Ten years later, in 1868, Neumann[4] and Bizozzero[5] independently proclaimed the bone marrow as the major source of blood cells in the adult, a controversial view that was finally accepted under the weight of Claude Bernard's[6] prestigious authority.

Further progress in the investigation of the structural and dynamic characteristics of the hemopoietic and nonhemopoietic cell lines in the marrow and their alterations in disease had to wait until 1929 when Arinkin[7] introduced the intravital bone marrow aspiration technique.

The last 50 years, under the weight of the great advances in microscopy, cytochemistry, immunology, biochemistry, molecular biology, tissue and cell culture, etc. have witnessed a veritable explosion of information on the origin of the blood cells in the bone marrow from the morphologically unrecognizable stem cells through the recognizable marrow elements to the mature blood cell elements and the role of the marrow microenvironment and the control mechanisms of marrow cellular proliferation and differentiation in both health and disease.

The purpose of the present monograph is to provide the clinician and student with a detailed account of our contemporary understanding of the structure and function of the bone marrow and how this knowledge may serve in the investigation of disease in the clinic. The underlying assumption of this volume is the basic dialectic unity of structure and function, and that the static morphologic information obtained from the commonly employed clinical techniques of examination of marrow aspirates can be transformed into its more dynamic physiologic counterpart which provides more meaningful insight into the clinical problem under study.

To this end the first half of the book has been devoted to the discussion of the anatomy, embryology of the marrow, and of the current concepts of the stem cells, their proliferation and differentiation in the marrow, and the ultimate delivery of mature elements into the circulation. Much of the knowledge of these aspects of the marrow has been derived from studies of laboratory animals and from in vitro cultures of both human and animal stem cells, chiefly the latter. Many gaps necessarily exist in our knowledge of this basic area of marrow function, and the animal studies do provide a useful framework and overall gestalt for understanding the mechanisms by which the human marrow produces the blood cell elements.

The latter half of this monograph deals with the morphological and physiological considerations of the recognizable elements of the bone marrow and their alterations in disease.

Since the overall aim has been the integration of information derived from different disciplines, some morphologic, some chemical, some immunologic, and not the compilation of images in the form of an atlas, photographs of normal and abnormal immature and differentiated cells of marrow and blood have been kept to a minimum. Photographs of the cells of the marrow and blood are abundantly available in many excellent published atlases to which the reader is referred.

REFERENCES

1. **Naegeli, O.,** *Blutkrankheiten und Blutdiagnostik,* Julius Springer, Berlin, 1923, 1.
2. **Hewson, W. and Johnson, J.,** *No. 72 Pauls Church Yard,* London, 1774; as reprinted in Yoffey, J. M. and Courtice, F. C., Eds., *Lymphatics, Lymph and Lymphmyeloid Complex,* 3rd ed., Harvard, Cambridge, 1970, 3.
3. **Virchow, R.,** *Cellular Pathology,* translated from the 2nd German edition by Chance, F., Dover Publ., New York, 1971, 258.
4. **Neumann, E.,** Ueber die Bedeutung des Knochenmarks fur die Blutbildung, *Cbl. Med. Wiss.,* 6, 659, 1868.
5. **Bizozzero, G.,** Sul midolo delle ossa, *Morgagni,* p. 465, 1869.
6. **Bernard, C.,** Du rôle de la moelle des os dans la function de sang, *C.R. Acad. Sci.,* 68, 1869.
7. **Arinkin, M. I.,** Die intravitale Untersuchung des Knochenmarkes, *Fol. Haematol.,* 38, 233, 1929.

Chapter 2

PRENATAL HEMATOPOIESIS IN HUMAN BONE MARROW AND ITS DEVELOPMENTAL ANTECEDENTS

Endre Kelemen and Wenceslao Calvo

TABLE OF CONTENTS

I. INTRODUCTION

The description of the development of the human hematopoietic organs as it appears in this chapter is based on the comparison of the available literature on this subject with the data obtained from the study of our material* which includes nearly 400 human embryos, fetuses, and newborn infants.[1]

The fertilization age of our samples, which is 2 weeks less than the so-called menstruation age frequently used by clinicians, was calculated according to Patten.[2] The estimation of the age of early embryos and fetuses is not very accurate. Data taken from the literature regarding the time of appearance of a cell type of function are sometimes in disagreement. Frequently, 2 or 3 weeks difference can be found in the estimation of certain phenomena. Blood cell formation in the human fetal marrow begins during the third month. The marrow is the third and definitive major site of hematopoiesis. It is preceded by liver hematopoiesis, which starts during the second month, and by diffuse hematopoiesis taking place in extra-embryonic and embryonic mesenchymal tissue from the beginning of the third week. In order to better understand the development of the marrow, we shall describe premarrow hematopoiesis first.

II. SOME ASPECTS OF PREMARROW HEMATOPOIESIS IN MAN

During early development, there is a primitive type of erythropoiesis that originates in extraembryonic and embryonic sites. This type is the first to appear, lasts until the 12th week, and is replaced by the definitive type of erythropoiesis originating first in the liver and continuing in the marrow.

*This material was made available to us by members of the Second Department of Gynecology and Obstetrics of the Semmelweis University of Budapest (Hungary) and the Department of Gynecology and Obstetrics of the University of Ulm (Federal Republic of Germany). Some samples were sent to us by Dr. Lucarelli (Pesaro, Italy) and by Dr. J. M. Vera (Castellón, Spain). We express our thanks to all our colleagues who made this study possible.

A. Primitive Hematopoiesis

Most of the primitive hematopoiesis is erythroid. It starts in extraembryonic areas such as the yolk sac, chorion, and body stalk. The predominant role of the yolk sac in primitive hematopoiesis has been generally accepted,[3] although this opinion is based on observations made in the development of animals. Investigating murine hematopoiesis, Metcalf[4] suggested that the development of intraembryonic hematopoiesis requires the presence of an intact yolk sac, and that the migration of stem cells from the yolk sac to the embryo is necessary to start intraembryonic hematopoiesis. Luckett[5] emphasized that blood islands are restricted to the yolk sac in 16- to 19-day-old human embryos. Some observations, however, do not support the predominant role of the yolk sac. There is, among others, the work of Dieterlen-Lievre,[6] Le Douarin, using quail-chick chimeras,[7] Symann et al. in the mouse,[8] Turpen in the frog,[9] Dandy,[10] Jägerroos in man,[3] and Mazanec.[11]

On the basis of studies by Le Douarin and her school, Latsis et al.[12] recently stated that the concentration of CFU-S (colony forming units in spleen) in the 48-hr-old quail embryo is 100 times higher than that of the yolk sac, both after 48 and 60 hr of incubation.

A very important milestone in the developmental process is the transition from precirculatory to circulatory stage in early intrauterine life. Although some ineffective heart contractions begin by day 22 in man, coordinated contractions of the heart resulting in a unidirectional flow begin by the end of the 4th week.[13] According to Gilmour,[14] it is certain that the umbilical circulation between the body stalk and the human embryo is established before the vitelline circulation connects the yolk sac to the embryo. There is no general agreement about the time and place of the beginning of hematopoiesis.* Several blood islands were described in the yolk sac of a 2-week-old human embryo,[15b] and other blood islands were found in the body stalk. Those of the body stalk were larger and more mature than those of the yolk sac.[16] Numerous primitive erythroblasts were found in the heart blood at a time when neither yolk sac nor chorionic circulation was demonstrable.[17] Blood island formation in the chorion preceeded yolk sac circulation.[10] According to Knoll,[156] extravascular blood cell clusters cannot be found after the 4th week in the human yolk sac, a finding not confirmed by Fukuda[18] or ourselves.[1]

There were three precirculatory samples in our material corresponding to the critical period of 3- to 3-1/2-week-old embryos. Differentiated primitive erythroblasts containing light microscopically demonstrable hemoglobin were found in the chorionic vessels in each of the embryos. The extravascular cell clusters of the yolk sacs consisted of differentiated mesenchymal cells, at a time when the predominant cell type of the chorionic vessels was a type-II embryonic erythroblast.[19] Yolk sac priority in the beginning of hematopoiesis was, therefore, not demonstrable in these few samples. However, negative findings such as this cannot be conclusive unless the entire material is sampled in serial sections, which was not the case with these embryos. Local formation of the earliest blood cells seems to occur in extraembryonic as well as in embryonic mesenchyme. The vascular endothelium was thought to be the primary source of hemocytoblasts, primitive erythroblasts, and phagocytes, whereas detachment of endothelial lining cells could furnish, thereafter, phagocytic cells only.[20]

Vessels arise from mesodermal cells independently in three areas: the yolk sac, the chorion (with the body stalk), and the embryo.[14] If the earliest blood cell clusters were formed locally, the contribution of the different areas should depend on the volume of the blood-cell-containing vessels. In human beings, the chorion has much more ex-

*In the young chicken blastoderm BFU-E becomes detectable at the primitive streak stage (16 to 18 hr) and amounts to 1.600/blastoderm at 48 hr.[15a]

traembryonic mesenchyme than the yolk sac. Therefore, one could conclude that the blood cell contribution of the chorion to primitive blood formation may exceed that of the yolk sac.

It is difficult to investigate the origin of the stem cells. However large the contribution of the chorion could be, the main question is to determine the site of origin of the pluripotent stem cell preceding primitive erythroblast formation. There is no firm standpoint on this question. Although the ability of stem cells to migrate via circulation and their capacity to seed is unquestionable, local stem cell formation appears to be possible. Using alkaline phosphatase reaction as a marker, it was shown that marrow regeneration in the shielded, evacuated, femur of an 8 Gy-irradiated mouse bearing a heterologous rat marrow transplant, was caused by mouse cells.[211]

1. Embryonic Macrophages and Presumed Monoblasts

Embryonic macrophages can be found in each yolk sac sample.[3] Their number could reach 10% of all intravascular cells. In addition, there were up to 2% presumed monoblasts in certain yolk sac smears. These cells were about 15 μm in diameter and had a large, irregularly shaped nucleus with light chromatin structure, with or without visible nucleoli. Their narrow, homogeneous cytoplasm was dark blue when stained with the May-Grünwald-Giemsa method. The connection between these cells and the macrophages is, at present, hypothetical.

2. Erythropoiesis

The early embryo produces a primitive red cell population which has a limited life span and which is substituted by a self-perpetuating red cell population of definitive type. A simple classification for the primitive erythroblasts was given in our *Atlas*.[1] Primitive erythropoiesis starts at the end of the third week and practically ceases at about the 9th week of gestation.

Intraembryonic primitive erythroblasts were first seen toward the end of the 4th week, at the time when circulation is established. There is no adequate explanation for the shift from primitive to definitive erythropoiesis and there is no agreement in the literature on whether definitive erythropoiesis starts from a new stem cell population or originates from a colonizing progenitor of the primitive stem cell pool.

3. Erythroblastic Islands

Groups of erythroblasts surrounding a macrophage (erythroblastic islands) were thought to be absent during intrauterine life in humans.[22] In our *Atlas*[1] we showed such islands in the marrow and in the liver of human fetuses, and one of us, in collaboration with Jánossa,[23a] succeeded in finding them not only in smears prepared from the yolk sac, liver, bone marrow, and circulating blood (heart), but also in sections of glutaraldehyde-fixed tissue. Therefore, the erythroblastic islands cannot be regarded as artifacts of the smear technique. They can be found even at the earliest stages of human erythropoiesis.[23b] Both primitive and definitive erythroblasts can produce "rosettes" with macrophages, although rosettes with primitive erythroblasts are very rare. Preferential attachment of early precursors to the central macrophage suggests that, besides the well known phagocytosis, an information flow may take place in these islands, probably in both directions, i.e., to and from the central macrophage.

4. Differential Counts for Primitive Erythroblasts

From all of our material, we investigated 31 semithin sections and 38 MGG-stained smears from the yolk sac, chorion, and embryo of 4-1/2- to 10-week-old samples. In the 4-1/2-week-old embryo, about 60% of all erythropoietic cells were of the very

Table 1
DIFFERENTIALS FOR INTRAVASCULAR PRIMITIVE ERYTHROBLASTS

May-Grünwald-Giemsa Stained Smears

Fertiliz. age (weeks)	Primitive erythroblasts, % Pre—I and I					II					III				
	Y	S	C	L	B	Y	S	C	L	B	Y	S	C	L	B
3—4	97[a]	78	32			3	20	67			0	2	1		
4—5	**62**		**63**	**42**		30		30	39		8		7	19	
5—6	**39**		**42**	**43**	**33**	37		39	42	55	24		19	15	12
6—7	20		21	24	19	**46**		**56**	**57**	**57**	34		23	19	24
7—8	12		19	17	9	**45**		**34**	**56**	**34**	43		47	27	57
8—9	7		10	3	5	22		22	16	18	**71**		**68**	**81**	**79**
9—10			0		1			2		9			**98**		**90**

Note: Y = Yolk sac, S = Body stalk, C = Chorion, L = Liver, B = Blood.

[a] Undifferentiated mesenchymal blood island cells. Each number represents 1 to 3 samples. The space separates precirculatory stage from circulatory stage.

early type, and less than 10% were mature, nucleated red cells. In the later stages of development, there was a continuing shift in the differential count from the very early to the later stages of primitive erythroblasts. In the 8- to 10-week-old fetus, there is a preponderance of mature, (type-III) primitive erythroblasts (Table 1). It is shortly after this stage of development of hematopoiesis, that these primitive erythropoietic cells disappear altogether from extraembryonic and embryonic tissues. The simultaneous investigation of different areas enables us to suggest that, at least from 4-1/2 weeks onward (i.e., at a time when circulation has already started), the stage of differentiation of the primitive erythroblasts is similar at each place (Figure 1). As already noted, precirculatory samples exhibit a different pattern: the yolk sac has numerous primordial mesenchymal cells, while other hematopoietic areas contain differentiated erythroblasts.[1,3,11] If we consider that the stage of hematopoietic pattern is different at simultaneously investigated different areas of the early bone marrow hematopoiesis, the seemingly sharp contrast between primitive and definitive hematopoiesis becomes apparent. There is no accepted proof to explain this discrepancy, and the only thing which appears to be valid is that at least one factor having an important role in primitive vs. definitive hematopoiesis is different. One possible explanation could be the relative uniformity of the microenvironment before organogenesis.

5. *Hemoglobins—Terminal Differentiation of Stem Cells*

The so-called embryonic hemoglobins (Gower I and II, Portland I) are present in the 5-week-old embryo and remain detectable up to the 12th week.[24] These embryonic hemoglobins are produced by the primitive erythroblasts formed overwhelmingly at extraembryonic sites. The hemoglobin which predominates in the blood during the hepatic phase is the fetal hemoglobin (F). The adult-type hemoglobin (A) starts to appear in the blood of the fetus at about the 8th to 10th week of gestation, it remains below 20% up to the 32nd week, it rises relatively quickly to 30 to 40% until birth and reaches nearly 100% at about the 28th postnatal week. Wood and Weatherall suggested that the

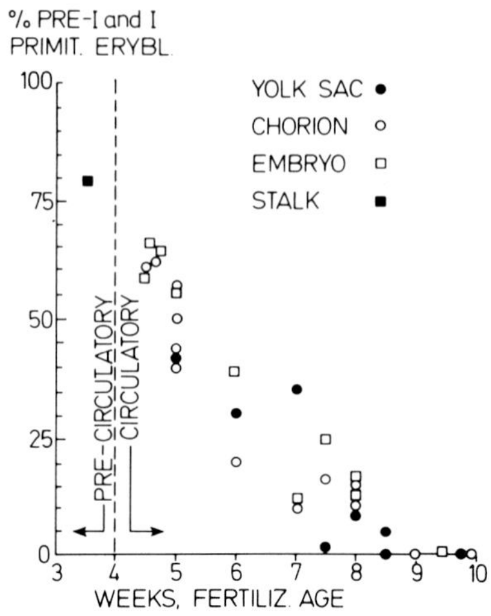

FIGURE 1. Percentage of pre-I and type-I primitive erythroblasts in the yolk sac, body stalk, chorion, and embryo according to age. (Clasification as outlined in Reference 1). The stage of differentiation of primitive erythroblasts is similar at each place, at least after circulatory contacts had been established between the different areas.

hgb-F and A production are under general control rather than the influence of local factors.[25] This means that there is no evidence of any difference in beta- and gamma-chain synthesis prior to or during the switch, i.e., this process is synchronous in all erythroid tissues. On the other hand, progenies of sheep fetal hematopoietic cells produced adult hemoglobin when transplanted into the adult animal at a time when predominently fetal hemoglobin would have been formed if the transplanted stem cells continued to express a predetermined development program.[26a] On the other hand, adult hemopoietic cells continue to produce red cells with adult hemoglobin when transplanted into the sheep fetus.[26b]

The reason the human embryo and fetus produce different red cell populations and different hemoglobins during development is unknown. In any event, each of the stages of differentiation of the erythroid stem cells contains a characteristic gamma- and beta-chain production program. Primitive BFU-E has a program that permits mostly gamma-gene expression, while the most differentiated BFU-E of the normal adult contains a developmental program that permits mainly beta-gene transcription. This means that gamma-gene is inversely related to the degree of differentiation of burst forming units.[27a] In this sense, during the fetal stage of development, terminal maturation may take place from erythroid stem cells that have only gone through the initial stages of erythroid stem cell differentiation. As pointed out,[27a] most instances of the reappearance of hgb-F (such as certain kinds of severe aplasia, certain types of leukemia, early regeneration following marrow transplantation, some types of severe erythropoietic stress) can be attributed to deviation from the normal process of differentiation of erythroid stem cells. Nevertheless, perinatal hemoglobin switching and the hemoglobin switching of cultured adult erythroid precursors do not appear to involve population changes in the precursors.[27b]

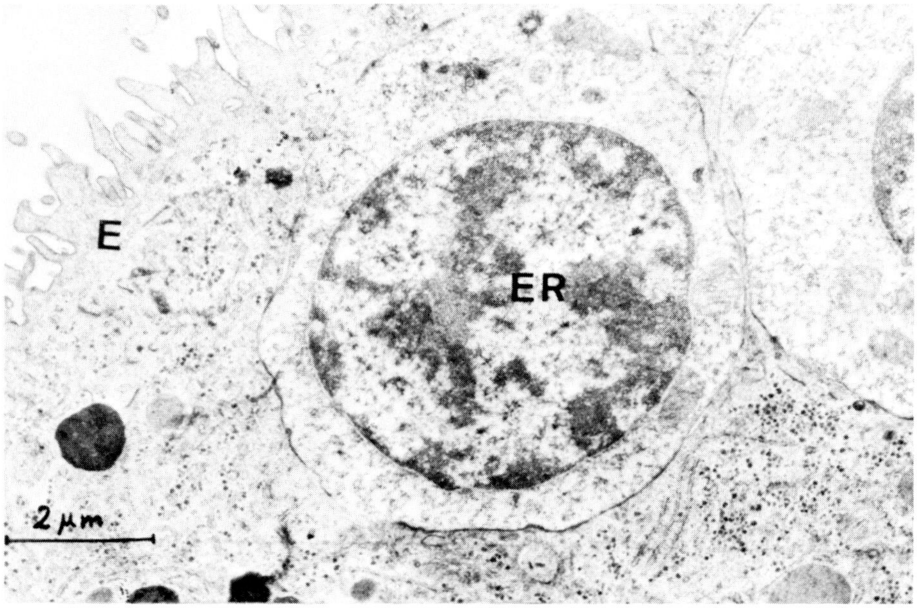

FIGURE 2. A proerythroblast (ER) is shown in contact with an endodermal cell of the yolk sac of a 7-week-old embryo. Observe the brush border of the endodermal cell (upper left) and the fact that this cell surrounds the erythroblasts completely.

It is tempting to speculate that a similar alteration in terminal differentiation could exist for the lymphocyte-producing systems, as well as for the granulocytic, macrophage, and megakaryocytic. It may be that the differences between embryonic and fetal or adult hematopoietic cell systems that we describe in this chapter are due to this factor, that is, early terminal differentiation in the earlier periods of intrauterine life.

6. Presumed Stem Cells

About 0.1% of nucleated cells found in smears of blood up to the 8th week, were unidentified lymphocyte-like cells. These cells were absent in the subsequent weeks, even when thousands of circulating cells were differentiated. However, these presumed stem cells were not found in semithin sections in either of the embryonic tissues which we investigated, even before the 8th week. The explanation for this discrepancy is not known.

7. The Role of the Yolk Sac Endoderm

Although the localization of embryonic hematopoietic cells in the endodermal epithelium of the human yolk sac was described several decades ago,[3] the nature and significance of the localization has remained obscure.[28]

The work of Fukuda,[18] as well as our ultramicrographs, demonstrated that there is an intimate contact between yolk sac endoderm and hematopoietic precursor cells (Figure 2). In addition to interdigitations, various types of intercellular contacts could be demonstrated. These contacts, especially the gap-like ones and those with associated electron dense cytoplasmic areas, suggest intercellular communication.[28] The presence of these contacts, however, does not mean that endodermal associations are indispensable for hematopoietic differentiation.

8. Yolk Sac Hematopoiesis

The hematopoietic cells of the early human embryo tend to be compartmentalized. Early hematopoietic precursors, including those that do not contain stainable hemoglobin, are located extravascularly, near to, or in the endodermal layer, whereas differentiated primitive erythroblasts with abundant eosinophilic cytoplasm are located mainly in the sinusoids or in the small vessels.[18,29]

The first clusters of hematopoietic cells in the yolk sac consist nearly exclusively of early primitive erythroblasts, but at the end of the 6th week at least one third of erythroblasts belong to the definitive series. These definitive erythroblasts appear to originate in the yolk sac, because only a few of them could be detected at this stage of development in the circulation.

Degenerative changes in the yolk sac were found in our material as early as the beginning of the 4th week. This confirms previous observations.[3] Numerous macrophages appeared to be present in certain specimens. Endodermal hematopoietic cell clusters were described,[1,18] but after the end of the 7th week it was difficult to find them in this location.

B. Definitive Hematopoiesis

It is difficult to precisely establish the time of appearance of the first blood cells of definitive type and their precursors in the parenchyma of the liver. The beginning of liver hematopoiesis can be traced to the end of the 4th week of gestation. Shortly after this, hematopoiesis of definitive type commences and this is almost exclusively erythropoietic. Liver hematopoiesis is, then, the major source of blood cells until the 5th or 6th month, when it begins to decline, leaving the marrow as the major and definitive site of hematopoiesis.

No "primitive" lymphopoiesis had, hitherto, been recognized. Lymphopoiesis, either primitive or definitive, also appears to start in the liver, where antigen-carrying T lymphocytes could be identified in the 5- to 6-week-old embryo.

1. Liver Hematopoiesis

The largest area of premarrow hematopoiesis is the liver. As previously mentioned, liver hematopoiesis starts at the end of the 4th week. During a short period of time (about a week), hematopoiesis is present in the liver sinuses but is not yet demonstrable within the liver parenchyme. At the end of the 5th week, groups of erythroblasts appear intermixed with hepatocytes, and from the 6th week on the number of the blood forming cells increases very rapidly. The proportion of hematopoietic cells during the 5th week is only ca. 10% of all cells found in the liver. They increase to 70% during the 8th week, and remain at about this level until the 21st week. Thereafter, hematopoietic cell representation slowly declines.

The weight of the embryonic liver is less than 0.1 g at the 8th week; 1 g during the 10th week; about 10 g at 16 to 18 weeks; about 100 g at 30 to 32 weeks; and around 130 to 190 g at term, depending on the weight of the fetus.

On the basis of 62 samples, the total hematopoietic cell mass has been estimated as follows: about 10^6 cells at the 6th week; 10^7 at the 7th week; 10^8 at 9 to 10 weeks; 10^9 at 13 to 15 weeks; and 10^{10} at 20 to 22 weeks. Only a few samples were obtained in good condition from the last trimester of fetal life, but the total cell mass of hematopoietic cells was calculated to be about 10^9 at term. Since the weight of the liver increases rapidly from the 22nd week until term, the decrease of the number of blood forming cells in one order of magnitude represents a drastic reduction in the proportion of hematopoietic cells in relation to the total cell population of the liver.

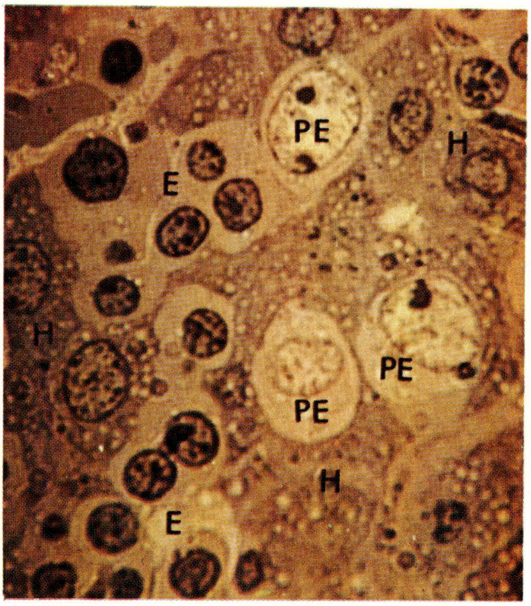

PLATE 1. Section of the liver at the 5th week of gestation. The erythroblasts (E) and hemocytoblasts-proerythroblasts (PE) are in contact with the endodermal derived hepatocytes (H). The relationship between the red cell precursors and the endodermal or endodermal derived cells is the same in the yolk sac and in the liver.

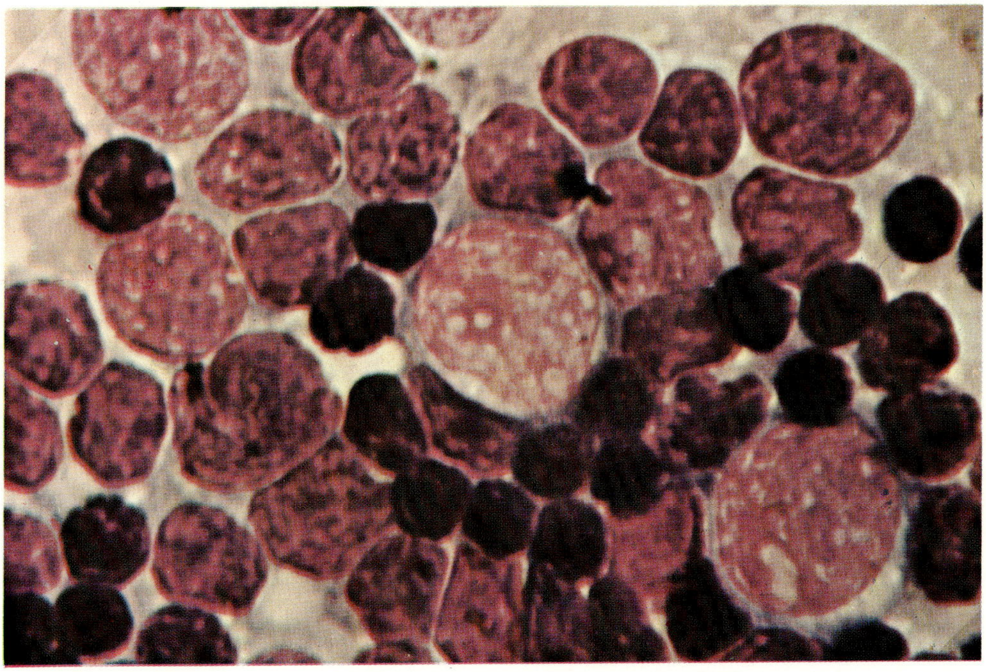

PLATE 2. Smear of the thymus at the 16th week of gestation. The figure shows small thymocytes with darkly stained nuclei and numerous precursor cells of various sizes and degree of chromatin density. (MGG stain; magnification × 2000.)

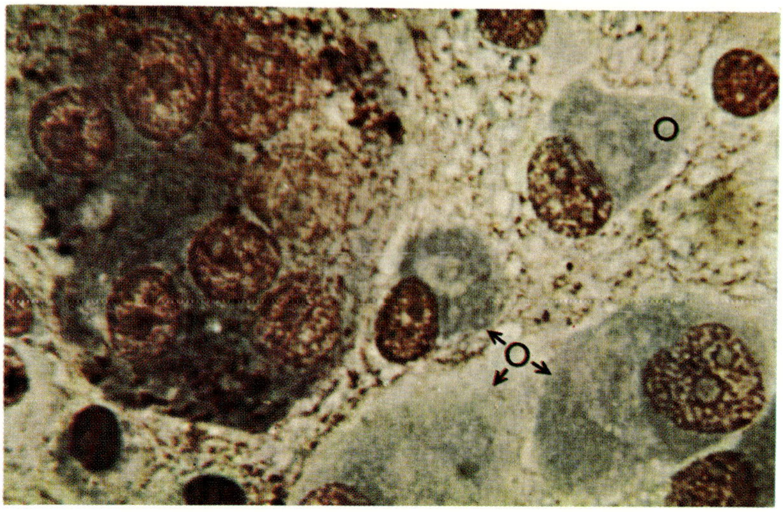

PLATE 3. Smear of the humerus of a 12-week-old fetus showing several osteoblasts (O). At the left is a large osteoclast with seven nuclei. In contrast to megakaryocytes, its nuclei are separated and each has a large nucleolus. (MGG stain; magnification × 2000.)

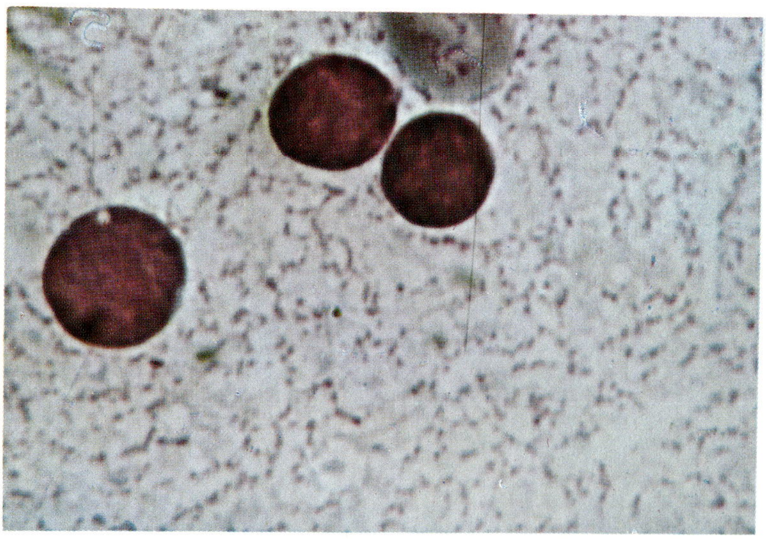

PLATE 4. Smear from the rib of a 9-week-old fetus, showing three small, lymphocyte-like cells with scanty cytoplasm (8 to 11 μm in diameter). Note the cytoplasmic vacuole in the largest cell.

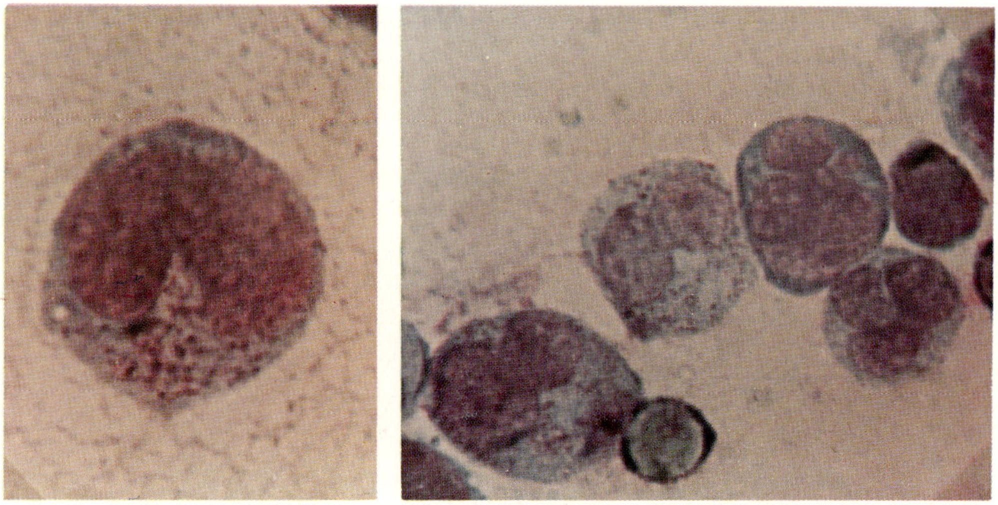

A B

PLATE 5(A). Ulnar smear from a 10-week-old fetus, showing a large fetal monocytoid granuloblast, 20 μm in diameter. Note the eccentric kidney-shaped nucleus, the concentration of azurophilic granules around the Golgi area, and the abundance of cytoplasm at that side of the cell. (B) Vertebral smear from a 13-week-old fetus. There is a group of early monocytoid granuloblasts. Note the variability of the nuclear shape in the cells, both with and without azurophilic granules.

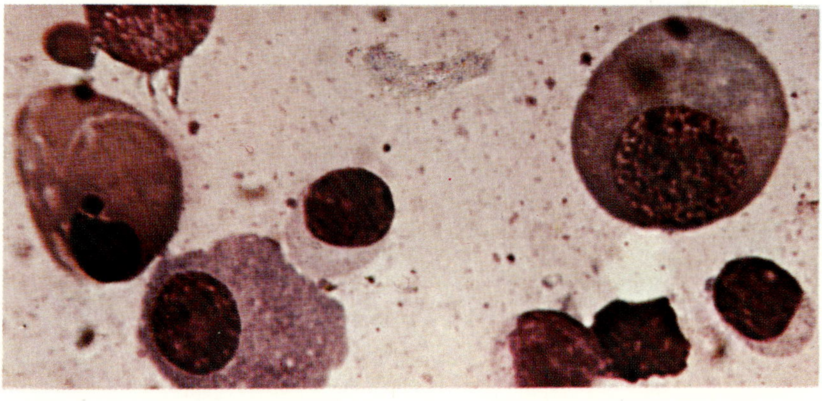

PLATE 6. Bone marrow smear from the blood of a 74-year-old untreated, seriously ill pernicious anemia patient. Note a type I primitive erythroblast at the right upper corner, and a type III primitive erythroblast with eccentric nucleus and abundant eosinophilic cytoplasma at the left corner.

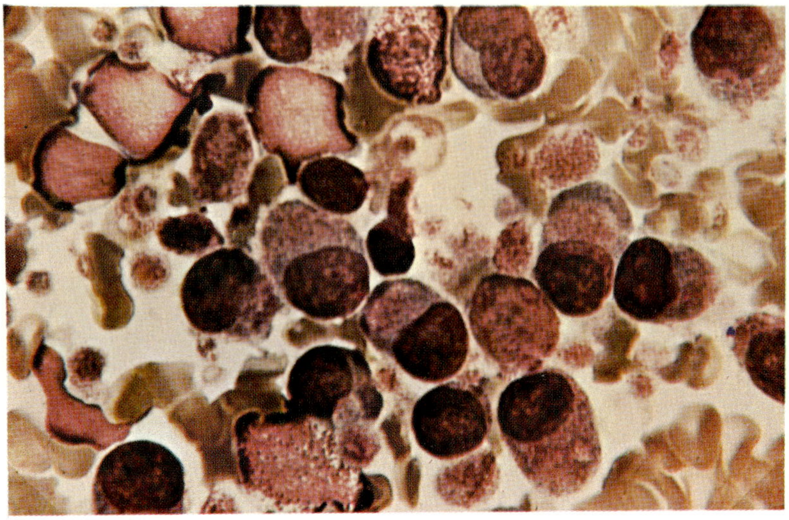

PLATE 7. The figure shows a micromegakaryocyte cluster at the lower half of the picture, found in the smear of blood of a recently splenectomized 53-year-old patient with myelofibrosis.

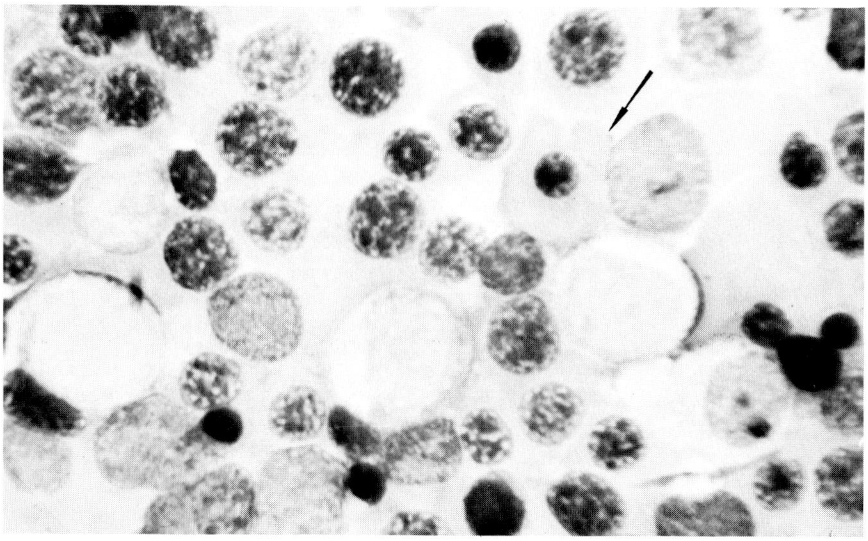

FIGURE 3. Smear of the liver of an 8-week-old fetus. The arrow shows a primitive erythrocyte with large, deeply stained cytoplasm and small compact nucleus. Most of the other cells in this figure are red cell precursors of definitive type in various stages of differentiation. The three large cells in the lower part of the figure, with pale nuclei and light blue cytoplasm seem to be of lymphoblastic type.

a. Hemocytoblasts and Macrophages

Large, lightly stained, benzidine-negative hemocytoblasts appeared in the course of the 5th week among the hepatocytes (endodermally originated cells), amounting to less than 5% of the extravascular cells (Plate 1). During the 7th week, their number reached 10% of the extravascular cells, and about 15% at the 9th week. Most of the hemocytoblasts differentiate into proerythroblasts and definitive erythroblasts, making the liver a hematopoietic organ with overwhelming erythropoiesis.[1] Figure 3 demonstrates the appearance of the liver smear at the 8th week of gestation.

Up to 70% of the free intravascular cells observed in semithin sections of the liver of a 4- and a 4-1/2-week-old embryo belonged to the macrophage series. At the 7th week the number of these cells in the sinusoids represented 10 to 50%. Groups of up to ten macrophages were detected in sections of liver in the early samples (Figure 4). The number of macrophages diminished abruptly during the weeks that followed, and at the 9th week, only 1% remained. The number of presumed macrophage precursors (presumed monoblasts-promonocytes) could reach 10 to 20% of the hematopoietic cells seen in smears. Numerous macrophages showed phagocytosed material demonstrable in electron micrographs of these cells.

MGG-stained smears from the liver of an embryo before, or at the time of the starting of extraembryonic-embryonic circulation, yielded the following differential percentages for free hematopoietic cells: 73.4 histiocytes, 22.4 blast cells, 2.4 small megakaryocytes, 1.4 erythroblasts, and 0.4 progranulocytes (500 cells counted). The paucity of primitive erythroblasts at this stage appears to exclude the circulatory origin of these histiocyte-macrophages. Only 15 to 20% of histiocytes appeared as phagocytic in smears.

On the basis of these observations, it was considered that the first differentiated definitive blood cells formed in the liver, or at least preferentially attracted to it, were

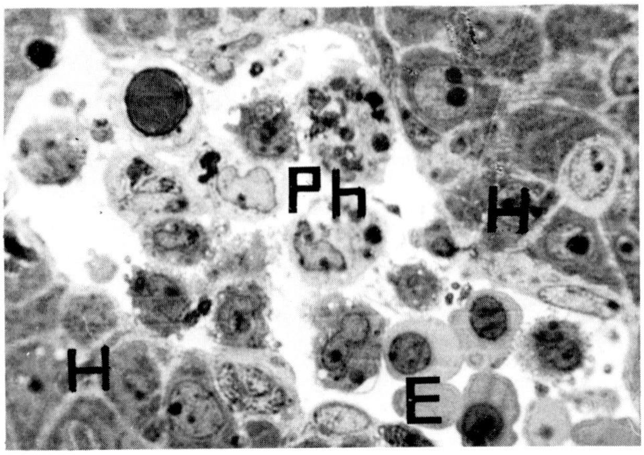

FIGURE 4. Group of phagocytes (Ph) found in a sinusoidal vein of the liver at the earliest stage of differentiation (4 to 5 weeks of gestation). In the same vein there are primitive erythroblasts (E). At both sides of the blood vessel there are hepatocytes (H) with large nucleoli.

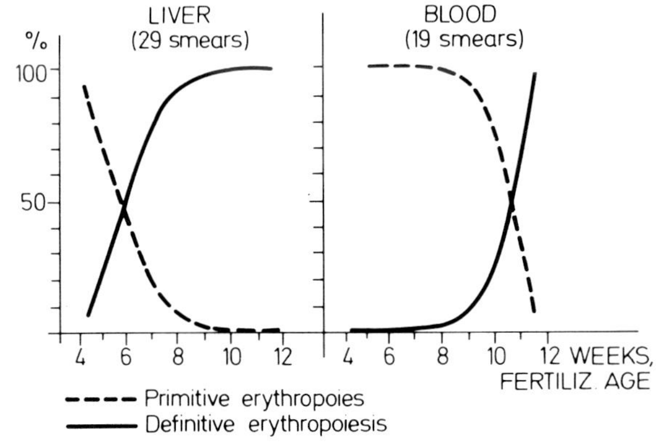

FIGURE 5. Changing pattern of primitive and definitive erythropoietic cells in the liver and blood during early stages of development. Note the delayed release of the early definitive erythroblast generations produced in the liver.

not only hemocytoblasts, but also macrophages.[30] It should be mentioned here, that mature (functioning) macrophages have been demonstrated in the yolk sac prior to the formation of the liver primordium.[14,31]

Although the main function of these macrophages may be the elimination of cells and debris from the sinusoidal spaces, the role of the macrophages in subsequent definitive hematopoiesis needs to be investigated. Occasional erythropoietic islands were found in the sinusoidal vessels of the liver from the 6th week onwards.

b. Erythroblasts

The variations in the content of primitive and definitive erythropoietic cells in embryonic and fetal liver, in comparison with the composition of the embryonic fetal blood, is shown in Figure 5. Primitive erythropoiesis was predominant in the 5th to

6th-week liver, but is was reduced to less than 50% at the 7th week. At 9th week, there were only a few primitive erythroblasts and they practically disappeared from smears prepared after 10th week. On the other hand, definitive nucleated red cells already predominated in the 6-week-old liver and constituted 90% of all erythroblasts at the end of 8th week. The total number of erythroblasts remained over 80% up to the 30th week.[32]

On the contrary, primitive erythroblasts predominated in the circulating blood up to the end of 10th week and disappeared from the circulation during the 12th week. Definitive erythroblasts only appeared in the circulating blood at about the 8th week, but they became rapidly predominant during the 11th week.

Nonnucleated erythrocytes were practically absent in the blood smears up to the 8th week, but there was a rapid increase in their number beyond the 8th week of gestation, and 90% of the circulating red cells were nonnucleated after the 10th week.

c. *Granulocytes*

Only a small number of granulocytes (less than 1%) were found in the liver smears or sections derived from the first trimester of gestation. Afterwards, their number increased (2 to 8%) in the material of Oguro et al.[32] Granulocytic cells were mainly located in the connective tissue. In the third trimester, both liver erythropoiesis and megakaryopoiesis diminished, whereas granulopoiesis reached a peak at the 7th month in the connective tissue of the capsule of Glisson.[33] Calvo and Carbonell[34] investigated the presence of granulopoietic cells in 8- to 32-week-old fetuses, and emphasized that, unlike erythropoietic cells that exhibit contacts with endodermally derived cells (hepatocytes), the granulocytes find their ecological niches in the portal spaces, among connective tissue fibers.

Nuclear pockets are often observed in electronmicroscopic photographs of neutrophils. Some of these cells are devoid of specific granules,[33] and, at least during the first trimester, they lack almost all alkaline phosphatase activity[35] not connected with the specific granules.

d. *Megakaryocytes*

Megakaryocytes are already present in the 4-week-old liver when histiocyte-macrophages predominate for a short period of time (see above). Up to the 21st week their percentage ranges between 0.2 to 1% of the free hematopoietic cells. Their numbers are rather scanty in the last preterm weeks.[14]

The size of embryonic/fetal megakaryocytes is smaller than in adults. The average size is 30 μm in smears[36] and about 14 μm in sections of formalin-fixed and paraffin-embedded preparations,[33] and many of them show only one or two nuclei or nuclear lobes. Micromegakaryocytes are frequent. The number of nuclei or lobes fails to correlate with the stage of differentiation of the individual cells. In adults, the average size of the megakaryocytes measured in smears is 40 μm[22] and about 20 μm in sections.[33] Recent results of Levine show that the diameter of isolated and highly purified human adult megakaryocytes ranges from 10 to 48 μm. The predominant ploidy class appears to be 8N.[37]

e. *Undefined Lymphocyte-Like Cells*

Some undefined lymphocyte-like cells could be found in early liver smears, reaching 5 to 8% of free hematopoietic cells in the course of the 5th and 8th weeks. The number of these cells became less than 2% after the 6th week, and from this time onward they were not found in several smears. A part of these cells could, perhaps, represent certain levels of hematopoietic stem cells and early T or pre-B lymphocytes. These cells, however, were not identified in semithin sections. The circulatory origin of these cells was not demonstrated.

f. Lymphocytes

Apart from the clinical significance of the total hematopoietic cell content of embryonic/fetal liver, as concerns therapeutic application of these cells such as in certain cases of bone marrow aplasia, their lymphocyte content may be important in relation to eventual graft vs. host activity of the transfused cell suspension.

Lymphocytes were not recognized in the liver smears up to the 7th week, but T-lymphocyte antigen-carrying cells appear earlier (see below). There is an apparent small abortive peak reaching about 0.3% of all hematopoietic cells around the 8th week, but a gradual increase in lymphocyte concentration only begins at the end of the first trimester. There are about 0.5% lymphocytes at the 12th week, about 1% around 15 to 16 weeks, and about 2% at 21 to 22 weeks. Other authors,[32] however, found them in a higher proportion (1 to 9% up to the 30th week and about 25 to 50% afterwards). There are approximately 10^5 lymphocytes in an 8 to 10-week-old liver, 10^6 lymphocytes at 12 weeks, 10^7 at 14 to 15 weeks, and as many as about 10^8 lymphocytes at 20 weeks. Previous calculations differ from our findings.[38] For some authors,[39] fetal liver derived lymphoid cells showed no evidence of thymic processing, or T lymphocyte differentiation, because they were unresponsive to PHA and Con-A and did not react in MLC. The cells appeared to be, therefore, functionally immature.

g. Dyserythropoiesis

The presence of morphologic changes in the nuclei of erythroblasts is a characteristic of dyserythropoiesis. In the normal liver of the human embryo, dyserythropoietic cells are less than 1% of the nucleated erythroid cells. In the later stages the proportion is somewhat higher (up to 5%). The percentage of damaged cells increases with the degree and with the duration of intrauterine metabolic injury. Nuclear changes of this type increase within a few hours up to 40% when fetal liver is left in vitro at 37°C, but fail to increase when the temperature is set at 4°C. The liver in the early stages is more resistant to these changes than one in more advanced stages of development. Nuclear damage in incubated liver samples can be inhibited during a few hours of continuous air flow oxygenation.[40] These observations suggest that high levels of nuclear changes similar to those found in dyserythropoiesis indicate severe injury of the fetus. This may be due to prolonged retention of a dead fetus; therefore, liver samples offered for transplantation may not be adequate if the proportion of "dyserythropoietic" nuclei surpasses 2% in the embryonic and 6% in the fetal liver. Nevertheless, some abnormal findings seen in dyserythropoietic anemia could be detected in embryonal and fetal erythroid cells when viewed at the electronmicroscopic level.[23h]

h. Colony Forming Units (CFU)

If one accepts that the CFU content of a cell suspension is an indicator for the presence of pluripotent stem cells, the fetal liver has to be considered as a rich stem cell source.[41] GM-CFU-C has been studied by several groups.[41-47] There were about 25 to 130 CFU-GM per 1×10^5 cells in the 11- to 19-week-old liver, with a peak of about 400 at the 21st week.[39] There were 20 to $100/10^5$ cells in the marrow of fetuses more than 12 weeks old, only a few colonies in the spleen, and none in the thymus. The CFU-C concentration appeared to amount to $1/10^2$ cells in the blood of the 16 to 18-week-old fetus, while it amounted to only $1/10^4$ cells in adult blood. We could say that CFU-C concentration in the liver is equivalent to that of adult marrow.

When compared to adult bone marrow cells, the BFU-E concentration per 10^5 cells of human fetal liver (more than 100 BFU-E per 10^5 cells between the 13th and the 24th week) was about five times that of the adult marrow.[48] Seven-day CFU-E (with erythropoietin) has been investigated.[49] Adult blood did not contain CFU-E at day seven. Cord blood contained 200 colonies per 0.1 mℓ, and 13- to 22-week-old fetal liver contained as many as over 1500 colonies per 0.1 mℓ. Fetal liver-derived BFU-E and CFU-E showed erythropoietin-independent growth in contrast to adult cells. In addition, they were responsive, or even more sensitive than adult CFU-E to erythropoietin, while CFU-E from early neonatal bone marrow showed an intermediate response to erythropoietin.[50,51]

In another study, CFU-TL/10^5 cells were found to be less than 10 in 15 to 17 week human fetal liver, as compared with about 150/10^5 cells in adult marrow.[52]

2. Development of Lymphopoiesis

The first lymphocytes which carry the T-cell antigen can be detected in the liver during the 5th week of gestation. Large lymphoid cells containing intracytoplasmic IgM (so-called pre-B cells) appear in the liver in the course of the 7th week. This is followed 1 to 2 weeks later by the appearance of surface IgM positive B lymphocytes.[53] Blood-born stem cells enter the epithelial ''Anlage'' of the thymus at 8 weeks, and thymic T lymphocytes appear during the following weeks. At the end of the first trimester, T lymphocytes appear in the bone marrow and spleen. Apart from the same territories, B lymphocytes can be found at the same time in the thymus and in the circulating blood. Cells with the morphology of lymphocytes are already present in the circulation at the 7th to 8th week. Presence of lymphocytes in the yolk sac at the 4th week have been reported,[38, 54] but confirmation with new specific methods is awaited.

Although experts accept[4] that the human fetus is neither immunologically inert nor does it exist in immunological isolation,[55] the presence of plasma cells in the normal fetus is debated.[32, 56, 57] In the course of the 13th to 14th week, plasma cells could be detected with special methods in the liver, spleen, bone marrow, and blood, whereas IgA positive plasma cells were also detected in the gut around the 20th week.[53] During embryonic development of the mouse, pre-B cells could be found both in the placenta and in embryonic blood before their appearance in the liver. Although fetal liver and yolk sac are connected with the placenta, and in contact with embryonic blood by circulation, they did not contain demonstrable numbers of pre-B cells.[58, 59]

Mixed lymphocyte reaction in the 8th week of gestation was reported but subsequent investigations failed to confirm this finding up to midgestation.[50]

Cell-mediated lympholysis (CML) was regarded as an in vitro model of graft rejection.[60] Marginal fetal CML-responses were detectable in some cases from the 14th week onwards, but high responses were not seen until the 16th week of gestation. Half of the samples were negative and a further quarter of them had borderline cytotoxic levels. On the other hand, CML response was fully mature at birth. As already noted, although the presence of different immunocytes and/or immunological functions has been demonstrated, Champlin et al.[39] concluded that up to 21 weeks of gestation, human fetal liver is a rich source of hematopoietic stem cells, but lacks readily detectable immunocompetent lymphocytes.

Suppressor T-cell activity has been demonstrated at 26 weeks of gestation,[61a] and fetal suppressor cells have been observed in vitro when untreated populations of maternal and neonatal lymphocytes were cultured together.[61b] There is little, if any, MHC expressed on any tissue during the first half of embryonic life.[61c] Development of natural killer cells was studied.[61d]

Percentage of rosetting T cells, lymphotoxin generation, complement component levels, neutrophil chemotaxis and phagocytosis all are reduced at birth and immunological memory appears to be absent.[61e]

a. Thymus

The thymus is the largest single lymphopoietic organ of the fetus. It originates from endodermal cells of the third and fourth pharyngeal pouch during the 6th week of gestation. During the next 2 weeks, buds of these cells intermix with the surrounding mesenchymal tissue of the retro-sternal area. At the 10th week, the primitive endodermal cells change their compact epithelial type structure into a meshwork of stellated cells which resemble the reticulum cells of the mesenchymal tissue.

After week 8, lymphocytes and their precursors populate the organ, and at the 12th to 14th week they are already very abundant. The thymus becomes a lobulated organ with a densely populated cortical area surrounding rather sparsely populated medullary regions. In the connective tissue separating the lobules, there are some groups of granulopoietic cells of neutrophilic and eosinophilic type. Occasionally, one can also find erythropoietic cells in this region. Basophils can be found in the capsule of the organ. Figure 6 demonstrates the structure of the fetal thymus at the 14th week of gestation. Plate 2 shows the smear.

The lymphocyte concentration in the thymus is over 96% at the 10th week and approaches 99% in the following weeks.[1] The weight of the thymus is about 0.1 g at the end of the first trimester, about 1 g at the beginning of the third, and 10 to 12 g at birth.[54,62]

Although Le Douarin and Jotereau[63] demonstrated that hemocytoblasts can be found in the thymic endodermal rudiment of avian interspecific chimeras before the vascularization of the thymic rudiment, the lymphoid cell population developing in the thymus seems to have an extrinsic orgin and is derived from stem cells that invade the rudiment during a precise and limited period of time.[64] The same is valid for the bursa. Tompkins et al.[65] proved the blood-born origin of thymic lymphopoiesis in frogs.

The stimulus for the differentiation and maturation of prothymocytes to thymocytes is presumed to originate from the thymic epithelial cells. Thymic epithelial products can induce differentiation of bone marrow stem cells into lymphocytes that bear recognizable T-cell markers.[66]

High thymidine incorporation of fetal thymus cells is well known.[67] In spite of this, very few mitotic figures could be found in the thymic smears, even if numerous prothymocytes were present and care was taken to prepare smears from a living embryo. Galili et al.[68] demonstrated that the concentration of thymocytes in a cell suspension regulated the rate of pro-thymocyte proliferation in human material. The question of intrathymic death of most thymocytes remains open.[69]

b. Lymph Nodes

Primary lymph node development and lymphopoiesis occur from the 10th to 12th week onward, whereas splenic lymphopoiesis, including both the T and the B series, starts at 12 to 15 weeks. Before the start of the lymphopoiesis in the nodes, small lymphocyte clusters can be found in the connective tissue of lymph plexuses (8 weeks).[14] During the third month of gestation, the clusters of lymphocytes associated with the loose mesenchymal tissue invade the lymphatic plexi of the neck, thorax, and abdomen, and become vascularized. The large lymphatic sacs flatten down to form the lymphatic sinuses of the nodes.

The developing lymph nodes contain not only lymphocytes, but also some granulocytes and undifferentiated lymphoid cells of "blast" type. Germinal centers appear

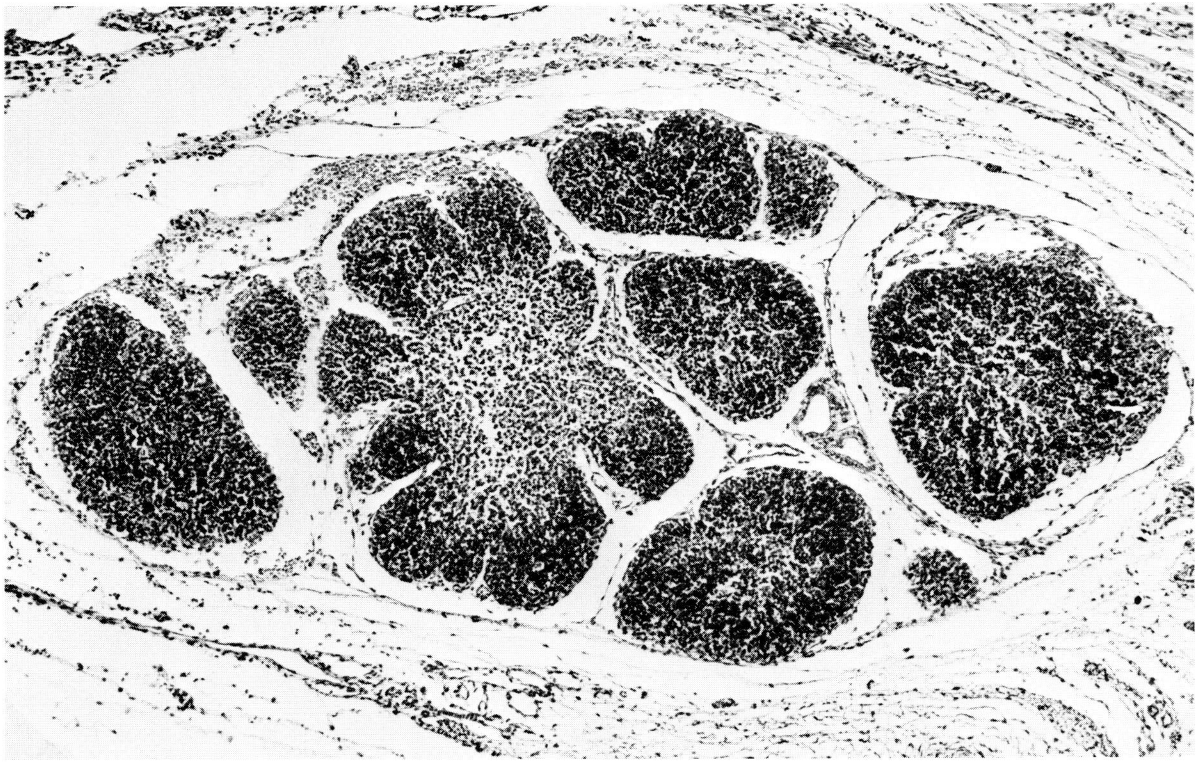

FIGURE 6. Low magnification of a sagittal section of the thymus of a 14-week-old fetus. The thymus is a large organ at this stage of development and shows a cortex containing closely packed small lymphocytes around a less populated medulla. (H and E stain; magnification × 80.)

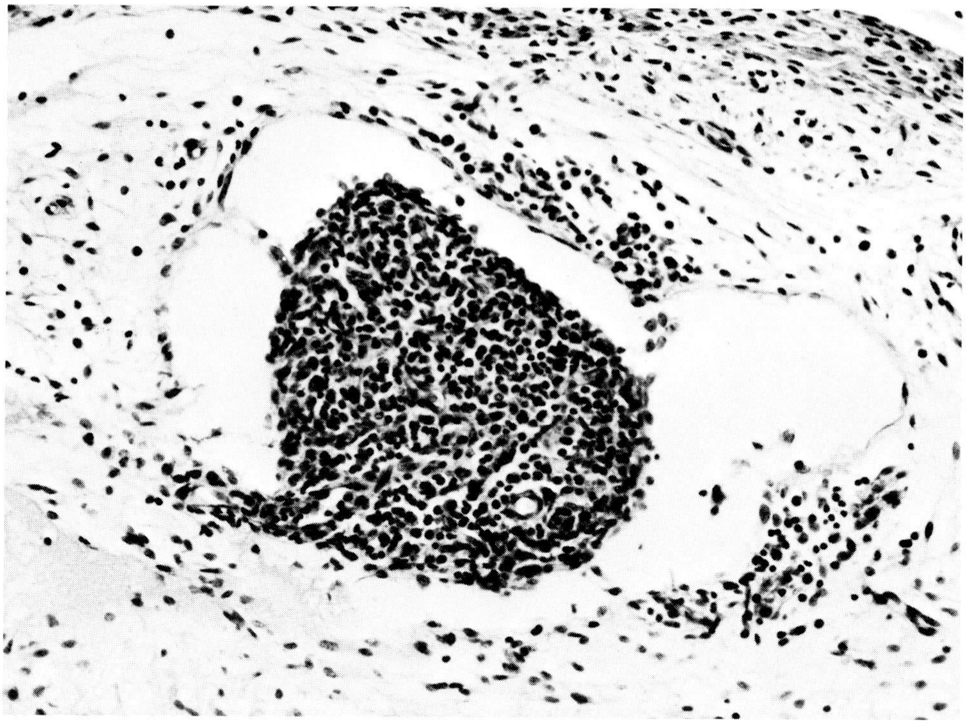

FIGURE 7. Section of a lymph node of a 14-week-old fetus. At this early stage of development, the lymph nodes consist of groups of lymphocytes contained in a meshwork of mesenchymal cells and fine blood vessels. The nodes are surrounded by large lymphatic sinuses. (H and E stain: magnification × 200.)

after birth. A section of a lymph node from a 14-week-old human fetus is shown in Figure 7.

c. Spleen

The spleen develops in the dorsal mesogastrium. At the beginning, the rudiment of the organ consists of a meshwork of vascularized connective tissue cells surrounded by a thin capsule. Occasionally primitive erythrocytes and some undifferentiated cells can be seen in dilated blood vessels during the prehematopoietic stage, which extends up to the 9th week of gestation. By the 12th to 14th week, small groups of erythroblasts, some megakaryocytes, and lymphocytes can be found.

The beginning of the formation of the white pulp can be observed at the 15th week of gestation, at which time the lymphocytes accumulate around arterial vessels. But until the 20th week, the periarterial cuffs of lymphocytes are sparsely populated.

Granulopoiesis, erythropoiesis, and megakaryopoiesis exist in the splenic red pulp during fetal life, but the contribution of the human spleen to hematopoietic activity is rather modest. There are only about 10^6 lymphocytes in the 12th to 13th week spleen, about 10^7 at the 15th week, about 10^8 at the 16th to 17th week,[38] about 10^9 lymphocytes around 24 to 25 weeks and about 7.5×10^9 at birth. The relative weight of the spleen is roughly 1/500 of the body weight in the newborn as well as in the adult. This is about one tenth of the marrow volume. A small hematopoietic contribution, other than lymphopoiesis, takes place in the spleen after the second trimester of pregnancy. There are about 30% erythroblasts at the 26th week, and less than 15% afterwards, when lymphocyte levels rise to two thirds of all hematopoietic cells. Ninety per cent of the

Table 2
FIRST APPEARANCE OF DIFFERENT BLOOD CELLS DURING HEMATOPOIETIC DEVELOPMENT IN MAN

	Extra-embryonic (yolk sac, chorion, and stalk)	Liver	Thymus	Spleen	Lymph node	Bone marrow	Blood
Lymphocyte-like cells with scanty cytoplasm	−5[a]	4—5	−8[a]	−8[a]	−9[a]	−8[a]	4—5
Monocytoid granuloblasts[b]	−6 (?)	−6 (?)				8—9	7—8
Osteoclasts	None	None	None	None	None	8—9	None
Primitive erythroblasts	3—4	4—5		8		8[c]	3—4
Definitive erythroblasts	5—6	4—5	10	8	11	8[c]	6—7
Granulocytes	3—4[d]	5	10	8	12	8[c]	6—8
Macrophages/histocytes	3—4	4—5	10	8	11	8—9[c]	3—4
Megakaryocytes	5	4—5	14	11		13—14	4—5
T lymphocytes		5—6	9—10			12	7—8
B lymphocytes		7—8	11—12	12		13—14	11—12

Note: Numbers mean fertilization age in weeks.

[a]These cells could be found in hematopoietic organs, *occasionally,* before hematopoiesis starts.
[b]For large, monocytoid granuloblasts, see Sec. III, A, 5. Monocytoid granuloblasts and osteoclasts precede intramarrow hematopoiesis.
[c]From the circulating blood: their presence does not mean intramarrow formation.
[d]Maternal origin could be considered.

cells are lymphocytes after the 30th week, while granulocytes are only 5 to 15% of the cells in the spleen.[1,32]

3. Delayed Release of Early Generations of Hepatic and Thymic Hematopoietic Cells

It has already been mentioned that large differences exist during a 2 to 3 week period between the composition of liver hematopoiesis and circulating blood cell differentials. The presence of overwhelming definitive erythropoiesis in the liver, while erythrocytic cells of the primitive type predominate in the blood up to the 10th week of pregnancy, was demonstrated in Figure 5. During this time, there are more than 70% reticulocytes among nonnucleated erythrocytes.[1] Therefore, one cannot speak of "ineffective" erythropoiesis. It is more likely that the release of differentiated red cells is inhibited during the aforementioned 2 to 3 weeks. In any event, the rate of proliferation, as measured by the expansion of hematopoietic cell counts, diminishes from the 9th week onward when total hematopoietic cell counts reached 10^8 cells per liver. One possible explanation of this pattern may be the presumption that until a certain level of growing cell mass is attained, the presence of numerous mature cells inhibits the release of differentiated red cells into the circulation. A similar suggestion was recently formulated.[68] An analogous discrepancy was found in the granulocytic series: a few granulocytic cells could be found in the 5-week liver, whereas these cells rarely appear in the circulation before the 8th week (see Table 2). The same is valid for thrombocytopoiesis: megakaryocytes are present in the 4-week-old liver sample and there is, in general, about one megakaryocyte in 200 hematopoietic cells, but the number of circulating platelets remains very low for several weeks (below 10,000/$\mu\ell$), at least during the first trimester. The explanation offered for the delayed release of the erythroid cells cannot be valid for the granulocyte and thrombocyte series, unless we presume that population pressure is the cause of the release of the red cells in the embryonic liver, and the minor cell populations are innocent bystanders.

The same discrepancy can also be found for lymphocytes. There is, again, about a 2-week period before the appearance of intrahepatic T lymphocytes, and about a 3-week period before the appearance of B lymphocytes in the circulating blood.[53,70] As already noted, the absence of significant T-lymphocyte release was explained by regulation through mature cell mass.[68]

4. Appearance and Definitive Location of Hematopoietic Cells

Table 2 summarizes the first appearance of different blood cell types in smears of hematopoietic organs and the circulating blood. It should be emphasized at this point, that in the course of the second month of development, the embryonic tissue is capable of forming practically all types of blood cells.[1,15,70] This is the reason for including in the chapter all these developmental antecedents before describing blood formation in the marrow as the definitive site of hematopoiesis in man.

III. DEVELOPMENT OF MARROW HEMATOPOIESIS IN MAN

Marrow hematopoiesis becomes predominant after the second trimester of gestation. On the basis of our quantitative data, we can confirm the already accepted notion that the total hematopoietic cell mass of the fetal marrow surpasses that of the liver after the 6th month of fetal life. For our calculation, the specific gravity of the fetal marrow was considered to be practically one, according to the studies of Hudson.[71]

In this part of the chapter, we begin with a description of the main events preceding marrow hematopoiesis in bones, to be followed by a description of the different cell types and marrow structures. The development of the bone marrow can be studied by dividing it into the following stages:

1. Prehematopoietic marrow
   a. Preosteoblastic stage
   b. Osteoblastic stage
2. Hematopoietic marrow
   a. Early, extrasinusoidal, hematopoietic cell clusters
   b. Marrow hematopoiesis

A. Prehematopoietic Marrow

The presence of chondroblasts, chondrocytes, and densely packed undifferentiated mesenchymal cells, characterize the preosteoblastic stage. Hematopoietic stem cells, osteoclasts, osteoblasts, and fibroblasts characterize the osteoblastic stage. The formation of the stromal matrix occurs during this period. Both cartilage and bone are derived from the mesenchyme.

1. Preosteoblastic Stage

In most skeletal parts where hematopoiesis will take place, chondroblasts and chondrocytes are the first specific cells. The ballooning effect of cartilage necrobiosis occurs shortly before penetration of blood vessels. During the time of establishment of the stromal matrix, fetal blood cells are seen within the vascular structures inside the bone cavity, but in the earliest bone samples it is difficult to find blood forming cells.

There are two main compartments in the developed hematopoietic marrow, and these are the hematopoiesis-supporting stroma and the hematopoietic-cell systems. Stromal elements have been described as fixed, and hematopoietic cells as free elements. The formation of the marrow stroma precedes hematopoiesis. In fact, it was reported[72] that human bone marrow fibroblasts CFUs (CFU-F) could not be found in peripheral blood with up to 10^8 cells per flask. On the other hand, according to Werts et al.[73] stromal cell migration precedes hematopoietic repopulation of the bone marrow in heavily irradiated mice. The generally accepted idea that hematopoietic stroma precedes the seeding of hematopoietic stem cells will be discussed in a subsequent part of this chapter.

2. Osteoblastic Stage

Osteoblasts (Plate 3) predominate and remain the most frequent cell type in smears of bones during the early stages of development. They represent about 30% of the cells in smears up to the 20th week. Large monocytoid granuloblasts (Plate 5) appear very early in certain bones but neither their origin nor their fate is known.

A section of the prehematopoietic stroma in the clavicula demonstrating the morphologic features of the primitive marrow, is shown in Figure 8.

3. Hematopoietic Stroma

For many years, the role of the hematopoietic stroma was not adequately emphasized. However, as a result of the work of Trentin,[74] Wolf,[75] and Friedenstein et al.,[76] the study of the stroma has gained in importance, and some authors even suggested that the total number of hematopoietic stem cells could be determined by the size of the stromal hematopoietic microenvironment rather than by the number of hematopoietic stem cells.[77]

Our embryonic heritage, Block wrote,[70] consists of a scaffolding of stellate mesenchymal cells in hematopoietic tissues. In the marrow, these cells may temporarily adopt morphological variations recognizable as reticular cells, fat cells, osteoblasts, fibroblasts, etc. The so-called reticulum cells cannot be considered as one class of cells, and their relationship to stromal cells in general,[78] or to monocytes, histiocytes, and macrophages[79] remains obscure. On the other hand, a transition of reticulum cells to hematopoietic cells, a notion defended even in recent publications, has not been proved. Human fibroblasts appear to be unrelated to hematopoietic stem cells. The stromal cells of the marrow tissue are a heterogeneous population including cells which are classified under a variety of names. The hematopoietic stem cells are supposed to precede hematopoiesis in the marrow. Hitherto, it was widely accepted that, as soon as the stromal matrix was ready to accept the seeding of stem cells, undifferentiated cells would appear, forming the center of developing hematopoietic cell colonies.[44] The first appearance of the hematopoietic cells and their early differentiation will be discussed later.

There is much evidence supporting the concept of regulation of hematopoiesis by stromal cells. Stromal cells may recognize hematopoietic stem cells and may participate in proliferation, differentiation, decay, and release of various kinds of hematopoietic cells. However, pertinent human data are not yet available.

4. Early Lymphocyte-Like Small Cells with Scanty Cytoplasm

Around the 8th week of gestation, several cells resembling small lymphocytes can be found in ossifying skeletal parts. These lymphocyte-like cells could amount to 10% of the smeared cells at a time when very few lymphocytes can be detected in the circulation (see Figure 15). The stem cell condition of similar lymphocyte-like cells was considered by several authors. Peak values for marrow lymphocytes were found in smears only after the end of the first trimester. Light microscopic morphology of these early mesenchymal cells is shown in Plate 4.

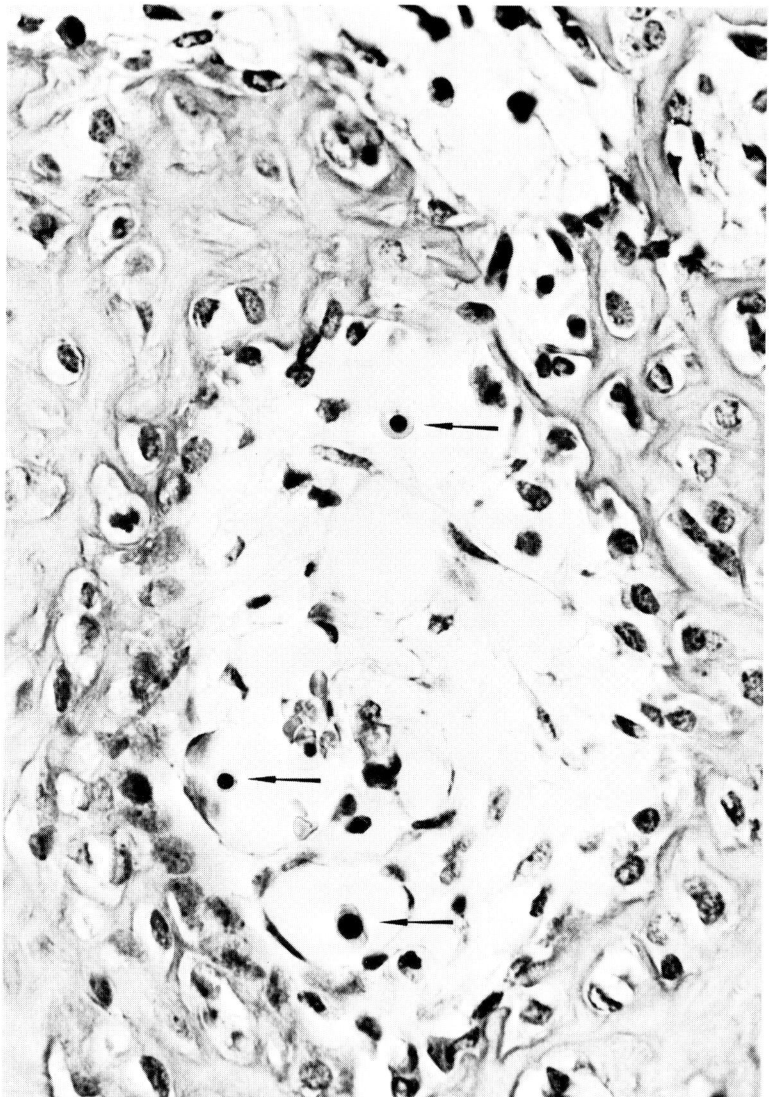

FIGURE 8. Clavicula of an 8-week-old fetus, showing a primitive stroma composed of loose connective tissue and large sinusoidal vessels containing nucleated erythrocytes and erythroblasts (arrows). There are no hemopoietic cells at this stage. (H and E stain; magnification × 500.)

5. Large Monocytoid Granuloblasts

Large progranulocytes which are not identical to any accepted hematopoietic precursor cell have been previously described. The presumed blast cells of this series were 14 to 24 μm in diameter, did not posses light microscopically detectable granulation, were pronouncedly basophilic, and had prominent nucleoli. Intermediate members of the series had bizarre nuclear shapes and some dispersed granules. The most characteristic type of these fetal granuloblasts (as they were called in the *Atlas of Human Hemopoietic Development*[1]), is a large cell, around 25 μm in diameter when measured in smears. This cell has an eccentric soya-bean-shaped nucleus containing two or more nucleoli and abundant basophilic cytoplasm with some large granules placed preferentially around the lap of the concave part of the nucleus (Plates 5A and B). Unlike the youngest representatives of these series, the mature members of this cell group showed peroxidase, Sudan black, and naphthol-AS-D chloroacetate esterase positivity in their granules. The presence of these cells in smears of various prehematopoietic bones has been reinvestigated. Figures 9A and 9B show the results in the long bones and vertebrae, respectively. Monocytoid progranulocytes were found in samples of long bones in the 9th to 10th week of gestation, in the 12th- to 13th-week ribs, and in the 9th- to 10th-week vertebrae. The appearance of the large granuloblasts in the long bones precedes hematopoiesis. In the vertebrae, where hematopoiesis develops slower than in the long bones, about 10% of the hematopoietic cells (including those derived from marrow vessels), belonged to the group of these cells as early as the 9th and 10th week, before osteoclasts could be detected in the same smears. The meaning of these early progranulocytes cannot be well understood at the present, but we do not think that they belong to the classic myeloblast-granulocyte series, as was formerly supposed.[1] One could instead hypothesize on the eventual connection between these cells and the monocyte-macrophage and/or the osteoclast system (cf. also References 32, 80).

6. Hematopoietic Stem Cell Origin of Osteoclasts

Although these cells were described in the *Atlas of Human Hemopoietic Development*[1] with the "nonhematopoietic cells in the bone cavities", the blood-born origin of osteoclasts is now accepted for several animal species. Formal proof for the origin of osteoclasts as deriving from hematopoietic stem cells was given by Ash et al.,[81] who used giant lysosomes as natural cytoplasmic cell markers of these cells. On the other hand, Testa et al.[82] succeeded in growing osteoclasts in vitro from cat, mouse, and even human marrow. If osteoclasts are derived from hematopoietic stem cells, their presence in marrow samples could be regarded as a rewarding "very early footprint" of these stem cells.[83a]

In our material, five different bone areas were investigated. May-Grünwald-Giemsa stained smears and serial sections were prepared with the purpose of studying the first appearance of the osteoclasts. It was found that they appeared in the clavicle during the 8th week, and in the course of the 9th week in the femora, humeri, radii, and tibiae. They were present in the ribs in the 10th week and in the course of the 13th week, appeared in the vertebrae (Table 3).

If one compares these results with those represented in Figure 10, one finds that the first appearance of osteoclasts coincides with the earliest stages of the development of the hematopoietic stromal matrix. Therefore, it may be suggested that hematopoietic stem cells, which must be present before their differentiation into osteoclasts, appear simultaneously with, or even before the formation of the stromal matrix. The number of osteoclast nuclei could increase by fusion of mononuclear cells. Since osteoclasts do not circulate, they might originate from a circulating precursor cell, or they could

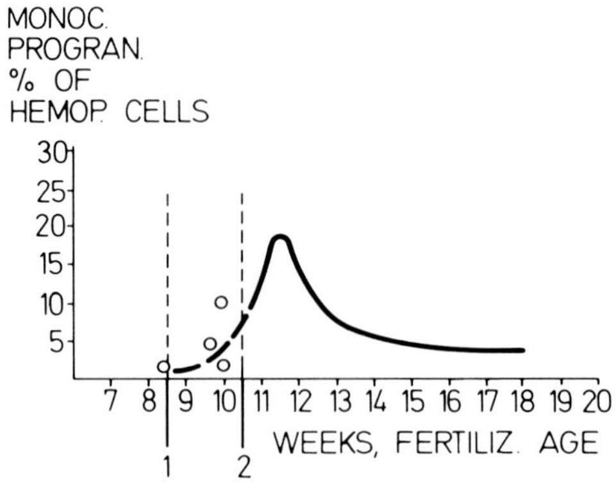

A

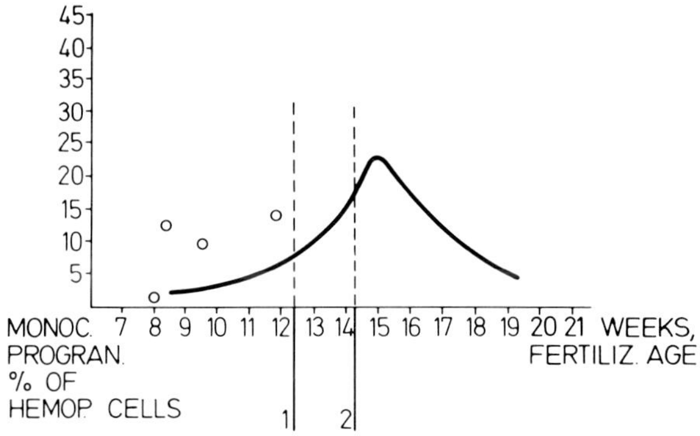

B

FIGURE 9. (A). Presence of large monocytoid progranulocytes (fetal granuloblasts) in 39 femoral and humeral smears. The line number 1 shows the time of appearance of osteoclasts and the line number 2 shows the onset of hematopoiesis in the same bones. A few early values for these progranulocytes have been selectively plotted, i.e., samples without large progranulocytes were not plotted. In these long bones, large monocytoid progranulocytes appeared at the same time as the osteoclasts. (B). Presence of large monocytoid progranulocytes (fetal granuloblasts) in 20 vertebral smears; these cells were present in about half of the samples before the 13th week, and in practically all samples thereafter. The line number 1 shows the time of appearance of osteoclasts and the line number 2 shows the onset of hematopoiesis. The four open circles were selected to demonstrate that these large progranulocytes could appear in smears before the osteoclasts.

be formed locally.* If the hematopoietic stem cells are the progenitors of osteoclasts, their differentiation into these cells could represent a good example of the influence of the microenvironment, because osteoclasts are not found outside the marrow.

*According to a recent review by T. J. Chambers (The cellular basis of bone resorption, *Clin. Orthopaed.*, 151, 283, 1980), the osteoclasts seem to be derived from the fusion of circulating cells of the mononuclear phagocyte system.

Table 3
FIRST APPEARANCE OF OSTEOCLASTS IN MGG-STAINED SMEARS AND SERIAL HISTOLOGICAL SECTIONS

Fertiliz. age (weeks)	Clavicle	Long bones of extremities	Ribs	Vertebrae	Sternum
7—8	±	−	−	−	−
8—9	+	±	−	−	−
9—10	+	+	±	−	−
10—11	+	+	+	−	−
11—12	+	+	+	−	−
12—13	+	+	+	±	−
13—14				+	−

Note: Ninety smears from 25 fetuses and 33 serial sections from other 25 fetuses. + means presence, − means absence of osteoclasts, and ± means that there were samples that did not contain osteoclasts. Solid lines show the onset of hematopoiesis in the appropriate bones.

	Fertilization age in weeks									
	7-8	9-10	11-12	13-14	15-16	17-18	19-20	21-22	25	31
Clavicula	--000 --000 --000	000++ 000++ 00+++	0++++ +++++	+++++ +++++ +++++	+++++ +++++ +++++	+++++ +++	+	++	+	+
Humerus	----- ----- ---00	0000+ 000++	+++++ +++++ +++++	+++++ +++++ +++++	+++++ +++++ +++++	++	+++	+++++	+	+
Radius	----- ----- -----	000++ +	+++++ +++++ +++++	+++++ +++++ +++++	+++++ +++++ ++	++++	++	+++++ +	+	+
Femur	----- ----- ----0	00000 000	+++++ +++++	+++++ +++++ ++	+++++ +++++ ++	+++++ ++	++	++++	+	+
Tibia	----- ----- ----0	00000	0++++ +++++	+++++ +++++ ++	+++++ +++++	+++++ +	++++	++++	+	+
Ribs	----- ----- ----0	----- --0	000++ 000++ 000+	0++++ +++++ +++++	00+++ +++++	+++++ +	+++	+++++	+	+
Vertebra	----- ----- -----	----- -----	00000 00000	--000 00000 00000	0000+ +++++	+++++ +	+	+++++ +++++ +	+	+
Sternum	----- ----- -----	---	----- ----- -----	----- ----- --	----- ----- ----0	0	0	0++++ +	+	+

FIGURE 10. Pattern of development of marrow hematopoiesis in eight different skeletal parts according to age. A + means presence of hematopoietic cells, a 0 represents prehematopoietic stroma, and − corresponds to the cartilagenous stage of development. The clavicula and the long bones of the extremities are the first and the sternum the last to begin hematopoietic activity.

Bone marrow matrix may recruit osteoclast-precursor monocytes.[83b] Although osteoclast formation from bone marrow mononuclear cells in osteoclast-free mouse bone has been reported,[83c] there is no definitive conclusion, and Tinkler et al.[83d] noted that even in the case of successful marrow grafts, the graft may have carried cells capable of restoring osteoclast function in the osteopetrotic recipient, while not acting as osteoclast-precursors themselves.

Another consideration appears to be pertinent here. As we pointed out before (see Section II.B.1.a), cells of the mononuclear phagocyte system were the first differentiated blood cells found in the liver during the earliest stage of hematopoietic development in this organ.[30] In the prehematopoietic marrow, the osteoclasts are among the first cells to be found in the bone cavities. If the osteoclasts are derived from the circulating cells of the mononuclear phagocyte system, then a parallel exists between the liver and the marrow respective to the first cells populating both organs during their earliest stages of development, prior to the appearance of differentiated hematopoietic cells. The above-mentioned cells seem to have a general pioneer role in the preparation of blood formation. An earlier study supports this suggestion.[83e] The nature of this role deserves to be investigated.

B. Hematopoietic Marrow

The onset of marrow hematopoiesis is related to the time each skeletal part begins the process of ossification, which spreads over several months of fetal development. Ossification starts in the clavicula at the end of the second month of gestation, and shortly after in the long bones of the extremities. The sternum remains in the cartilagenous stage until the end of the 4th month. The development of the marrow in these bones appears, therefore, in the same sequence (Figure 10).

The pattern of events leading to the formation of hematopoietic marrow can be followed in serial sections of bones of fetuses at different stages of development. The prehematopoietic marrow stroma is originated by the migration of mesenchymal cells from the peri-chondral-periosteal membrane into the cavities left by the decaying cartilage during the initial stage of ossification.

Blood vessels and nerves penetrate together with the mesenchymal cells through openings produced in the ossifying membrane. The bone cavities enlarge and the venous vessels dilate, forming thin-walled sinuses containing abundant blood. The nutrient vessels consist of arterioles and fine capillaries sprouting along the primitive marrow cylinder. Between the vessels and the newly formed bone trabeculae extends a network of fine reticulin fibers containing reticulum cells. Numerous osteoblasts and osteoclasts form and remodel bone trabeculae, while the bone cavities continually enlarge. As already mentioned, it takes about 2 weeks to develop such a vascularized stromal matrix before the first differentiated hematopoietic cells can be recognized in the primitive marrow. Figure 8 illustrates the morphologic characteristics of the prehematopoietic marrow in the clavicula of an 8-week-old human fetus.

The beginning of the hematopoietic activity occurs in the long bones of the extremities as early as the 3rd month of fetal development. The first differentiated hematopoietic cells appear in small groups of extrasinusoidal cells (Figure 11). At this early stage of marrow development, one can see isolated groups of erythroblasts and small areas of granulocytopoiesis, as well as some megakaryocytes. Shortly after, the areas occupied by each cell line extend and intermix in such a way that it becomes difficult to distinguish the limits of each cell line. During the 5th month, most of the bones contain a very active hematopoietic tissue in which all cell lines are represented. Figure 12 illustrates the abundant cellularity of the femoral marrow of a 22-week-old human fetus.

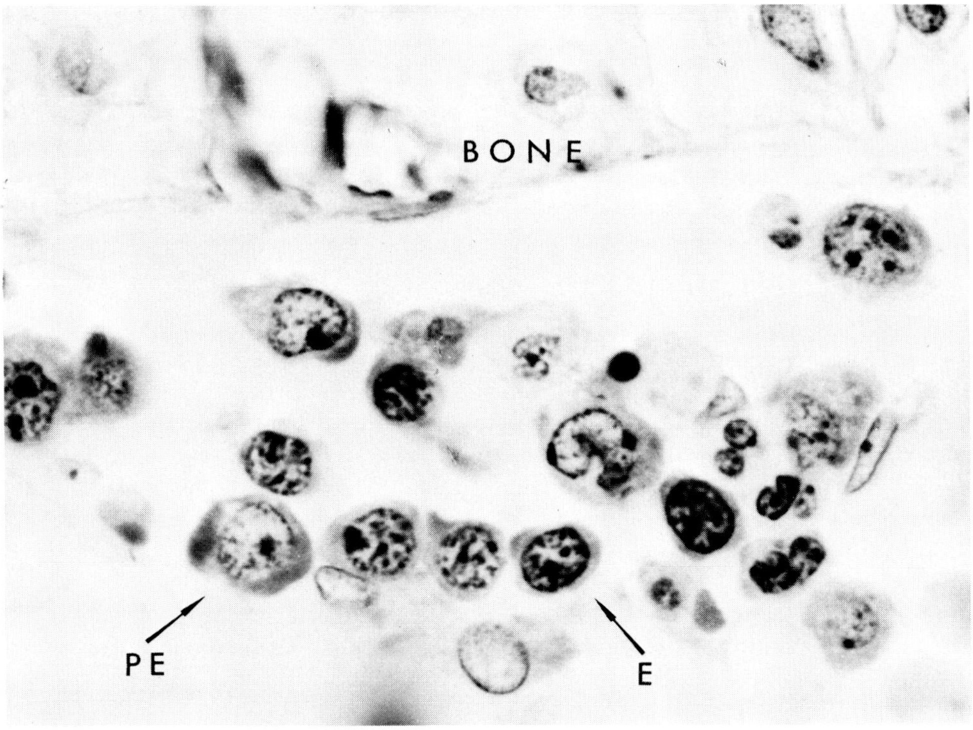

FIGURE 11. Marrow of the humerus of a 14-week-old fetus. A group of hematopoietic cells can be seen located at the subendosteal area of the diaphysis of the bone. The arrows point to a row of red cell precursors in various stages of maturation. Proerythroblast (PE) initiates the row which ends with one erythroblast (E). (Methacrylate embedded tissue stained with Giemsa; magnification × 1250.)

1. Quantitative Aspects

The percent of hematopoietic cells in the total number of marrow cells (relative hematopoietic cell concentration) was investigated in smears. Figure 13 shows the increase in the proportion of hematopoietic cells in the course of marrow development. After the 18th week of gestation their number is above 90% of all cells found in the marrow. The figure also shows the marrow volume given in milliliters. The volume of the marrow is only 2 to 3 mℓ at the 18th week. It increases to about 10 mℓ at the end of the second trimester and to about 45 mℓ at delivery.[71] Somewhat larger volume (67 mℓ at delivery) has been reported by Wetzel.[84] The total volume of the red marrow is about 1/50 of the body weight in the newborn, which is similar to that of the adult.

Large variations exist in the proportion of hematopoietic cells present in different bones of fetuses of the same age. For instance, in the radius of an 11-week-old fetus there are only 7% while in the corresponding humerus 60% of all nucleated cells are hematopoietic. Presumably, the size of the bone cavity is responsible for such variations.

Contradictory data can be found in the literature with respect to the absolute number of marrow cells. It seems that there are some 10^{10} hematopoietic cells in the newborn. From the 29th week to birth the proportion of hematopoietic cells in different body areas has been reported to be about 30% in the cranium, 47% in the limbs, and about 23% in the trunk.[71]

Kelemen and Jánossa estimated cell counts for the whole marrow organ in 22 samples (from 12 weeks to term) with the following results:

Fertilization age	Approx. cell count for the whole marrow organ
12–14	10^8
15–17	$1–2 \times 10^8$
18–20	$4–6 \times 10^8$
21–22	$7–8 \times 10^8$
23–25	$1–4 \times 10^9$
26–32	$5–8 \times 10^9$
32–38	$1–1.5 \times 10^{10}$
Term	$1.5–2.5 \times 10^{10}$

As already mentioned, at about the end of the second trimester the hematopoietic cell concentration reaches its peak. From this time onward, the volume of the bone marrow is approximately the same as the total volume of hematopoietic cells.[71] Furthermore, as noted in *Smith's Blood Diseases of Infancy and Childhood*[85], the only way the fetus and the newborn can significantly increase their hematopoietic output and reserve is at the expense of reactivated or persistent extramedullary hematopoiesis.

2. Fat Cells

In the adult, medullary adipose tissue is interspersed with the hematopoietic cells, and both are contained in the rigid, nonexpansive confines of the bone. A reciprocal relationship exists between the two elements: hematopoiesis is only able to expand at the expense of the elimination of adipose tissue, and vice versa.[83] Fat cells as found in the normal pattern of the marrow in adults were not present in our fetal material. We are aware of the remarkable vulnerability of the fat cells in the course of the preparation of smears,[87] but the large fat cells so characteristic of the adult marrow were absent in the histologic sections of fetal marrow. The absence of such cells reflects the high proliferation rate of the developing marrow.

There were giant fat cells with an apparent nursing or feeder function which seem to be responsible for the long-term stem cell maintenance in bone marrow culture.[88] Lipid-loaden adipocytes appeared to be essential for long term hematopoiesis.[89] On the other hand, the marrow smears prepared with material from the 11th to the 16th week of gestation contained 0.5 to 5% vacuolated histiocytes, about 35 μm in diameter, showing up to 100 small and regular vacuoles which were Sudan black-negative.

3. Erythropoiesis

During the earliest stage of marrow development and for a short period of time, one can find primitive erythroblasts inside the blood vessels. These cells disappear after the 13th week. Marrow erythropoiesis is of definitive type. Erythropoietic cells amount to 30 to 50% up to the 18th week; thereafter, as a consequence of the expanding granulopoiesis, the proportion declines to 14 to 27%. This value is comparable to that of adults.

The rate of red cell formation during fetal life is greater than in adults. Red cell survival is about 60 to 80 days in the premature and 80 to 100 days at term, which is shorter than in adults. The blood volume is about 100 mℓ in a fetus of 1 kg body weight and 85 mℓ/kg at term, with a venous hematocrit level of 57%.

The differential counts for the first two trimesters of fetal life, in percent of all hematopoietic cells are:

1. Proerythroblasts: 1 to 4%
2. Basophilic normoblasts: 3 to 19%

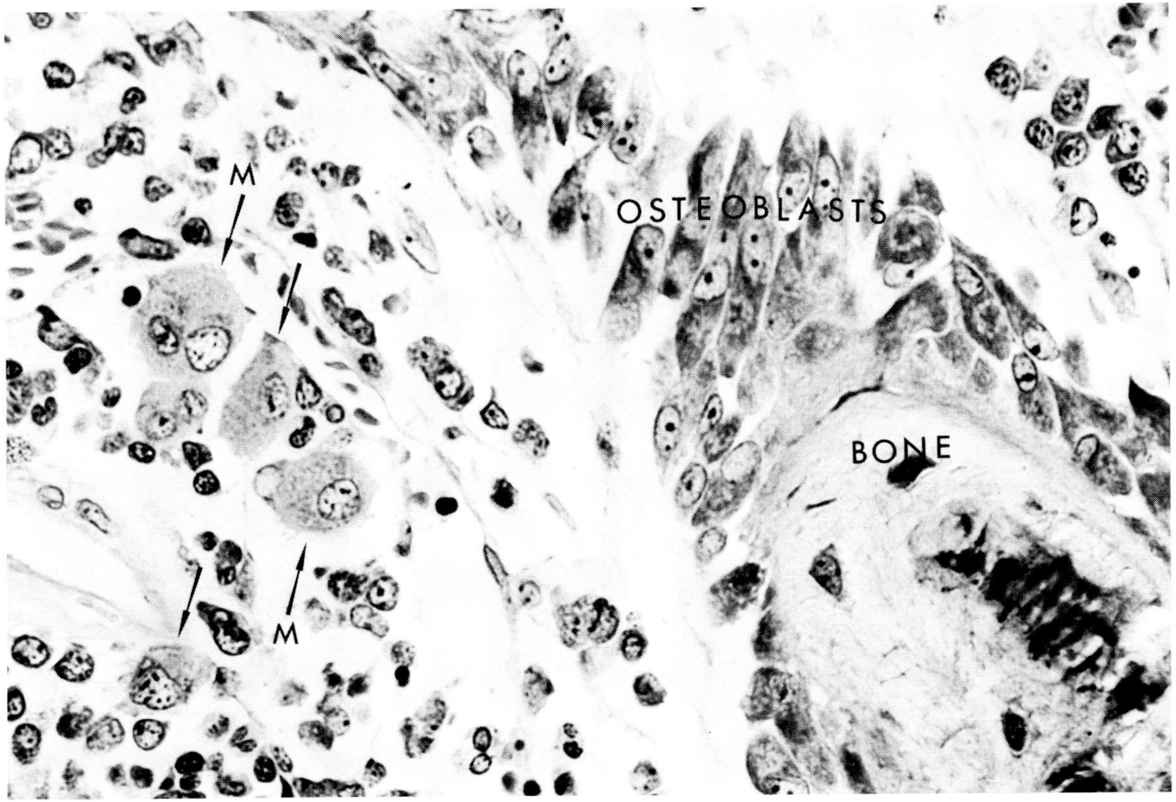

FIGURE 12. Humeral marrow of a 22-week-old fetus. At this stage of development, most of the bones contain a very cellular marrow in which all cell lines are represented. At the right of the figure, there is a bone trabecula surrounded by osteoblasts. At the left, there are megakaryocytes (arrows) and numerous hematopoietic cells. (Methacrylate, Giemsa; magnification × 500.)

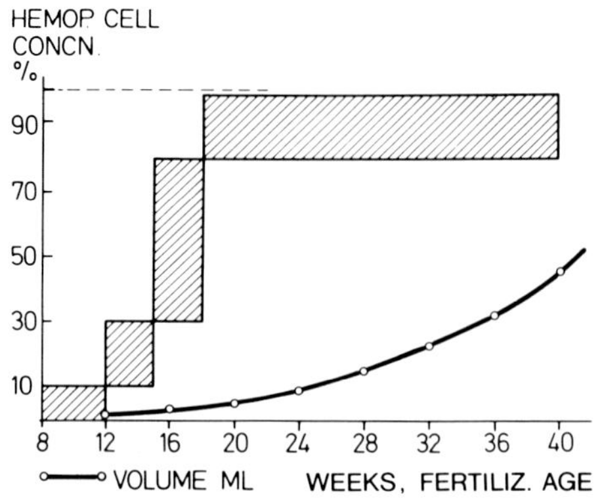

FIGURE 13. Hematopoietic cell concentration in smears, as percent of all free cells (hatched areas) and the corresponding changes in the total bone marrow volume in the course of marrow development. Note that hemopoietic cell concentrations have reached levels around 90% already after the 18th week.

3. Polychromatophilic normoblasts up to the 12th week: 30 to 45%; thereafter: 10 to 25%
4. Orthochromatic normoblasts: 1 to 5%

Similar counts were reported by Oguro et al.[32] for the second trimester.

4. Granulopoiesis

In contrast to liver, marrow hematopoiesis is predominantly granulopoietic and rich in lymphocytes. The G/E ratio is about 2 to 3 after the 17th week, when the marrow volume begins to increase rapidly. The different cell lines predominate in different territories: marrow granulocytes and lymphocytes appear more frequently in the connective tissue around the arterial vessels, while erythroid cells and megakaryocytes are formed around the sinusoids.[91] Among the granulopoietic cells, the neutrophils are about 30 to 50% of all hematopoietic cells, the eosinophils 1 to 2% until the 16th week, and 3 to 8% thereafter. Basophils are under 1% of hematopoietic cells. Lower numbers of granulocytes (8 to 34%) were counted by Oguro et al.[32] in samples from the second trimester.

Findings in some blood diseases such as severe agranulocytosis, as well as in vitro cloning experiments, suggest that there is a distinct eosinophilic cell line (CFU-Eo). This could explain the occasional finding of eosinophil clusters in the fetus.[92] Several samples over 20 weeks of gestation (both in the literature and in our own material) were from fetuses suffering from disease and/or head injury. Nevertheless, normal cases appear to form the basis of cell counting in the literature,[93,98] including the differential counts for full-term, healthy children.

Up to the 22nd week of gestation, 35% of the granulocytes belonged to the proliferative (capable of division) compartment. A slight reduction of this compartment (about 20 to 25%) can be observed thereafter. We present here data from 14- to 20-week-old samples in the phase of the extending marrow hematopoiesis. Table 4 compares early granulopoiesis with that of full-term infants.

It seems that the rate of granulocyte production in the fetus is higher than in adults. This presumption is based on the following data: the total marrow volume is about 1

Table 4
DIFFERENTIAL COUNTS FOR EARLY FETAL BONE MARROW GRANULOPOIESIS IN MAN

	Fertilization age (weeks)					
	13—14	15—16	17—18	19—20	21—22	Full term
Myeloblasts	2	2.5	2.5	2.5	2	0.5—4
Promyelocytes	11.5	8	17—24	18	20	1—8
Neutrophil myelocytes	15—23	10—18	10	19.5	15—30	4—24
Neutrophil metamyelocytes	15—29	11.5	13—20	15	13	8—40
Neutrophil bands	12—16	8—17	16	11	6—12	8—48
Neutrophil segments	16—21	6—28	15—30	7—25	9—28	16—56
Eosinophils, early	1—3	2.5	3	7	5—12	1—3
Eosinophils mature	1—2	3—6	3	5—15	7—19	1—5
Basophils	0—2	0—1.5	0.5—1	0—0.25	0.5	0—1
Number of samples (500 granulocytes per sample)	2	2	2	2	2	5

mℓ at the 13th week, 10 to 15 mℓ at the 26th week, and 45 mℓ or more at 39 weeks; the hematopoietic cellularity is already 75% or more from the 18th week onward, with values over 90% in the third trimester. The number of circulating granulocytes rises sharply from $10^2/\mu\ell$ of blood in the first trimester, around 10^3 during the second and up to $10^4/\mu\ell$ during the third trimester.[99]

5. Macrophages and Monocytes

Unlike adult macrophages, early embryonic/fetal macrophages cannot originate from the bone marrow, because there are numerous macrophages in the yolk sac and in the embryonic liver several weeks before the initiation of marrow hematopoiesis.[30] Marrow-derived macrophages must represent a different cell population, unless they originate from liver macrophages that seeded the primitive marrow.

Classic monocytes were found in the marrow smears of the first trimester. During this time, they amounted to about 2 to 4% of hematopoietic cells. Later samples contained less than 1% monocytes. Oguro et al.[32] found 3 to 7% in the 30th week.

6. Megakaryocytes and Platelets

In our material, the megakaryocytes appeared in smears of a 12 week sample. Haas[96] did not find these cells until the 26th week. The increase in marrow megakaryopoiesis coincides with the decline of megakaryocyte content in the liver. We do not know the mechanism governing the shift from one organ to the other.

Twenty-four randomized marrow samples from 13- to 32-week-old fetuses were used to investigate the presence of megakaryocytes, differentiating 2000 hematopoietic cells per smear. The number of megakaryocytes ranged between 0.02 and 0.4% of hematopoietic cells. Samples having a high degree of nuclear changes (dyserythropoiesis) did not contain megakaryocytes. These "negative" samples were mostly from spontaneous abortions. Therefore, absence of megakaryocytes in smears suggests that the fetus had suffered from a process leading to necrobiotic injury involving mature erythroblasts as well as early megakaryocytes. Adequate evaluation of such parallel changes are not found in the literature. Osteoclasts, on the other hand, were found even in smears from pathologic cases.

The circulating platelet count was less than $10^4/\mu\ell$ in seven samples of fetuses up

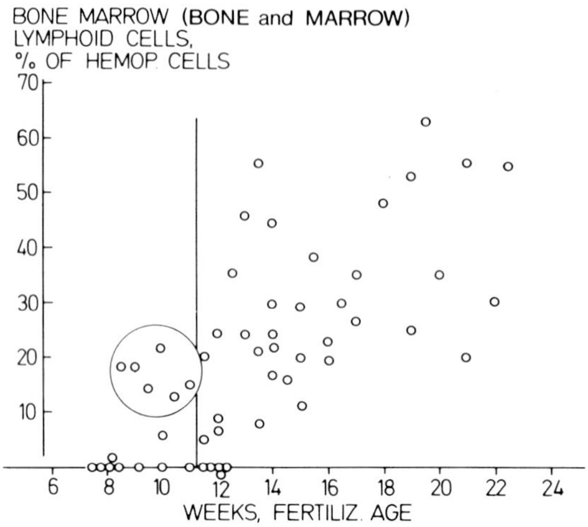

FIGURE 14. Bone and marrow lymphoid cell concentration in smears as percent of hematopoietic cells. The vertical line shows the beginning of hematopoiesis in most of the bones. Encircled points show that the corresponding percent values could be as high as about 20, i.e., substantial ammounts of lymphocyte-like cells might be found in some samples before hematopoiesis starts. The origin and significance of these cells remains to be proved. As Figure 15 shows, these cells hardly originated from the circulating blood.

to the 10th week of gestation. In three samples of the 12th to 16th week, there were about 2 to 5 $\times$ 10^4. Afterwards, there was a rapid rise in the number of blood platelets,[100] (up to 3 $\times$ $10^5/\mu\ell$ during the 20th week). The normal adult level platelet count can be found during the third trimester of fetal life.[101,102] The sudden rise in the number of circulating platelets coincides in time with the expansion of marrow megakaryopoiesis. Unlike liver megakaryocytes, those of the marrow seem to release platelets into the blood without appreciable delay.

For information on pathophysiology of neonatal coagulation, see Buchanan.[103]

7. Lymphocytes

Generation of diversity is one of the main characteristics of cells produced by lymphoid progenitors of the marrow. The hierarchy of hypothetical lymphoid progenitors was discussed.[104a] The key step in the generation of diversity, however, takes place in a cell that does not produce Ig and which thus, at present, we have no direct means of identifying.

Figure 14 shows marrow lymphocyte concentration in 58 samples of the first two trimesters of pregnancy. The finding of lymphocytes in smears of the marrow during the first trimester is somewhat irregular. They were absent in some cases while other samples from the 9th week contained up to 20% of all cells. From the second trimester to term, the lymphocyte representation increased, showing values of 30 to 60% of marrow cells. Using the Barka-Anderson method for acid phosphatase which marks T lymphocytes, 76 to 94% of fetal marrow lymphocytes behaved as non-T cells (in the first half of pregnancy).

Figure 15 serves to compare the above marrow values with those of circulating lymphocytes. It appears that there are already some lymphocytes in the prehemopoietic and

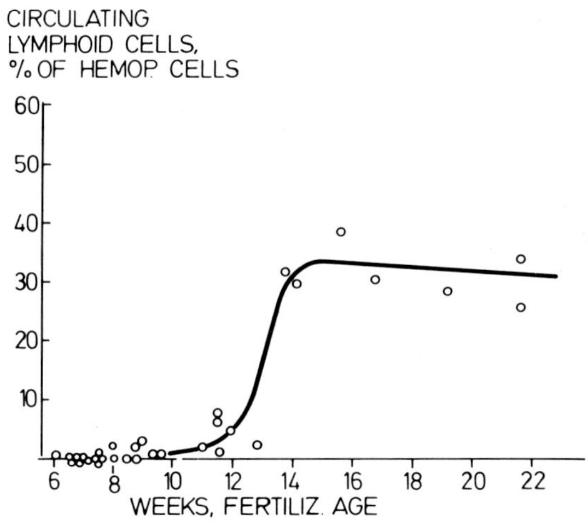

FIGURE 15. Percent of lymphoid cells present in smears of blood at different times after fertilization. A rapid increase in the proportion of these cells occurs after the 12th week of gestation.

early hematopoietic marrow at a time when there are only very few lymphocytes in the circulating blood. The appearance of remarkably high levels of lymphocytes in the blood coincides with a rapid rise in the number of marrow lymphocytes.

Although the inherent functional immaturity of neonatal B cells is well known, by the 12th week all of the major Ig isotopes are expressed by B cells. Thus, well before mid-gestation all of the genetic events necessary for generation of antibody diversity, intraclonal isotope switching, and synthesis of secretory antibody products have been initiated.[104b]

8. *Mast Cells*

Mast cells can be found in very small numbers in the portal spaces of the liver, in the capsule and interlobular septa of the thymus, and only rarely in the marrow.

9. *Mitosis*

Mitotic figures were counted and 0.1 to 1.2% of the hematopoietic cells were found in mitosis, but because the period of time that had elapsed between abrasion or delivery and the preparation of smears was sometimes from 10 to 30 min, the actual number of cells in mitosis could have been higher. An apparently important but frequently overlooked factor should be considered: the number of cells that die per unit of time. Even the knowledge of the number of cells in mitosis along with its duration could not predict growth unless *the growth fraction* and *the rate of cell loss* are known. Pertinent data are scanty for the developing human hematopoietic cell systems, and it is only suspected that both might be higher than in adult life.

10. *Colony Forming Cells*

For information on colony forming cells of the marrow, see Section II.B.1.h.

C. Cytochemical Observations

In the following paragraphs we discuss material which is somewhat connected with

Table 5
NEUTROPHIL GRANULOCYTE ALKALINE PHOSPHATASE ACTIVITY IN HUMAN EMBRYONIC AND FETAL LIVER, BONE MARROW, SPLEEN, AND PERIPHERAL BLOOD

Source of material	Fertil. age (weeks)	No. cases	Number of AP: Negative	+ to ++	+++ to ++++	Score
Liver	5—8	21	396	9	0	3
	9—13	7	306	13	1	6
	18—20	4	185	139	26	82
	21	1	29	48	23	152
Bone marrow	10—16	6	577	21	2	6
	18—22	9	1743	250	8	19
Spleen	15—20	8	628	296	27	54
	21	1	5	69	26	192
Peripheral	18—20	4	196	97	7	53
Blood	22—32	5	50	423	127	169
	21	1	9	49	42	225
	Term	7	175	949	376	183

Note: Neutrophil bands and segments are scored from 0 (negative) to ++++ positive and the score is given for 100 cells.

antenatal conditions. The use of cytochemical methods provides interesting information about differences in the reactivity of primitive and definitive cell types. The cytoplasm of *primitive erythroblasts* was diffusely greenish-yellow in peroxidase preparations, whereas the cytoplasm of definitive erythroblasts did not give this reaction. Slight, diffuse PAS-positivity occurred in some early precursors in both series. Mature cells were mostly PAS-negative; however, occasional granular positivity was found in some type-III primitive erythroblasts (primitive erythrocytes of Custer).

Early members of the *large monocytoid granuloblast* series (our fetal granuloblasts), were chloroacetate esterase and Sudan black-negative. These cells did not show cytoplasmic granules when observed with the light microscope. On the contrary, the cells of this series that possessed large primary granules were positive for peroxidase and chloroacetate esterase reaction, as well as for Sudan black. Each member of this series was alkaline phosphatase negative and either PAS negative or slightly, diffusely positive. Even granulated cells were acid-phosphatase negative.

The *osteoclasts* were chloroacetate esterase negative, and exhibited slight, diffuse PAS-positivity. Occasional coarse PAS-positive material was present on their surface, preferentially in cells with one or two nuclei. (PAS-positivity of megakaryocytes was stronger than that of osteoclasts; it was partly diffuse, partly patchy.) Their nonspecific esterase reaction was moderate to strong. Their positivity diminished only slightly after treatment with fluoride. They exhibited peroxidase negativity. These cells showed a slight AP-positivity, which is a cytochemical difference with the megakaryocytes. On the other hand, osteoclasts are strongly and diffusely acid phosphatase positive.

On the other hand, *osteoblasts* did not stain for acid phosphatase. Their nonspecific esterase reaction was slightly positive. Alkaline phosphatase reaction, however, was always negative.

Neutrophil granulocyte alkaline phosphatase (AP) reaction of fetal cells was also different from the corresponding cells of adults. Table 5 shows the AP reaction of granulocytes in our material. Only a small percentage of AP positive cells could be found during the first trimester of gestation. Occasional cells with a strong AP reaction appeared in the second trimester. Neutrophil AP positivity increased greatly in the third trimester, and newborn children had a somewhat higher than normal AP activity in their circulating neutrophils. In contrast with the AP negativity of the earliest developed neutrophils, these cells were chloroacetate esterase, peroxidase, and PAS positive.

It seems that strong neutrophil reactivity is related to gestation age rather than to the site of granulopoiesis. It starts at about the same time in the cells originating in the liver, marrow, spleen, and those circulating in the blood. However, bone marrow values are lower, and the score is around 20 at the 18th to 22nd week, when the corresponding values are over 50 in other areas. This observation confirms earlier work of Trubowitz et al.[105]

Histiocytes-macrophages had a tendency to exhibit precipitates of nonspecific esterase positive material, but this positivity diminished moderately in fluoride-treated smears. PAS-positivity was rather regular. Peroxidase, chloroacetate esterase, Sudan black, and alkaline phosphatase were negative. According to Cawley and Burns,[106] peroxidase and acid phosphatase were present in monocytic cells from their earliest identifiable stages, but later no peroxidase activity could be found in the endoplasmic reticulum, and nonreactive cytoplasmic granules began to appear in the cells.

During the last few years, several publications have reported the possibility of distinguishing members of the T and B *lymphocyte lines* by a nonspecific esterase test. We did not succeed in demonstrating unequivocal differences because practically all apparently mature lymphocytes originating in different sites, including bone marrow, tended to exhibit slight granular positivity. On the other hand, T lymphocytes exhibited a regular dot-like acid phosphatase positivity by the Barka-Anderson method.

D. Regulation of Hematopoietic Systems—Physiological and Pathological Samples

Little is known about the regulation of prenatal hematopoiesis. The bone marrow stroma is a vascularized and innervated connective tissue with a fine network of reticulin fibers that serve as support for the blood forming cells. One of us[92] studying the innervation of the human marrow during development found that nerves could be demonstrated in the marrow of the tibia of a 15-week-old fetus. These nerves begin to differentiate myelin sheaths during the 7th month of gestation and at the time of birth 10% of the nerve fibers are already myelinated. The presence of such fibers among the blood forming cells, as well as the existence of nonmyelinated fibers in the wall of the nutrient vessels, suggests that the nerves of the marrow may play a direct role in the regulation of hematopoiesis at the local level.

Microenvironmental aspects were discussed in another part of this chapter (see Section III.A.6). Stimulatory and inhibitory factors, as well as recognized hemopoietins are discussed elsewhere in this book.

The most frequent injury which seriously threatens the life of the fetus is severe infection, especially common in spontaneous abortion. Studying 28 samples, we tentatively concluded that there is no uniform pattern in marrow differential counts in these conditions. In some cases the G/E ratio was as high as 30. Sometimes mature granulocytes were lacking or lymphoid representation was very low. In other cases, large numbers of eosinophils were present, and sometimes it was difficult to find megakaryocytes. Classic plasma cells were exceptional even in these cases. The single morphological alteration which appeared rather regularly was dyserythropoiesis (see Section II.B.1.g), characterized by nuclear changes present in normoblasts. These changes were present in 20 to 50% of erythropoietic cells among fetuses that were dead at spontaneous abortions. It is proper to emphasize that an important source of discrepancies lies in the fact that several data of the literature are at least 'contaminated' with the inclusion of pathological samples.

For neonatal hematological abnormalities associated with maternal disease, see Lukens.[107]

Certain functional differences from part of the lymphoid system were already mentioned. Knowing the susceptibility of newborn infants to bacterial infections, it is not surprising to find deficiencies of both the humoral and cellular components in certain responses of the neutrophil granulocytes[108] and macrophages.[109]

E. Reappearance of Embryonic/Fetal Characteristics in Certain Disorders

The observation that some embryonic fetal characteristics of different hematopoietic cell systems reappear in certain blood disorders deserves special comment. Postnatal marrow contains undifferentiated mesenchymal cells of similar potential to those found at early stages of fetal marrow development.[110] Reappearance of apparent primitive erythroblasts (Plate 6), which is nowadays exceptional, was frequently seen more than 50 years ago in cases of severely "decompensated" pernicious anemia. We recently observed an extremely serious case in which many of the marrow megaloblasts resembled primitive embryonic erythroblasts and, according to preparations treated with the Betke-Kleihauer method, members of these series contained fetal or embryonic hemoglobin.

Presence of alkaline phosphatase negative neutrophils is a characteristic of early embryonic/fetal granulopoiesis[34] (see Section III.C). A similar pattern characterizes most cases of chronic granulocytic leukemia.

The megakaryocytes of the hematopoietic liver are small and have one to four nuclear lobes only. The so-called micromegakaryocytes are frequent in the fetal liver.[36] The presence of such cells is a well-known phenomenon in certain myeloproliferative disorders and in preleukemia. Plate 7 shows micromegakaryocytes in the blood of a patient with myelofibrosis.

Finally, the authors of this chapter would like to point out that, although abundant new data are included in the text, human development hematology is based on classical morphologic studies. Modern functional techniques developed during the last 20 years for cytokinetic studies have not yet been extensively applied to human material. The present chapter should be regarded as an up-to-date account of the structure and function of the blood forming cells during intrauterine development. The kinetic studies and the interest in the blood stem cells are areas of research in a rapidly expanding process and one can expect that great progress will be made here.

REFERENCES

1. **Kelemen, E., Calvo, W., and Fliedner, T. M.,** *Atlas of Human Hemopoietic Development,* Springer-Verlag, Berlin, 1979.
2. **Patten, B. M.,** *Human Embryology,* McGraw-Hill, New York, 1968, 142.
3. **Bloom, W.,** Embryogenesis of mammalian blood, in *Handbook of Hematology,* Vol. 2, Downey, H., Ed., Hoeber, New York, 1938, 863.
4. **Metcalf, D. and Moore, M. A. S.,** *Haemopoietic Cells,* North-Holland, Amsterdam, 1971, 264.
5. **Luckett, W. P.,** Origin and differentiation of the yolk sac and extraembryonic mesoderm in presomite human and Rhesus monkey embryos, *Am. J. Anat.,* 152, 59, 1978.

6. **Dieterlen-Lievre, F.,** Yolk sac erythropoiesis, *Experientia,* 34, 284, 1978.
7. **Le Douarin, N. M.,** Dependence of myeloid and lymphoid organ development on stem cell seeding: investigations on mechanisms in cell marker analysis, in *Mechanisms of Cell Exchange,* Ebert, J. D. and Okada, T. S., Eds., John Wiley & Sons, New York, 1979, 293.
8. **Symann, M., Anckaert, M. A., Cordier, A., Rodhain, J., and Sokal, G.,** Murine yolk sac hematopoiesis studied with the diffusion chamber technic, *Exp. Hematol.,* 6, 749, 1978.
9. **Turpen, J. B.,** Early embryogenesis of hematopoietic cells in Rana pipiens, in *Development and Differentiation of Vertebrate Lymphocytes,* Horton, J. D., Ed., Elsevier, Amsterdam, 1980, 15.
10. **Dandy, W. W.,** A human embryo with seven pairs of somites measuring about 2 mm in length, *Am. J. Anat.,* 10, 85, 1910.
11. **Mazanec, K.,** *Blastogenese des Menschen,* G. Fischer, Jena, 1959, 109.
12. **Latsis, R. V., Deryugina, E. I., and Drize, N. I.,** Colony forming capacity of different hemopoietic organs of the quail embryo, *Bjull. Ekszp. Biol. Med. Moskva,* 88, 214, 1980.
13. **Moore, K. L.,** *The Developing Human,* 2nd ed., W. B. Saunders, Philadelphia, 1977, 262.
14. **Gilmour, J. R.,** Normal haemopoiesis in intra-uterine and neonatal life, *J. Pathol. Bacteriol.,* 52, 25, 1941.
15a. **Samarut, J. and Bouabdelli, M.,** In vitro development of CFU-E and BFU-E in cultures of embryonic and post-embryonic chicken hematopoietic cells, *J. Cell. Physiol.,* 105, 553, 1980.
15b. **Knoll, W.,** Die Entwicklung des blutbildenden Gewebes und des Blutes beim Menschen, in *Handb. gesamt. Hämatologie,* Heilmeyer, L. und Hittmair, A., Eds., Urban-Schwarzenberg, München, 1957, 36.
16. **Stieve, H.,** Ein 13 1/2 Tage altes, in der Gebärmutter erhaltenes und durch Eingriff gewonnenes menschliches Ei, *Z. Mikrosk. Anat. Forsch.,* 7, 195, 1926.
17. **Stieve, H. and Strube, I.,** Über die Entwicklung des Dottersackkreislaufes beim Menschen, *Z. Mikrosk. Anat. Forsch.,* 32, 107, 1933.
18. **Fukuda, T.,** Fetal hemopoiesis. I. Electron microcopic studies on human yolk sac hemopoiesis, *Virchows Arch. B.,* 14, 197, 1973.
19. **Kelemen, E.,** Extraembryonic haemopoiesis in man, in *Antenatal Development of Human Blood Cells,* 28th Congr. I.U.P.S. Symp., Pergamon Publ. and Publishing House of Hungarian Academy of Science, Budapest, 1981, 45.
20. **Maximow, A.,** Untersuchungen über Blut und Bindegewebe I. Die frühesten Entwicklungsstadien der Blut- und Bindegewebszellen beim Säugetierembryo, bis zum Anfang der Blutbildung in der Leber, *Arch. Mikrosk. Anat.,* 73, 444, 1909.
21. **Fong, P. L., Maloney, M. A., and Patt, H. M.,** Origin of repopulating cells in a mechanically depleted medullary cavity as determined by studies with marrow transplants, *Blood,* 37, 413, 1971.
22. **Bessis, M.,** *Blood Smears Reinterpreted,* Springer-Verlag, Berlin, 1977, 38.
23a. **Jánossa, M. and Kelemen, E.,** Erythroblastic islands in human extraembryonic and embryonic tissue, in symposium on *Antenatal Development of Human Blood Cells,* 28th Congr. I.U.P.S. Symp., Pergamon Publ. and Publ. House of Hung. Acad. Sci. Budapest, 1981, 81.
23b. **Fukuda T.,** Ultrastructure of fetal hemopoiesis, *Acta Haematol. Jpn.,* 41, 1204, 1978.
24. **Wickramashinge, S. N.,** *Human Bone Marrow,* Blackwell Scientific, Oxford, 1975, 36.
25. **Wood, W. G. and Weatherall, D. J.,** Hemoglobin synthesis during human fetal development, *Nature,* 244, 162, 1973.
26a. **Zanjani, E. D., McGlave, P. B. and Stamatoyannopoulos, G.,** Fetal to adult transplant in sheep, in *Fetal Liver Transplantation,* Lucarelli, G., Fliedner, T. M. and Gale, P. R., Eds., Excerpta Medica, Amsterdam, 1980, 108.
26b. **McGlave, P. B., Zanjani, E. D., and Stamatoyannopoulos, G.,** Use of hematopoietic stem cell transplants in the study of the regulation of hemoglobin switching in sheep, *Clin, Res.,* 38, 729A, 1980.
27a. **Stamatoyannopoulos, G. and Papayannopoulou, T.,** Fetal hemoglobin and the erythroid stem cell differentiation process, in *Cellular and Molecular Regulation of Hemoglobin Switching,* Stamatoyannopoulos, G. and Nienhuis, A. W., Eds., Grune & Stratton, New York, 1979, 323.
27b. **Terasawa, T. and Ogawa, M.,** Hemoglobin biosynthesis in individual bursts from human adult peripheral and umbilical cord blood: analysis of the relative rates of synthesis of G and A globin chains, *J. Cell. Physiol.,* 105, 483, 1980.
28. **Kelemen, E. and Balogh, I.,** Intimate contact between human yolk sac endoderm and haemopoietic precursor cells, *Acta Morphol. Acad. Sci. Hung.,* 24, 71, 1976.
29. **Kelemen, E.,** Compartmentalization of haemic cells in human yolk sac, *Acta Med. Acad. Sci. Hung.,* 28, 113, 1975.
30. **Kelemen, E. and Jánossa, M.,** Macrophages are the first differentiated blood cells formed in human embryonic liver, *Exp. Hematol.,* 8, 996, 1980.

31. **Deimann, W. and Fahimi, H. D.,** Peroxidase cytochemistry and ultrastructure of resident macrophages in fetal rat liver: a developmental study, *Dev. Biol.,* 66, 43, 1978.
32. **Oguro, M., Koizumi, F., and Sasagawa, S.,** Blood cells in the peripheral blood and hematopoietic organs of the human fetus during hepatic hematopoiesis, *Acta Haematol. Jpn.,* 41, 1231, 1978.
33. **Ohkita, T. and Enzyn, H.,** Morphological studies on the hepatic hematopoiesis of human fetuses, in *Antenatal Development of Human Blood Cells,* 28th Congr. I.U.P.S. Symp., Pergamon Publ. and Publ. House of Hung. Acad. Sci., Budapest, 1981, 53.
34. **Calvo, W. and Carbonell, F.,** The development of liver granulopoiesis in the human fetus, in *Fetal Liver Tranplantation,* Lucarelli, G., Fliedner, T. M., and Gale, R. P., Eds., Excerpta Medica, Amsterdam, 1980, 14.
35. **Kelemen, E., Gulya, E., and Vass, K.,** Ontogeny of human neutrophil granulocyte alkaline phosphatase, *J. Cell. Physiol.,* 95, 553, 1978.
36. **Kelemen, E.,** Small megakaryocytes in human embryonic liver, *Blood Cells,* 5, 101, 1979.
37. **Levine, R. F.,** Isolation and characterization of normal human megakaryocytes, *Br. J. Hematol.,* 45, 487, 1980.
38. **Carr, M. C., Stites, D. P., and Fudenberg, H. H.,** The numerical development of lymphoid cells during human embryogenesis, *Transplantation,* 20, 410, 1975.
39. **Champlin, R., Niskanen, E., and Gale, R. P.,** Hematopoiesis and immune reactivity of human fetal liver cells, in *Fetal Liver Transplantation,* Lucarelli, G., Fliedner, T. M., and Gale, R. P., Eds., Excerpta Medica, Amsterdam, 1980, 117.
40. **Kelemen, E. and Pajor, A.,** Human prenatal dyserythropoiesis in the liver: a temperature-dependent danger-signal of normoblasts, Abstr., Int. Congr. European Hematol., Hamburg, August 16 to 18, 1979, 78.
41. **Fliedner, T. M. and Calvo, W.,** Hematopoietic stem cell seeding of a cellular matrix: a principle of intitiation and regeneration of hematopoiesis, in *Differentiation of Normal and Neoplastic Hematopoietic Cells,* Clarkson, B., Marks, P. A., and Till, J. E., Eds., Cold Spring Harbor Laboratory, New York, 1978, 5.
42. **Moore, M. A. S., and Williams, N.,** Analysis of proliferation and differentiation of foetal granulocyte-macrophage progenitor cells in haemopoietic tissue, *Cell Tissue Kinet.,* 6, 461, 1973.
43. **Dresch, C. and Faille, A.,** Granulocyte-monocyte colony forming cells from bone marrow, blood, cord blood and foetal liver in normal man, in *Cell Lineage, Stem Cells and Cell Determination,* Le Douarin, N. M., Ed., North-Holland, Amsterdam, 1979, 191.
44. **Fliedner, T. M., Calvo, W., Nothdurft, W., and Grilli, G.,** Fetal liver: a transitory site for hemopoietic stem cell replication and selective differentiation, in *Fetal Liver Transplantation,* Lucarelli, G., Fliedner, T. M., and Gale, R. P., Eds., Excerpta Medica, Amsterdam, 1980, 5.
45. **Gerasimova, L. P.,** Colony forming capacity of hemopoietic and lymphoid organs in human embryo- and fetogenesis, *Probl. Hematol. Perel. Krovi (Moskva),* 25/5, 45, 1980.
46. **Barak, Y., Karov, Y., Levin, S., Soroker, N., Barash, A., Lancet, M., and Nir, E.,** Granulocyte-macrophage colonies in cultures of human fetal liver cells: morphologic and ultrastructural analysis of proliferation and differentiation, *Exp. Hematol.,* 8, 837, 1980.
47. **Porcellini, A., Manna, A., Izzi, T., Delfini, C., and Lucarelli, G.,** In vitro culture of granulocytic colonies from liver, spleen and bone marrow of human fetuses, in *Fetal Liver Transplantation,* Lucarelli, G., Fliedner, T. M., and Gale, R. P., Eds., Excerpta Medica, Amsterdam, 1980, 45.
48. **Shadduck, R. K., Pigoli, G., Waheed, A., and Boegel, F.,** Characterization of hemopoietic progenitor cells in fetal liver, in *Fetal Liver Transplantation,* Lucarelli, G., Fliedner, T. M., and Gale, R. P., Eds., Excerpta Medica, Amsterdam, 1980, 29.
49. **Hassan, M. W., Lutton, J. D., Levere, R. D., Rieder, R. F., and Cederquist, R. D.,** In vitro culture of erythroid colonies from human fetal liver and umbilical cord blood, *Br. J. Haematol.,* 41, 477, 1979.
50. **Gale, R. P.,** Concepts of fetal liver transplantation in man, in *Fetal Liver Transplantation,* Lucarelli, G., Fliedner, T. M., and Gale, R. P., Eds., Excerpta Medica, Amsterdam, 1980, 247.
51. **Kubanek, B., Heit, W., and Rich, I.,** Fetal erythropoiesis, in *Fetal Liver Transplantation,* Lucarelli, G., Fliedner, T. M., and Gale, R. P., Eds., Excerpta Medica, Amsterdam, 1980, 71.
52. **Löwenberg, B.,** Take of fetal liver transplants, in *Fetal Liver Transplantation,* Lucarelli, G., Fliedner, T. M., and Gale, R. P., Eds., Excerpta Medica, Amsterdam, 1980, 157.
53. **Hijmans, W. and Vossen, J. J.,** The development of the B and T cell systems in humans, in *Antenatal Development of Human Blood Cells,* 28th Congr. I.U.P.S. Symp., Pergamon Publ. and Publ. House of Hung. Acad. Sci., Budapest, 1981, 69.
54. **Chandra, R. K. and Matsumura,** Ontogenic development of the immune system and effects of fetal growth retardation, *J. Perinat. Med.,* 7, 279, 1979.

55. **Handzel, A. T., Levin, S., et al.,** Immune competence of newborn lymphocytes, *Pediatrics,* 65, 491, 1980.
56. **Jones, W. R.,** Fetal and neonatal immunology, in *Immunology of Human Reproduction,* Scott, J. S. and Jones, W. R., Eds., Academic Press, London, 1976, 127.
57. **Taylor, R. B. and Skinner, J. M.,** Evidence for significant hematopoiesis in human thymus, *Blood,* 47, 305, 1976.
58. **Melchers, F.,** Three waves of B-lymphocyte development during embryonic development of the mouse, in *Cell Lineage, Stem Cells and Cell Determination,* Le Douarin, N. M., Eds., North-Holland, Amsterdam, 1979, 281.
59. **Melchers, F. and Abramczuk, J.,** Murine embryonic blood between day 10 and 13 of gestation as a source of immature precursor B cells, *Eur. J. Immunol.,* 10, 763, 1980.
60. **Rayfield, L. S., Brent, L., and Rodeck, C. H.,** Development of cell-mediated lympholysis in human fetal blood lymphocytes, *Clin. Exp. Immunol.* 42, 561, 1980.
61a. **Hayward, A. R. and Kurnick J.,** Newborn T cell suppression: early appearance, maintenance in culture and lack of growth factor suppression, *J. Immunol.,* 126, 50, 1981.
61b. **Toivanen, P. and Granberg, C.,** Mother/child MLR: is it depressed?, *Immunol. Today,* 1, 76, 1980.
61c. **Klein, J.,** Demystifying the MHC, *Immunol. Today,* 2, 166, 1981.
61d. **Toivanen, P., Uksila, J., Leino, A., et al.,** Development of mitogen responding T cells and natural killer cells in the human fetus, *Immunol. Rev.,* 57, 89, 1981.
61e. **Pabst, H. F. and Kreth, H. W.,** Ontogeny of the immune response as a basis of childhood disease, *J. Pediatr.,* 97, 519, 1980.
62. **Schulz, D. M., Giordano, D. A., and Schulz, D. H.,** Weights or organs of fetuses and infants, *Arch. Pathol.,* 74, 244, 1962.
63. **Le Douarin, N. M. and Jotereau, F. V.,** Tracing of the avian thymus through embryonic life in interspecific chimeras, *J. Exp. Med.,* 142, 17, 1975.
64. **Le Douarin, N. M.,** Ontogeny of hematopoietic organs studied in avian embryo interspecific chimeras, in *Differentiation of Normal and Neoplastic Hematopoietic Cells,* Clarkson, B., Marks, P. A., and Till, J. E., Eds., Cold Spring Harbor Laboratory, New York, 1978, 5.
65. **Tompkins, R., Volpe, E. P., and Reinschmidt, D. C.,** Origin of hemopoietic stem cells in amphibian ontogeny, in *Development and Differentiation of Vertebrate Lymphocytes,* Horton, J. D., Ed., Elsevier, Amsterdam, 1980, 25.
66. **Touraine, J. L., Incefy, G. S., Touraine, F., Rho, Y. M., and Good, R. A.,** Differentiation of human bone marrow cells into T lymphocytes by in vitro incubation with thymic extracts, *Clin. Exp. Immunol.,* 17, 151, 1977.
67. **Parkman, R. and Merler, E.,** Discontinuous density gradient analysis of the developing human thymus, *Cell. Immunol.,* 8, 328, 1973.
68. **Galili, U., Polliack, A., Okon, E., Leizerovitz, R., Gamliel, H., Korkesh, A., Shenkar, J. G., and Izak, G.,** Human prothymocytes. Membrane properties, differentiation patterns, glucocorticoid sensitivity, and ultrastructural features, *J. Exp. Med.,* 152, 796, 1980.
69. **McPhee, D., Pye, J., and Shortman, K.,** The differentiation of T lymphocytes. V. Evidence for intrathymic death of most thymocytes, *Thymus,* 1, 151, 1979.
70. **Block, M. H.,** *Text-Atlas of Hematology,* Lea & Febiger, Philadelphia, 1976, 14.
71. **Hudson, G.,** Bone marrow volume in the human foetus and newborn, *Br. J. Haematol.,* 11, 446, 1965.
72. **Castro-Malaspina, H., Gay, R. E., Resnick, G., et al.,** Characterization of human bone marrow fibroblast CFCs/CFU-F/ and their progeny, *Blood,* 56, 289, 1980.
73. **Werts, E. D., Gibson, D. P., Knapp, S. A., and deGowin, R. I.,** Stromal cell migration preceded hemopoietic repopulation of the bone marrow after irradiation, *Radiat. Res.,* 81, 20, 1980.
74. **Trentin, J. J.,** Hemopoietic inductive microenvironments, in *Stem Cells of Renewing Cell Populations,* Cainnie, A. B., Lala, P. K., and Osmond, D. G., Eds., Academic Press, New York, 1976, 255.
75. **Wolf, N. S.,** The haemopietic microenvironment, *Clin. Hematol.,* 8, 469, 1979.
76. **Friedenstein, A. J., Chajlakjan, R. K., Latzinik, N. V., Pansjuk, A. F., and Keiliss-Borok, I. V.,** Stromal cells responsible for transferring the microenvironment of the hemopoietic tissues. Cloning in vitro and retransplantation in vivo, *Transplantation,* 17, 331, 1974.
77. **Chertkov, J. L., Gurevitch, O. A., and Udalov, G. A.,** Role of bone marrow stroma in hemopoietic stem cell regulation, *Exp. Hematol.,* 8, 770, 1980.
78. **Biermann, A. and von Keyserlingk, D.,** Ultrastructure of reticulum cells in the bone marrow, *Acta Anat.,* 100, 34, 1978.

79. **Lumb, J. R.,** Perspectives on the in vivo location of cellular interactions in the humoral immune response, *Ann. Rev. Microbiol.,* 33, 439, 1979.
80. **Anderson, N. A., Colyer, R. A., and Riley, R. H., Jr.,** Skeletal changes during prolonged external irradiation: alterations in marrow, growth plate and osteoclast populations, *Johns Hopkins Med. J.,* 145, 73, 1979.
81. **Ash, P., Loutit, J. F., and Townsend, K. M. S.,** Osteoclasts derived from hematopoietic stem cells, *Nature,* 283, 669, 1980.
82. **Testa, N. G., Allen, T. D., Suda, T., Onions, D., and Jarrett, O.,** Generation of Osteoclasts in Vitro, *Ann. Rep. Paterson Labor. Medical Oncol.,* 1979/80, 130.

83a. **Kelemen, E. and Calvo, W.,** First appearance of human fetal osteoclasts coincides with the formation of prehematopoietic stroma, Abstr. 10th Congr. Int. Soc. Hematol., Munich, *Exp. Hematol. Suppl.* 9, 104, 1981.

83b. **Malone, J. D., Teitelbaum, S. L., et al.,** Recruitment of osteoclast precursors by purified bone marrow matrix constituents, *J. Cell Biol.,* 92, 227, 1982.

83c. **Ko, J. S., and Bernard, G. W.,** Osteoclast formation in vitro from bone marrow mononuclear cells in osteoclast-free bone, *Am. J. Anat.,* 161, 415, 1981.

83d. **Tinkler, S. M. B., Linder, J. E., et al.,** Formation of osteoclasts from blood monocytes during 1α-OH Vit-D-stimulated bone resorption in mice, *J. Anat.,* 133, 389, 1981.

83e. **Chen, L., and Weiss, L.,** The development of vertebral bone marrow of human fetuses, *Blood,* 46, 389, 1975.

84. **Wetzel, G.,** Die blutbildenden Organe. Das Knochenmark, in *Hanbd. Anat. des Kindes,* Bergmann, München, 1, 140, 1938.
85. **Pearson, H. A.,** Origin and development of blood cells and coagulation factors, in *Smith's Blood Diseases of Infancy and Childhood,* 4th ed., C. V. Mosby, St. Louis, 1978, 3.
86. **Tavassoli, M.,** Ultrastructural development of bone marrow adipose cell, *Acta Anat.,* 94, 65, 1976.
87. **Mendelow, B., Grobicki, D., et al.,** Characterization of bone marrow stromal cells in suspension and monolayer cultures, *Br. J. Haematol.,* 46, 15, 1980.
88. **Allen, R. D. and Dexter, T. M.,** Cellular interrelationships during in vitro granulopoiesis, *Differentiation,* 6, 191, 1976.
89. **Gartner, S. and Kaplan, H. S.,** Long-term culture of human bone marrow cells, *Proc. Natl. Acad. Sci. U.S.A.,* 77, 4756, 1980.
90. **Mollison, P. L., Veall, N., and Cutbush, M.,** Red cell volume and plasma volume in newborn infants, *Arch. Dis. Child.,* 25, 242, 1950.
91. **Demmler, K. and Burkhardt, R.,** Gefäßveränderungen im Knochenmark bei Bluterkrankungen, *Med. Klin. Munich,* 75, 238, 1980.
92. **Calvo, W.,** Bone marrow haemopoiesis in human foetuses, in *Antenatal Development of Human Blood Cells,* 28th Congr. I.U.P.S. Symp., Pergamon and Publ. House of Hung. Acad. Sci., Budapest, 1981, 65.
93. **Gairdner, D., Marks, J., and Roscoe, J. D.,** Blood formation in infancy. I. The normal bone marrow, *Arch. Dis. Child.,* 27, 128, 1952.
94. **Kalpaktsoglou, P. K. and Emery, J. L.,** Human bone marrow during the last three months of intrauterine life. A histological study, *Acta Haematol. (Basel),* 34, 228, 1965.
95. **Opitz, H. and Weicker, H.,** *Das Blut. Biologische Daten für den Kinderarzt,* Springer-Verlag, Heidelberg, 1954.
96. **Haas, R. J.,** in *Das Knochenmark. Morphologie, Funktion, Diagnostik,* Quiesser, W., Ed., Georg Thieme, Verlag Suttgart, 1978, 70.
97. **Shapiro, L. M. and Bassen, F. A.,** Sternal marrow changes after the first week of life, *Am. J. Med. Sci.,* 202, 341, 1941.
98. **Warninghoff, G. und Hausmann, K.,** Die Morphologie der embryonalen Hämatopoese des Menschen im Vergleich zu postfetalen Blutbildungsstörungen, *Acta Haematol. (Basel),* 14, 273, 1955.
99. **Thomas, D. B. and Yoffey, J. M.,** Human foetal haemopoiesis. I. The cellular composition of foetal blood, *Br. J. Haematol.,* 8, 290, 1962.
100. **Homberg, L., Henrksson, P., et al.,** Coagulation in the human fetus, *J. Pediatr.,* 85, 860, 1974.
101. **Aballi, A. J., Puapondh, Y., and Desposito, F.,** Platelet counts in thriving premature infants, *Pediatrics,* 42, 685, 1968.
102. **Fogel, B. J., Arias, D., and Kung, F.,** Platelet counts in healthy premature infants, *J. Pediatr.,* 73, 108, 1968.
103. **Buchanan, G. R.,** Neonatal coagulation: normal physiology and pathophysiology, *Clin. Haematol.,* 7, 85, 1978.

104a. **Schrader, J. W.,** Stem cell differentiation in the bone marrow, *Immunol. Today,* 2, 7, 1981.

104b. **Gathings, W. E., Kubawaga, H., and Cooper, M. D.,** A distinctive pattern of B cell immaturation in perinatal humans, *Immunol. Rev.,* 57, 107, 1981.
105. **Trubowitz, S., Feldman, D., Benate, C., and Hung, V. M.,** The alkaline phosphatase content of the human polymorphonuclear leukocyte in blood and marrow, *Am. J. Clin. Pathol.,* 31, 481, 1959.
106. **Cawley, J. C. and Burns, G. F.,** The cytochemistry of human lymphoreticular subpopulations, *Immunol. Today,* 1, 85, 1980.
107. **Lukens, J. N.,** Neonatal hematological abnormalities associated with maternal disease, *Clin. Haematol.,* 7, 155, 1978.
108. **Miller, M. E.,** Chemotactic function in the human neonate: humoral and cellular aspects, *Pediatr. Res.,* 5, 487, 1971.
109. **Blaese, R. M. and Lawrence, E. C.,** in *Development of Host Defenses,* Cooper, M. D. and Dayton, D. H., Eds., Raven Press, New York, 1977, 201.
110. **Ashton, B. A., Allen, T. D., Howlett, C. R., Eaglesom, C. C., Hattori, A., and Owen, M.,** Formation of bone and cartilage by marrow stromal cells in diffusion chambers in vivo, *Clin. Orthoped.,* 151, 294, 1980.

Chapter 3

THE BONE MARROW MATRIX

Sidney Trubowitz and Stephen Davis

TABLE OF CONTENTS

I. INTRODUCTION

The human bone marrow is one of the larger organs of the body and is housed in the interior spaces of the skeleton. Its weight has been estimated at 3.4 to 5.9% of the total body weight.[1] In the adult it acquires a weight of some 3000 g of which half, the yellow marrow, is essentially adipose tissue and found in the distal portions of the long bones. The red, hemopoietically active marrow occupies the spaces in the proximal parts of the long bones and of the axial skeleton, the skull, vertebrae, pelvis, and ribs. Half of the total mass of the red marrow is adipose tissue. Since fat at body temperature is an oil, the marrow has a soft paste-like quality with no inherent gross architectural characteristics other than those imposed by the shape of the bony space itself.

At first glance, the structure of the bone marrow is not impressive and offers little insight into its enormous functional capacity to produce and maintain a constant flow of large numbers of red cells, white cells, and platelets. However, if we were to examine a particle of marrow such as is found in an aspirate of human marrow under a stereo-microscope at about 30 diameters, we would be struck by its rather superficial resemblance to an aggregate of small fish or frog eggs, namely embryonic structures, spread over the surface of yolk sac (Figures 1, 2). At this magnification the marrow appears to consist of a spherical pack of fat cells whose surfaces are covered with the proliferating hemopoietic cells. At slightly higher magnification and with appropriate staining the vascular channels can be identified coursing over and between the fat cells. Under higher magnification a loose syncytium of reticulum cells and macrophages can be identified intercalated between the vascular sinus and the hemopoietic cells (Figure 2). Thus, during normal hemopoietic activity, the human marrow, similar to the marrow of rabbits,[2,3] guinea pigs, and birds consists of a mass of differentiating cells proliferating, like cells in a tissue culture flask, over the surfaces of fat cells. The vascular sinusoids course over and between the fat cells and a system of reticulum cells is spread between the sinusoids, the fat cells, and the hemopoietic cells. The marrow matrix is this collection of sinusoids, reticulum cells, and fat cells, whose topological and functional relationships to each other and to the differentiating hemopoietic cells are the consideration of this chapter.[4-8]

II. MARROW FAT

Recognition of fat as a major constituent of the marrow came with the very early discovery, made independently by Bizzozero[9] and Neumann,[10] that the bone marrow is the site of blood cell production. Indeed, Neumann pursued the relationship of fat to hemopoiesis and in 1882 reported on the conversion of the red hemopoietically active, distal bone marrow to a yellow, fatty marrow in the growing child.[11]

Adipose cells occupy about half of the red marrow volume.[12] In the normal rabbit the isolated marrow fat cells possess a mean diameter of 50 μm; their mean cell volume is about one fifth the mean volume of the extramedullary fat cells isolated from the perinephric and subcutaneous sites. Except for size, the marrow fat cell is morphologically indistinguishable from its counterpart in the extramedullary sites, and both cells show the same fatty acid turnover per cell as measured by palmitate-1-^{14}C incorporation.[13]

Studies of the fatty acid composition of bone marrow fat have shown relatively small differences from the compositional characteristics of other adipose tissues.[14-16] Zach and Shafrir[17] demonstrated the interspecies differences in the fatty acid composition of fat taken from identical adipose sites, but rather consistent similar fatty acid composition of the different adipose sites, including marrow, in the same animal. In the rabbit,

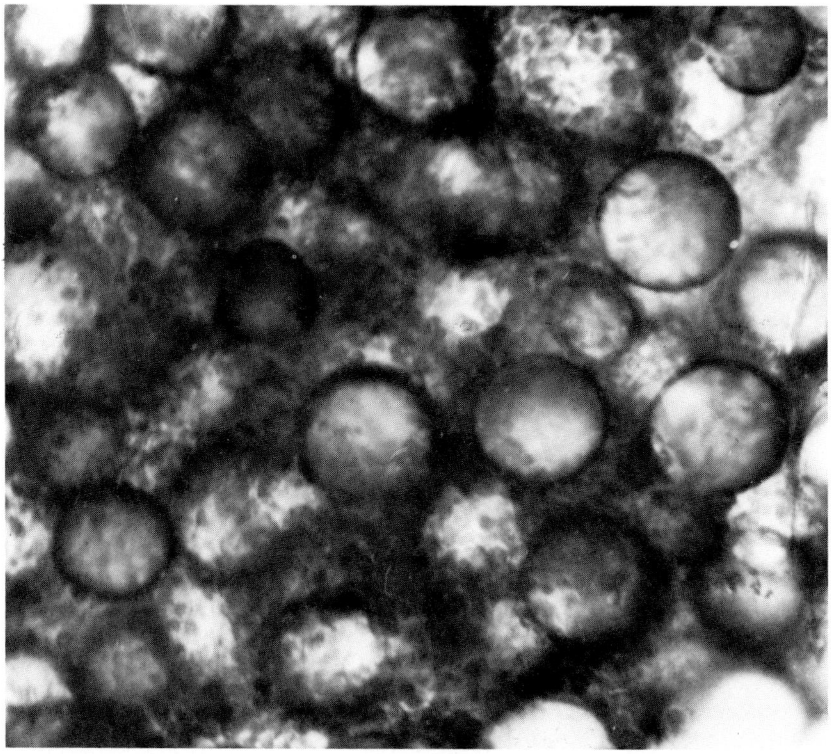

FIGURE 1. Bone marrow particle, human aspirate; toluidine blue stain, whole mount. (Magnification ca × 150).

only small differences exist between the fatty acid composition of the yellow and red marrow fat. The yellow marrow is somewhat richer than the red marrow in palmitoleic acid.[18] There appears to be a somewhat higher concentration of total unsaturated fatty acids in the fat of the red marrow than in the fat of the extramedullary regions.[18] Tavassoli[19] identified a population of fat cells in the hemopoietically active marrow, and not in the yellow marrow, which stained positively with performic acid-Schiff reagent. No differences were found with the lipid stains: oil red, Sudan black, Nile blue sulfate, and acid hematin. Since the performic acid—Schiff reaction is based on the oxidation of ethylene groups in unsaturated lipids, the difference in staining characteristics between the yellow and red marrow may be in part due to the slightly higher concentration of unsaturated fatty acids in the red marrow.

The origin of the marrow fat cells has been ascribed to the adventitial cell of the sinusoidal wall,[6] the parasinusoidal reticulum cell. The bone marrow adipocyte first begins to develop in the 2-week-old rabbit and appears to be associated with the sinus endothelium and the adventitial cell. Unlike the extramedullary fat cell,[20–24] the marrow adipocyte is not associated with collagen and does not contain an abundantly organized rough endocytoplasmic reticulum. The extramedullary fat cell is said to arise from a ''fibroblast-like'' cell.[25] Zucker-Franklin et al.[26] have shown that under appropriate in vitro conditions, monocytes could transform into fat cells. However, the lipid in the monocytes remained divided in multiple compartments and did not coalesce to form the large lipid mass so characteristic of fat cells. Whether the transformation of monocytes into fat cells is an important physiological event is debatable. Similar cells, namely large reticular macrophages with eccentrically displaced nuclei and multiple

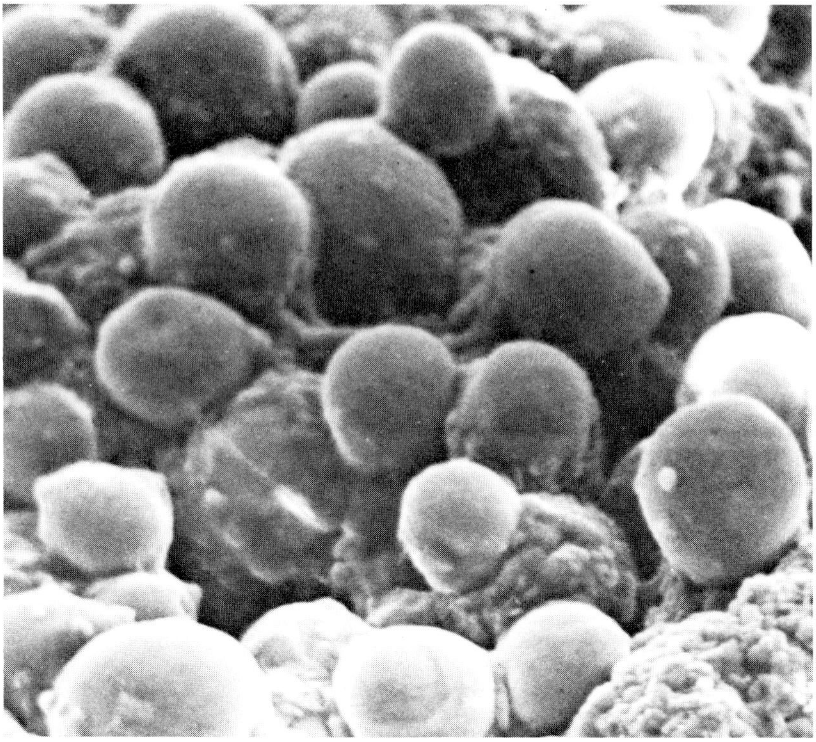

FIGURE 2. Bone marrow particle, human aspirate. Scanning electron microscope. (Magnification ca. × 300.)

lipid droplets, may be seen in normal human marrow aspirates. Whether these cells are in the process of becoming fat cells or whether these cells merely function as agents for the transfer of fat from the fat cells to the neighboring proliferating hemopoietic cells is not known.[27]

Recently, an in vivo culture system has been developed for the long-term culture of hemopoietic cells. Maintenance of the culture is dependent on the development of an adherent layer of cells consisting of a heterogeneous population of cells, reminiscent of the bone marrow matrix: endothelial cells, reticular cells, giant, fat containing cells, and macrophages.[28−33] The fat cells appear to be particularly important for stem cell maintenance and for granulopoiesis; the differentiating granulocytic cells are found selectively clustered in and around areas of fat cell aggregation.[34]

Prevailing opinion holds that the marrow fat cells serve only as passive space fillers and accomodate, within the fixed confines of the bone, to hemopoietic demands by altering their volume or number. According to this view, heightened hemopoiesis causes the fat cells to shrink—the fat is said to be squeezed out by the expanding hemopoietic mass; or in reverse, a decreased marrow activity leads to an expansion of the fat cell volume and number.[35,36] A minority view however holds that the marrow fat cells may be actively involved in the hemopoietic process, serving as a direct metabolic support tissue rather than as a purely passive mechanical filler.[37,38] Tavassoli et al.[39−42] concluded from a series of studies on both red and yellow marrow that an inherent (epigenetic) determinant of marrow cellularity exists in the different sites, and that the epigenetic determinant can be modified to a certain extent by environmental factors and physiological stimulation. The epigenetic determinant appears to reside in the adipose cells of the marrow.

In general, the adipose tissues form a large energy storage system. In the fed state they synthesize fatty acids and glycerol from glucose and esterify the free fatty acids which reach them from the liver and the intestines. In the fasting state the stored triglycerides are hydrolyzed and the fatty acids and glycerol released for the total energy needs of the body. Fat then is a metabolically active tissue centrally involved in the stabilization of the animal's fuel requirements.

For the most part, investigations on adipose tissue have assumed a functional unity for all of the widely dispersed fat depots. However, compelling evidence has accumulated to suggest that different adipose sites respond differently to lipolytic stimuli,[43] and that some fat areas such as the periorbital fat may assume purely structural, essentially nonmetabolic roles.[44] The metabolic activity of structural support fat appears to be lower than of those depots concerned primarily with energy conservation.[45]

The introduction of a technique for the isolation of individual fat cells from adipose tissue[46] and the development of sizing procedures[47] have been largely responsible for the expansion of information on the physiology and metabolism of the fat cell. The determination of fat cell size has been a dominant theme in the investigations of adipose tissue because of the postulated relationship between cell size, metabolic rate, and insulin sensitivity.[48–53] These relationships are sharply modified by other variables such as age, nutrition, and animal species.

The isolated fat cells of the red marrow of the rabbit are consistently smaller than the isolated fat cell from the perinephric or subcutaneous adipose tissue. In the young adult animal the ratio of marrow fat cell volume to extramedullary fat cell volume is about 1:5.[13] As the animals increase in weight, the extramedullary fat cells show a significant increase in cell volume; no corresponding increase in marrow fat cell volume is noted. Regardless of size, the fatty acid turnover per cell for both the marrow and extramedullary fat cells is the same in vivo. In vitro, the isolated extramedullary fat cells show a five to ten times greater response to hormonally (adrenocorticotrophin, ACTH; growth hormone; beta melanocyte stimulating hormone, βMSH) induced lipolysis than the marrow fat cells, suggesting that cell size may play some role in the regulation of the response of the marrow adipose tissue to systemic hormonal stimulation.[54]

Perturbations of hemopoiesis, particularly an increase in activity, have a profound effect on the marrow fat cells. As early as 1882, Neumann[10] observed that following bleeding there is an extension of the red marrow in a peripheral direction, that is in the direction of the yellow fatty marrow. It was subsequently shown that upon stimulation, hemopoiesis begins in the subendosteal parts of the fatty marrow. Barth and Kados[55] reported the presence of a serum factor that transforms fatty marrow into an active erythropoietic organ following bleeding.

Temperature[56] and low oxygen pressure[57] have also been proposed as significant factors in the conversion of the fatty marrow into an active red marrow.

The intense hemolysis induced by phenylhydrazine administration transforms the yellow fatty marrow into an erythropoietically rich, red marrow[58] and probably does so through stimulation of erythropoietin synthesis.[59] At the marrow level attention has been paid to the disappearance of fat and the appearance of vessels during the transformation to erythroblastic hyperplasia. Hyperemia, proliferation of capillaries, and sinusoidal formation were considered prerequisites for the increased erythropoietic activity.[60] Saterborg[61] postulated that the newly formed capillaries, which appeared in response to the phenylhydrazine induced hemolysis, were formed by the marrow fat cells and that these capillaries finally appeared as sinusoids. Tavassoli and Crosby[40] suggested that the conversion of fatty to red marrow takes place by means of an invasion of capillaries from the adjacent red marrow.

Few studies have dealt directly with the response of marrow fat to increased hematopoiesis. Evans et al.[62] noted a 60 to 70% decrease in the total fat content of the femoral marrow of rabbits following 30 days of phenylhydrazine administration. They also noted a preferential release of the polyunsaturated fatty acids and postulated that the expanding erythropoietic mass forced the fat out of the marrow cavity. The same investigators[63] found similar changes after bleeding and concluded that the marrow fat was primarily a storage depot. Cohen and Gardner[64] reported a striking reduction in the percent content of fat in the marrow of rabbits treated with phenylhydrazine. They pointed out that the physiological role of marrow fat had not been elucidated and suggested the possibility that the release of fatty acids following the phenylhydrazine administration was a primary event to serve the local needs of the actively proliferating and differentiating red cells. Tavassoli et al.[65] observed rapid mobilization of fat from the proximal bones (red marrow) and only moderate response from the yellow marrow of the distal bones after phenylhydrazine administration or bleeding. Further, they noted a more rapid disappearance of those marrow fat cells which reacted positively to the performic acid Schiff reaction.[19] Bathija et al.[66] demonstrated a striking reduction in the volume of the marrow fat cell of the rabbit, following a sustained burst of increased erythropoiesis stimulated by phenylhydrazine-induced hemolysis. Similar but less dramatic results were seen in chronically bled animals. The marrow fat cell volumes decreased to 50% of control; the esterification capacity, despite the intense lipolysis, remained unaltered from the control state and there appeared to be a preferential release of unsaturated fatty acid. The isolated fat cells of extramedullary sites of the phenylhydrazine-treated rabbits showed no change in volume, esterification capacity, or fatty acid composition.

The factors that control the vascular, hemopoietic, and adipose cell activities in the bone marrow during normoblastic hyperplasia are largely unknown. Emphasis has been centered on erythropoietin which promotes the differentiation of the stem cells to normoblasts.[67] Erythropoietin has been reported to stimulate vasoproliferation[68] and the amplification of committed stem cells.[69,70] No evidence has been presented to indicate that erythropoietin can stimulate lipolysis. The factors that do trigger lipolysis in the marrow fat cell are presumably of local origin and as yet unidentified. Similarly, the function of the released lipid has not been elucidated. The marrow fat cell lipids may serve the local nutrition needs of the rapidly proliferating hemopoietic cells but may also play some role in the maturation process itself. A lipid soluble factor capable of stimulating erythropoiesis was isolated from the plasma of anemic animals.[70] It has been suggested[71] that this erythrocytosis stimulating factor may be identical or closely related to batyl alcohol, $CH_3(CH_2)_{17}$-O-CH_2-CH(OH)-CH_2(OH). It has been known for some time that large doses of batyl alcohol can induce an increase in all of the blood cell elements and produce erythrocytosis, leukocytosis, and thrombocytosis. Potter and Wright[72] found a threefold increase in the neutral glycerol ether lipids in the marrow of mice subjected to phenylhydrazine-induced hemolysis immediately preceding a twofold increase in the recognizable red cell precursors, which suggested to them a role for fat in erythropoiesis.

Bone marrow fat has been viewed as a passive tissue accomodating to the proliferative activity of the hemopoietic cells and thereby maintaining the constancy of the marrow volume.[73] Thus the marrow fat cells should grow smaller with increased hemopoiesis, which they do, and grow larger when hemopoiesis is curtailed. Indeed, Ehrlich[74] emphasized the fatty nature of the marrow in his early description of aplastic anemia in 1888. This morphological characteristic of the hypocellular marrow has been repeatedly observed and interpreted to mean an increase in either number or size of the marrow fat cells, a replacement of the hemopoietic compartment by fat.[75–77]

Pathophysiologically, aplasia of the bone marrow may be viewed as the result of an abnormality of the stem cell or of a defect in the stromal cells, i.e., an altered microenvironment.[78] Knospe and Crosby[79] reasoned that the aplasia that follows local X-irradiation is the result of a disordered sinusoidal circulation of the bone marrow. Further evidence to support the importance of the microenvironment in regeneration was provided by Patt and Maloney[80] in their studies on the changes following the mechanical disruption of the marrow cavity. Bond and Brecher, quoted by Stohlmann,[78] utilized a deuterium beam to produce a pencil-thin aplasia of the bone marrow of mice. Active hemopoiesis existed in the area adjacent to the beam target. These findings were interpreted to indicate that the aplasia was the result of local disturbances in the microenvironment. Tavassoli et al.[41,42] demonstrated that marrow could be transplanted to extramedullary sites. They compared the histogenesis of active red and inactive yellow fatty marrow transplants. Both transplants underwent similar regeneration of sinusoidal stroma and formed hemopoietic nodules. However, the yellow marrow transplant rapidly involuted, hemopoiesis ceased, and the nodule reverted to fat tissue. These findings were thought to be indicative of an intrinsic predetermined (epigenetic) difference between the microenvironments of yellow and red marrow.

Since X-irradiation can reliably produce hypoplasia of the bone marrow it has become a common experimental tool for the study of this state.[81] The results of such studies, namely, the effect of irradiation on bone marrow fat, have yielded conflicting data. Dietz and Steinberg[75] reported an increase in bone marrow lipid and a decrease in both water and lipid free solids immediately after an exposure of 3000 rad to the limb of a rat. Elko and DiLuzio[82] found no significant changes in either the total amount of lipid or in lipid composition of the marrow after 1000 rad of whole body irradiation. In a series of papers, Snyder and co-workers,[83–86] found that the triglycerides of the femoral marrow of the mouse increased from 5 to 50% of the marrow wet weight within a week after total body irradiation of 800 rad. They also suggested that following total body irradiation of 800 rad there appeared to be an increase in the number of fat cells, judged morphologically, and a stimulation of triglyceride synthesis. An increased biosynthesis of fatty acid esters and a decrease of fatty acid oxidation were postulated as the major mechanisms for the accumulation of triglycerides in the marrow.

For the most part these early studies were concerned with the acute effects of X-irradiation on the marrow adipose tissue, and the results were expressed principally as percent change in marrow lipid content. The absolute quantities of fat were not determined and one cannot be certain that the reported changes were due to a real increase in fat or a decrease in the non adipose elements of the marrow. In an attempt to arrive at some absolute figures, Bathija et al.[87] exposed the femur of a rabbit to a single dose of 8000 rad. The opposite unirradiated limb served as a control. When aplasia in the irradiated limb was well established, they isolated the fat cells of both femoral marrows, the overlying subcutaneous fat as well as the fat cells from the perinephric adipose tissues. They found no change in cell number, cell volume, or esterification capacity of the fat cells of the irradiated aplastic marrow when compared with the control limb. They did not identify the material or mechanism that compensated for the loss of the hemopoietic tissue.

The effects of starvation on the extramedullary fat depots are indeed well known. The effects of starvation on marrow fat cells are less clear. The remarkable transformation of the bone marrow in advanced states of cachexia and inanition did not escape the attention of the early students of the bone marrow.[88] Certainly, throughout human history famine and war gave ample opportunity to observe effects of semistarvation on the bone marrow of man.[89-91] In advanced inanition, the marrow assumes a gelatinous character most marked in the inactive fatty marrow. Jolly[92] gave a detailed description in his text on hematology. He described fat cells completely devoid of lipid which appeared like fibroblasts submerged in a homogeneous material resembling mucin. The transformation was much less severe in the red marrow but nevertheless present. Marked hyperemia and congestion imparted a bright red color to the hemopoietic marrow. The disappearance of the fat cells masked the atrophy of the hemopoietic cells which thus appeared to be more abundant in the sections of the marrow. In reality, the disappearance of fat from the marrow was followed by a decrease in hemopoietic activity.

Gelatinous degeneration of the marrow has been observed in the self-induced inanition of anorexia nervosa,[93-95] as well as in the cachexia associated with other chronic illnesses.[96-98] Tavassoli et al.[99] found hypoplasia of the hemopoietic cells, fat atrophy, and characteristic gelatinous transformation in a group of individuals who had suffered from severe and prolonged self-induced starvation. The gelatinous substance appeared amorphous and stained pink with the Romanowsky stains. The material was shown to be an acid mucopolysaccharide, localized in the extracellular ground substance. They suggested that the increase in acid mucopolysaccharide synthesis in all tissues in the starved state[100] served to compensate for the loss of volume of the hemopoietic tissue and was possibly responsible for the observed inhibition of erythropoietic activity. The process was reversible with restoration of marrow structure and function on refeeding.

In contrast to the clinical situation, where prolonged semistarvation is the rule, most experimental studies are acute, short-term, and based on total food deprivation. In their early classical investigations on pigeon marrow, Doan and co-workers[37] found that following acute starvation and a loss of 25 percent of body weight, the marrow became hypoplastic and fatty. On resumption of feeding and just prior to resumption of hemopoietic activity they noted rapid mobilization of fat, presumably for local utilization in the hemopoietic process. This interpretation has been criticized and the preparatory mobilization of fat attributed to starvation rather than to blood cell formation.[35] Newlin and McKay[101] concluded from their studies on starvation in rabbits that ''the marrow provides the animal body with a unique storage space for reserve nutrients without increase in the bulk of the body.'' Evans et al.[102] studied the composition and quantity of marrow fat of starved rabbits. Their findings led them to conclude that the absolute quantity of the saturated fatty acid component of marrow fat was unaffected by starvation and that the polyunsaturated fatty acids of the marrow were transported elsewhere for utilization or discard. Similary, Dietz and Steinberg[103] found that after 25 days of total starvation, rabbits lost 50% of their body weight, and that the liquid content of the marrow fell to less than 5%.

Cohen and Gardner[64] reinvestigated the effects of starvation on marrow fat and reported that the distal (yellow) marrow defended itself against total starvation whereas the proximal (red) marrow fat was mobilized as readily as extramedullary fat. Tavassoli[104] looked at the distal tibial marrow of acutely starved rabbits and found no histologic evidence of fat mobilization despite marked shrinkage of the cells of the epididymal fat pad. He proposed that the marrow adipose tissue is functionally distinct from the extramedullary fat tissue and that its primary function is regulation of the intensity of hemopoiesis rather than conservation of energy. Bathija et al.[105] subjected rabbits to acute starvation for 21 days with a subsequent loss of some 30% of body weight. They found no change in the volume of fat cells isolated from the femoral red marrow. The extramedullary fat cells shrank to about 17% of control values. The esterification capacity of the marrow fat cells was unchanged from that of the fed state. The esterification capacity of the extramedullary fat cells fell sharply, in keeping with the well-established observations that the esterification capacity of adipose tissue is influenced by the nutritional state of the animal.[106–108] Bathija et al.[105] concluded that the adipose cell of the red marrow behaves metabolically, as judged by esterification capacity,[41] like cells from adipose sites concerned with energy storage and release, but unlike such fat depots, in the starved state it continues to compete for the available free fatty acids despite the animal's urgent need for fuel.

In summary, fat is a major component of the active red marrow of man and many animals. The marrow fat cells display unique behavior, apparently attuned to hemopoietic activity rather than the total energy need of the animal. The marrow fat cells are considerably smaller than the extramedullary fat cells, but cell for cell show equal metabolic activity. The role of the marrow fat cell in hemopoiesis is in dispute, but there is growing evidence to suggest that it may supply surface, believed to be essential for differentiation and maturation of the hemopoietic cells, as well as nutritional support, and possibly hemopoietic growth factors. The marrow fat cell is thought to arise from the reticulum cell either by synthesis or storage of fat.

III. MARROW CIRCULATION

The extraordinary extent and unusual characteristics of the vasculature of the mammalian marrow were immediately appreciated by early investigators. Bizzozero[9] commented on the large vascular component of the marrow which he estimated to occupy about half the marrow volume. He[9] and others[109–112] were struck by the large sinusoidal network and relative paucity of arterial vessels. A fairly comprehensive and valid picture of the general vascular architecture of the marrow emerged from these early studies in the latter half of the 19th century. The fine details of the marrow circulation eluded the early investigators whose studies were based primarily on injection and corrosion specimens (Figure 3). Jolly,[111] following his description of the then available information on the sinusoidal structures of the marrow, pointed to the fact that "the true nature of the wall of these sinuses and its relationship to the hemopoietic tissue is difficult to determine."

The femur of the rabbit, guinea pig, and rat as well as birds and amphibians has received major attention as a model of the marrow vasculature. Perfusion techniques utilizing India ink or silicone rubber have been most often employed in these efforts in which specimens were studied by the clearing method described by Spalteholz,[113] and by light microscopy of thick and thin section.[60,114–122] Branemark[123,124] introduced a new approach, vital microscopy, to the investigation of bone marrow circulation in the living rabbit. This technique unfortunately disrupted the periosteal blood supply and afforded only modest resolving power in the examination of this poorly accessible organ (Figure 4).

In the picture that emerges from these many studies the nutrient artery is described as the major blood supply of both bone and marrow. The vessel enters the bone through a nutrient foramen. A vessel of small caliber, it penetrates to the center of the marrow where it divides into an ascending and descending branch. The branches of the nutrient artery run generally in a direction parallel to the long axis of the bone. The total arterial arborization of the nutrient artery forms a strikingly small compartment relative to the voluminous sinusoidal network. Furthermore, connections between the arterial capillaries and the venous sinusoids are difficult to find. Connections between the marrow vessels and the Haversian canalicular system have been recognized but are not considered significant. Doan et al.[37] believed that a system of intersinusoidal capillaries was inserted between the nutrient arterial plexus and the sinusoidal network. They thought

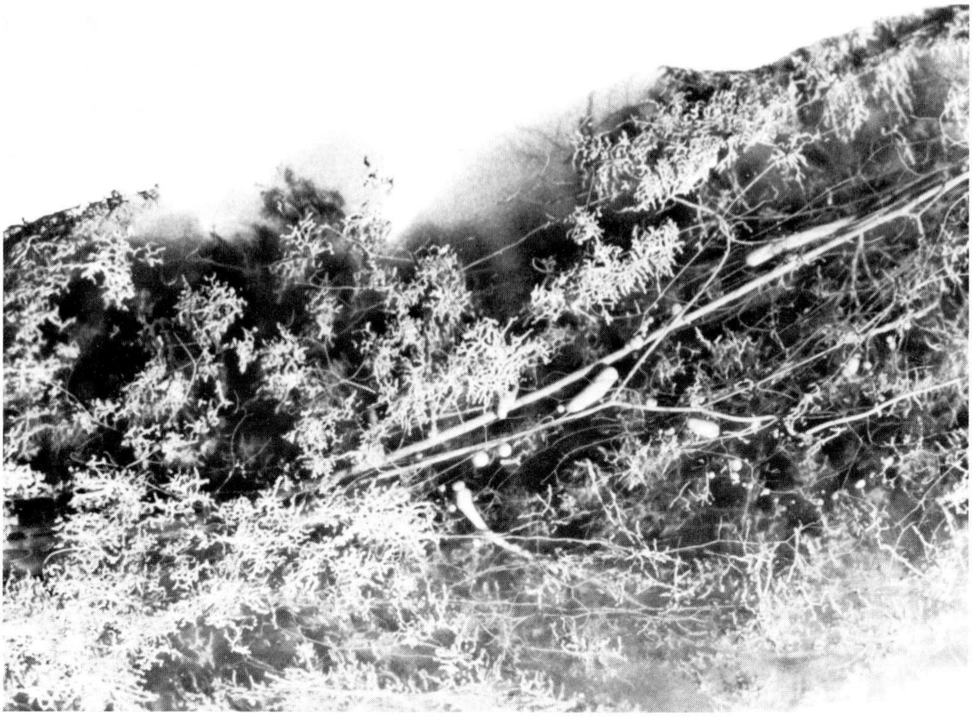

FIGURE 3. Silicone rubber cast of rabbit femur, cleared. Note branching of nutrient artery and the large sinusoidal system.

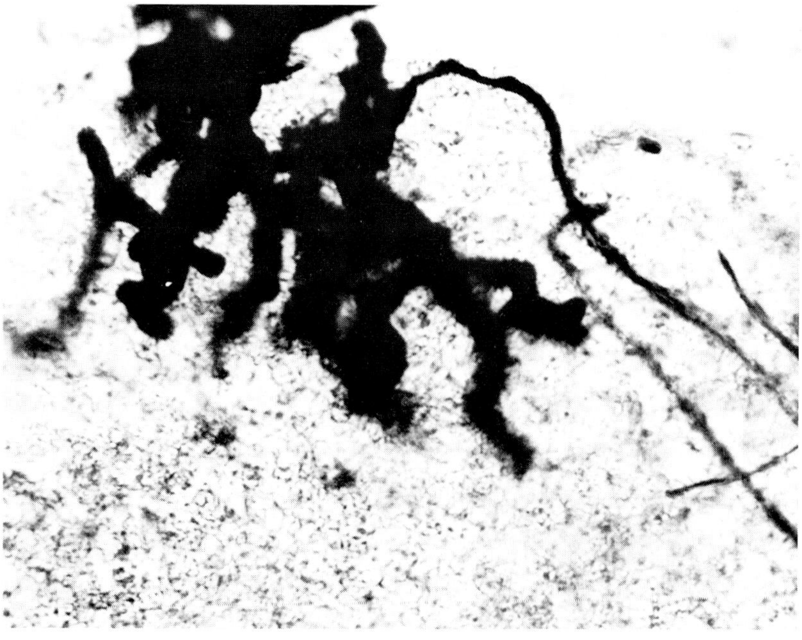

FIGURE 4. Silicone rubber cast, rabbit femoral marrow, showing arteriole and sinusoidal structures. (Magnification ca. × 200.)

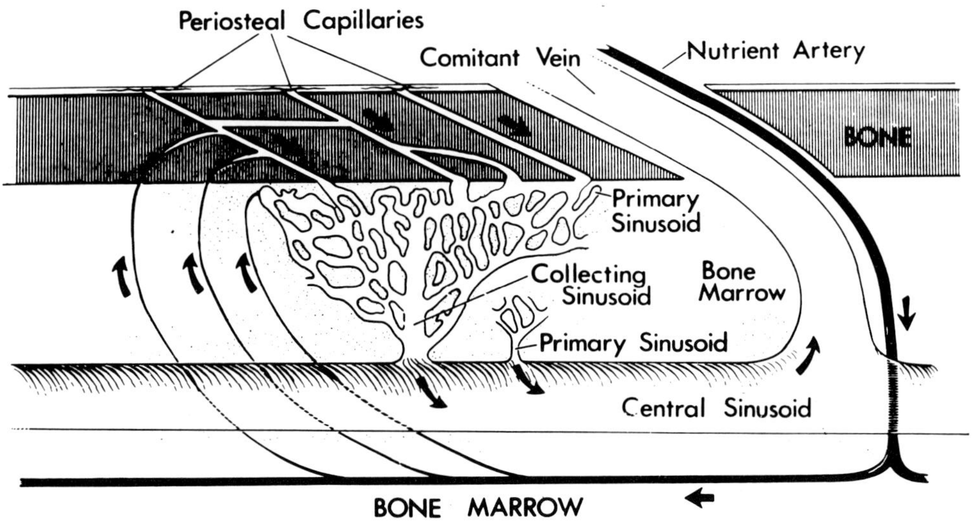

FIGURE 5. From De Bruyn with approval.

that erythrocyte maturation took place intravascularly in the intersinusoidal capillaries. In the absence of erythropoietic activity the capillaries were presumed collapsed and hence invisible.

Much attention and speculation were focused on the nature of the sinusoidal system. For many, the morphologic appearance of the sinusoidal wall suggested an "open" circulation, supported by the appearance of the suspensions and colloids of the employed perfusion mixtures which were found widely dispersed in extravascular sites. Drinker et al.[121] and Maximow[125] held, on the other hand, that the marrow circulation was essentially a "closed" system, the reticulocytes escaping through small gaps which appeared in the sinusoidal wall when the erythroblastic cells reached maturity.

Reinvestigation of the microcirculation by de Bruyn et al.[126] in 1970 confirmed the overall general description of the vasculature of the mammalian marrow but with some new insights. The major blood supply to the sinusoids is contained in the perforating vessels in the osteal canals. The surface of any long bone, stripped of its periosteum is indeed pitted by numerous small holes spaced some 100 μm apart. The periosteal capillary network sends small branches, the transosteal vessels, through these foramini. The transosteal vessels are composed of a single layer of endothelium and their diameters are, on an average, three times larger than the periosteal capillaries. These vessels widen at the osteomyeloid junction to form the sinusoids whose lumen is now about twice that of the transosteal vessel (Figure 5).

The arterial system, formed by the nutrient artery, consists of fine branches which gradually curve towards the periphery of the marrow. Most of the centrifugally running branches enter the bony shaft as capillaries of very narrow lumen, to empty into the transosteal vessels. A small number of the terminal branches of the nutrient artery may enter the sinuses directly at the osteomyeloid junction.

The sinusoids form an extensive and abundantly anastomosing structure of thin-walled vascular channels. These vessels course over and between the fat cells to assume geometric patterns imposed upon them by the obtrusive adipocytes. The sinusoids drain in this fashion more or less perpendicularly to the long axis of the bone to enter the larger collecting sinusoids, and these in turn enter the central venous sinus. Primary sinusoids may also drain directly into the central venous channel rather than through the intermediary collecting sinusoids. The central venus sinus runs in the center of the marrow, along with the nutrient artery, parallel to the long axis of the bone to exit through the nutrient foramen.

In a physiologic sense the vascular system of the bone marrow is a portal system. The blood in the sinusoidal system has already traversed both the periosteum and the bone, and a small amount of arterial blood is introduced through the direct entry of the capillaries of the nutrient artery. Whether this portal system is important to marrow function is not known, but there has been some speculation on the possible flow of hemopoietic growth or regulating factors from bone to marrow (Figure 5).

IV. THE SINUSOIDAL WALL

The rich sinusoidal network of the marrow vasculature attracted the attention of early investigators who were particularly impressed with the unusual quality of these vessels: their relatively large size and markedly attenuated, thin vessel walls. They thought that the lining cells were phagocytic and sufficiently different from typical endothelial cells to warrant the appellation "reticular" to denote a more primitive cell. The modest resolving power of the techniques of the period was not able to reveal the true nature of the sinusoidal wall; the greater resolving power of the electron microscope was required.

In a series of studies Pease[127,128] and Zamboni and Pease[129] examined the ultrastructural characteristics of the guinea pig marrow. The walls of the sinusoids were found to be lined with extremely flattened cells whose cytoplasmic sheets simply butted against each other with only occasional overlapping. The cytoplasm of these cells showed no particular features except for evidence of considerable pinocytotic activity. The lining cells were thought to be reticular cells and highly distinctive of sinusoidal structure. Fat droplets were occasionally seen in the cytoplasm and a relationship was postulated to a slightly differentiated fat cell. They did not detect any basement membrane, desmosomes, or terminal bars. Few and only occasional collagen fibrils were detected, usually associated with a flocculent precipitate, probably a mucopolysaccharide. They concluded that the contacts between neighboring lining cells were labile, constantly changing the sinusoidal pattern in response to the dynamic state of the marrow to allow free passage of blood cells from the parenchyma to the systemic circulation and the free and rapid passage of colloids from blood to parenchyma. De Bruyn et al.,[130] in a similar study on guinea pig marrow, demonstrated that the lining cells were continuous, if fixation artifact was kept to a minimum.

Weiss,[5,6,131,132] based on an extensive ultrastructural examination of the rat marrow, depicted the vascular sinus as a single layer of endothelial cells of variable thickness. The endothelial cells contained many vacuoles, expressive of active pinocytosis, a moderate number of lysosomes and mitochondria, and were occasionally phagocytic. An attenuated and defective basement membrane, composed of some granular material, probably glycoprotein, and a few filaments could be identified. Adventitial cells, morphologically similar to the endothelial cells, lay against the basement membrane or, in absence of the basement membrane, against the abluminal side of the endothelial cell. The adventitial cell cover was incomplete and subject to abrupt and irregular variation in volume, density, and vesiculation. The cells contained rough endoplasmic reticulum, vesicles, and filaments or tubules, particularly in their perisinusal processes. The adventital cell projected many processes into the adjacent hemopoietic compartment where they contacted the individual erythrocytic and myelocytic cells. The adventitial cells could take on fat and became adipocytes.

In birds, pigeons, and chickens,[133] the sinus wall is formed by extremely thin flat cells which contain mitochondria, free ribosomes, profiles of rough endocytoplasmic reticulum, lipid droplets, and phagosomes. Pinocytotic vesicles are frequent on both the internal and external surfaces. No basement membrane is present. Cells are held together by tight junctions; often the long segment of one adjoining cell overlaps another to form a wall two cell layers thick. The lining cells are frequently closely associated with fat cells from which they are separated by a 200 Å wide space filled with electron-dense material. The wall of the sinus is continuous except at sites where blood cells are passing through them. Membrane-associated pores are found only in association with blood cells in transit. Collagen fibrils are absent.

The lining cells of the sinus of the hemopoietic marrow of the frog, *Rana pipiens,* are flattened cells with thin cytoplasmic extensions from the sinus wall. The cytoplasm contains mitochondria, rough endoplasmic reticulum, free ribosomes, and microtubules, but no phagosomes or lysosomes. Adjacent membranes of overlapping cells are separated by a variable space ranging from apparent fusion to an intercellular separation of 200 Å. The overlapping cells often enclose maculae occludentes. Collagen fibrils are observed near lining cells, but no basement membrane is present. The lining cells form a continuous layer; openings occur only in association with migrating blood cells.[134]

Thus the overall structure of the sinus of the marrow of mammalian and nonmammalian species appears to be quite similar. All are lined by flattened, continuous cells which are phagocytic in some (mammals) but not in other animal (amphibian) species. A basement membrane and adventital cells form an incomplete cover of the abluminal side of the lining cells in rats but not in guinea pigs, birds, and frogs. Few or no collagen fibrils are present and membrane pores are associated with the transmigration of blood cells from the hemopoietic parenchyma to the blood stream.

V. THE RETICULAR CELLS

A. Definition and Classification

The term ''reticulum cell'' or ''reticular cell'' in the bone marrow or in lymphoreticular tissue refers to a group of cells which characteristically form a reticulum or syncytium, a cytoplasmic network.[135] In the bone marrow these branched cells, associated with reticular fibers, form a three-dimensional meshwork which holds the vascular sinuses and the hemopoietic elements. The cells are in close apposition to the sinusoidal lining cells and extend into the marrow parenchyma. The reticular cells possess an abundant cytoplasm and a large ovoid nucleus, occasionally with prominent nucleoli. The cytoplasm is pale, often lacy, and may contain a variety of tingeable material. The cells may be metalophilic and may be associated with reticulum, an argyrophilic, precollagenous fibril. The cells tend to be cohesive and form a loose and incomplete syncytium.

The designation, reticular cell, as used by Aschoff[136] refers to those cells in the marrow and elsewhere which ingest intravenously administered vital dyes. Based on patterns of tissue uptake of the intravital dyes, Aschoff divided the cells into four groups. Groups I and II demonstrated weak staining and included the endothelial cells of blood and lymphatic vessels as well as fibroblasts. Group III consisted of the reticular cells of the spleen and lymph nodes, and Group IV, the cells lining the sinusoids of the liver, bone marrow, and lymph nodes. The lining cells of the sinusoids and the reticulum cells formed the structural components of Aschoff's reticuloendothelial system.

The origin of the reticulum cell as well as its identification are clouded in ambiguity.

Lack of precise morphologic definition and functional concepts have burdened us with a confusing array of names: clasmatocyte, adventitial cell, histiocyte, rhagiocrine, etc. a "chaotic miasma."[137] More recently these cells have been included in the larger framework of mechanocytes along with the fibroblasts, osteoblasts, and chondrocytes.[138,139] The tissue macrophages or histiocytes which include the resident and free macrophages of the peritoneum and pleura, the alveolar macrophages, the Kupfer cells, the inflammatory macrophages, the marrow macrophages, etc. are all thought to be of bone marrow origin, a continuum of marrow monocytopoiesis. The concept of a monocyte-macrophage system of marrow origin has been introduced to replace the system of cells elaborated by Aschoff as the reticuloendothelial cells.[140,141] What then are the reticulum cells of the marrow? These ill-defined cells are known to proliferate slowly and constitute the major cellular component of the bone marrow stroma. There is little evidence for the previously held view that the reticulum cells are synonymous with the hemopoietic stem cells.[142]

B. Phagocytic and Nonphagocytic Reticular Cells

Ultrastructural studies of the reticulum cells of the marrow reveal morphologic heterogenity according to which the cells are classified as phagocyte reticulum cell and undifferentiated nonphagocytic reticulum cells of types I and II.[143]

The phagocytic reticulum cell[144,146] has an irregular outline with long marrow cytoplasmic processes that follow the contours of the adjacent cells. The broad cytoplasmic mass contains many vesicles and lysosomes and a Golgi complex. With iron loading, ferritin aggregates are found diffusely but more noticeably about the Golgi zone. Small elements of endoplasmic reticulum, partially loaded with ribosomes, are scattered throughout the cytoplasm. The nucleus is large with many nuclear pores and scattered chromatin. The cell is seen associated with erythroblasts,[147] lymphocytes, and other marrow elements.

The undifferentiated reticulum cell is described by Caffrey et al.[142] by light microscopy as a cell with an oval nucleus, a sharp nuclear outline and delicate chromatin. The cytoplasmic margins are indistinct, the cytoplasm pale. On electron microscopic observation, the nuclear membrane is somewhat irregular with a dense band of chromatin at the margin. The cytoplasmic content is scanty, poor in ribosomes, with an underdeveloped Golgi apparatus and a few smooth-edged and coated vesicles. A stringy network of filaments coats the surface, attached preferentially to the cytoplasmic processes. The cells are not phagocytic and have no intracytoplasmic filaments.

The filamentous cell type I contain bundles of cytoplasmic filaments in thin cytoplasmic processes. The filaments are 4 to 8 mm in diameter and join to form dense bodies. The cells in human marrow characteristically border the blood sinuses, are separated from the endothelial cell by a basal lamina, and are not phagocytic.[148]

The fibrous reticulum cell type II resembles the phagocytic reticulum cell but is not phagocytic. It may contain globules of fat and 10-nm filaments. The cells are in contact with the reticulum fibers.

Two broad groups of reticulum cells have been distinguished on the basis of their phagocytic capacity. The phagocytic reticulum cell is a macrophage, observed most prominently as the central reticular cell in the erythroid islands.[149] The nonphagocytic cell is thought to arise from a progenitor cell different from the hemopoietic stem cell and capable of producing fibroblast colonies in culture, the CFU-F.[150] Another cell, probably a member of the population of cells grouped under the CFU-F, capable of transferring the hemopoietic microenvironment has been identified recently.[151] The term "reticular" may include a number of additional cells whose origin, function, and characteristics have not been precisely determined.

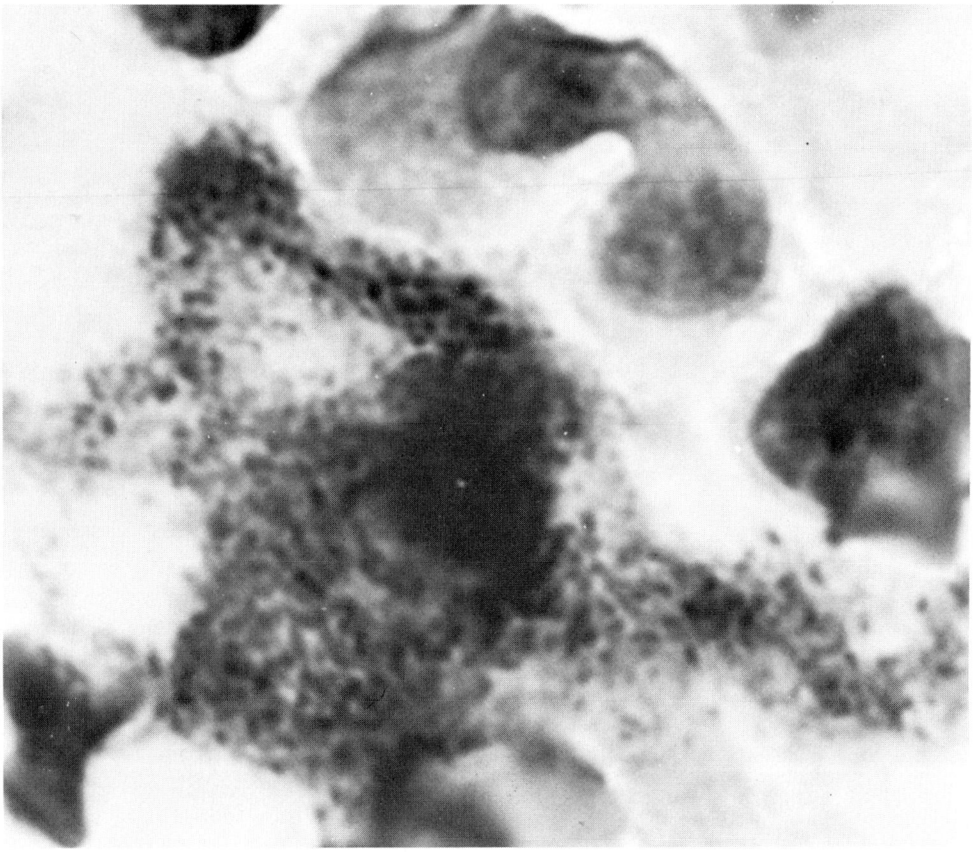

FIGURE 6. Nonphagocytic reticulum cell. Human marrow alkaline phosphatase reaction. (Magnification ca. × 2000.)

C. Morphology and Cytochemistry

The nonphagocytic reticular cells stain intensely on cytochemical examination for alkaline phosphatase activity (Figure 6) as well as for adensosine mono-, di-, and triphosphatase. The arterioles and capillaries are also visualized by the reaction product of the alkaline phosphatase reaction. An extensive capillary network is thus revealed coursing between and around the large fat cells. The heavily stained reticulum cells are scattered between and on the fat cell surfaces in close approximation to but separate from the endothelial cells (Figure 7). Reaction product is also present about the individual hemopoietic cells forming a hexagonal network.[152] These reticulum cells do not stain with the PAS, esterase, or acid phosphatase reactions.[152] Following the injection of India ink into the femoral artery of the rabbit, the carbon particles assume a position about the individual hemopoietic cells in a manner remarkably similar to the alkaline phosphatase reaction product. These findings suggested a possible transport role for the nonphagocytic, alkaline-positive reticular cells (Figure 8).[152]

The sinusoidal lining cells of the rat bone marrow have been shown to be permeable to carbon.[153]

Phosphatase activity has been associated with the enzymatic mechanisms of transport.[154] Phosphatase activity has also been demonstrated in the pinocytic vesicles of the endothelial cells.[154] Hyman and Paldino[156] assigned a protein transport role to the reticuloendothelial system. They saw the reticulum cell as a ‘‘window’’ built into the vascular

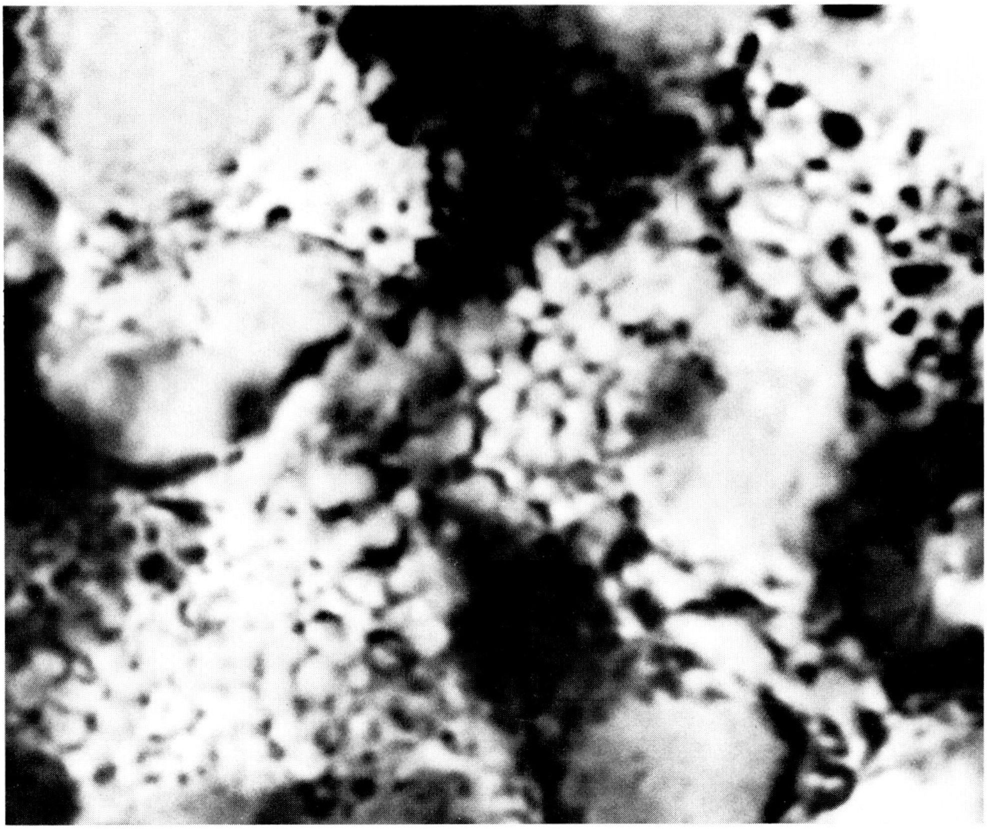

FIGURE 7. Particle of human marrow; alkaline phosphatase reaction, whole mount. Note intense reaction between individual cells on the fat cell surfaces. (Magnification ca. × 1000.)

wall to allow the transfer of protein molecules from the lumen to the parenchymal cells. Some investigators[156,158] found evidence for a lipid transfer role of the reticuloendothelial system; others[159] found a broad transport function involving the movement of material to and from the blood to the extravascular spaces.

Westen and Bainton[160] in their study of the stroma of the hemopoietic microenvironment by combined light and electron histochemistry identified twó different types of reticulum cells: a fibroblast type of reticulum cell characterized by alkaline phosphatase associated with its plasma membrane (the alkaline positive reticulum cell) and a macrophage type of reticulum cell characterized by its abundance of lysosomal acid phosphatase. The alkaline phosphatase-positive reticulum cell was found throughout the marrow but concentrated chiefly near the endosteum in close association with the granulocytic precursors, particularly the myeloblasts and promyelocytes. The macrophage type of reticulum cell was distributed uniformly throughout the marrow associated mainly with the erythroid precursors. Weston and Bainton[160] also detected alkaline phosphatase activity in the small arterioles and capillaries of the bone marrow localized in the pinocytic vesicles, the intravascular lumina, and portions of the basement membrane as well as between adjacent endothelial cells.

The reticular cell and its surrounding erythroblasts are considered a function-unit, the erythroblastic island, in which the central reticular cell has three main functions. The reticular macrophage ingests old red blood cells and possibly transfers its stored

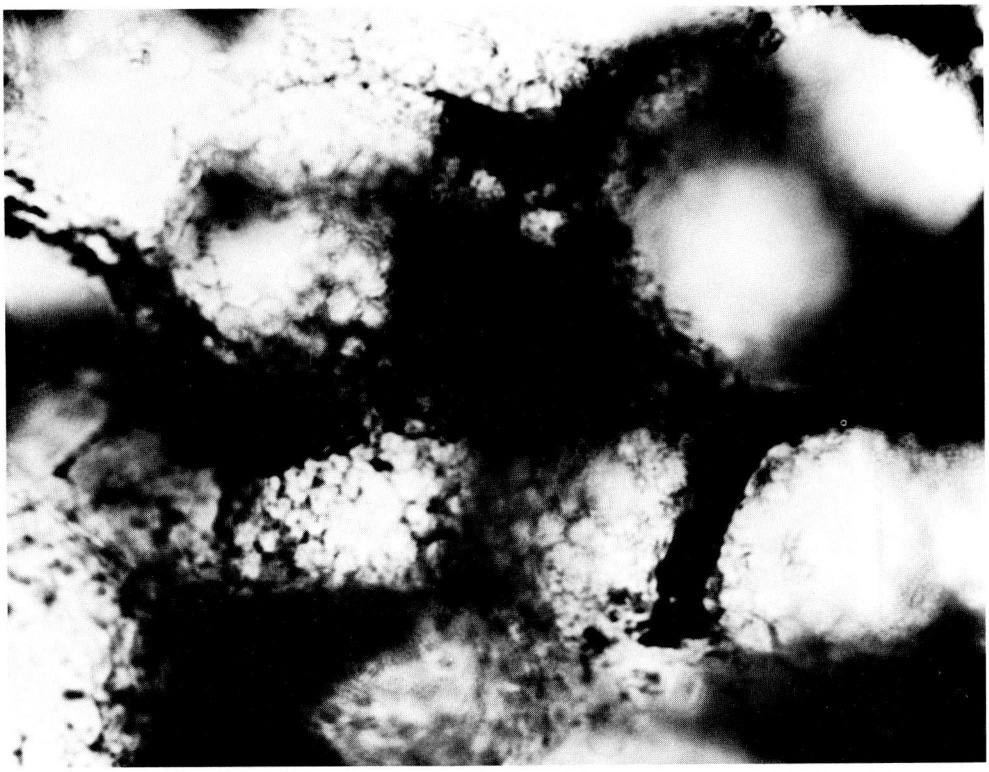

FIGURE 8. Femoral marrow, rabbit intrarterial. India ink injection; note sinusoids coursing over the fat cells and carbon particles surrounding the individual hemopoietic cells lying on surface of the fat cells. (Magnification ca. × 1000.)

iron to the developing red cells.[161] It is also actively involved in the engulfment of the extruded nuclei of the normoblasts.[149]

The functions of the intricate network of phagocytic and nonphagocytic reticulum cells have yet to be clarified, but there is little question that these cells together with the sinusoids create the environment for hemopoietic activity in the bone marrow.

VI. HEMOPOIETIC MICROENVIRONMENT

Under conditions of normal blood cell demand, the hemopoietic tissues display great capacity for differentiation and proliferation which under periods of stress can increase many-fold. To maintain this capacity for self-renewal the system must contain stem cells, namely, cells capable of division to maintain a population of daughter cells identical to themselves and also capable of differentiation to mature, nondividing red cells, leukocytes, and platelets for delivery to the peripheral blood.

The exact structure and nature of the hemopoietic stem cell (see chapter on stem cells) is not known but the concept of a hemopoietic stem cell has been central to all speculations on the origin and development of the blood cells in the hemopoietic tissues. The adherents of a monophyletic theory proposed a common stem cell, a pluripotential cell, from which all the blood cells were derived.[162] The polyphyletists[163] suggested a distinct stem cell, a unipotential cell, for each of the blood cell elements. Present-day evidence supports both schools of thought. The experimental data obtained from hemopoietic spleen colonies in mice support the existence of pluripotent and unipotent stem cells in murine hemopoiesis.[164] In vitro culture of murine[165,166] and human marrow[168] support the presence of unipotent stem cells in both mouse and man. The presence of the Philadelphia chromosome in the precursor cells of erythrocytes, granulocytes, and megakaryocytes in chronic myelocytic leukemia lends indirect evidence for the existence of a common pluripotent stem cell in man.[169]

The classic studies of Till and McCulloch[170–172] in the 1960s provided the experimental model for the operational, functional, and quantitative approach to the investigation of the hematopoietic precursor cells. They injected isolated murine marrow cells into heavily irradiated (1000 R) syngeneic mice and found discrete colonies of erythroid, granulocytic or megakaryocytic cells in the spleens of these animals. During the first 8 to 10 days the spleen colonies were predominantly clonal, committed to a single line of cell differentiation. After 8 to 10 days the colonies became mixed, developing a second line of hemopoietic differentiation. The cell capable of forming a colony has been termed a CFU-S (colony forming unit-spleen) and is believed to be pluripotential because of the heterogeneity of the colonies formed from a single CFU-S.[173] Self-renewal of the CFU-S was shown by producing colonies of all cell types on retransplantation of the isolated cells of a pure colony into an irradiated host.[172–174]

The mechanism which direct the conversion of the pluripotential cell to a unipotential stem cell are largely unknown. The direct action of a hormone such as erythropoietin had been suggested, but it is now known that erythropoietin acts on a committed cell, a step away from the pluripotent stem cell.[175–179] A stochastic model has been proposed in which differentiation depends on a chance or random interaction with unknown regulatory factors.[180–182] A third model suggests that the local hematopoietic stroma of marrow and spleen dictates the direction of differentiation of the pluripotential cell. This environmental influence is referred to as the hemopoietic inductive microenvironment.[183–186] Wolf and Trentin[187,188] suggest that both marrow and splenic stroma contain four types of microenvironmental compartments each dictating a distinctive type of hemopoiesis—erythrocytic, neutrophilic, eosinophilic, or megakaryocytic. The ratios of the microenvironments differ in marrow and spleen and, on transplantation, each organ maintains its distinctive microenvironmental characteristics.

As indicated, splenic colonies formed in the irradiated mouse following the injection of marrow cells tend to be clonal for the first 8 to 10 days and remain essentially committed to a single line of hemopoietic differentiation. Of such colonies 60% are erythroid, 20% neutrophilic, 15% megakaryocytic, and about 1% eosinophilic. The erythroid colonies are the largest and fastest growing; the neutrophilic are the next largest but grew more slowly; the eosinophilic colonies are barely visible, and the megakaryocytic are not seen grossly. After 8 to 10 days as the colonies enlarge, a second line of differentiation arises from the same clone of pluripotential cells. For example, as an erythroid colony enlarges, its peripheral margins may take on granulocytic or megakaryocytic differentiations as it presumably encroaches on a colony of another microenvironment.[187–190]

The spleen colonies have a rather distinctive distribution: about half are on the surface and of these 80% are erythroid. Neutrophilic colonies tend to localize along the trabeculae and below the capsule. Further, on suppression of erythroid colony growth by hypertransfusion of the recipient mouse, the colonies remain small and undifferentiated. They do not undergo neutrophilic differentiation although they contain pluripotent cells, suggesting again that microgeography is important in differentiation of the stem cell.[190,193]

Erythroid colonies outnumber the granulocytic colonies in the spleen by a factor of three (E/G colony ratio ~3). Of the hemopoietic colonies forming in the marrow the granulocytic colonies are twice as numerous as the erythrocytic (E/G colony ratio ~0.5).[177] The different propensities for differentiation are determined by the local environment, not by the injected cells. Thus, when bone marrow cells are injected into an irradiated mouse and the cells are recovered from the mouse's marrow a day later and reinjected into a second irradiated recipient, the ratio of colonies in the spleen was found to be 2.5 and in the marrow 0.6.

Bone marrow fragments transplanted into an isogeneic spleen give rise to hemopoietic colony ratios distinctive of marrow, whereas the spleen maintained its E/G colony ratio of about 3. At the junction of the marrow and the spleen, the colonies were mixed, granulocytic towards marrow and erythroid towards the spleen.[180]

Further evidence for a possible role of the microenvironment in differentiation is provided by transplantation studies on the Sl^1/Sl^d mutant mouse. This mutant mouse has normal stem cells and erythropoietin but defective stromal elements. W/W^v anemic mice have defective stem cells but normal stroma. Transplantation of the marrow of these two strains can each correct the anemia of the other.[192,193]

The concept of a hemopoietic inductive microenvironment has been strengthened by a host of transplantation experiments;[201] by the reaction of mice to granulopoietic stress[203–205] where the spleen becomes an erythroid organ and the marrow granulocytic; by a host of observations on the regeneration of marrow following curettage and mechanical depletion;[80,206–211] and by the long-term cultures of bone marrow developed by Dexter.[28,34] The concept of a hematopoietic inductive environment which activates the hemopoietic stem cells and regulates their proliferative behavior is an attractive hypothesis backed by considerable convincing indirect evidence, but still lacks formal proof.

The reticular cells of marrow and spleen have been singled out as the most likely single most important structural representatives of the hemopoietic environment.[141,186] Fridenstein et al.[150,212–214] obtained fibroblast colonies in monolayer cultures of bone marrow spleen, thymus, and lymph nodes of a variety of animals and of man. On passage of the cultures on monolayers the cells did not differentiate and maintained their fibroblast character. When the fibroblasts were retransplanted into diffusion chambers they formed reticular tissue and when transplanted under the kidney capsule the fibroblasts reformed the stromal tissues of their origin. Thus the fibroblasts derived from marrow produced bone and a bone marrow. Fibroblastic character of the CFU-F and their progeny has been confirmed by the demonstration of Type I and III collagen in these cells.[215]

VII. BLOOD CELL EGRESS—THE MARROW BLOOD BARRIER

Not only must the bone marrow matrix provide the environmental conditions for normal hematopoiesis, it must also provide an efficient and selective mechanism for the release of the mature cellular products of hematopoiesis. It is now well appreciated that mammalian hematopoiesis takes place in the extravascular spaces of the marrow and that the marrow circulation is closed. How the mature hemopoietic cell navigates its passage from its birthplace past the sinus wall barrier to its final abode is still unknown. The special properties of the maturing cell such as deformability, surface charge, migratory potential, motility, and surface receptors, as well as the special properties of the sinus wall have received particular attention in the effort to elucidate the nature of the cell-sinusoid interaction.

The sinus endothelium is continuous and contains no preformed aperture. The blood cells of the marrow migrate through the sinus wall, through the cytoplasm of the endothelial cell.[216–223] A transient transcellular aperture is formed on contact of the migrating cell with the endothelial cell through a mechanism still unknown.[216–220] Weiss[218] showed that 65% of the abluminal surface of the sinus wall of the marrow is covered by adventitial reticular cells. Following release of the marrow granulocyte reserve pool by endotoxin, there was a lifting away of the adventitial cover which presumably allowed passage for the increased flow of granulocytes from the marrow. Chamberlain et al.[221] found that following erythropoietin administration to mice there was a marked increase in the number of apertures in the sinus wall, an increased number of reticulocytes and leukocytes in transit, and a sharp decline in the adventitial cell cover. Tavassoli[222,223] reported a marked reduction in the adventitial cover, coincident with the reticulocyte response, following the removal of 25% of the calculated blood volume of rabbits. Thus the adventitial cell seems in some fashion to regulate the number of red or white cells leaving the marrow. Weiss[218] proposed that the change in adventitial cover may be purely passive, secondary to the press of large numbers of cells attempting to gain access to the endothelial cells. Tavassoli[222,223] suggested that the process may be active and mediated by the contraction of microfilaments in the cell's cytoplasmic projections.

Meuret and Heibges[224] studied the marrow egress of neutrophils in patients with polycythemia vera. The cells were pulse labeled with ^{3}H-thymidine and the labeling indices of segmented and band forms of the neutrophils obtained. The data in no way differed from that found in individuals with normal granulocytic activity and the investigators concluded that the factors controlling cell egress from the marrow in polycythemia vera functioned normally. De Bruyn et al.[225] found an intact sinus lining in rats made leukemic. The abnormal leukemic blast cells migrated transcellularly through apertures in a fashion no different from normal, mature cells. Mature cells were, however, not present in the sinusoids. De Bruyn et al.[225] concluded that the massive flow of blast cells to the peripheral blood was due to some intrinsic characteristic of the cell rather than to a breakdown in the sinus wall itself. Other studies[226–228] have reported degeneration of the sinusoidal wall allowing free access of the leukemic blast cells into the peripheral circulation. This discrepancy may be related to the state of the illness: in the early stages, the blast cells breach an intact sinus wall; in the advanced stages of disease, the wall gives way.[223]

Ultrastructural alterations of the sinusoidal wall of the liver have been reported in allergic liver injury,[229] poisoning,[230] and hepatitis.[231] Lindblad and Bjorkman[232] observed marked fragmentation of the endothelial cytoplasm as well as complete loss of the endothelium of the bone marrow sinusoids of dogs infected with a canine hepatitus virus.

Giordano and Lichtman[233] have looked into some of the properties of the migrating cell and considered motility and deformability[234–236] as central features in the cell's interaction with the sinus wall. Ackerman and Waksal[237] noted a sharp decrease in concanavalin A binding sites with maturation of the hemopoietic cells. During neutrophil maturation in the human marrow, the changes in membrane differentiation of the cells were particularly prominent in the late forms and seemed parallel to the changes in elasticity and locomotion noted by Lichtman and Weed.[236] Skutelsky and Farquhar[238] revealed similar changes in the red cells, namely, decreasing concanavalin A binding sites with maturation, but increasing concentrations of ferric oxide binding sites with differentiation. Lichtman et al.[239] reviewed the various factors concerned with cell egress: degree of maturation of the cell, the state of the sinus wall, the presence of releasing factors, and neutrovascular factors which may control the rate of sinusoidal blood flow. They suggested that the mechanisms of release for the different cell types may be different.

The different hemopoietic cells assume different topological relationships to the sinus wall. The megakaryocytes are in close apposition to the endothelial cell with no interposed basal membrane or adventitial cell. The erythroblasts and their associated reticular cell—the erythroblastic island—form the next closest group and the proliferating myeloid cells are the most distinct.[240] The platelet, thus, has the shortest path, the neutrophil, the longest, to the sinus. The megakaryocyte, because of its intimate contact with the sinus endothelium can send thin cytoplasmic processes through the endothelial cytoplasm. The processes detach and undergo further fragmentation into individual platelets in the circulation.[241] The large megakaryocyte size prevents leakage through the endothelial aperture.[242] Indirect evidence that the rate of blood flow through the sinus may also be a determinant of marrow cell release was presented by Chamberlain et al.[243]

VIII. BONE AND MARROW BLOOD FLOW

The high grade vascularity of the bone marrow was well appreciated by former generations of physicians who employed the intramedullary cavity as a site for parenteral administration of blood or medication when direct venous routes were denied them. Tocantins and O'Neill[244] demonstrated the rapid appearance of blood, plasma, medication, and diagnostic agents in the systemic circulation following their injection into the marrow. They reported that fluids can be infused at a rate of 0.4 to 2.5 mℓ/min into the marrow, probably an underestimation of the peak capacity of the marrow for the clearance of the fluids.

Physiological studies of bone marrow circulation have lagged behind anatomical investigations, due in large measure to the peculiarity of the architecture of the marrow vasculature, the difficulty of separating bone flow from marrow flow, and the relative inaccesibility of the organ. Large gaps exist in the available information on marrow circulation; much has yet to be learned of such fundamental events as the arterio-venous difference for gases, metabolic substrates, and the products of hematopoiesis, the red cells, white cells, and platelets.

An early attempt to study the physiology of the bone marrow circulation was made by Drinker and Drinker[245] in 1916, and later in 1922 they extended it considerably in collaboration with Lund.[121] Utilizing perfusion and dye injection techniques, they established the existence of vasoconstrictor nerves in the marrow, as well as the rate of flow of perfusing blood for a variety of laboratory animals. Utilizing a similar technique, namely the injection of a dye into the nutrient artery of a rabbit femur and collecting the venous effluent, Cummings[246] was able to measure the marrow blood flow. He was impressed with the rapidity of the marrow flow, 0.51 mℓ/g/min compared with the rate of flow through resting muscle, 0.038 mℓ/g/min, and for the brain, 0.54 mℓ/g/min. He also reported that hypoxia and hypercapnia produced a reflex vasodilatation and that adrenalin and noradrenalin produced vasoconstriction in the bone marrow. The high rate of blood flow through the marrow is in keeping with the reported high rate of metabolism of the rabbit red marrow.[247,248]

In further study, Cummings and Nutt[248] determined the mean rate of blood flow through the rabbit marrow and simultaneously measured the cardiac output. Basing their calculations on a figure of 1.7% of body weight for the marrow volume of rabbits[249] they concluded that the marrow receives 7.6% of the cardiac output.

Measurement of bone marrow blood flow in cats by use of a heated thermocouple and of intramarrow pressure simultaneously by a transducer led Shaw[250] to conclude that marrow flow can change independently of systemic blood pressure, but that there was a direct relationship between intramarrow pressure and blood flow. Occlusion of the nutrient artery did not produce a fall in bone marrow blood flow or marrow pressure. Both acetylcholine and adrenalin cause a fall in marrow blood flow and pressure.

The introduction of radiopharmaceutical techniques opened new possibilities for the study of bone and marrow flow. Impressed by the high rate of capillary circulation in the red marrow of a rabbit as measured by the effluent method,[240] Brown-Grant and Cummings[251] developed and applied a radioisotope depot clearance technique. Intramedullary installation of ^{131}Na as well as ^{26}NaCl were cleared with a half time of 20 to 30 sec, a value compatible with the high average rate of flow determined by direct measurement. Again, intravenous infusion of adrenalin caused a slowing of the clearance rate. They concluded that the depot technique is valid for the study of gross changes in blood flow of this somewhat inaccessible tissue. Najean and Clement[252] injected ^{51}Cr in an isotonic solution into the sternum of normal men and measured the arrival of the isotope in the inguinal region. They obtained a 2-phase washout curve: the first was very rapid and corresponded to a direct intravenous injection, indicating a rapid medullary flow; the second curve was exponential and due to the equilibration of the isotope with body fluids. Trubowitz et al.[253] introduced ^{22}NaCl, ^{131}I human serum albumin and ^{131}I-hippuran, directly into the sternal marrow of hematologically normal men and measured the clearance of the radioisotopes. They noted a rapid clearance, a half-time of 21 to 24 sec, independent of ion or molecular size. A delay in clearance was observed in the sternal marrow of patients previously exposed to therapeutic doses of X-rays in the course of treatment for carcinoma of the lung.[254]

Anger and Van Dyke[256] made a major advance in the study of bone blood flow and marrow distribution with their application of the positron scintillation camera utilizing radio fluoride as a bone blood flow indicator and radio iron to map the erythropoietic marrow. They were particularly impressed with the striking similarity between the distribution of bone blood flow and distribution of the active erythropoietic marrow. In the normal adult man both the ^{18}F and the ^{52}Fe were concentrated in coincident patterns in the spine, pelvis, sternum, ribs, and proximal portions of the extremities. In patients with myelofibrosis and polycythemia vera the extension of the red marrow into distal sites of the skeleton showed comparable distribution patterns of both ^{18}F—bone blood flow, and of ^{52}Fe—the erythropoietic marrow. The conincidence of increased bone blood flow and the marrow activity was thought to be evidence in support of the conjecture that the bone-bone marrow portal system may be important in the promotion of marrow growth. Considerations of vascular flow from bone to marrow have led to the speculation of the possible transport of local regulatory factors from bone to the neighboring hemopoietic sites.[257] Further support for this concept was derived from observations on chamber studies of marrow.[258] Increased hemopoietic activity and increased cellularity were associated with increased vascularity and resorption of bone. The intimate relationship between bone, hemopoietic cells, and sinusoids was deemed highly suggestive for a role of bone derived factors in hemopoiesis.[260,261]

In early studies, Huggins and Blocksom[262] showed that the fatty, aplastic marrow of terminal vertebrae of a rat's tail resumed active hematopoiesis following abdominal implantation. The authors attributed the conversion of the yellow marrow to increased vascularity brought about by the increased temperature of the intraabdominal site. This speculation was confirmed by Van Dyke[263] who was able to demonstrate a threefold increase in bone blood flow in the implanted tail of the Huggins preparation.

The ideal tracer for organ clearance measurement of bone and marrow has not been found, and no good method exists for measuring bone blood flow and marrow flow separately. ^{18}F has been useful and a minimum "bone blood flow" value can be obtained if appropriate leakage corrections are made. Measurements with ^{18}F in man have given a bone blood flow value of 3.3% of cardiac output[264] and of 4.3% in the rat.[265] Jones[266] estimated a minimum blood flow through the erythropoietic marrow of 7% of the circulating blood volume from data obtained from the uptake of radiocolloid. The distribution of ^{99m}Tc-labeled colloids in the reticuloendothelial system is also strikingly similar to the distribution of the active erythropoietic marrow.[267–269] Iron has not been a useful tracer for flow studies.

Van Dyke et al.[270] have explored the application of the washout method for the measurement of local bone and marrow flow. The washout technique can be performed either by nutrient artery or intramedullary injection. In carefully controlled studies in dogs Van Dyke et al.[270] were able to show rapid clearance of an intramedullary instilled radioisotope for the active red marrow, but, surprisingly, in many instances for the yellow, fatty marrow as well. Washout for protein bound as well as for diffusible isotopes was rapid and identical, confirming permeability to molecules the size of albumin. The findings also suggest that the extracellular fluid space and the plasma compartment of the marrow are essentially the same.

Another approach to the study of bone blood flow in experimental animals has been the intravascular injection of materials such as radiopotassium labeled microspheres which are presumably removed by all organs in proportion to their fraction of the cardiac output.[271,272] Again, the common circulation of bone marrow presents difficulties in the use of this technique.

IX. NERVE SUPPLY

Although nerve fibers have been described in the bone marrow in the middle 1800s there has been a surprising lack of interest in this area. Myelinated and nonmyelinated nerves enter the marrow cavity through the nutrient foramen.[273,274] Single myelinated fibers were found in direct association with parenchymal cells of the marrow. Ottolenghi[275] described a group of fibers that form a plexiform network between the adventitia and media of the arterioles, fibers which surround the capillaries, and fibers associated with and surrounding the parenchymal cellular elements. Rossi[276] described similar relationships to blood vessels and described, in addition, fibers, not related to vessels, that end as small brushes, buttons, or rings of filaments in the parenchyma. Foa[277] demonstrated a vasomotor function for some of the fibers. Kuntz and Richins[278] showed abundant sympathetic and afferent nerve fibers. They thought the afferent fibers were imbedded in the parenchyma and concluded that the pain induced by bone marrow aspiration was carried by these afferent fibers.

Calvo[279] studied the innervation of the marrow of the long bones of a variety of laboratory animals: the normal adult mouse, rat, rabbit, and monkey. He found, as had been previously demonstrated, that a nerve enters the nutrient foramen in close association with the nutrient artery. The nerve can be traced from its origin in the region of the spinal cord that corresponds to the territory in which the foramen is located, until its final termination in the periosteum and the marrow. The periosteal nerve branches from a network over the surface of the bone from which nerve fibrils enter the marrow in company of the small arterioles through the perforating ostia. The medullary branch of the nerve enters via the nutrient foramen and follows a path roughly parallel to the distribution of the nutrient artery. The nerve pattern is thus strikingly similar to the arterial supply. The innervation of the circular layers of muscle in the initial part of arterial branches is plentiful, suggesting a nerve control for sphincter-like action of these muscles. The finer vascular branches, the arterioles and capillaries, are accompanied by a single naked fiber. The sinusoids are poorly innervated. The nerve fibers curve and bend to conform to the shapes of the larger structures in their path, such as the sinusoids and fat cells. The fibers ultimately become very thin and disappear among the cells of the parenchyma or in contact with the endothelial cells of the sinusoids. The morphological characteristics of the different animals examined appear to be quite similar and conform in general to the description given. The nerve fibers of the bone marrow are both myelinated and nonmyelinated. The myelinated fibers are thicker and less numerous and are believed to be afferent fibers. The nonmyelinated fibers are intimately associated with the arterioles and believed to be autonomic in nature.

In a subsequent study Calvo and Forteza-Vila[280,281] demonstrated the presence of Schwann cells in the bone marrow which are morphologically identical to the cells in peripheral nerves. The differentiation of Schwann cell structure begins toward the end of the second postnatal week. The cells separate the bundles of numerous axons by means of cytoplasmic extensions, followed later by the formation of myelin. It is of interest that the regulation of erythropoiesis in the neonatal rat is different from that of the adult. The newborn rat does not respond to humoral stimulation[282] or to starvation or hypoxia[283] during the first 2 weeks of life. Since morphologic differentiation of the marrow nerves is completed just at this period transition to the adult marrow response, the speculation has been raised that adult hemopoietic control may involve neural as well as hormonal mechanisms. Evidence has also been presented for a role of the sympathetic nerves in the release of cells from the marrow. Stimulation of lumbar sympathetic trunks in the rat resulted in the release of reticulocytes and neutrophils.[284]

Beta adrenergic receptors have been demonstrated on both pluripotential stem cells and immature erythroid cells. The beta adrenergic receptors are distinct from the receptors for erythropoietin and in the erythroid cells of birds and mammals are linked to adenylcyclase. The addition of beta adrenergic agonists to cultures of canine marrow cells enhances erythroid colony formation. The beta adrenergic antagonist, propanalol, blocked the reaction.[283–288] The beta adrenergic agents, isoproterenol and salbutamol, produce a marked stimulation of erythropoiesis in the polycythemic mouse.[289] Salbutamol was, however, ineffective in stimulating erythropoiesis in an in vivo culture of rabbit bone marrow cells. Salbutomol was found to increase plasma erythropoietin in the intact rabbit and this mechanism was invoked to explain the enhanced erythropoiesis stimulated by the beta-adrenergic agonists.[290] More study is required to reconcile these differences and more precisely define the mechanisms involved.

Little need be said about lymphatics of the bone marrow. Lymphatic vessels have never been demonstrated.

REFERENCES

1. **Mechanik, N.,** Untersuchungen uber das Gewicht des Knochenmarkes des Menschen, Z. Anat. Entwicklungsgesch., 79, 53, 1926.
2. **von Herrath, E.,** Morphology of the reticuloendothelial system, *Z. Alla Pathol. (Jena)*, 90, 493, 1953.
3. **Fleicher, J.,** The normal bone marrow picture in the rabbit, *Hematologia*, 79, 89, 1962.
4. **Fliedner, T. M., Calvo, W., Hass, P., et al.,** Morphologic and cytokinetic aspects of bone marrow stroma, in *Hemopoietic Cellular Proliferation*, Stohlman, F., Ed., Grune and Stratton, New York, 1970, 67.
5. **Weiss, L.,** Structure of the bone marrow. Functional interrelationships of vascular and hemopoietic compartments in experimental hemolytic anemia, *J. Morphol.*, 117, 467, 1965.
6. **Weiss, L.,** The histology of the bone marrow, in *Regulation of Hematopoiesis*, Vol. 1, Gordon, A. S., Ed., Appleton-Century-Crofts, New York, 1970, 79.

7. **Trubowitz, S., Broers, A., and Pease, R. F. W.,** Surface ultrastructure of the human marrow: a brief note, *Blood*, 35, 112, 1970.
8. **Trubowitz, S. and Masek, B.,** Structural organization of the human marrow matrix in thin sections, *Am. J. Clin. Pathol.*, 53, 908, 1964.
9. **Bizzozero, G.,** Sulla funzione ematopoietica del midolla delle ossa, *Gazz. Med. Ital. Lombardia*, 28, 381, 1968.
10. **Neumann, E.,** Ueber die Bedeutung des Knochenmarks fur die Blutbildung, *Zentralbl. Med. Wiss.*, 6, 689, 1868.
11. **Neumann, E.,** Das Gesetz der Verbreitumg des gelbem und roten Markes in den Extremitatenknochen, *Zentralbl. Med. Wiss.*, 20, 321, 1882.
12. **Rohr, K.,** Dan menschliche Knochenmark, George Thieme Verlag, Stuttgart, 1960, 29.
13. **Trubowitz, S. and Bathija, A.,** Cell size and palmitate-1-^{14}C turnover of rabbit marrow fat, *Blood*, 49, 599, 1977.
14. **Dietz, A.,** Composition of normal blood marrow in rabbits, *J. Biol. Chem.*, 165, 505, 1946.
15. **Dietz, A.,** Chemical composition of normal bone marrow, *Arch. Biochem. Biophys.*, 21, 21, 1949.
16. **Lund, P., Abadi, D., and Mathies, J.,** Lipid composition of human normal bone marrow by column chromatography, *J. Lipid Res.*, 3, 95, 1962.
17. **Zach, E. and Shafrir, E.,** Composition of bone marrow adipose tissue in relation to body fat depot in various species, *Isr. J. Med. Sci.*, 10, 1541, 1974.
18. **Shore, L. S.,** Bone Marrow as an Adipose Tissue, Thesis, Hahnemann Medical College, Philadelphia, 1960.
19. **Tavassoli, M.,** Marrow adipose cells. Histochemical identification of labile and stable components, *Arch. Pathol. Lab. Med.*, 100, 16, 1976.
20. **Napolitano, L.,** The differentiation of the white adipose cell: an electron microscopic study, *J. Cell. Biol.*, 18, 663, 1963.
21. **Napolitano, L. and Fawcett, D.,** The fine structure of brown adipose tissue in newborn mouse and rat, *J. Biophys. Biochem. Cytol.*, 4, 685, 1958.
22. **Chase, W. H.,** Fine structure of rat adipose tissue, *J. Ultrastruct. Res.*, 2, 283, 1959.
23. **Cushman, S. W.,** Structure-function relationships in the adipose cell, *J. Cell Biol.*, 46, 326, 1970.
24. **Salvin, B. G.,** The cytophysiology of mammalian adipose cells, *Int. Rev. Cytol.*, 33, 297, 1972.
25. **Tavassoli, M.,** Ultrastructural development of bone marrow adipose cell, *Acta Anat.*, 94, 65, 1976.
26. **Zucker-Franklin, D., Grusky, G., and Marcus, A.,** Transformation of monocytes into "fat" cells, *Lab. Invest.*, 38, 620, 1978.
27. **Trubowitz, S. and Masek, B.,** A histochemical study of reticuloendothelial system of human marrow—a possible transport role, *Blood*, 32, 610, 1968.
28. **Dexter, T. M. and Lajtha, L. G.,** Proliferation of hemopoietic stem cells and development of potentially leukemic cells in vitro, in Comparative Leukemia Research, Clemmensen, J. and Yohn, D. S., Eds., S. Karger, Basel, 1976, 1.
29. **Dexter, T. M., Allen, T. D., and Lajtha, L. G.,** Conditions controlling proliferation of haemopoietic stem cells in vitro, *J. Cell. Physiol.*, 91, 335, 1977.
30. **Dexter, T. M., and Moore, M. A. S.,** In vitro duplication and "cure" of haemopoietic defects in genetically anemic mice, *Nature*, 269, 412, 1977.
31. **Dexter, T. M., Wright, E. G., Krizsa, F., and Lajtha, L. G.,** Regulation of haemopoietic stem cell proliferation in long term bone marrow cultures, *Biomedicine*, 27, 334, 1977.
32. **Dexter, T. M., Allen, T. D., Lajtha, L. G., et al.,** In vitro analysis of self renewal and commitment of haemopoietic stem cells, in, *Differentiation of Normal and Neoplastic Haemopoietic Cells*, Clarkson, R. T., Marks, D. R., and Till, J. E., Eds., Cold Spring Harbor Laboratory, New York, 1978, 63.
33. **Allen, T. D.,** Ultrastructural aspects of in vitro haemopoiesis, in *Stem Cells and Tissue Homeostasis*, Lock, B. I., Potter, C. S., and Cole, R. S., Eds., Cambridge University Press, London, 1978, 217.
34. **Allen, T. D. and Dexter, T. M.,** Cellular interrelationships during in vitro granulopoiesis, *Differentiation* 6, 191, 1976.
35. **Erslev, A. J.,** Medullary and extramedullary blood formation, *Clin. Orthop.*, 52, 25, 1967.
36. **Ascenzi, A.,** Physiological relationship and pathological reference between bone tissue and marrow, in *The Biochemistry and Physiology of Bone*, Vol. 4, Bourne, G. H., Ed., Academic Press, New York, 1976, 403.
37. **Doan, C. A., Cunningham, R. S., and Sabin, F. R.,** Experimental studies on the origin and maturation of avian and mammalian red blood cells, *Contrib. Embryol. Carnegie Inst. Wash.*, 16, 163, 1925.
38. **Krause, R. E.,** Changes induced by anemia in bone marrow lipids of cats, *J. Biol. Chem.*, 149, 395, 1943.

39. **Maniatis, H., Tavassoli, M., and Crosby, W. H.,** Factors affecting the conversion of yellow to red marrow, *Blood*, 37, 581, 1971.
40. **Tavassoli, M. and Crosby, W. H.,** Transplantation of marrow to extramedullary sites, *Science*, 161, 54, 1968.
41. **Tavassoli, M. and Crosby, W. H.,** Bone marrow histogenesis: a comparison of fatty and red marrow, *Science*, 169, 291, 1970.
42. **Tavassoli, M., Maniatis, A., and Crosby, W. H.,** Induction of sustained hemopoiesis in fatty marrow, *Blood*, 43, 33, 1974.
43. **Renold, A. B. and Cahill, G. F.,** in preface of Handbook of Physiology, Section 5, American Physiological Society, Washington, D.C., 1968, 1.
44. **Werheimer, H. E.,** in introduction of Handbook of Physiology, Section 5, American Physiological Society, Washington, D.C., 1965, 5.
45. **Aronovsky, E., Levari, R., Kornblueth, W., and Wertheimer, E.,** Comparison of metabolic activities of orbital fat with those of other tissues, *Invest. Opthalmol.*, 2, 259, 1963.
46. **Rodbell, M.,** Metabolism of isolated fat cells. I. Effect of hormones on glucose metabolism and lipolysis, *J. Biol. Chem.*, 239, 375, 1964.
47. **Hirsch, J. and Gallian, R.,** Method for the determination of adipose cell size in man and animals, *J. Lipid Res.*, 9, 110, 1968.
48. **Bjorntorp, P.,** Studies on adipose tissue from obese patients with or without diabetes mellitus. II. Basal and insulin-stimulated glucose metabolism, *Acta Med. Scand.*, 179, 229, 1966.
49. **Zinder. O., Arad, R., and Shapiro, B.,** Effect of cell size on metabolism of isolated fat cells, *Isr. J. Med. Sci.*, 3, 787, 1967.
50. **Bjorntorp, R. and Karlsson, M.,** Triglyceride synthesis in human subcutaneous adipose tissue cells of different size, *Eur. J. Clin. Invest.*, 1, 112, 1970.
51. **Smith, U.,** Effect of cell size on lipid synthesis by human adipose tissue in vitro, *J. Lipid Res.*, 17, 65, 1971.
52. **Bjorntorp, P. and Sjostrom, L.,** Composition and metabolism of adipose cells of different sizes, *Eur. J. Clin. Inves.*, 2, 78, 1972.
53. **Salans, L. B., Knittle, J. L., and Hirsch, J.,** Role of adipose cell size and adipose tissue insulin sensitivity in carbohydrate tolerance of human obesity, *J. Clin. Invest.*, 47, 153, 1965.
54. **Miller, W. and Trubowitz, S.,** Unpublished data.
55. **Barth, I. and Kados, I.,** The role of marrow fat in the development and recovery of anemia, *Z. Ges. Inn. Med.*, 14, 594, 1959.
56. **Huggins, C. and Blockson, B. H.,** Changes in outlying bone marrow accompanying local increase of temperature within physiological limits, *J. Exp. Med.*, 64, 253, 1936.
57. **Tribukait, B.,** Experimental studies on the regulation of erythropoiesis with special reference to the importance of oxygen, *Acta Physiol. Scand.*, 58, (Suppl. 208), 1, 1963.
58. **Bodansky, M., Marr, W. L., and Brindley, P.,** An experimental study of the action of phenylhydrazine and acetylphenyl hydrazine, with reference to their use in the treatment of polycythemia vera, *Am. J. Clin. Pathol.*, 2, 391, 1932.
59. **Jacobsen, E. M., Davis, A. K., and Alpen, E. L.,** Relative effectiveness of phenylhydrazine treatment and hemorrhage in production of erythropoietic factor, *Blood*, 11, 937, 1956.
60. **Sabin, F. R.,** Bone marrow, *Physiol. Rev.*, 8, 191, 1928.
61. **Saterborg, N. E.,** Bone marrow abnormalities after phenylhydrazine induced hemolysis in rabbits, *Acta Radiol.* Ther. (Stockholm), 13, 345, 1974.
62. **Evans, J. D., Baker, J. M., and Oppenheimer, M. J.,** Alterations of rabbit marrow fat in anemia from phenylhydrazine, *Am. J. Physiol.*, 181, 504, 1955.
63. **Evans, J. D. and Oppenheimer, M. J.,** Effect of bleeding on rabbit marrow polyunsaturated fatty acids, *Am. J. Physiol.*, 181, 509, 1955.
64. **Cohen, P. and Gardner, F. H.,** Effect of massive triamcinolone administration in blunting the erythropoietic response to phenylhydrazine hemolysis, *J. Lab. Clin. Med.*, 65, 88, 1965.
65. **Tavassoli, M., Maiatis, A., and Crosby, W. H.,** Effects of phenylhydrazine induced hemolysis on the behavior of regenerating stroma, *Br. J. Haematol.*, 23, 707, 1972.
66. **Bathija, A., Davis, S., and Trubowitz, S.,** Marrow adipose tissue: response to erythropoiesis, *Am. J., Hematol.*, 5, 315, 1978.
67. **Morse, B. S., Renricca, N. J., and Stohlman, R.,** Relationship of erythropoietic effectiveness of the regenerative cycle of erythroid precursor cell, *Blood*, 35, 287, 1970.
68. **Felippa, A. E., Meinicke, H. A., and Mc Gluskey, R. S.,** Studies on transplanted hemopoietic tissue utilizing a modified back chamber. I. Vasoproliferation following erythropoietin stimulation, *Scand. J. Hematol.*, 8, 86, 1971.

69. **Reissmann, K. R. and Samorapoomichit, S.,** Effect of erythropoietin on proliferation of erythroid stem cells in absence of transplantable colony forming units, *Blood*, 36, 287, 1970.
70. **Linman, J. W., Bethell, F. H., and Long, M. J.,** Studies on the nature of the plasma erythropoietic factor(s), *J. Lab. Clin. Med.*, 51, 8, 1958.
71. **Linman, J. W., Long, M. J., Korst, D. R., and Bethell, F. H.,** Studies on the stimulation of hemopoiesis by bathyl alcohol, *J. Lab. Clin. Med.*, 54, 335, 1959.
72. **Potter, J. E. R. and Wright, E. G.,** Bone marrow lipids in normal and anemic mice, *Am. J. Hematol.*, 8, 361, 1980.
73. **Rohr, K.,** Das menschliche Knochenmark, Georg Thieme Verlag, Stuttgart, 1960, 35.
74. **Ehrlich, P.,** Ueber einen fall von Anamie mit Bemerkungen über regenerative Veranderungen des Knochenmarks, Charite—Ann., 13, 309, 1888.
75. **Dietz, A. A. and Steinberg, B.,** Chemical composition of irradiated bone marrow, *Arch. Biochem.*, 23, 222, 1949.
76. **Harris, J. W. and Kellermeyer, R. W.,** *The Red Cell*, Harvard University Press, Cambridge, 1970, 707.
77. **Te Velde, J. and Kaak, H. L.,** Aplastic anemia. Histological investigation of methacrylate embedded bone marrow biopsy specimens: correlation with survival after conventional treatment in 15 adult patients, *Br. J. Haematol.*, 35, 61, 1977.
78. **Stohlmann, F. J.,** Editorial: aplastic anemia, *Blood*, 40, 282, 1972.
79. **Knospe, W. H. and Crosby, W. H.,** Aplastic anemia: a disorder of the bone marrow sinusoidal microcirculation rather than stem-cell failure?, *Lancet*, 1, 20, 1971.
80. **Patt, H. A. and Maloney, M. A.,** *Hematopoietic Cellular Proliferation*, Stohlman, F. J., Ed., Grune and Stratton, New York, 1970, 56.
81. **Knospe, W. H., Blum, J., and Crosby, W. H.,** Regeneration of locally irradiated bone marrow. I. Dose dependent, long term changes in the fat, with particular emphasis upon vascular and stromal reaction, *Blood*, 28, 398, 1966.
82. **Elko, E. E. and DiLuzio, N. R.,** Effect of irradiation on plasma, liver and bone marrow lipids of the rabbit, *Radiat. Res.*, 11, 1, 1959.
82. **Snyder, F. and Cress, E. A.,** Bone marrow lipids in rats exposed to total body radiation, *Radiat. Res.*, 19, 129, 1963.
84. **Snyder, F.,** Fatty acid oxidation in irradiated bone marrow, *Nature*, 206, 733, 1965.
85. **Snyder, F. and Wood, R.,** Deposition of triglycerides of increased carbon number in irradiated rat marrow, *Radiat. Res.*, 33, 142, 1968.
86. **Snyder, F.,** Triglyceride biosynthesis in irradiated bone marrow, *Radiat. Res.*, 27, 375, 1966.
87. **Bathija, H., Ohanian, M., Davis, S., and Trubowitz, S.,** The marrow fat cell: response to X-ray induced aplasia, Life Sci., 25, 921, 1979.
88. **Bizzozero, G.,** Ueber die Atrophie der Fettzellen des Knochenmarks, *Archiv. Mikr. Anat. Bonn*, 33, 247, 1889.
89. **Keys, A., Brozek, J., Heschel, A., Michelsen, O., and Taylor, H. L.,** *The Biology of Human Starvation*, University of Minnesota Press, Minneapolis, 1950.
90. **Kelweg-Larsen, P., Hoffman, H., Kieler, J., et al.,** Famine disease in concentration camps, complications and sequels, *Acad. Med. Scand. Suppl.*, 274, 170, 1952.
91. **Szejnman, M.,** Le sang dans la maladie de famine, in *Maladie de Famine*. Recherches Cliniques sur la Famine Executees dans le Ghetto de Varsovie en 1942, Apfelbaum, E., Ed., American Joint Distribution Committee, Warsaw, 1946, 227.
92. **Jolly, J.,** Traite Technique D'Hematologie, A. Maloine, Paris, 1923, 678.
93. **Pearson, H. A.,** Marrow hypoplasis in anorexia nervosa, *J. Pediatr.*, 71, 211, 1967.
94. **Finkel, H. E. and Mitus, W. J.,** Gelantinous degeneration of the bone marrow (Abstr.), 12th Congr. Int. Soc. Hematol., New York, 1968, 145.
95. **Mant, M. J. and Faragher, B. S.,** The hematology of anorexia nervosa, *Br. J. Haematol.*, 23, 737, 1972.
96. **Adami, J. G.,** *Principles of Pathology*, Vol. 1, Lea and Febiger, Philadelphia, 1972, 905.
97. **Meyer, A. W.,** Some morphological effects of prolonged inanition, *J. Med. Res.*, 3, 31, 1917.
98. **Michael, P.,** Gelatinous degeneration of the bone marrow, *J. Pathol. Bacteriol.*, 53, 533, 1930.
99. **Tavassoli, M., Eastland, T. D., Yam, L. T. et al.,** Gelatinous transformation of bone marrow in prolonged self-induced starvation, *Scand. J. Haematol.*, 16, 311, 1976.
100. **Manthorpe, R., Helin, G., Kofod, F., and Lorenzen, I.,** Effects of glucocorticoids on connective tissue of aorta and skin in rabbits, *Acta Endocrinol.*, 77, 310, 1972.
101. **Newlin, A. E and McKay, C. M.,** Bone marrow for fat storage in rabbits, *Arch. Biochem.*, 17, 125, 1948.

102. **Evans, J. P., Riemenschneider, R. W., and Herb, S. F.,** Fat composition and in vitro oxygen consumption in marrow from fed and fasted rabbits, *Arch. Biochem. Biophys.*, 53, 157, 1954.
103. **Dietz, A. H. and Steinberg, B.,** Chemistry of bone marrow. VII. Composition of rabbit bone marrow in inanition, *Arch. Biochem.* 45, 10, 1953.
104. **Tavassoli, M.,** Differential response of bone marrow and extramedullary adipose cells to starvation, *Experientia*, 30, 424, 1974.
105. **Bathija, A., Davis, A., and Trubowitz, S.,** Bone marrow adipose tissue: response to acute starvation, *Am. J. Hematol.*, 6, 191, 1979.
106. **Bragdon, J. H. and Gordon, B. S., Jr.,** Tissue distribution of palmitate C^{14} after intravenous injection and labeled chylomicrons and esterified fatty acids in the rat, *J. Clin. Invest.* 37, 574, 1958.
107. **Olivecrona, T.,** The metabolism of 1-C^{14}-palmitic acid labeled chylomicrons in rats, *Acta Physiol. Scand.*, 55, 170, 1962.
108. **Jeanrenaud, B.,** Aspects of adipose tissue metabolism: a review, *Metabolism*, 10, 535, 1961.
109. **Palladino, J.,** Ueber die Histologie des Knochenmarkes, *Ebl. Med. Wiss.*, 7, 513, 1869.
110. **Hoyer, H.,** Zur Histologie des Knochenmarkes, *Ebl. Med. Wiss.*, 7, 257, 1869.
111. **Jolly, J.,** Traite Technique d'Hematologie, A. Maloine, Paris 1923, 646. (Contains a summation of the information on marrow circulation through the first quarter of the 20th century.)
112. **Bargmann, W.,** Ueber den Feinbau der Knochenmarkskapillaren, *Z. Zellforsch. Mikrosk. Anat.*, 11, 1, 1930.
113. **Spalteholz, W.,** Das "Durchsichtigmache" als biologische arbeitsmethode, in *Handbuch Biologische Arbeitsmethoden*, Aberhalden, W. Ed., 9(1), 1932, 408.
114. **Brookes, M. and Harrison, R. G.,** The vascularization of the rabbit femur and tibiafibula, *J. Anat.*, 91, 61, 1957.
115. **Ecoiffier, J., Prot, D., Friffie, R., and Catach, D..** Etude du reseau veineux dans les os longs du lapin, *Rev. Chir. Orthop.*, 43, 29, 1957.
116. **Hashimoto, M.,** Ueber das Kapillareblutgefäss system des Kaninchenknockenmarks, *Trans. Soc. Pathol. Jpn.*, 26, 300, 1936.
117. **Morgan, J. D.,** Blood supply of the growing rabbit's tibia, *J. Bone J. Surg.*, 418, 185, 1959.
118. **Yoffey, J. M.,** A note of thick walled and thin walled arteries of bone marrow, *J. Anat.*, 96, 425, 1962.
119. **Lewis, O. J.,** Blood supply of developing long bones with special references to the metaphysis, *J. Bone J. Surg.*, 38, 928, 1956.
120. **Doan, C. A.,** The circulation of the bone marrow, *Carnegie Inst. Washington Contrib. Embryol.*, 14, 27, 1925.
121. **Drinker, C. K., Drinker, K. R., and Lund, C. C.,** The circulation of the mammalian bone marrow, *Am. J. Physiol.*, 62, 1, 1922.
122. **Hurley, L. A. and Miller, C. W.,** Demonstration of the marrow vascular space (macrocanalicular system) of bone, *Arch. Pathol.*, 68, 615, 1959.
123. **Branemark, P. I.,** Vital microscopy of bone marrow in rabbit, *Scand. J. Clin. Lab. Invest.* Suppl. 38, 2, 1959. (Contains in addition an extensive historical review of early investigations on marrow circulation.)
124. **Branemark, P. I.,** Experimental investigation of microcirculation in bone marrow, *Angiology*, 12, 93, 1961.
125. **Maximow, A., Bindegewebe und blutbildende Gewebe,** in *Handbuch der mikroskopischen Anatomie des Menschen*, Mollendorf, Ed., Springer-Verlag, Berlin, 1927, 232.
126. **de Bruyn, P. P. H., Breen, P. C., and Thomas, T. B.,** The microcirculation of the bone marrow, *Anat. Rec.*, 168, 55, 1970.
127. **Pease, D. C.,** Marrow cells seen with the electron microscope after ultrathin sectioning, *Rev. Hematol.*, 10, 300, 1955.
128. **Pease, D. C.,** Electron microscopic study of the red bone marrow, *Blood*, 11, 501, 1956.
129. **Zamboni, L. and Pease, P. C.,** The vascular bed of the red bone marrow, *J. Ultrastruct. Res.*, 5, 65, 1961.
130. **de Bruyn, P. P. H., Thomas, T. B., and Michelsen, S.,** Fine structure of the vascular components of the guinea pig bone marrow, *Anat. Rec.*, 154, 499, 1966.
131. **Weiss, L.,** *The Cells and Tissues of the Immune System*, Prentice-Hall, Englewood Cliffs, N.J., 1972.
132. **Weiss, L.,** An electron microscopic study of the vascular sinuses of the bone marrow of the rabbit, *Bull. Johns Hopkins Hosp.*, 108, 171, 1961.
133. **Campbell, F.,** Fine structure of the bone marrow of the chicken and pigeon, *J. Morphol.*, 123, 405, 1967.
134. **Campbell, F.,** Ultrastructure of the bone marrow of the frog, *Am. J. Anat.*, 129, 329, 1970.

135. **Williams, W. J., Beutler, W. J., Erslev, A. J., and Rundles, R. W.,** *Hematology*, McGraw-Hill, New York, 1972, 902.
136. **Aschoff, L.,** Das reticuloendotheliale system, *Ergeb. Inn. Med. Kinderheilkd.*, 26, 1, 1924.
137. **Gall, E. A.,** The reticulum cell, the cytological identity and interrelation of mesenchymal cell of lymphoid tissue, *Ann. N.Y. Acad. Sci.*, 78, 120, 1958.
138. **Willmer, E. W.,** *Cytology and Evolution*, Academic Press, New York, 1960.
139. **Fridenstein, A. J.,** Precursor cells of mechanocytes, *Int. Rev. Cytol.*, 47, 327, 1976.
140. **Van Furth, R., Cohn, Z. A., Hirsch, J. G. et al,** Mononuclear phagocytic system: a new classification, *Bull. WHO*, 46, 845, 1972.
141. **Van Furth, R., Langervoort, H. L., and Schaberg, A.,** Mononuclear phagocytes in human pathology—proposal for an approach to improved classification, in *Immunity, Infection and Pathology*, Van Furth, R., Ed., Blackwell Scientific, Oxford, 1975, 1.
142. **Caffrey, R. W., Everett, N. B., and Rieke, W. O.,** Radio-autographic studies of reticular and blast cells in hemopoietic tissues of the rat, *Anat. Rec.*, 155, 41, 1966.
143. **Biermann, A. and von Keyserlingk, D. G.,** Ultrastructure of reticulum cells in the bone marrow, *Acta Anat.*, 100, 34, 1978.
144. **Berman, J.,** The ultrastructure of the erythroblastic island and reticulum cells in bone marrow, *J. Ultrastruct. Res.*, 17, 291, 1967.
145. **Bessis, M.,** *Living Blood Cells and Their Ultrastructure*, Springer-Verlag, Berlin, 1973.
146. **Seki, M. and Shirasawa, N.,** Role of reticular cells during maturation process of the erythroblast, *Acta Pathol. Jpn.*, 15, 387, 1965.
147. **Bessis, M.,** Lilot erythroblastique, unite functionelle de la moelle osseuse, *Rev. Hematol.*, 13, 8, 1958.
148. **Tanaka, Y.,** An electron microscopic study of non phagocytic reticulum cells in human bone marrow. I. Cells with intracytoplasmic fibrils, *Acta Haematol. Jpn.*, 32, 275, 1969.
149. **Ben-Ishay, Z.,** Reticulum cells, stem cells and lymphocytes, *Isr. J. Med. Sci.*, 10, 1379, 1974.
150. **Fridenstein, A. J., Challakayan, R. K., Latsinik, N. V., et al.,** Stromal cells responsible for transferring the microenvironment of the hemopoietic tissue, *Transplantation*, 17, 331, 1974.
151. **Chertkov, J. L. and Gurevitch, O. A.,** Radiosensitivity of progenitor cells of the hemopoietic environment, *Radiat. Res.*, 79, 177, 1979.
152. **Trubowitz, S. and Masek, B.,** A histochemical study of the reticuloendothelial system of human marrow—its possible transport role, *Blood*, 32, 610, 1968.
153. **Bankston, P. W. and de Bruyn, P. P. H.,** The permeability to carbon of the sinusoidal lining cells of the embryonic rat liver and rat bone marrow, *Am. J. Anat.*, 141, 281, 1974.
154. **Post, R. L. and Sen, A. K.,** An enzymatic mechanism of active sodium and potassium transport, *Histochem. Cytochem.*, 13, 105, 1965.
155. **Marchesi, V. T. and Barnett, R. J.,** The demonstration of enzymatic activity in pinocytotic vesicles of blood capillaries with the electron microscope, *J. Cell Biol.*, 17, 547, 1963.
156. **Hyman, C. and Paldino, R. L.,** Possible role of reticuloendothelial system in protein transport, *Ann. N.Y. Acad. Sci.*, 88, 232, 1960.
157. **Byers, S. O.,** Lipids and reticuloendothelial system, *Ann. N. Y. Acad. Sci.*, 88, 240, 1960.
158. **Di Luzzio, N. R.,** Lipid composition of Kupfer cells, *Am. J. Physiol.*, 196, 884, 1959.
159. **Janeso, M.,** as cited by **Zweifach, B. W.,** in *Vascular Endothelium in the Arterial Wall*, Lansing, A. L., Ed., Williams & Wilkins, Baltimore, 1959.
160. **Westen, H. and Bainton, D. F.,** Association of alkaline-positive reticulum cells in bone marrow with granulocytic precursors, *J. Exp. Med.*, 150, 919, 1979.
161. **Bessis, M. and Breton-Gorius, J.,** Incorporation de granvules ferrugineux par les erythroblastes. Observees au microscope electronique, *C. R. Soc. Biol.*, 150, 1903, 1956.
162. **Maximow, H. A.,** Relation of blood cells to connective tissue and endothelium, *Physiol. Rev.*, 4, 533, 1924.
163. **Sabin, F. R., Miller, F. R., Smithburn, K. C., et al.,** Changes in the bone marrow and blood cells of developing rabbits, *J. Exp. Med.*, 64, 97, 1936.
164. **Boggs, D. K. and Chervenick, P. A.,** *Hematopoietic Stem Cells in Formation and Destruction of Blood Cells*, Greenwalt, T. J. and Jamieson, G. A., Eds., Lippincott, Philadelphia, 1970, 240.
165. **Bradley, T. R.,** Aspects of stimulation of bone marrow colony growth in vitro, *Aust. J. Exp. Biol. Med. Sci.*, 46, 335, 1968.
166. **Boyum, A. and Bergstrom, R.,** The concentration of granulocytic stem cells in mouse bone marrow determined with diffusion chamber technique, *Scand. J. Haematol.*, 7, 294, 1970.
167. **Chervenick, P. A. and Boggs, D. R.,** In vitro growth of granulocytic and mononuclear cell colonies from blood of normal individuals, *Blood*, 37, 131, 1971.

168. **Pike, B. and Robinson, W. A.,** Human bone marrow culture in agar gel, *J. Cell. Physiol.*, 76, 77, 1970.
169. **Whang, J., Frei, E., III, Tijo, J. H., et al.,** The distribution of the Phildelphia chromosome in patients with chronic myelocytic leukemia, *Blood*, 22, 664, 1963.
170. **Till, J. E. and McCulloch, E. A.,** A direct measurement of the radiation sensitivity of normal mouse bone marrow cells, *Radiat. Res.*, 14, 213, 1961.
171. **Till, J. E. and McCulloch, E. A.,** Early repair proecesses in marrow cells irradiated and proliferating in vivo, *Radiat. Res.*, 18, 96, 1963.
172. **Till, J. E. and McCulloch, E. A.,** Proliferation of hematopoietic colony-forming cells transplanted into irradiated mice, *Radiat. Res.*, 22, 383, 1964.
173. **Wu, A. M., Till, J. E., Siminovich, L., and McCulloch, E. A.,** A cytological study of the capacity for differentiation of normal hematopoietic colony forming cells, *J. Cell. Physiol.*, 69, 177, 1967.
174. **Lewis, J. P. and Trobaugh, F. E., Jr.,** Haemopoietic stem cells, *Nature*, 204, 589, 1964.
175. **Juraskova, V. and Tkadlecek, L.,** Character of primary and secondary colonies of haematopoiesis in the spleen of irradiated mice, *Nature*, 206, 951, 1965.
176. **Bruce, W. K. and McColloch, E. A.,** The effet of erythropoietic stimulation on the hemopoietic colony-forming cells of mice, *Blood*, 23, 216, 1964.
177. **Fried, W., Martinson, D., Weisman, M., et al.,** Effect of hypoxia on colony forming units, *Exp. Hematol.*, 10, 22, 1966.
178. **Schooley, J. C.,** The effect of erythropoietin on the growth and development of spleen colony-forming cells, *J. Cell. Physiol.*, 68, 249, 1966.
179. **Till, J. E., Siminovich, L., and McCulloch, E. A.,** The effect of plethora on growth and differentiation of normal hemopoietic colony forming cells transplanted in mice of genotype W/W^v, *Blood*, 29, 102, 1967.
180. **Marks, P. A., Cantor, L., Cooper, M., et al.,** *Control of Proliferation of Cells*, Vol. 1, Clarkson, Baserea Eds., Cold Spring Harbor Laboratory, New York, 1974, 853.
181. **Kork, A. P., Henkelman, R. M., O'Hensmeyer, F. P., and Till, J. E.,** Investigations of stochastic model of hemopoiesis, *Exp. Hematol.*, 1, 362, 1973.
182. **Till, J. E., McCulloch, E. A., and Siminovich, L.,** A stochastic model of stem cell proliferation based on the growth of spleen colony-forming cells, *Proc. Natl. Acad. Sci. U.S.A.*, 51, 29, 1964.
183. **Till, J. E., Price, G. B., Mak, T. W., and McCulloch, E. A.,** Regulation of blood cell differentiation, *Fed. Proc.*, 34, 2279, 1975.
184. **Trentin, J. J.,** Influence of hematopoietic organ stroma (hematopoietic inductive microenvironment) on stem cell differentiation, in *Regulation of Hematopoiesis*, Vol. 1, Gordon, A. S., Ed., Appleton-Century-Crofts, New York, 1970, 161.
185. **Trentin, J. J.,** Hemopoietic microenvironments transplant, *Transplant. Proc.*, 10, 77, 1978.
186. **Wolf, N. S.,** The hemopoietic microenvironment, *Clin. Haematol.*, 8, 469, 1979.
187. **Wolf, N. S. and Trentin, J. J.,** Hemopoietic colony studies. V. Effect of hemopoietic organ stroma on differentiation of pluripotent stem cells, *J. Exp. Med.*, 127, 205, 1968.
188. **Wolf, N. S. and Trentin, J. J.,** Linearity of counts of endogenous and exogenous colonies on mouse bone marrow, *Exp. Hematol.*, 3, 54, 1975.
189. **Nowell, P. C., Hersch, B. E., Fox, D. H., et al.,** Evidence for the existence of multipotential lympho-hematopoietic stem cells in the adult rat, *J. Cell. Physiol.*, 75, 151, 1970.
190. **Trentin, J. J.,** Determination of bone marrow stem cell differentiation by stromal hemopoietic inductive microenvironments (HIM), *Am. J. Pathol.*, 65, 621, 1971.
191. **Curry, J. L. and Trentin, J. J.,** Hemopoietic spleen colony studies. I. Growth and differentiation, *Dev. Biol.*, 15, 395, 1967.
192. **Curry, J. L., Trentin, J. J., and Wolf, N. J.,** Hemopoietic spleen colony studies. Erythropoiesis, *J. Exp. Med.*, 125, 703, 1967.
193. **Jenkins, V. K., Trentin, J. J., Speirs, R. S., et al.,** Hemopoietic colony studies. VI. Increased eosinophil containing colonies obtained by antigen pretreatment of irradiated mice reconstituted with bone marrow cells, *J. Cell. Physiol.*, 79, 413, 1972.
194. **McCulloch, E. A., Siminovich, L., Till, J. E., et al.,** The cellular basis of genetically determined hemopoietic defects in anemic mice sl/sl^d, *Blood*, 26, 399, 1968.
195. **Bernstein, S. E.,** Tissue transplantation as an analytic and therapeutic tool in hereditary anemias, *Am. J. Surg.*, 119, 448, 1970.
196. **Wolf, N. S.,** Dissecting the hemopoietic microenvironment. I. Stem cell lodgements and commitment and the proliferation and differentiation of erythropoietic descendents in sl/sl^d mice, *Cell Tissue Kinet.*, 7, 89, 1974.
197. **Wolf, N. S.,** Dissecting the hemopoietic microenvironment. II. The kinetics of the erythron of the sl/sl^d mouse and the dual nature of its anemia, *Cell Tissue Kinet.*, 11, 325, 1978.

198. **Wolf, N. S.,** Dissecting the hemopoietic microenvironment. III. Evidence for a positive short-range stimulus for cellular proliferation, *Cell Tissue Kinet.*, 11, 335, 1978.
199. **Kitamura, Y., Kawata, R., Suda, O., et al.,** Changed differentiation pattern of parental colony-forming cells in Fi hybrid mice suffering from graft versus host disease, *Transplantation*, 10, 455, 1970.
200. **Rauchwerger, J. M., Gallagher, M. T., and Trentin, J. J.,** Role of the hemopoietic inductive microenvironments (HIM) in xenogenetic bone marrow transplantation, *Transplantation*, 15, 610, 1973.
201. **Seki, M.,** Hemopoietic colony formation on a macrophage layer provided by intraperitoneal insertion of cellulose acetate membrane, *Transplantation*, 15, 544, 1973.
202. **Meck, R. A., Haley, H., and Brecher, G.,** Hematopoiesis versus osteogenesis in ectopic marrow implants, *Blood*, 42, 661, 1973.
203. **Twentyman, R. P.,** Effects of repeated doses of endotoxin on erythropoiesis in the normal and splenectomized mouse, *Br. J. Haematol.*, 22, 169, 1972.
204. **Quesenberry, P., Halperin, J., Ryan, M., et al.,** Tolerance to the granulocyte-releasing and colony-stimulating factor elevating effects of endotoxin, *Blood*, 45, 789, 1975.
205. **Quesenberry, P. J., Levin, J., Zuckerman, K. et al.,** Stem cell migration induced by erythropoietin or hemolytic anemia; the effect of actinomycin and endotoxin contamination of erythropoietin preparations, *Br. J. Haematol.*, 41, 253, 1979.
206. **Branemark, P. L., Breine, U., Johansson, B., et al.,** Regeneration of bone marrow, a clinical and experimental study following removal of bone marrow by curettage, *Acta Anat.*, 59, 1, 1964.
207. **Patt, H. M. and Maloney, M. A.,** Bone marrow regeneration after local injury: a review, *Exp. Hematol.*, 3, 135, 1975.
208. **Sick, H., Oberling, F., and Fricker, J. P.,** La regeneration de la vascularisation de la moelle osseuse du femur de lapin apres curettage, *Arch. Anat. Histol. Embryol. Norm. Exp.*, 57, 229, 1974.
209. **Brecher, G., Tijo, J. H., Smith, W. W., and Haley, J. E.,** Marrow regeneration after mechanical depletion, *Blood*, 48, 679, 1976.
210. **Patt, H. M. and Maloney, M. A.,** Regulation of stem cells after local bone marrow injury: the rise of an osseous environment, in *Stem Cells of Renewing Cell Population*, Cairnie, A. B., et al., Eds., Academic Press, New York, 1976, 239.
211. **Sahebekhtian, H. A. and Tavassoli, M.,** Studies on bone marrow histogenesis: morphometric and autoradiographic studies of regenerating marrow stroma in extramedullary autoimplants and after evacuation of marrow cavity, *Cell Tissue Res.*, 192, 437, 1978.
212. **Fridenstein, A. J. and Lalykina, K. S.,** Lymphoid cell populations are competent system for induced osteogenesis, *Calcif. Tissue Res.*, Suppl. 4, 105, 1970.
213. **Fridenstein, A. J., Deriglasova, U. V., Kulagina, N. N., et al.,** Precursors for fibroblasts in different populations of hemopoietic cells as detected by the in vitro colony assay method, *Exp. Hematol.* (Copenhagen), 2, 83, 1974.
214. **Fridenstein, A. J., Gorskaja, J. F., and Kulagina, N. N.,** Fibroblast precursors in normal and irradiated mouse hemopoietic organ, *Exp. Hematol.*, 4, 267, 1976.
215. **Casto-Malaspina, H., Gay, R. E., Resnick, G., et al.,** Characterization of human bone marrow fibroblasts colony-forming cells (CFU-F) and their progeny, *Blood*, 56, 289, 1980.
216. **de Bruyn, P. P. H., Michelsen, S., and Thomas, T. B.,** Migration of blood cells of the bone marrow through the sinusoidal wall, *J. Morphol.*, 133, 417, 1971.
217. **Campbell, F. R.,** Ultrastructural studies of the transmural migration of blood cells in the bone marrow of rats, mice and guinea pigs, *Am. J. Anat.*, 135, 521, 1972.
218. **Weiss, L.,** Transmural cellular passage in vascular sinuses of rat bone marrow, *Blood*, 36, 189, 1970.
219. **Muto, M.,** A scanning and transmission electron microscopic study on rat bone marrow sinuses and transmural migration of blood cells, *Arch. Histol. Jpn.*, 39, 51, 1976.
220. **Irino, S.,** Stereo microvascular architecture and transmural migration of blood cells in the bone marrow as revealed by scanning electron microscopy, *Acta Haematol. Jpn.*, 38, 647, 1975.
221. **Chamberlain, J. K., Leblond, P. F., and Weed, R. L.,** Reduction of adventitial cell cover: an early direct effect of erythropoietin on bone marrow ultrastructure, *Bone Cells*, 1, 655, 1975.
222. **Tavassoli, M.,** Adaptation of marrow sinus wall to fluctuation in the rate of cell delivery: studies in rabbits after blood letting, *Br. J. Haematol.*, 35, 25, 1977.
223. **Tavassoli, M.,** Annotation: the marrow blood barrier, *Br. J. Haematol.* 41, 297, 1979.
224. **Meuret, G. and Heibges, M.,** Neutrophil marrow egress in polycythemia vera, *Blut*, 34, 19, 1977.
225. **de Bruyn, P. P. H., Beker, R. P., and Michelson, S.,** The transmural migration and release of blood cells in acute myelogeneous leukemia, *Am. J. Anat.*, 149, 247, 1977.
226. **Mladenov, Z., Heine, U., Beard, D., and Beard, J. W.,** Strain MC29 avian leukosis virus, Myelocytoma, endothelioma and renal growths: pathomorphological and ultrastructural aspects, *J. Natl. Cancer Inst.*, 30, 251, 1967.

227. **Chen, L., Handler, E. E., Handler, E. S., and Weiss, L.,** An electron microscopic study of the bone marrow of the rat in an experimental myelogenous leukemia, *Blood*, 39, 99, 1972.
228. **Campbell, F.,** Ultrastructure of the sinus wall of murine bone marrow in myelogenous leukemia, *Am. J. Anat.*, 142, 319, 1975.
229. **Steiner, J. W.,** Investigations of allergic liver injury, *Am. J. Pathol.*, 38, 411, 1961.
230. **Rouiller, C. and Simon, G.,** Contribution de la microscope electronique au progres de nos connaissances en cytologie et an histopathologie hepatique, *Rev. Int. Hepatol.*, 12, 167, 1962.
231. **Miyai, K., Stusner, R. J., and Huebner, B. H.,** Viral hepatitis in mice: an electron microscopic study, *Exp. Mol. Pathol.*, 2, 464, 1963.
232. **Lindblad, G. and Bjorkman, Nils,** Ultrastructural alterations in sinusoidal endothelim of liver and bone marrow in dogs with experimental hepatitis contagiosa canis, *Acta Pathol. Microbiol. Scand.*, 62, 155, 1964.
233. **Giordano, G. F. and Lichtman, M. A.,** Marrow cell egress: the central interaction of barrier pore size and cell maturation, *J. Clin. Invest.*, 52, 1154, 1973.
234. **Lichtman, M. A.,** Cellular deformability during the maturation of the myeloblast possible role in marrow egress, *N. Engl. J. Med.*, 283, 943, 1970.
235. **Le Blond, P. F., La Celle, P. L., and Weed, R. I.,** Cellular deformability: a possible determinant of the release of maturing erythrocytes from the bone marrow, *Blood*, 27, 40, 1973.
236. **Lichtman, M. A. and Weed, R. I.,** Alterations of the cell periphery during granulocyte maturation. Relationship to cell function, *Blood*, 39, 310, 1972.
237. **Ackerman, G. A. and Waksal, S. D.,** Ultrastructural localization of concavalin A binding sites on the surface of differentiating hemopoietic cells, *Cell Tissue Res.*, 150, 331, 1974.
238. **Skutelsky, E. and Farquhar, M.,** Variations in distribution of con A receptor sites and anionic groups during red blood cell differentiation in the rat, *J. Cell Biol.*, 71, 218, 1976.
239. **Lichtman, M. A., Chamberlain, J. K., and Santillo, P. A.,** Factors thought to regulate the egress of marrow cells, in *The Year in Hematology 1978*, Gordon, A. S., Silber, R., and Lobue, J., Eds., Plenum Press, New York, 1978.
240. **Weiss, L. and Chen, L.,** The organization of the hematopoietic cords and vascular sinuses in the bone marrow, *Blood Cells*, 1, 617, 1975.
241. **Lichtman, M. A., Chamberlain, J. K., Simon, W., and Santillo, P. A.,** Parasinusoidal location of megakaryocytes in marrow: a determinant of platelet release, *Am. J. Hematol.*, 4, 303, 1975.
242. **Becker, R. P. and de Bruyn, P. P. H.,** The transmural passage of blood cells into myeloid sinusoids and the entry of platelets into the sinusoidal circulation: a scanning electron microscopic investigation, *Am. J. Anat.*, 145, 183, 1976.
243. **Chamberlain, J. K., Weiss, L., and Weed, R. L.,** Bone marrow sinus cell packing: a determinant of cell release, *Blood*, 46, 91, 1975.
244. **Tocantins, L. M. and O'Neill, J. F.,** Infusions of blood and other fluids into the general circulation via the bone marrow, *Surg. Gynecol. Obstet.*, 73, 281, 1941.
245. **Drinker, C. K. and Drinker, K. R.,** A method of an artificial circulation through the tibia of a dog with a demonstration of the vasomotor control of the marrow vessels, *Am. J. Physiol.*, 40, 514, 1916.
246. **Cummings, J. D.,** A study of the blood flow through the bone marrow by a method of venous effluent collection, *J. Physiol.*, 162, 13, 1962.
247. **Orr, J. W. and Strickland, L. H.,** The metabolism of bone marrow, *Biochem. J.*, 32, 567, 1938.
248. **Cummings, J. D. and Nutt, M. E.,** Bone marrow blood flow and cardiac output in rabbits, *J. Physiol.*, 162, 30, 1962.
249. **Nye, R. N.,** Bone marrow volume in rabbits, *Proc. Soc. Exp. Biol.*, 29, 34, 1931.
250. **Shaw, N. E.,** Observations on intramedullary blood flow and marrow pressure in bone, *Clin. Sci.*, 24, 311, 1963.
251. **Brown-Grant, K. and Cummings, J. D.,** A study of the capillary blood flow through the bone marrow by the radio-isotope technique, *J. Physiol.*, 162, 21, 1962.
252. **Najean, Y. and Clement, F.,** Etude de la circulation medullaire chez L'Homme par une technique isotopique, *Nouv. Rev. Fr. Hematol.*, 3, 133, 1963.
253. **Trubowitz, S., Strauss, H., and Small, M. J.,** Sternal marrow circulation by the radioisotope clearance technique, *J. Nucl. Med.*, 5, 864, 1964.
254. **Trubowitz, S., Strauss, H., and Small, M.,** Effect of X-rays on human sternal marrow circulation, *Radiology*, 88, 140, 1967.
255. **Van Dyke, D., Anger, H. O., Yano, Y., and Bozzini, C.,** Bone blood flow shown with 18-F and the positron camera, *Am. J. Physiol.*, 209, 65, 1965.
256. **Anger, H. O. and Van Dyke, D. C.,** Human bone marrow distribution shown in vivo by 52 Fe and positron scintillation camera, *Science*, 144, 1587, 1964.
257. **Van Dyke, D.,** Similarity in distribution of skeletal blood flow and erythropoietic marrow, *Clin. Orthop.*, 52, 37, 1967.

258. **Rohlich, K.,** On the relationship between bone substance and hemopoiesis in the bone marrow, *Z. Mikrosk. Anat. Forsch.*, 49, 425, 1941.
259. **Petrakis, N. L.,** Some physiological and development considerations of the temperature gradient hypothesis of bone marrow distribution, *Am. J. Phys. Anthropol.*, 25, 119, 1966.
260. **McCluskey, K. S., McClugage, S. G., Jr., and Younker, W. J.,** Microscopy of living bone marrow in situ, *Blood*, 38, 87, 1971.
261. **McClugage, S. G., Jr., McCluskey, R. S., and Meinecke, H. A.,** Microscopy of living bone marrow in situ. II. Influence of the microenvironment on hemopoiesis, *Blood*, 38, 96, 1971.
262. **Huggins, C., and Blocksom, B. H., Jr.,** Changes in outlying bone marrow accompanying a local increase of temperature within physiological limits, *J. Exp. Med.*, 64, 253, 1936.
263. **Van Dyke, D., Anger, H. O., Parker, H., et al.,** Markedly increased bone blood flow in myelofibrosis, *J. Nucl. Med.*, 12, 506, 1971.
264. **Van Dyke, D., Anger, H. O., Yano, Y., et al.,** Bone blood flow shown with F-18 and the positron camera, *Am. J. Physiol.*, 209, 65, 1965.
265. **Shim, S. S.,** Physiology of blood circulation of bone, *J. Bone Joint Surg.*, 50A, 812, 1968.
266. **Jones, H. B.,** cited in *Medical Physics,* Vol. 2, Glaser, O., Ed., Yearbook Publishers, Chicago, 1950, 860.
267. **Edwards, C. L., Andrews, E. A., Sitterson, B. W., and Knisely, B. M.,** Clinical bone marrow scanning with radioisotopes, *Blood,* 23, 741, 1964.
268. **Greenberg, M. L., Atkins, H. L., and Schiffer, L. M.,** Erythropoietic and reticulo-endothelial function of bone marrow in dogs, *Science,* 152, 526, 1966.
269. **Nelp, W. B., Larson, S. M., and Lewis, R. J.,** Distribution of the erythron and the RES in the bone marrow organ, *J. Nucl. Med.*, 8, 430, 1967.
270. **Van Dyke, D. Dobson, E. L., and Parker, H. I., et al.,** Radiopharmaceutical techniques for the study of bone and marrow blood flow, in *Radiopharmaceuticals,* Subramian, G., Rhores, B. A., and Cooper, J. F., et al., Eds., *Society of Nuclear Medicine,* New York, 1975, 329.
271. **Kane, W. J., and Grim, E.,** Blood flow to canine hind limb, bone, muscles, and skin: a quantitative method and its validation, *J. Bone Joint Surg.*, 51A, 309, 1960.
272. **Lunde, P. K., and Michelson, K.,** Determination of cortical blood flow in rabbit femur by radioactive microspheres, *Acta Physiol. Scand.*, 80, 39, 1970.
273. **Gros, M.,** Note sur les nerfs des os, *C.R. Acad. Sci.*, 23, 1100, 1846.
274. **Variot, G., and Remy, G.,** Sur les nerfs de la moelle des os, *J. Anat. Physiol.*, 6, 273, 1880.
275. **Ottolenghi, D.,** Sur les nerfs de la moelle des os, *Arch. Ital. Biol.*, 37, 73, 1902.
276. **Rossi, F.,** Linnervazione del midollo osseo, *Arch. Ital. Anat. Embriol.*, 29, 539, 1932.
277. **Foa, P. P.,** Studies on the innervation of the bone marrow. II. Physiology, *Univ. Hosp. Bull. Ann Arbor, Mich.*, 9, 19, 1943.
278. **Kuntz, A. and Richins, C. A.,** Innervation of the bone marrow, *J. Comp. Neurol.*, 83, 213, 1945.
279. **Calvo, W.,** The innervation of the bone marrow in laboratory animals, *Am. J. Anat.*, 123, 315, 1968.
280. **Calvo, W. and Forteza-Vila, J.,** Schwann cells of the bone marrow, *Blood*, 36, 180, 1970.
281. **Calvo, W. and Forteza-Vila, J.,** On the development of bone marrow innervation in new born rats as studied with silver impregnation and electron microscopy, *Am. J. Anat.*, 128, 355, 1969.
282. **Garcia, J. C. and Van Dyke, D. C.,** Response of rats of various ages to erythropoietin, *Proc. Soc. Exp. Biol. Med.*, 106, 585, 1961.
283. **Lucarelli, F., Porcellini, A., Carnevali, C., et al.,** Fetal and neonatal erythropoiesis, *Ann. N.Y. Acad. Sci.*, 149, 544, 1968.
284. **Di Pace, D. M., and Webber, R. H.,** Electrostimulation and morphologic study of the nerules of the bone marrow of the albino rat, *ACTH Anat.*, 93, 1, 1975.
285. **Byron, J. W.,** Evidence for a B-adrenergic receptor initiating DNA synthesis in haemopoietic stem cells, *Exp. Cell Res.*, 71, 228, 1972.
286. **Gauger, D., Kaiser, E., Quiring, K., and Palm, D.,** The B-adrenergic receptor-adenyl-cyclase system of rat reticulocytes effect of adrenergic stimulants and inhibitors, *Naunyn Schmiedeberg Arch. Pharmacol.*, 289, 379, 1975.
287. **Brown, E. M., Fedak, S. A., Woodward, C. J., et al.,** B-adrenergic receptor interactions. Direct comparison of receptor interactions and biological activity, *J. Biol. Chem.*, 251, 1239, 1976.
288. **Brown, J. E. and Adamson, J. W.,** Modulation of in vitro erythropoiesis. The influence of B-adrenergic agonists on erythroid colony formation, *J. Clin. Invest.*, 60, 70, 1977.
289. **Fink, G. D. and Fisher, J. W.,** Stimulation of erythropoiesis by Beta adrenergic agonists. I. Characterization of activity in polycythemic mice, *J. Pharmacol. Exp. Ther.*, 202, 192, 1977.
290. **Fink, G. D. and Fisher, J. W.,** Stimulation of erythropoiesis by Beta adrenergic agonists. I. Mechanisms of action, *J. Pharmacol. Exp. Ther.*, 202, 199, 1977.

Chapter 4

HEMATOPOIETIC STEM CELLS*

Hal E. Broxmeyer

TABLE OF CONTENTS

*Supported by Public Health service grant CA-23528 from the National Cancer Institute, grant CH-138 from the American Cancer Society, The Gar Reichman Foundation, and a Scholar award from the Leukemia Society of America.

I. INTRODUCTION AND DEFINITION OF STEM CELLS

The morphologically recognizable and functionally capable cells circulating in blood include erythrocytes, neutrophilic, eosinophilic, and basophilic granulocytes, B-, T-, non-B, non-T lymphocytes and platelets. These mature and in most cases end stage cells derive from and are replaced, on demand, by morphologically recognizable dividing precursor cells for the respective cell lineages. These are in turn derived from morphologically unidentifiable progenitor cells committed to differentiation within specific cell lineages. Maintaining this pool of lineage specific progenitor cells are hematopoietic pluripotential and totipotential stem cells. Among the aims of a recent workshop on experimental hematopoiesis was a clarification of concepts and definitions of terms used in the research of hematopoietic stem cells.[1]

The definitions of stem and progenitor cells are operational and depend on functional, rather than on morphological, criteria. Stem cells are defined as cells with extensive self-renewal or self-maintenance capacity. The necessity for self-renewal is apparent as an absence or depletion of these cells would result eventually, after continuous demand for functional end stage cells, in the complete depletion of one or more cell lineages, a catastrophic event which would lead within a short time to disease and death of the individual.

Some of these stem cells have the capacity to differentiate upon need, but other stem cells or their daughter cells must maintain this precious pool of cells. The pluripotential hematopoietic stem cell is capable of differentiating into several sublines of progenitor cells. The progenitor cells are members of a cell population with little or no self-renewal capacity which are capable of proliferating and differentiating into one (e.g., granulocytes) or more than one of the differentiation pathways (e.g., granulocytes and macrophages). The multitude of pathways open to the pool of progenitor cells is not as large as that which is available for the stem cells (e.g., granulocytes, macrophages, erythrocytes, platelets, and lymphocytes). The progenitor cell compartment feeds eventually into a more mature or unipotent progenitor cell compartment committed to one line of differentiation (e.g., granulocytes or macrophages) which then differentiates into a specific precursor cell compartment such as the myeloblast, promonocyte, and proerythroblast which have morphological and cytochemical features recognizable as belonging to the nonproliferating end stage cells (e.g., granulocytes, macrophages, or erythrocytes). Short term and rapid amplication of the absolute number of end stage cells can be achieved within the progenitor and precursor cell compartments, but continuous and long-term replenishment of cells requires movement from an intact and maintained pool of pluripotential or totipotential hematopoietic stem cells.

The concept of hematopoietic stem cells has been around for a long time, but it is only within the past 10 to 20 years that we have had at hand functional assays which allow detection of clonal expansion from a single cell that meets the criteria for a stem or progenitor cell. The assays for stem cells had been confined to studies on murine cells with analysis of stem cells of humans being indirect via analysis of progenitor cells. This situation is now changing as will be described below.

Phenotypic characterization of stem and progenitor cells have been attempted based on light and electron microscopic analysis.[2–4] These are described in the chapter on lymphopoiesis. However, under usual conditions, less than one cell in one thousand in bone marrow, and even fewer in spleen and peripheral blood, can be considered to fit into stem and progenitor cell categories based on a comparison with functional assays. The use of cell enrichment procedures has increased the percentage of such cells within a sample preparation of cells. The lack of complete purity of cell type, the heterogeneity of these cells with regards to density, size, and cycling characteristics, which would also result in morphological heterogeneity within subpopulations of these cells as they "mature" and move through these compartments, has not allowed a definitive description of these cells morphologically. While the presence of a definitive classification of stem and progenitor cells on morphological grounds might be of help to clinicians for diagnosis and prognosis of various hematological diseases it is probably not necessary and might in actuality be a hinderance to understanding the classification and characteristics of disease progression. In the first place the morphological characteristics of these cells might be modified during disease, but more importantly a knowledge of the unique characteristics of these cells which encompass self-renewal capacity and differentiation ability would not be distinguishable in a static light or electron microscopic picture. This situation might be considered analogous to the detection of molecules biochemically or immunologically which might not distinguish between the functionally active or inactive species of those molecules.

The advent of in vivo studies in intact mice and in vitro studies in cell cultures in combination with cell separation procedures and biochemical purification of cell-derived molecules has allowed for rapid advances and new leads into an understanding of the kinetics and regulation of blood cell formation.

This chapter will be devoted to hematopoietic pluripotential stem cells as defined above with information on progenitor, precursor, and mature cells discussed in other chapters within this book.

It is the aim of this chapter to focus mainly on the new and very exciting advances recently being made in the area of stem cell kinetics and its regulation during health and disease. An extensive literature exists on past studies of pluripotential stem cells for the granulocyte, erythroid, and megakaryocytic lines in cells of the murine system. This information, which has been reviewed already in an extensive manner by others,[5–7] will be mentioned briefly in order that the reader unfamiliar with this literature be informed enough to understand the more recent advances which have focused on the regulation of stem cell production, differentiation, and renewal capacity. It is hoped that the interested readers will avail themselves of the opportunity to refer to the cited references of the original communications since a review cannot hope to cover all the intricacies of the primary investigations.

II. FUNCTIONAL ASSAYS TO DETECT STEM CELLS IN ANIMALS

A. Production of Erythrocytes, Granulocytes, Monocytes-Macrophages, and Platelets from a Single Cell

There is now overwhelming evidence that cells of the erythrocytic, granulocytic, macrophagic, and megakaryocytic lineages are derived from a common ancestral cell. The original studies involved repopulation kinetics, then clonal assays in vivo, and more recently, clonal assays in vitro.

1. Repopulation Studies in Vivo

Studies of irradiation and its influences on the hematopoietic system began after World War II and the explosion of the atom bomb. The repopulating capacity of cells given to animals who had been given what should have been lethal dosages of irradiation were evaluated.[8–15] Using sensitivity to irradiation as an end point, a radiation survival curve was plotted and the D_o, or dose required to decrease the numer of viable cells to 37% of control values, was calculated as 105 ± 24 rad whether the cells were irradiated in vivo or in vitro.[14]

2. Exogenous Spleen Colony Assay in Vivo

It became apparent that nodules, containing hematopoietic cells, arose on the spleens of mice injected with bone marrow cells after dosages of lethal irradiation. There was a direct relationship between the number of cells inoculated into the mice and the number of nodules which formed suggesting that each nodule, containing thousands of cells, was derived from one injected bone marrow cell.[16] The cells giving rise to these nodules were termed colony forming units-spleen (CFU-S) and a measurement of the radiation sensitivity of these cells irradiated in vitro gave a D_o of 115 ± 8 which compared favorably with the previous studies on survival of mice.[14] A comparative survival curve for CFU-S was noted when those cells were irradiated in vivo and then injected into lethally irradiated mice.[17] The single cell derivation of these colonies (nodules) was substantiated by karyotypic analysis of unique radiation-induced chromosome markers of the injected bone marrow cells,[18] and the CFU-S were found to be relatively in a noncycling state within the mice.[19]

The transplanted CFU-S did not proliferate in the irradiated recipients during the first day, but then increased in number in an exponential manner for approximately the next 7 days with a doubling time of 20 to 25 hr.[20] During reseeding experiments, wherein cells from a spleen colony were inoculated into secondary recipient mice, it became apparent that not all of these cells seeded to the spleen. A seeding efficiency or f-factor was calculated and found to be 0.17 or 17% of the injected colony forming cells formed colonies on the spleen. The f-factor has been discussed[21] and various agents have been shown to influence the seeding efficiency of CFU-S.[22] A major factor determining the seeding and ultimate retention of CFU-S in the spleens of recipient mice was considered to be the size of the spleen.[23] In addition, CFU-S in cycle manifested a 50% decrease in seeding to the spleen when compared to normal bone marrow or to noncycling CFU-S separated by velocity sedimentation from cycling CFU-S. This led the authors to suggest that the spleen colony assay would underestimate the number of CFU-S in an inoculum by a factor which was related to the number of CFU-S in cycle.[24] CFU-S fulfilled the criteria for a hemopoietic stem cell as they demonstrated extensive self-renewal capacity[25] as well as capability of giving rise to many hematopoietic cell types. It has been demonstrated that CFU-S also seed to and form colonies in bone marrow, and that microscopic analysis of spleen and bone marrow is necessary to determine the actual number of colonies formed and the type of cells within the colony.[26]

A histological analysis of spleen colonies as reported in the literature has been summarized (see pages 77 and 78 of Reference 6). Few eosinophils are noted in spleen colonies, but antigenic stimulation of the recipient mice increased the number of eosinophil-containing colonies, presumably by affecting cells other than the CFU-S.[27] Overlap errors in the counting of spleen colonies have been discussed[28] as have the accuracy of counts.[29] Evidence for a pre-CFU-S cell surviving treatment in mice with 5-fluorouracil has also been given.[30] These cells give rise to colonies containing large numbers of CFU-S and appear as spleen colonies earlier than cells from mice not treated with the drug.

The question of whether any kind of treatment that causes depletion of CFU-S in the spleen of a host would provide an environment suitable for the production of colonies by transplanted CFU-S was investigated.[31] Allogeneic lymph node cells were used as a means to remove CFU-S,[32] and mixtures of lymph node and bone marrow cells from C57B1 mice were injected into F_1 hybrid mice that had not been treated previously. Hematopoietic colonies were detected in these mice, and the number increased linearly with increased number of bone marrow cells injected. CFU-S were shown to be of donor origin and erythroid colonies predominated over granulocytic colonies. In comparison to detection of spleen colonies in previously irradiated mice after 6 days, it took more than 16 days to detect spleen colonies in the nonirradiated recipients. Other studies[33] had suggested that permanent colonization by donor cells required not only triggering CFU-S into cycle but the emptying of ''niches'' normally occupied by endogenous CFU-S.

3. Endogenous Spleen Colony Assay in Vivo

When mice recovered sublethal dosages of irradiation spleen colonies could be detected.[34] The regrowth of these cells began almost immediately after irradiation in comparison to the 1- to 4-day delay in growth of transplanted CFU-S.[35,36] It was found that in contrast to transplantable CFU-S, which were mainly noncycling, endogenous CFU-S were in a more rapid proliferative state.[37] It was not clear if two different stem cell compartments were being manifested or if the endogenous CFU-S represented the cycling portion of the exogenous CFU-S compartment. Endogenous bone marrow colony forming cells have been detected also.[38]

4. Multipotential Cell Assay in Vitro

Semisolid culture medium systems which allow clonal growth are available and detect populations of progenitor cells committed to one (e.g., granulocytes) or two (e.g., granulocytes and macrophages) lines of differentiation.[39,40] Progenitor cells are recognized by the formation of colonies containing the progeny of the progenitor cells. The progenitor cell assays for granulocytes and macrophages are discussed in detail in the chapter on granulopoiesis. It is only recently that in vitro assays have become available for cells demonstrating multipotentialities.[41–43] This includes cells with capacity for generating erythrocytes and megakaryocytes,[41] erthyrocytes, megakaryocytes and macrophages,[42] and erythrocytes, neutrophilic and eosinophilic granulocytes, macrophages, and megakaryocytes.[43] The latter[43] were first seen when fetal liver cells from CBA mice gave rise to these mixed colonies after stimulation with culture medium conditioned by pokeweed mitogen stimulated mouse spleen cells. Erythroid colonies were detected but perhaps more importantly one third to one half of these erythroid colonies contained in addition neutrophils, macrophages, and, to a lesser extent, megakaryocytes and/or eosinophils. Interestingly, the spleen cell conditioned medium failed to demonstrate the presence of erythropoietin, a presumed humoral regulator of erythropoiesis, when assayed in polycythemic mice.

Single cell cloning studies were performed to eliminate the possibility that the observed erythroid colony formation resulted from the production of erythropoietin by other fetal liver cells in the culture dish since fetal mouse liver cells have been shown to produce erythropoietin.[44] The influence of trace amounts of erythropoietin in the serum in the culture system could not be ruled out and definitive evidence for the influence of erythropoietin in this assay will probably have to await the use of serum-free culture medium. The single cell cloning experiments were also necessary in order to demonstrate that these colonies containing mixtures of hematopoietic cells were derived from single cells. The numbers of these erythroid colony forming cells declined with advancing fetal age, being highest in day 11 and 12 fetal livers, with low numbers detected in adult bone marrow. It was suggested that these colony forming cells might be members of the multipotential stem cell compartment in hemopoietic tissues.[43]

Peripheral blood and all hematopoietic organs, except the thymus, contained cells capable of forming these erythroid colonies during fetal development, but in the immediate postnatal period the bone marrow was the only organ containing these cells.[45] CBA fetal livers demonstrated the highest frequency of cells forming these mixed colonies of the various mouse strains assayed.

Cells giving rise to mixed-erythroid colonies were characterized by various parameters.[45] The fetal peripheral blood cells had a buoyant density of 1.056 to 1.069 g/cm^3 with a peak buoyant density of 1.058 to 1.060 g/cm^3 noted for the 12-day-old CBA fetal liver cells. The erythroid colony forming cells from 12-day-old fetal liver sedimented at 6 to 9 mm/hr as a broad single peak whereas older day 18 fetal liver colony forming cells sedimented at 3 to 9 mm/hr with peaks at 5 to 7 mm/hr. The colony forming cells appeared to be nonadherent, nonphagocytic and were radiosensitive with a D_0 of approximately 110 rad. The use of high specific activity tritiated thymidine or hydroxyurea killed more than 50% of the colony forming cells demonstrating that this was relatively a quickly cycling population of cells.

The cells within the mixed-erythroid colonies which derived from the colony forming cells were also analyzed.[46] The wide range of hematopoietic cells present within a single colony was confirmed by electron microscopy. Cells at all stages of morphologically recognizable maturity were seen within the colonies but the majority of the cells had features of incomplete differentiation. Lymphocytes and plasma cells have not been detected in these colonies.

In order to analyze the self-renewal capacity of the original colony forming cells, individual colonies derived from 12 day CBA fetal liver cells in vitro were transferred to other medium, the cells dispersed, and then recultured using spleen conditioned medium as the necessary stimulus for colony formation.[46] The reseeded culture plates were then analyzed for the occurrence of secondary colonies. Approximately one colony forming cell was found per 1000 colony cells; the size of the recloned colonies was small. Some contained up to 1500 cells, but the majority contained fewer than 200 cells which contrasted with the size of up to 10,000 cells from the original donor colonies. The majority of recloned colonies contained neutrophils but in 8 of the 76 secondary colonies other cell types were detected. This was in contrast to recloning from colonies derived from granulocyte-macrophage progenitor cells which gave mainly small colonies of macrophages. B-lymphocyte colonies were not detected on recloning from the mixed-erythroid colonies. When cells from the mixed-erythroid colonies were assessed for their capacity to form spleen colony forming cells (CFU-S) there were 0.76 spleen colony forming cells per in vitro colony, as calculated from an assumed seeding efficiency of 0.2.[46] The spleen colonies were mainly erythroid. Karyotypic analysis using the T6T6 marker chromosome demonstrated that five of nine colonies contained karyotypes of the donor-injected cells. These data allowed the suggestion that at least some of the cells forming mixed colonies in agar culture could be categorized as hematopoietic stem cells.

It was originally determined that approximately 70 mixed-erythroid colony forming cells were present per 10^5 12-day fetal liver cells but only two to three of these colony forming cells were detected per 10^5 adult marrow cells.[46] Modifications in culture conditions increased the apparent cloning efficiency of these cells in adult marrow, thus allowing characterization of the adult cells and comparison with the fetal cells.[47] Optimal adult colony numbers were noticed when cultures contained 20% fetal calf serum, in comparison to human serum used for fetal cells, and spleen cell conditioned medium which had been concentrated. The highest frequency of mixed-erythroid colonies was found in cultures of CBA and DBA adult mouse bone marrow cells (20 to $25/10^5$ cells) with lower numbers detected in other mouse strains. Added erythropoietin did not change the number of colonies or the degree of hemoglobinization of the cells within the colonies. In the CBA adult mice, the erythroid colony forming cells were only reduced by 12.5% after incubation of the cells with hydroxyurea or high specific activity tritiated thymidine, suggesting a slowly cycling population of cells. The erythroid colony forming cells sedimentated with a peak rate of 4.5 mm/hr compared to CFU-S which sedimented at 4.25 mm/hr. A correlation coeficient of $r = 0.93$ was assessed for the number of erythroid colony forming cells and CFU-S in 90 individual spleen colonies, suggesting a close relationship between the two cell types. The various characteristics of these cells indicated that the erythroid colony forming cells expressing multiple hematopoietic differentiation steps were members of the hematopoietic multipotential stem cell compartment.[47]

Characterization of the cells involved in the production of the stimulatory activity for mixed-erythroid colony formation suggested that the cells producing the activity might be T lymphocytes, but collaborative interactions between adherent (possibly macrophage) cells were necessary.[48] The factor producing cells were restricted to lymphoid organs, were radiosensitive ($D_0 = 154 \pm 32$ rad), slowly sedimenting cells (3.5 to 5.0 mm/hr), and of low density (density, <1.075 g/cm^3).

As will be described in the chapter on granulopoiesis, triggering and maintenance of the proliferation and differentiation of granulocyte-macrophage progenitor cells requires the continued presence of granulocyte-macrophage colony stimulatory factors (GM-CSF).[39,40] Interestingly, purified GM-CSF was able to support, at least temporarily, the survival and/or initial proliferation of at least some of the cells forming the mixed-erythroid colonies, but was unable to stimulate the formation of these colonies.[49] When purified GM-CSF from mouse lung conditioned medium was used as an initial stimulus during the first 2 days of culture of mouse fetal liver cells and then spleen cell conditioned medium added, up to 50% of the mixed-erythroid colonies in cultures stimulated at the beginning of culture by the spleen cell conditioned medium were detected.[50] No erythroid colonies were detected if the cultures were started with erythropoietin or saline. The GM-CSF responsive cells could not be discriminated from the total number of mixed erythroid colony forming cells on the basis of cell cycle analysis or after separation of the cells by velocity sedimentation.[50] The concentration of GM-CSF necessary to permit the proliferation of mixed-erythroid colony forming cells was two to fivefold higher than that required for stimulation of granulocyte-macrophage progenitor cells. Cell transfer experiments demonstrated that GM-CSF stimulated the proliferation rather than only the survival of these cells and that the action of GM-CSF was directly on the colony forming cell itself rather than via an indirect action on other cells within the culture. GM-CSF itself could not support the continued proliferation and maturation of mixed-erythroid colonies.

The availability of a multipotential and probably stem cell assay in vitro in terms of a clonal assay now makes feasible experiments designed to understand the regulation of this cell compartment during health and disease in a way which was not possible before.

B. Production of Erythrocytes, Granulocytes, Monocytes, Megakaryocytes, and Lymphocytes from a Single Cell

The existence of one cell capable of giving rise, under the appropriate conditions, to cells which could repopulate the myeloid and lymphoid lineages has been suggested by numerous works.[51,52] The same radiation-induced chromosome markers were detected in lymphoid organs and bone marrow after the spontaneous recovery of some mice from sublethal dosages of whole-body irradiation.[53] Also, repopulation of functional myeloid and lymphoid cells in irradiated mice was possible with bone marrow cells from adult mice,[54] and cells derived from some individual spleen colonies, which were themselves presumably derived from a single cell, could repopulate irradiated mice with cells of the myeloid and lymphoid systems.[55,56] Cells with similar radiation-induced chromosomal markers were found in both spleen colonies and in the thymus.[57] Moreover, it was noted that in bone marrow from repopulated lethally irradiated mice, chromosome markers allowed detection of similarly marked cells in the spleen colonies containing erythroid cells and in blood lymphocytes triggered to proliferate in both a mixed leukocyte reaction and in response to several different histocompatibility isoantigens.[58] Cells which bound sheep red blood cells and formed rosettes were found also to contain the same chromosome marker as cells repopulating the myeloid system.[59]

These latter studies[59] were accomplished by inducing unique chromosome markers in individual bone marrow stem cells and injecting these cells into mice of the genetically anemic w/w^v mouse strain. The mice whose hematopoietic systems were repopulated were immunized with sheep red blood cells and spleen cell suspensions made at the peak of the secondary immune response. The rosette forming cells were purified by velocity sedimentation and included apparently all the antibody-producing cells, demonstrating by functional analysis that these purified cells, which had the same karyotypic marker as myeloid cells, were antibody producing cells.

Evidence for a totipotent stem cell giving rise to lymphoid and myeloid cells as well as for a pluripotential stem cell, giving rise to myeloid cells or a cell restricted to a subset of lymphocytes was given based on an elegant series of experiments.[60] Radiation-induced chromosomal marked stem cells were injected in limiting dilutions into the stem-cell deficient strain of mice, w/w^v. From 3 to 11 months after bone marrow inoculation, the bone marrow, spleen, and thymus cells were examined, and in some cases bone marrow cells from the primary recipients injected into secondary recipients in order to determine if the marker could be detected on CFU-S and if the tissue distribution of marked cells could be propagated. Three patterns of stem cell regeneration were found. One included the observation of a unique chromosome marker in CFU-S and in PHA- and LPS-stimulated cultures suggesting a totipotent cell for the myeloid and lymphocyte series. Another included the observation of more restricted stem cells for myeloid but not B and T lymphocytes or for T cells only. Each of these patterns of toti- or restricted-stem cells remained consistent when the cells were injected into the secondary recipient. In another set of experiments,[61] cells with some properties of stem cells were removed from a continuous marrow culture system, described in Section V of this chapter, and found mainly to repopulate the lymphoid system. It was suggested that the bone marrow might contain lymphoid-restricted stem cells which might be able to maintain a selective advantage in vitro over totipotent and myeloid-restricted stem cells.[61] It was emphasized, however, that there was no definitive proof given that these lymphoid precursors were actually stem cells, but if it proved to be a stem cell it would be the first designation of a lymphoid stem cell restricted to B and T cells.[61]

Evidence for repopulation of mice with restricted lymphoid cells which are not necessarily very closely related to the stem cell described[61] have been given by others.[62–64] Bone marrow cells, depleted of T cells, were capable of repopulating the spleens of irradiated mice with T cells.[62] The progenitors of T cells were different from T cells in that they were not able to respond to alloantigenic stimulation, were resistant to treatment with antibody to theta-antigen, and banded in a lower density region than T cells after separation of the cells by equilibrium density-gradient centrifugation. Moreover, the profile of the progenitor T cells was different from the myeloid restricted stem cells (CFU–S) in that they banded in a heavier density region of the gradient than CFU-S.

In addition, in an interesting set of experiments, evidence was presented that a committed progenitor pool for B lymphocytes existed which formed early in embryonic development and constituted the major pool of cells for the generation of lymphocytes.[63,64] B-lymphocyte precursor cells in mice were noted which did not seem to be closely related to CFU-S.[63] CBA/H-T6T6 cells were injected into unirradiated CBA/N mice taking advantage of the finding that CBA/N mice don't have B lymphocyte colony forming cells, but have a microenvironment which will support the differentiation of B cells from precursors of normal CBA/H-T6T6 mice.[65,66] The cells generating B lymphocytes during the first 6 weeks after transplantation, and perhaps afterwards, sedimented at 4.5 to 6.0 mm/hr, lacked surface immunoglobulin, and were found in adult bone marrow and in liver from fetal mice from day 12 onwards. The pre-B cells were notably different from CFU-S as they were not found in yolk sac, were not correlated with numbers of CFU-S or repopulating capacity of CFU-S, and were inhibited from reconstituting the B cell lineage after treatment with a monoclonal antibody which did not recognize CFU-S.

III. CHARACTERISTICS AND ISOLATION OF STEM CELLS

There is little definitive evidence for the morphological characteristics of the pluripotential hematopoietic stem cell (see Section I of this chapter). However, various physical, immunological, and pharmacological criteria have elucidated some of the phenotypic characteristics of this population of cells and have allowed their isolation and separation from other hematopoietic cells. These procedures have also elucidated subpopulations of stem cell. It is emphasized that the stem cells discussed in this section do not include those considered to give rise to lymphocytes also.

A. Physical Methods

Mouse bone marrow cells were separated on the basis by cell density by equilibrium density gradient centrifugation with bovine serum albumin or on the basis of size by velocity sedimentation through a gradient of fetal calf serum at unit gravity.[67] The CFU-S had a peak sedimentation range of 1.071 to 1.078 g/cm^3, but were in most cases separable from the granulocyte macrophage progenitor cells which formed colonies in semisolid medium in the presence of medium conditioned by mouse L cells and which had a heavier density distribution. As will be seen in the chapter on granulopoiesis, the subpopulation of granulocyte-macrophage progenitor cells which will proliferate and differentiate depends on the specific stimulus applied.

Separation of some stem cells from progenitor cells was also accomplished by size as many of the CFU-S had a slower sedimentation rate with a peak range of 4.0 mm/hr as compared to the granulocyte-macrophage progenitor cells. Separation of these two cell populations has also been noted by others[68,69] using density separation. Separation of CFU-S by velocity sedimentation also revealed heterogeneity in capacity for self-renewal, a methodology requiring a double transplant.[70] Cell suspensions prepared from single spleen colonies were assayed for their content of CFU-S by inoculation into a secondary irradiated recipient. A trend was detected that demonstrated that slowly sedimenting or smaller cells had a greater capacity for self-renewal than the larger and more quickly sedimenting cells. The number of CFU-S per colony were 14.4 $\pm$ 1.4, 23.2 $\pm$ 2.2, 24.6 $\pm$ 2.0, 18.9 $\pm$ 4.0, 0.5 $\pm$ 0.5, 3.4 $\pm$ 0.8, and 1.6 $\pm$ 0.6 for the following respective sedimentation rates (in millimeters per hour) = 2.0, 2.4, 2.7, 3.0, 6.2, 6.9, and 7.7 to 8.4.

Other evidence for the inherent capacity of individual CFU-S to self-renew differently has been presented.[71] Bone marrow cells in mitosis were eliminated by 1 mg vinblastine per mouse. The surviving 5 to 10% of CFU-S were slowly or noncycling cells which produced colonies with a greater portion of CFU-S per spleen. The self-replication capacity of CFU-S separated by density was assessed in normal marrow and marrows from mice pretreated with vinblastine.[71] Density separation did not demonstrate populations of CFU-S differing in self-renewal capacity in normal marrow; however, separation of CFU-S from marrows of mice pretreated with vinblastine demonstrated a greater self-renewal capacity in the lower density CFU-S. It was suggested that the low density slowly or noncycling CFU-S were similar to those reported by others.[4] It was also suggested[71] that the ability to exhibit extensive self-renewal capacity may be related to the stage of cycle of the CFU-S at the moment of localization in the spleen and that such capacity may be transitory.

Separation of proliferating from nonproliferating CFU-S of mouse bone marrow was accomplished using a single injection of hydroxyurea which stimulated recruitment of a large fraction of slowly or noncycling CFU-S into cycle.[72] This population of cells, which then contained rapidly and noncycling mixtures of cells, was separated by velocity sedimentation into those sedimenting at 4.2 mm/hr which appeared to be the noncycling population and those sedimenting at 4.3 to 5.0 mm/hr which were apparently the more rapidly cycling cells.

Further evidence for separation of cycling and slowly- or noncycling CFU-S was provided by studies in which cells from normal and regenerating marrow were separated by velocity and subsequently subjected to treatment with high specific activity tritiated thymidine which is only picked up by cells in S-phase and which will sterilize these cells so that they cannot proliferate.[73] The majority of CFU-S from the marrows of untreated mice sedimented at 4.0 mm/hr with CFU-S noted to 7.5 mm/hr. Exposure of these separated cells to tritiated thymidine killed the more rapidly sedimenting cells which were in cycle but did not affect the majority of cells which sedimented at 4.0 mm/hr. CFU-S from marrows of mice recovering from radiation damage had a faster sedimentation rate than those from marrows of untreated mice and these cells were shown to be in cell cycle. Using separation of CFU-S by density gradient separation, it was noted that the resting (slowing cycling) and cycling stem cells had model densities, respectively, of 1.070 and 1.075 g/cm^3. The noncycling CFU-S were considered to be homogeneous population of cells with a diameter of 7.0 $\pm$ 0.4 μm while the subpopulation of cycling CFU-S varied from 7.3 $\pm$ 0.4 to 9.2 $\pm$ 0.5 μm depending on the phase of the cell cycle.

Heterogeneity in content of CFU-S of spleen colonies was seen also from yolk sac and early fetal liver.[74] These CFU-S were in rapid cycle, were a relatively homogeneous population of low density cells, and high self-renewal capacity of the embryonic CFU-S could not be correlated with the small size and slowly or noncycling state of adult CFU-S having a similar capacity for self-replication. At the earliest stage of liver hematopoiesis (10½ days gestation), the CFU-S were found in a marrow density region of 1.057 to 1.059 g/cm^3.[75] As the age of the liver increased, CFU-S with higher densities were seen, and by day 18 gestation the CFU-S had a density profile overlapping that found with adult bone marrow. Using a two dimensional separation procedure[73] it was found that adult marrow CFU-S of a density of 1.0565 to 1.0585 g/cm^3 had a major population of volume 260 mμ^3 and a minor population of 430 mμ^3 whereas fetal liver CFU-S of similar density revealed major populations of 820 and 1000 mμ^3 demonstrating that embryonic CFU-S were probably larger than the equivalent adult CFU-S.

Separation of CFU-S and their apparent heterogeneity has also entailed combinations of techniques including buoyant density gradients and adherence[76] and velocity sedimentation in an isokinetic gradient of Ficoll.[77] It has been noted that the modal sedimentation velocity of erythropoietin sensitive cells (6.5 to 7.7 mm/hr) assessed by the response of heme synthesis of mouse fetal liver cells to erythropoietin in vitro, was greater than CFU-S from mouse fetal liver (4.9 to 6.3 mm/hr).[78] Mouse spleen cells have been separated by a discontinuous gradient of dextran into fractions containing CFU-S with repopulating capacity which were at least partially separable from heavier fractions containing immunocompetent cells capable of mounting a graft vs. host reaction.[79]

A combination of procedures has been used to enrich for mouse CFU-S.[80] A three-step procedure was used. Bone marrow cells were first freed of erythroid cells and lymphocytes by culturing the cells for several weeks. Macrophages and adherent mature granulocytes were then removed by adherence to plastic. Most of the PMN and more immature granulocytes were removed by neutral density centrifugation or by differential centrifugation after rosette formation with sheep erythrocytes coated with immunoglobulin (EA-rosettes). This population of cells included 1 to 3% CFU-S which was based on a seeding efficiency of 0.06.

Light scattering properties have also been used to enrich and study the CFU-S compartment.[81,82] The light-scattering properties of CFU-S were examined in a fluorescence-activated cell sorter (FACS) II (Bectin and Dickinson, Sunnyvale, Calif.). Forward light scatter (FLS) intensity as measured in this instrument with a fully opened diameter gave a measure of cell size, and perpendicular light scatter (PLS) intensity gave a measure of the degree of folding of the cell and nuclear membrane and/or the presence of inclusions in the cytoplasm. It was considered that the characteristics of CFU-S most closely paralled that of large lymphocytes. When the forward and perpendicular light scatter signals of CFU-S were compared to those of cells with a known morphology, the CFU-S had a low perpendicular scatter which suggested a spherical shape and few cytoplasmic inclusions. The CFU-S appeared to measure 7.2 μm in diameter which agreed with calculations based on separation of CFU-S by density gradient and velocity sedimentation analysis. The recovery of CFU-S was in the order of 70 to 90% and a fivefold increase in CFU-S concentration was obtained although no mention was made of correcting for seeding efficiency.

B. Immunological Methods

Extensive work on the differentiation of the lymphoid cell series has established the acquisition of selected functional abilities of morphologically nondistinguishable cells with distinct phenotypes.[83,84] It has been mentioned that because of the limited evidence for specific markers on stem cells that they were considered to be "null" cells.[85] It was suggested that "a characteristic of stem cells may be the presence of a multiplicity rather than a paucity of markers".[85] It is highly likely that stem cells will be shown to contain specific surface markers or at least differing levels of antigenic determinants than on other more mature cells of the potential lineages. Some work has already been done suggesting the presence of antigens on stem cells, and this area will no doubt flourish with the recent advent of the production of monoclonal antibodies using the hybridoma technology[86–88] in combination with the technique of fluorescence activated cell sorting utilizing the monoclonal antibodies.

An antigen shared with CFU-S was found in mouse brain and an antiserum made against the antigen.[89] The brain-associated stem cell specificity was different from brain-associated theta[90] and brain-associated erythroid cells.[91] This antigen was not found on granulocyte-macrophage progenitor cells[92,93] or on late erythroid progenitor cells.[94] A rabbit antimouse brain sera not only impaired the capacity of marrow cells treated with it in the presence of complement to repopulate the marrow and spleen with CFU-S, but also impaired restoration of erythrocytes, survival, and in addition, reduced the number of macroscopic spleen colonies to the same extent as the number of macroscopic colonies.[95] However, one problem with treating cells with an antiserum and complement and looking for inhibition of colony formation as an end result is that it might be an accessory or helper cell, rather than the colony forming cell, which is killed. Several lines of evidence suggest that this might in some cases be the case with the rabbit antimouse brain sera. In mice pretreated with potassium carrageenan 1 day before lethal irradiation, the number of colonies resulting from the antibody plus complement-treated cells increased from 8 to 65% of control.[96] Moreover, pretreating mice with poly-2-vinylpyridine-*N*-oxide, a macrophage-stabilizing agent, prior to treatment with carrageenan, decreased the number of colonies rescued by carrageenan by approximately 33%, which supported the hypothesis that it was the effect of carrageenan on macrophages that effected the rescue. The suppression of CFU-S activity after incubation with rabbit-antimouse brain sera could be reversed by incubating the antibody coated cells with papain.[97] The authors suggested that if the effect of the antisera of CFU-S was caused by a cytotoxic antibody, papain should not have been able to rescue the CFU-S after treatment with complement and that the anti CFU-S activity might have been caused by noncytotoxic antibodies.[97] However, changes in an accessory cell pool could also have been considered. Other evidence for an action on an accessory cell was presented when injection of thymus cells simultaneously with or within 1 day of the injection of mouse bone marrow cells previously treated with a rabbit antimouse brain sera plus complement restored spleen colony formation to control values, but this effect appeared to involve only a subpopulation of CFU-S.[98]

Significant positive enrichment for stem cells has been accomplished using fluorescence-activated cell sorting with rabbit antihuman brain sera,[99] and it may be that only a subpopulation of CFU-S is recognized by the rabbit antihuman or antimouse brain sera. It has been suggested that there are differences in the expression of rabbit antimouse brain determinants between circulating CFU-S with different capacities for self-renewal.[100]

Using inhibition of spleen colony formation as an end result, it has been shown that CFU-S may express $H\text{-}2^K$ and $H\text{-}2^D$ antigens but lack Thy 1 antigens.[101] In this case, however, the results may actually suggest that these antigenic determinants are on CFU-S since the fluorescence distribution of CFU-S after labeling with anti H-2 and anti Thy-1 sera demonstrated that CFU-S were very high in H-2 density, but did not contain detectable amounts of Thy-1.[81]

Use of complement dependent cytotoxicity testing and fluorescence-activated cell sorting has failed to detect Ia antigens on CFU-S.[102–104] Moreover, Ia antigens appear to be absent on mouse progenitor cells for the granulocyte-macrophage lineage.[103] This is interesting and suggests species differences, since while Ia antigenic determinants are apparently absent on probable human pluripotential stem cells, they are present on human progenitor cells for the granulocyte-macrophage and erythroid lineages.[105] This maturation sequence of human stem and progenitor cells will be discussed in the chapter on granulopoiesis. Use of a fluorescence activated cell sorter has also implicated the presence of determinants recognizing a human antihuman system and mouse antimouse F9 sera (which recognizes embryonic determinants).[104]

A series of serologically defined cell-surface antigens termed Qa are encoded by genes in the Tla region which is distal to the H-2D end of the major histocompatibility complex of the mouse. The use of complement dependent cytoxicity assays have shown Qa antigens to be potential antigens on subpopulations of CFU-S; Qa negative CFU-S were also seen.[106]

Surface antigens on CFU-S which show cross-reactivity with antisera against differentiated hemopoietic cell surfaces have been described.[107,108] Antisera against CBA mouse lymph node lymphocytes, thymocytes, peritoneal macrophages, and platelets cross-reacted with CFU-S as determined by inhibition of spleen colonies in lethally irradiated mice. Antisera against erythrocytes showed little cross-reactivity. Exogenous complement treatment of bone marrow cells previously incubated with the antisera had no influence on the assay, and the means of inhibition was not known but did not appear to be due to masking cell surface components which might have prevented the seeding of CFU-S to the spleen. Absorption of the antisera with hemopoietic cells other than those used to prepare the antisera or in most cases with nonhematopoietic tissues such as brain, liver, kidney, or testis has little or no influence on the antistem cell activity, and the antibodies did not appear to be recognizing histocompatibility antigens. It was suggested that nucleated hematopoietic cells and platelets retained cell line specific antigens in common with CFU-S, and that the continued expression of these antigens during maturation might be involved in the differentiation process.[107] This class of antigens appeared to be distinct from those such as Ia, Fc receptors, Thy-1, and immunoglobulin.[108]

While Thy-1 antigens are not expressed on mouse CFU-S, there is now evidence that Thy-1 antigens are expressed on rat CFU-S.[109] CFU-S from fetal liver, neonatal spleen, and adult bone marrow of rats did not form spleen colonies in lethally irradiated rats when these cells were pretreated with antibodies to Thy-1 antigen (heteroantisera and alloantisera). The inhibitory effect of the antibodies was absorbed out with purified Thy-1 antigen. Additionally, all hemopoietic stem cell activity was recovered after fluorescence activated cell sorting in the Thy-1-positive population of cells. By double immunofluorescence, co-capping, and differential absorbtion studies it was also shown that Thy-1 and rat bone marrow lymphocyte antigen, which has anti-stem cell activity, were parts of the same molecule. The use of anti Thy-1, fluorescence-activated cell sorting, and cortisone pretreatment allowed a 320-fold enrichment of rat CFU-S.[110] This enrichment was possible since the CFU-S were strongly positive for Thy-1 antigen, had light-scattering properties between those of bone marrow lymphocytes and granulocyte-macrophage progenitor cells, and were relatively resistant to cortisone. It was estimated that CFU-S might constitute 80% of the cells in the CFU-S rich fraction. Moreover, two populations of accessory cells were distinguished: putative helper cells which were strongly Thy-1 positive and cortisone sensitive and putative suppressor cells which were weakly Thy-1 positive and cortisone resistant.

The use of selective agglutination by lectins has been used also to isolate CFU-S.[111,112] Sequential fractionation of spleen cells from SWR mice by soybean agglutinin and peanut agglutinin, or single fractionation by soybean agglutinin of spleen cells from Balb/c mice gave rise to a fraction of cells that reconstituted lethally irradiated (Balb/c $\times$ C57B1/6)F_1 mice, and no complications due to graft-vs.-host reaction were apparent.[111] Further studies[112] demonstrated that the stem cell rich fraction contained 1% contaminating T cells in the singularly agglutinated soybean agglutinin fraction. This could be removed by a second agglutination step suggesting that a minor population of T cells didn't bear receptors for soybean agglutinin. It was found that the twice agglutinated fractions, with soybean and peanut agglutinin or soybean agglutinin alone, contained prothymocytes,[112] but these fractions did not produce delayed graft vs. host disease when transplanted into allogeneic recipients.[111]

C. Pharmacological Methods

On the basis of pretreatment studies of bone marrow cells in vitro or in vivo, at least four mechanisms in the initiation of the cycling of previously noncycling CFU-S have been elucidated. These include β-adrenergic receptor stimulation, cholingeric-receptor stimulation, histamine-receptor stimulation, and stimulation by steroids.[113–119] These studies suggested the appropriate receptors for these agents on CFU-S.

Increased sensitivity of CFU-S to the killing action of high specific activity tritiated thymidine was noted 6 hr after a single subcutaneous injection of testosterone.[115] Moreover, by 1 hr after exposure in vitro to 2 to 4 $\times$ 10^{-8} *M* testosterone, CFU-S became more sensitive to the tritiated thymidine kill as well as to the cytotoxic action of another S-phase drug, 10^{-3} *M* hydroxyurea.[116] Dibutyryl cyclic AMP, but not 5′-AMP, also placed the CFU-S into cycle suggesting that the adenyl cyclase system played a role in the regulation of the proliferation of CFU-S.[117] Isoproterenol, a stimulator of β-adrenergic receptors, was similarly active, but initiation of CFU-S cycling by this drug could be abrogated by the antagonistic action of 10^{-6} *M* propanolol, a specific blocker of β-adrenergic receptors.[118] Most interesting is that the near maximal effect seen with 10^{-14} *M* isoproterenol represents only one to two molecules per cell. Since much higher concentrations of two agents that act primarily on β_2-adrenergic receptors (salbutamol and orciprenaline) were required to increase the cycling of CFU-S, it was suggested that the active site for isoproterenol might be a β_1-adrenergic receptor.[118] The β-adrenergic receptor is closely associated with the adenyl cyclase system. Cholinergic mechanisms have also been involved.[119] Carbamylcholine, or acetylcholine, in the presence of an inhibitor of cholinesterase, triggers CFU-S into DNA synthesis. Again, only a few molecules of acetylcholine per cell trigger the spleen colony forming cell into cycle. The effect of carbamylcholine was blocked by *d*-tubocurarine and this blockage was reversed by increasing the carbamylcholine. The effect of carbamylcholine was not blocked by the β_1-adrenergic receptor blocking agent propanolol, and the effect of isoproterenol was not blocked by *d*-tubocurarine, suggesting separate actions on separate receptors: β_1-adrenergic and cholinergic. Dibutyryl cyclic GMP also increased the cycling status of CFU-S. The action of acetycholine was most effective when neostigmine, an inhibitor of cholinesterase, was used.[119] It was suggested that cyclic GMP mediated in the cell cycle action of the cholinergic agents.[119] Methylazoxymethanol acetate, a potential chemical carcinogen triggered CFU-S into cycle via its conversion after hydrolysis to methylazoxymethanol or other metabolites.[120] Acetylcholinesterase was needed but the action was not mediated via β_1-adrenergic or cholinergic receptors.[120]

Histamine H_2-receptors have also been implicated as being on CFU-S.[121,122] The increased cycling of CFU-S by 4-methyl histamine, a stimulator of histamine H_2 receptors, but not by 2-methylhistamine, a stimulator of histamine H_1-receptors, and the antagonism of the effects of 4-methyl histamine by metiamide, a histamine H_2-receptor blocking agent suggested histamine H_2-receptors on CFU-S.[121] Exposure of bone marrow cells to inhibitors of histamine catabolism or to known histamine releasing agents increased the cycle status of CFU-S. Cimetidine, a more potent histamine H_2-receptor blocking agent than metiamide, antagonized the action of 4-methyl histamine and this antagonism was reversed by increasing the concentrations of 4-methylhistamine.[122] This latter study is of interest since both metiamide and cimetidine administration have been associated with cases of bone marrow suppression and the association may be causal rather than temporal.[122]

Low concentrations of PGE_2 have been shown to trigger CFU-S into cycle,[123] but the increase in the number of CFU-S in S-phase in vivo was not followed by a rise in femoral CFU-S content or in an increase in differentiation.[124] It was thus suggested that hemopoiesis after PGE-induced CFU-S stimulation was ineffective.

Another drug with an effect on CFU-S is Ouabain which at 10^{-9} *M* inhibits spleen colony formation by in vitro treated cells by more than 95%.[125] The authors suggested that Ouabain at concentrations below that (10^{-6} *M*) considered necessary to inhibit membrane-bound $Na^+ K^+$ ATPase could influence the proliferation of mouse stem cells.

Many chemotherapeutic drugs are known to influence hematopoietic stem and progenitor cells. The accumulated knowledge in this area up to the year 1976 has been summarized in an extensive and in depth review article.[126] In a study of the sensitivity of stem and progenitor cells to treatment with myleran[127] it was noted that the drug destroyed both, but the effect on CFU-S was tenfold more severe than on granulocyte-macrophage progenitor cells. The drug indirectly enhanced the seeding efficiency of CFU-S and directly impaired the capacity of the cells to self-renew and to generate granulocytic spleen colonies. Myleran influenced those CFU-S which had low density distributions, after density gradient centrifugation, and the surviving CFU-S were contained in a minor, higher density peak of cells which demonstrated a high potential for generating erythroid colonies in the spleen.[128]

IV. KINETICS OF STEM CELL MAINTENANCE AND REPOPULATION IN VIVO

One of the prevalent views in developmental hematopoiesis suggests that hematopoietic stem cells develop *de novo* in the blood islands of the yolk sac where they proliferate and migrate to the developing lymphoid organs such as the thymus and bursa of Fabricius, or its equivalent tissue in mammals, and the fetal liver, spleen, and then the bone marrow.[129,130] Both hematopoietic stem (CFU-S) and progenitor cells have been detected in yolk sac islands at 7 to 8 days of gestation, in the circulation by 9 to 10 days and in embryonic liver by 10.5 days.[6] In vivo grafting studies substantiated in vitro organ culture observations that yolk sac-derived stem cells had colonized the hepatic rudiment of the mouse embryo at about the 28-somite stage of development.[131] It has been shown that yolk sac contained many precursors of CFU-S which could not be detected by immediate grafting, but which could be seen after a prior cultivation of yolk sac cells in vitro.[132] As much as an 84-fold increase of CFU-S was detected after 48 hr in culture, but the reason(s) for this enhancement in numbers was not known. Differences in physical characteristics between fetal and adult CFU-S have been given in Section III.A and it has been suggested that stem cells in fetal liver have a higher intrinsic capacity for self-renewal than those in adult bone marrow.[133] Chromosome markers were used and fetal-liver cells, although starting at lower numbers of stem cells than for adult bone marrow, rapidly increased their numbers in myeloid and lymphoid tissues for a period of over several weeks.

A hypothesis was proposed that stem cells were organized for use on the basis of their generation age.[134] A young stem cell was considered to be one that had undergone few generations since its birth and its capacities for self-renewal and production of progenitors would be greater than an older stem cell which had undergone more generations. Data to substantiate the hypothesis were presented later.[135] A younger population of stem cells whose capacity for stem cell generation was three- to fourfold greater than normal untreated cells was noted after kill by phase specific drugs of older stem cells from adult bone marrow and 13-day fetal liver. Additionally, stem cell generative capacity declined eightfold after continuous irradiation to the mice; serial retransplantation and stem cell generative capacity of circulating cells was one quarter to one fortieth that of normal adult marrow stem cells. A model of the stem cell compartment as a continuum of cells with decreasing capacities for self-renewal and increased chance for differentiation was suggested by others[136] based on decreased self-renewal capacity with serial transplantation and continued production of differentiated cells. It was noted also that the probability of stem cell renewal was decreased after apparent recovery from busulphan treatment. Progression in one direction was not reversible. The self-maintenance capacity of CFU-S was studied and it was found in general that treatments such as cytotoxic drugs or irradiation resulted in a lowering of capacity for self-renewal of CFU-S and a shortening of the cell cycle time of CFU-S.[137] It was speculated that those CFU-S with high self-renewal probability were the more primitive stem cells. Another hypothesis[138] suggested that under normal conditions CFU-S remained in a G_o, or out of cycle, state and this restored them to full self-reproductive capacity. CFU-S modified by certain experimental maneuvers spent less time in G_o and thus had less time to rejuvenate themselves and demonstrated a decrease in self-maintenance capacity. Studies on endogenous colony formation of CFU-S using irradiation[36] and various foreign substances[139] which increased the endogenous pool of CFU-S have demonstrated that self-replication began soon after a reduction in the compartment size, and that the onset of differentiation was linked to the size of the stem cell pool.

For long-term replacement of cells the most important stem cells would be those that were the least differentiated and had maximum ability to proliferate and repopulate. However numbers of CFU-S did not always correlate with long-term functional capacities, and thus a competitive repopulation assay for long-term stem cell functional capacity was designed.[140] Marrow cells from two types of donors with distinguishable hemoglobin were mixed and the mixtures given to lethally irradiated recipients. The results were given by the percentage of erythrocytes in the recipient descended from stem cells of each donor type as measured by the percentage of hemoglobin of each donor type.

The relative spatial distributions of stem and progenitor cells in the femurs of normal mice have been elucidated.[141,142] The concentration of CFU-S increased from the femoral axis to the bone surface in approximately a square-law relationship;[141] CFU-S near the bone surface were found to be a more rapidly proliferating population of cells than CFU-S more distant from the surface of the bone.[141] More rapidly proliferating cells have been detected in the subendosteal region[143] in which the more rapidly proliferating CFU-S were detected.[141] Others have detected a uniform spatial distribution of CFU-S across the diameter of the femoral medullary cavity, but suggested that spatial parameters may be important determinants of hemopoiesis.[144]

Direct experimental procedures substantiated the belief that cell migration from a shielded marrow was responsible entirely for the 30 day recovery of marrow irradiated with 1000 rad.[145] However, regeneration of damaged bone marrow involved a significant contribution from extrinsic stem cells only after high dosages of radiation[146] which might be explained by removal of endogenous CFU-S from the areas[31,33] before new stem cells could seed into the appropriate spaces. A study of movement of stem cells from a shielded marrow to an irradiated spleen demonstrated a constant rate of migration during the first 24 hr after irradiation.[147] The low concentration of CFU-S in the blood stream was indicative of a greatly increased blood turnover of CFU-S.

The properties of circulating hematopoietic stem cells have been investigated. In comparison to bone marrow CFU-S, the blood CFU-S had a lower radiosensitivity (D_o of 140 rad), a higher seeding efficiency, and more cells in cycle, but both had a 21-hr doubling time even though the blood CFU-S demonstrated a longer lag period before exponential growth.[148] The turnover of circulating CFU-S was investigated by short term parabiosis of male and female mice of the CBA/CaJ strain.[149] A half time of 1.7 hr in the blood was detected, and these CFU-S were equilibrated with a subpopulation of marrow CFU-S which had a disappearance half time of 9.5 hr. Splenectomy did not influence the apparent rate of disappearance from the blood. Stem cells in the blood have been shown not to be a random sample of those in bone marrow, but a population which in general manifests low proliferative potential and low self-renewal capacity[150] and may be the older generated CFU-S.[134–137] Serial transfer studies have shown cells from yolk sac, fetal liver, and neonatal liver to have greater renewal capacity than adult marrow cells, but older and younger adult mice had similar capacity for serial transfers.[6,151–153] It was calculated that immediate stem cell proliferative capacities decline more after one serial transplantation than after a lifetime of normal function.

Bacterial endotoxin has been shown to have various influential capacities with regard to increasing CFU-S numbers and the migration trend of CFU-S from marrow to spleen. It was considered that *S. typhosa* endotoxin increased CFU-S numbers in marrow and spleen by a genetically controlled regulatory mechanism since the increase was prevented by colecemid and did not occur in mice of the Sl/Sl^d strain which contain a defective microenvironment for the proliferative cycle.[155] Irradiation resistant microenvironmental factors in the spleen determined the accumulation of CFU-S after endotoxin, and the rise of blood CFU-S numbers at this time was shown to be independent of the spleen.[156] After injection of *B. pertusis* vaccine (killed, but intact bacteria) it was observed that splenic CFU-S increased due at first to proliferation *in situ* and then later to proliferation in the marrow with subsequent migration to the spleen via the blood.[157] In addition to endotoxin, trypsin, proteinase, zymosan, phytohemagglutinin, concanavalin A, di-isopropylfluorophosphate-inhibited trypsin and pyran copolymer, a divinyl-ether maleic anhydride, mobilized CFU-S into the blood although the rates of mobilization varied with the agents.[158–160] The complement system was linked to the early mobilization of CFU-S.[159,161] Pretreatment of mice with the complement-activating factor of cobra venom, which lowered serum C3 levels, completely prevented mobilization of CFU-S by high doses of cobra venom, *S. typhosa* endotoxin, inulin, zymosan, proteinase, and trypsin.[161] Mobilization induced by dextran sulphate and the copolymer of polymethacrylic acid and styrene was not influenced to any great extent, suggesting that certain agents mobilized CFU-S via the complement system while others involved a system independent of complement components.[161] Interestingly, the mobilization effects of injected preparations of erythropoietin on CFU-S were found to a significant extent to be secondary to the presence of endotoxin in the preparations of erythropoietin.[162]

V. MAINTENANCE OF STEM CELLS IN VITRO

A. Normal Maintenance

The capacity to maintain pluripotential hematopoietic stem cells and progenitor cells in liquid culture for many weeks was an extremely important advance in the area of experimental hematology. Until the initial report in 1973,[163] it was possible to maintain stem and progenitor cells in suspension culture or in diffusion chambers implanted into mice[164] only for days. This did not allow detailed studies on the self-maintenance and differentiation capacity of this pool of cells. Initially, coculturing of bone marrow cells with thymus cells was necessary for maintenance of the production and differentiation of cells.[163] At this time granulocytes in all stages of differentiation could be maintained in culture for 2 weeks with stem and granulocyte-macrophage progenitor cells maintained for this time period at 10 to 15% of the level of the original number placed into culture.

Modifications of the culture conditions resulted in a prolongation of the maintenance of stem, progenitor, and more mature cells.[165] After 7 to 9 weeks in culture, hematopoietic pluripotential stem cells (CFU-S) were able to protect lethally irradiated mice from hematopoietic death. Further modifications of this culture system maintained proliferation of stem and progenitor cells for months.[166] Among the modifications were removal of half the culture medium every few days and an incubation temperature of

33°C rather than the usual 37°C. The cultures consisted of populations of adherent and nonadherent cells. The adherent population containing phagocytic mononuclear cells, "epithelial" cells, and "giant fat" cells, appeared to be a necessity for stem cell maintenance. The cultures showed initially extensive granulopoiesis followed by an accumulation of blast cells, and eventually phagocytic mononuclear cells predominated. Much work has gone into characterizing the adherent population of cells.[167,168]

Without the formation of aggregations of epithelial cells swollen to enormous proportions by the presence of numerous lipid-containing vacuoles, granulocyte production was not maintained beyond an initial period. Healthy cultures showed a characteristic clumping of granulocytes around these aggregates. Epithelial cells formed a layer over some of the attached cells and pinocytic vesicles, and gap junctions were observed between the adjacent membranes of undifferentiated granulocytes and epithelial cells themselves. A quantitative assessment of the formation of adherent cell colonies in bone marrow cell cultures has been reported.[169] In reports from another laboratory[176] it was demonstrated that the marrow-derived adherent cells included some cells with esterase I activity and complement 3 receptors; Fc receptors were not detected. Collagen types I and III and fibronectin were seen and staining for epithelial basement membrane proteins (collagen types IV and V and laminin) was negative. Few fat containing cells were noted in the study and it was concluded that the vast majority of the cells were fibroblasts and that these fibroblasts were necessary for support of granulopoiesis.[170] This is in contradistinction to reports which suggested that the formation of fibroblast-like cells were coincident with a loss of maintenance of granulopoiesis within the cultures.[171]

As originally described,[166] cultures were allowed to form a suitable adherent layer and after approximately 3 weeks all culture medium was removed and an inoculum of fresh bone marrow cells in culture medium added to the established adherent layer. Several modifications have since been made on this system,[172,173] and at this time it appears as if the correct culture conditions from the time of first marrow inoculation into the culture flasks allows extensive maintenance of cells for over a year without need for complete cell depopulation and addition of a secondary marrow sample. The addition of hydrocortisone[173] apparently was involved in the maintenance of the fat cells, which appeared to be necessary for continuous cell proliferation within this culture system and may have substituted for poor batches of serum. An extensive study of lipids in the bone marrow of six strains of normal mice was undertaken.[174] Of total lipids 60 to 75% was accounted for by cholesterol and phospholipid. The rest of the lipids were composed of triglyceride and neutral glyceryl ether lipids. A comparison was made between bone marrow cells and cells maintained in the adherent populations of long-term bone marrow cultures. In cultures of $B6D2F_1$, bone marrow, the adherent layers contained the same lipids as freshly aspirated bone marrow.

The crucial role of the adherent layer of cells in maintenance of stem and progenitor cells was evaluated using the W/W^v and Sl/Sl^d mice.[175,176] The lesion in W mice is considered to be due to a defect in the stem cells, while that in Sl mice is believed to be due to a defect in the hemopoietic microenvironment. Adherent layers from bone marrow of Sl/Sl^d mice did not support the proliferation of Sl/Sl^d progenitor cells, and the W/W^v adherent layers did not support proliferation of W/W^v progenitor cells. However, the W/W^v adherent layer did support proliferation of Sl/Sl^d progenitor cells. No gross defect was detected in the adherent marrow population of Sl/Sl^d.[175,176] However, it has been noted that the lipid content of the adherent layers differed from normal bone marrow particularly in the absence of ether-containing lipids.[174]

In a study designed to test the maintenance of hemopoietic stem cells and production of differentiated progeny in allogeneic and semiallogeneic bone marrow chimeras in vitro,[177] it was found that bone marrow-derived adherent cells from a particular mouse strain could sustain the growth of cells from syngeneic as well as genetically incompatible mice. Production was not compromised in semiallogeneic or allogenic bone marrow combinations. It was suggested that the reactive cells responsible for host transplantation resistance and for graft vs. host disease in vivo were lost or suppressed in these cultures. Interestingly, natural killer cells are lost from these cultures after a short time.[178] It has, however, been demonstrated that maintenance of cell proliferation varies when bone marrow cells from different strains of mice are used.[177,179]

A survey of the functional capacities of cells maintained within the cultures[172] has shown that polymorphonuclear neutrophils derived from these cultures were similar to primary bone marow neutrophils in that they had complement 3 and IgG receptors and actively phagocytosed foreign substances. Moreover, the granulocyte-macrophage progenitor cells were similar to those from primary marrow in their response to stimulation in semisolid medium and to their rate of sedimentation after separation by cell size.

Interestingly, the first reports suggested that the colony stimulatory factors necessary for the stimulation of granulocyte-macrophage progenitor cells could not be found in cultures of long-term marrows,[166,180,181] and moreover that conditioned medium containing these factors actually decreased the maintenance of cellular proliferation and differentiation in these cultures.[166,181] Two later reports using purified preparations of these factors demonstrated that they did not run the system down nor did they appear to influence granulopoiesis within the cultures.[182,183] The results were interpreted cautiously and suggestions made that the possibility still exists that these factors could have a role in these cultures, but that it would have to be at a very local level with contact between effector and responder cell populations perhaps necessary.

In addition to granulocytes and macrophages, the proliferation of other cell lineages in maintained within these cultures. Megakaryocytes and their progenitor cells have been sustained in culture for many weeks.[184] The megakaryocytes were identified by cytoplasmic acetylcholinesterase and by electron microscopic analysis and the progenitor cells by their capacity to form colonies of megakaryocytes in semisolid culture medium. No inductive regulator of the colony forming cells was found in the supernatants from the long-term marrow cultures. Early erythroid progenitors cells (BFUe) were also detected in these cultures[185] as were even more immature erythroid progenitors with the capacity to give rise also to megakaryocytes.[186] At this time the more mature erythroid progenitor cells, CFUe, and recognizable erythroid cells were not detected in these cultures.[183] Modifications of the system utilizing addition of erythropoietin to the cultures allowed detection of a more mature early erythroid progenitor.

Maturation of these cells into mature late erythroid progenitors and nonnucleated erythroid cells was possible by mechanical agitation of the cultures or by transfer of the cells to dishes where attachment of cells to surfaces was prevented.[187] Nonadherent cells harvested from long-term cultures showed detectable levels of antibody dependent lysis and phagocytosis of erythrocyte targets.[188] At later times when macrophages predominated in these cultures the cells were highly active, particularly in the phagocytosis of erythrocyte targets. Considerable antibody-dependent lysis and phagocytosis of erythrocytes was also detected in cells from the adherent layers. While T and B lymphocytes have not been detected after the first week of culture,[178] cells capable of repopulating irradiated hosts with T and B lymphocytes have been detected.[189] The repopulated lymphocytes were functional and there was no evidence that these lymphocytes contained a gross restriction of their receptors. Moreover, the cultured cells reconstituted irradiated semiallogeneic hosts with no graft vs. host disease being evident.

This study along with the others already reported[177,178] suggests the potential usefulness of this system for the culture of donor marrow prior to bone marrow transplantation in humans when tissue matching is incomplete. It has been noted[190] that long-term marrow cultures contained colony forming cells that produced Thy 1-positive progeny after stimulation by culture medium conditioned by human leukocytes in the presence of phytohemmagglutinin. These colony forming cells could be maintained in continuous cultures supplemented with hydrocortisone. Cells from the individual colonies lacked precursors for cytotoxic lymphocytes, but they could provide nonspecific help required for the generation of cytotoxic lymphocytes.

It has been demonstrated that bone marrow cells (CFU-S) removed from long-term cultures are capable of forming spleen colonies when injected into lethally irradiated mice and can save these mice from death.[166] The self-renewal capacity of pluripotential hematopoietic stem cells obtained from the nonadherent and adherent portions of long-term cultures and evidence for a structured variation in self-renewal capacity was suggested.[191] CFU-S within the adherent stromal layer demonstrated a significantly greater capacity for self-renewal than did nonadherent CFU-S. At initiation, the self-renewal capacity of adherent CFU-S decreased as the total number of CFU-S increased. After 3 weeks there was stabilization of the self-renewal capacity of adherent cell derived CFU-S. It was suggested that in order to increase the primitive stem cell pool size there was a proliferation early in time of stem cells with a high self-renewal capacity. This population of cells then maintained themselves once this pool was established.

Modulation of hematopoiesis within long-term cultures by lithium was attempted in order to understand the influence of lithium, a compound known to increase production of granulocytes under certain circumstances.[192] After a week of incubation with 1 mmol lithium carbonate per liter there was noted a significant increase in pluripotential stem cells, granulocyte-macrophage progenitor cells, granulocytes and megakaryocytes, respectively, to 232, 218, 125, and 246% of control values. However, prolonged exposure to lithium for 3 to 12 weeks was associated with a decline in numbers of stem and progenitor cells. It was suggested that lithium enhancement of granulopoiesis might be due to a primary stimulation of the pluripotential stem cell and that prolonged stress might deplete the stem cell reserve. It should be noted that initial increases in cell numbers were associated with transient rises in levels of stimulatory activities for granulocyte-macrophage progenitors. It has previously been reported that lithium might exert its effect by increasing the production and/or release of these factors or by counterbalancing the inhibition by lactoferrin of the production of the stimulatory activities.[39,193] It was not yet clear whether the early stem cell enhancing activity of lithium in the long-term cultures was due to a direct effect on the stem cells or on other accessory or helper cells.[192]

B. Viral and Chemical Modification of Maintenance

The interaction between viruses and cells within the continuous marrow culture has been investigated in order to shed some light on the interactions involved in leukemogenesis. The influence of murine leukemia virus on proliferation of pluripotential stem cells and on differentiation of these cells as studied using two virus variants: the Moloney strain of lymphatic leukemia virus (Mol-MuLV) and the erythroleukemia Friend virus complex (FLV) which includes the lymphoid leukemia helper virus and the defective spleen focus-forming virus (SFFV).[194] Infection of cultures with Mol-MuLV and its sarcoma vs. pseudotype, MSV (Mol-MuLV), yielded viral replication, but stem cells were lost rapidly and there was a change in populations to cells of the mononuclear phagocyte series. However, infection with FLV induced prolonged survival of stem and progenitor cells. Production of SFFV was maintained for more than 40 weeks, but no late erythroid progenitor cells (CFUe) or hemoglobulin-producing cells were detected. Instead, there was a hyperproliferation of the granulocytic series.

It could not be determined whether FLV infection and replication occurred in all cell types or whether there was a particular target cell for viral replication.

Cultures infected with an nb-tropic Friend strain of helper C-type virus (F-MuLV) free of spleen focus forming units began to deviate significantly from control cultures after 10 to 11 weeks.[195] The change was eventually marked by an increase in cell production with increased immature granulocytic elements. Cultures infected with F-MuLV plus spleen focus forming virus did not demonstrate the high incidence and phenotypic changes seen in the F-MuLV-infected cultures, but by 19 weeks cell production was tenfold greater than in control cultures with a predominance of immature granulocytes. In contrast, significant changes in hematopoiesis were observed within 3 weeks of infection with Kirsten-MSV pseudotype when a conversion of the cultures to a macrophage morphology was noted. Stem cells declined rapidly and cells when placed into semisolid medium formed large numbers of three to five cell macrophage clusters. Cluster formation required exogenously added colony stimulatory activities.

Evidence for spontaneous leukemia transformation, without addition of exogenously added virus, has been obtained in continuous marrow culture.[176] In vitro transformation was noted in a number of cultures of allogeneic combinations of CBA and BDF_1 bone marrow and in a syngeneic coculture of CBA marrow and day 15 gestation CBA fetal liver cells. Colonies of blast cells negative for Fc and complement receptors, surface and cytoplasmic immunoglobulin, and lysozyme production were detected. Colony formation did not require addition of exogenously added colony stimulatory activities. Cytogenetic analysis showed marked aneuploidy and a unique spectrum of metacentric and minute marker chromosomes. Continuous lines were established from these cells after colony formation in semisolid culture medium, and the cells produced rapidly growing tumors in nude and syngeneic mice after subcutaneous injection.

Injection of continuous cultures with FLV has induced the occurrence of myelomonocytic leukemia cells which have been established as a cell line, 427E-MC.[196] This cell line contained cells with the morphology of blasts, promyelocytes, and myelocytes. No differentiation to mature granulocyte cells was detected. The cells produced colony stimulatory activity for granulocyte macrophage progenitor cells and lymphatic leukemia helper virus but not spleen focus-forming virus. The line demonstrated a 10 to 30% cloning efficiency in semisolid culture medium which did not require colony stimulatory activity addition, a replating efficiency of 10 to 15%, and caused leukemia when injected into neonatal and adult mice. The production of producer cell lines was also established after infection of cultures with Abelson murine leukemia virus.[197] The infection led to transformation of cells in the early B-lymphocyte lineage. An IgM negative and IgM producing cell population were found in the uncloned population. The IgM negative cells could be induced to synthesize IgM. Various other cell lines have been induced after infection of long-term cultures with the anemia-inducing strain of Friend leukemia virus and Abelosn virus.[198]

Treatment of bone marrow cells with the chemical leukemogen, methylnitrosourea, has also resulted in leukemia cell transformation after culture in vitro.[199] Apparently normal pluripotential stem cells were detected for the first 10 to 12 weeks, but later the spleen colonies formed from the cultured cells contained undifferentiated blast cells. These cells produced a transplantable leukemia and contained no detectable theta antigen or surface immunoglobulin.

In addition to the production of tumor cell lines there has also been a report of a cell line which has a diploid complement of chromosomes, is not tumorigenic, is bipotent, and which can under the appropriate conditions protect mice from potentially lethal irradiation.[200] The cell line was isolated from a long-term culture of (C57Bl/6 $\times$ DBA/2)F_1, female bone marrow cells, which had been infected with NB-tropic, polycythemia-inducing Friend leukemia virus. The cells were designated 416B and the majority were undifferentiated blast cells and "promyelocytic" cells. In addition, larger multi-lobed cells resembling megakaryocytes were noted. When injected into irradiated mice, spleen colonies containing granulocytes and megakaryocytes were detected. While the block in differentiation could be overcome in vivo it could not be abrogated in vitro even after treatment with agents known to promote differentiation of other cell lines.

VI. EVIDENCE FOR HUMAN HEMATOPOIETIC STEM CELLS

The evidence for the presence of human hematopoietic stem cells was mainly indirect due to the absence of an assay as in mouse, that could at the same time document single cell origin, extensive self-replicating or renewal capacity, and differentiative direction for the myeloid and/or lymphoid lineages. The original evidence for human stem cells was based on marker analyses of cells, but this information is being substantiated by newer cell culture procedures which allow continuous marrow cell growth and differentiation in suspension culture or clonal growth of cells with multipotentialities in semisolid medium. This information is presented below.

A. Marker Analysis: Philadelphia Chromosome, Glucose-6-Phosphate Dehydrogenase (Isoenzymes) and Antigenic Characterization of Cell Surfaces

For the most part, marker analysis has utilized disease states and the clonality of cell lines to establish multipotenciality and its derivation from a single cell.[201] One of the first pieces of evidence for the common derivation of myeloid cells from a single cell came when the Philadelphia (PH^1) chromosome was found in cells of the erythrocytic, megakaryocytic, granulocytic, and monocytic lines.[202,203] The PH^1 chromosome was discovered in the bone marrow of patients with chronic myeloid leukemia and was noted as a deletion in the long arm of one of the group G chromosomes.[204] It was later found that the PH^1 chromosome involved a balanced reciprocal translocation between the long arms of chromosomes 22 and 9[205] or 22 and other chromosomes.[206] Background information on the PH^1 chromosome and its correlation to disease is discussed elsewhere.[207]

A marker for cell clonality which has been used more recently is dependent on X-chromosome inactivation mosaicism using the glucose-6-phosphate dehydrogenase locus as the X-linked marker.[208] The theory behind the use of this procedure is explained in detail elsewhere.[208] In general, this marker is useful because it is polymorphic in certain ethnic groups, and the locus undergoes inactivation with only one of the two genes for glucose-6-phosphate dehydrogenase being active in somatic cells of females.[209] Therefore, certain women heterozygous for the usual B gene and a variant allele can have two populations of cells with one expressing a B-type isoenzyme and the other an A-type isoenzyme. Tumors deriving from more than one cell will contain cells of B and A types, whereas a clonally derived tumor will contain cells all with only one isoenzyme, either A type of B type being expressed.[209] Such isoenzyme studies corroborated those with the PH^1 chromosome which showed that chronic myeloid leukemia was a stem cell disorder with the clonal origin of granulocytes, macrophages, erythrocytes, and platelets, but were additionally able to demonstrate clonality extending to a subpopulation of lymphocytes also.[210–212] Several reports had already suggested a correlative link between the myeloid and lymphoid series[201] which included finding lymphoid cells during the blastic phase of chronic myelogenous leukemia, which had been considered previously to be composed entirely of myeloblasts, and the documentation of the PH^1 chromosome in some patients with acute lymphoblastic leukemia without an apparent phase of chronic myelogenous leukemia.

When the technique of glucose-6-phosphate dehydrogenase locus inactivation was used to study three patients with chronic myeloid leukemia it was found that skin tissue contained both A and B enzymatic expression, but the myeloid cells and a population of B lymphocytes or non-T, non-B lymphocytes showed only one isoenzyme.[212] Cells of the T-lymphoid series from these patients expressed both A and B isoenzymes. These studies suggested the common ancestral origin of myeloid cells and at least some cells of the lymphoid series. Interestingly, lymphocytes responding to stimulation by phytohemmaglutinin and pokeweed mitogen which had manifested single enzyme phenotypic expression and which therefore were considered to have been derived from a single myeloid-lymphoid stem cell generally lacked the PH^1 chromosome. It was suggested, as one alternative interpretation, that some cells, such as these lymphocytes, were clonally derived, but that the acquisition of the PH^1 chromosome may have occurred later in time or development.[212]

There is a report also of a patient with acquired idiopathic sideroblastic anemia who demonstrated one isoenzyme type in erythrocytes, granulocytes, platelets, macrophages, and B and T lymphocytes, whereas skin fibroblasts and salivary epithelial cells contained A and B isoenzymes.[213] Further evidence for B-cell derivation from a myeloid-lymphoid stem cell comes from the discovery of pre-B-lymphocytic phenotypes in the blastic phase of PH^1 chronic myeloid leukemia using membrane markers and enzyme assays as a means to detect these pre-B-lymphocytes.[214] Twenty-six cases of PH^1 positive acute leukemia or the blastic phase of chronic myeloid leukemia were investigated. Nineteen had the same ''lymphoid'' phenotype as PH^1 negative common acute lymphoblastic leukemia, and three patients with chronic myeloid leukemia in blastic crisis had leukemia cells with a pre-B phenotype. In two other cases a minority population of leukemia cells had a similar pre-B phenotype.

Clonal evolution of cells has also been investigated in polycythemia vera, agnogenic myeloid metaplasia with myelofibrosis, and acute myeloid leukemia.[209,215] While normal stem cells could be detected in polycythemia vera[215] no evidence for residual normal stem cells were detected in PH^1 negative chronic myeloid leukemia[216] or during the stable ''remission'' phase of PH^1-positive chronic myeloid leukemia. Single-enzyme glucose-6-phosphate dehydrogenase phenotypic expression persisted at that time.[217,218] However, intense chemotherapeutic treatment had removed, at least temporarily, the PH^1 clone and resulted in a true remission for some of these patients.[217] Prior to treatment only the type B-phenotype was detected in the patients erythrocytes, granulocytes, and platelets and all unstimulated marrow metaphases demonstrated the PH^1 chromosome.[219] After four cycles of chemotherapy, 76% of the marrow cells were PH^1-negative and about 80% of the granulocytes were nonclonal, suggesting the restoration of a nonclonal and presumably nonneoplastic cell line.[219]

B. Maintenance of Probable Human Stem Cells in Vitro

Continuous proliferation in culture of cells other than from mouse strains was accomplished with exceptional success using cells from *Tupaia glis,* the tree shrew, a member of the family Tupaiidae, considered to be one of the most primitive living prosimians, bridging the gap between insectivores and primates.[195,220] With a single inoculum of bone marrow these cultures have been maintained for over 1 year. Ultrastructurally, a complex interrelationship of sheets of pavement endothelial cells, fat-containing cells, macrophages, and hematopoietic elements were seen. With *Tupaia* cells the areas of fat cells were predominant, the lipid droplets in these cells did not coalesce to the extent seen in mouse cultures, and numerous myelin-figure-like inclusions were present. The *Tupaia* immature granulocytes had a more dendritic shape than mouse cells and basophils were more numerous.

The first report on adaptation of the continuous marrow culture system for human cells used an established adherent cell layer and a second inoculum of autologous bone marrow cells.[195] Cultures were maintained at 37°C which for human marrow appeared superior to the 33°C conditions found optimal for culturing of mouse cells. Production of granulocytes was maintained for 5 weeks, but by the 6th week 10% of the cultures converted to a lymphoblastoid morphology, and continuous EBV-positive, Ig-positive B cell lines developed. The rest of the cells maintained a macrophage morphology for many more weeks. Morphologically detectable erythropoiesis persisted for 2 to 3 weeks and small lymphocytes (2 and 22%) persisted throughout the culture. Granulocyte-macrophage progenitor cells were produced for 5 to 6 weeks and their colony size, morphology, and responsiveness to colony stimulatory activity were similar to the noncultured cells. Further characterization of these cultures[105] demonstrated that between the second to fourth week of culture a complex adherent population of bone marrow cells becomes established. These contained focal areas of macrophages, endothelial cells, hemopoietic cells, and infrequent lipid-containing cells. Initially, the interfocal areas contained a monolayer of well spread macrophages, but fibroblasts predominated at later times. With weekly removal of half the suspension cells, granulocytic differentiation was detected for 6 weeks and granulocyte-macrophage and early erythroid progenitor cells were apparent for 5 weeks. A small but significant improvement in the extent and duration of myelopoiesis was seen when a secondary autologous marrow was added to an established adherent cell layer than when the cultures were established from a single marrow inoculum. The addition of a second, unrelated marrow sample did not support growth as well as with a single marrow inoculum.

Other studies on human cells[221] demonstrated maintenance of granulocyte-macrophage progenitor cells and late erythroid progenitor cells for 4 to 9 weeks with morphologically recognizable granulocytes apparent for 4 to 6 weeks and erythroid cells seen for 1.5 to 2.5 weeks. Functional T lymphocytes were detected for 5 weeks. The adherent population was composed of macrophages, fibroblast-like cells, and flat pavement-like cells. Fat-containing cells were not prominent.

Modifications of the culture conditions have now allowed granulocytic proliferation in excess of 20 weeks.[222,223] As with murine cells, the adherent layer contained mononuclear phagocytes, endothelial cells, and lipid containing adipocytes.[222,223] The adipocytes appeared essential for long-term hematopoiesis. The best growth conditions utilized McCoy's medium plus fetal bovine serum, horse serum, hydrocortisone, and incubation at 33°C.[222] Horse serum plus hydrocortisone appeared necessary for the growth of adipocytes.[222] Addition of a second inoculum of marrow cells did not enhance maintenance of proliferation of cells and in some cases decreased proliferation.[222] Similar results were obtained by others,[223] but in this case horse serum, fetal calf serum, and hydrocortisone were used. Delayed removal of red blood cells after the adherent layer was formed was necessary for continued proliferation of cells.[223] Granulocytes generated in the cultures appeared to have normal functional capability for ingestion of particles, respiratory burst activity, and degranulation.[223]

Results[105] to be presented in greater detail in the chapter on granulopoiesis have demonstrated the absence on probable pluripotential cells of certain antigenic determinants present on early and late granulocyte-macrophage and erythroid progenitor cells. This antigenic determinant is a human Ia-like molecule. The 28,000 to 37,000 dalton complex isolated from human B-cell line membranes and produced by genes mapping in the major histocompatibility complex[224] is biologically and chemically homologous to the murine I-region antigen system (Ia). It appears as if the human Ia-like antigens are absent on a probable human pluripotential stem cell recognized in prolonged culture, is gained rapidly as commitment to the various progenitor cell types occurs, and is subsequently lost as these cells undergo differentiation towards the more mature morphologically recognizable cells within the marrow. It has been suggested that these Ia-like antigenic determinants may be involved in the regulation of myelopoiesis,[105,225] and evidence has already appeared that a subpopulation of human monocytes[226] and mouse peritoneal macrophages[227] bearing Ia antigens are involved in the negative feedback regulation of myelopoiesis by lactoferrin. These interactions and their relevance to myelopoiesis will be considered in detail in the chapter on granulopoiesis.

C. Multipotential Cell Assay in Vitro

The development of in vitro clonal assays for detection of multipotential cells in mice[41–43,45–50] has been extended and is now available also for human cells.[228–231] The original report demonstrated that colonies containing granulocytes and erythropoietic cells could form from cells in human bone marrow, peripheral blood, and cord blood.[228] When these cells were placed into methylcellulose, a semisolid culture medium, for 4 to 5 days in the presence of a culture medium conditioned by human peripheral blood leukocytes in the presence of phytohemagglutinin, some of these colonies contained granulocytes after another 9 to 10 days of incubation. If, however, erythropoietin was added by day 4 or 5 of culture, erythroid bursts were detected. Some of these latter colonies contained cells positive for hemoglobin as well as cells positive for myeloperoxidase or chloroacetate esterase. In 15 of 19 bone marrows, these mixed granulocyte-erythroid colonies were seen at a ratio of 1/2 to 3×10^5 nucleated cells plated. The same frequency was noted for six of eight peripheral blood samples and one cord blood sample yielded one colony per 2×10^5 nucleated cells. These colony forming cells sedimented at 4 to 4.5 mm/hr, and the colonies were determined to have arisen from a single cell after analysis of the presence or absence of Y-bodies. A total of 14 colonies from female donors showed no Y-chromatin bodies in any of the cells while 11 colonies from male donors demonstrated the Y-chromatin in 60 to 70% of the cells within the colonies. The Y-chromatin bodies were seen in both cells of the erythroid or granulocyte series.

A later communication reported that mixed granulocyte-erythroid colonies could also contain eosinophils, megakaryocytes, and/or macrophages, suggesting a true multipotential cell.[229] In some of the mixed colonies cells representing four lineages were seen, but none of the colonies assessed contained all five of these cell types. Erythroblasts were more often found associated with granulocytes than with megakaryocytes. One difference between the growth of multipotential cells from murine[43,45–50] and human sources[229] was that the human cells required erythropoietin while the murine cells didn't appear to need it.

The cycling status of the human mixed erythroid colony forming cells from normal donors and patients recovering from bone marrow transplantation was assessed with pulse exposure of cells to high specific activity tritiated thymidine.[230] Zero to 25% of the colony forming cells from bone marrow of normal donors were killed by this procedure suggesting that these cells were in a relatively noncycling state when compared to progenitor cells for the granulocyte-macrophage or erythroid lineages. This is similar to the low cycling rate of mixed-erythroid colony forming cells from adult murine bone marrow.[42,47] In contrast to the low cycling rate of human mixed-erythroid colony forming cells from normal donors, the cycling status of these cells was increased when analyzed from bone marrow cells of bone marrow transplant recipients during the early phase post transplantation. This implied that this cell population was actively involved in regeneration of the bone marrow cells.

It has been suggested that numerical correlations between classes of cell types might provide information on the relationships of one cell lineage to another.[232] Examination of data from 133 patients demonstrated a high correlation between the multipotential colony forming cell and the erythroid progenitor cell, but not between the multipotential colony forming cell and the granulocyte-progenitor cell.[231] These data suggested a closer lineage relationship between the erythroid progenitor cells and the multipotential cells than between the granulocyte progenitor cells and the multipotential cells.

The self-renewal capacity of these multipotential cells was checked by replating the cells from individual colonies containing several cell lineages.[231] Preliminary evidence for secondary replating capacity was attained. In cultures derived from two mixed colonies, erythroid bursts, granulocyte colonies, and secondary mixed colonies were identified, suggesting that at least some of the multipotential cells detected had self-renewal capacity.[231]

Analysis of fetal hemoglobulin was compared in progeny cells from multipotential cells and erythroid progenitor cells.[231] These appeared to be a higher proportion of fetal hemoglobulin positive cells in the colonies derived from multipotential cells as compared to those derived from the erythroid progenitor cells.

An investigation of multipotential colony forming cells in patients was undertaken.[231] Polycythemia rubra vera is considered to be a clonal disorder involving pluripotential stem cells.[233] Mixed-erythroid colonies have been detected without exogenous erythropoietin in three such patients.[231] This suggested the possibility that these colony forming cells may have belonged to an abnormal clone of cells. In preliminary correlative studies with disease progression during bone marrow hypoplasia,[231] it was found that 11 patients with hypoplastic states demonstrated heterogeneity with respect to mixed-erythroid colonies and six patients demonstrated little or no growth. Two patients in the former group recovered while none of the patients in the latter group demonstrated spontaneous recovery. It was emphasized, however, that more patients and longer follow-up periods were necessary before definitive correlations could be made.

One of the weaknesses of this assay system had been the apparent low cloning efficiency of the multipotential colony forming cells. Modifications in culture conditions and scoring have now increased the apparent cloning efficiency so that more than 20 mixed-erythroid colonies can be observed per 2×10^5 nucleated bone marrow cells.[234] The modifications included use of Iscove's modified Dulbecco's medium with 2-mercaptoethanol and scoring of colonies using dark field illumination which increased the contrast between hemoglobinized and translucent cells.

VII. REGULATION OF STEM CELL PROLIFERATION AND DIFFERENTIATION

A. Models

1. Stochastic

The stochastic model is based on the probability of chance interactions between CFU-S and unspecified regulatory mechanisms that might determine the possibility of differentiation along a particular pathway.[85,235,236] This model was suggested by the heterogenous distribution of spleen colony forming cells within individual spleen colonies.[25] Each spleen colony is considered to be derived from a single cell as discussed in Section II.A of this chapter. After well-separated spleen colonies were removed and each assayed separately for their content of CFU-S, it was seen that some colonies contained few or no CFU-S while others contained thousands of CFU-S. This distribution suggested that self-renewal of CFU-S varied widely from colony to colony.

2. Hematopoietic Inductive Microenvironment

An alternative model to the postulated stochastic or random one is that a specific local environment exists for stem cell proliferation and differentiation. Many excellent reviews exist which describe the experiments leading to the development of this model system.[26,237–240] Sequential microscopic analysis of hematopoietic colonies developing in the spleen and bone marrow after inoculation of bone marrow cells into mice given a potentially lethal dosage of irradiation demonstrated that at first colonies containing one cell lineage developed after which colonies containing more than one cell lineage were found. Cells derived from colonies containing only one cell lineage were able to, upon reassay for CFU-S, give rise to colonies containing cells other than or in addition to cells of the original lineage. Moreover the ratio of erythroid to granulocytic colonies differed in the spleen where it was approximately 3 from that of the marrow where it was 0.5. When marrow stroma was transplanted into the spleen it was noticed that when colonies containing mixtures of erythroid and granulocytic cells were growing across both the spleen and marrow segments those cells within the spleenic domain were mainly erythroid while those cells in the marrow domain were mainly granulocytic.[26] The readers are referred to the review articles[26,237–240] and the primary papers quoted in these reviews for an extensive look at the experimental maneuvers which formed the basis for this theory.

While many studies concentrated on the effects of irradiation and drugs to the stem cell pool, it became clear that these treatments could also influence the environment into which these cells had seeded. The hematopoietic stromal cells have been assayed by transplantation of intact hematopoietic organs.[241–247] It has been shown that implantation of femoral marrow subcutaneously is followed in progressive fashion by loss of cells, proliferation of primitive mesenchymal tissue, formation of sinusoids, and the reconstitution of blood cell formation. The blood cells were believed to have been derived from the host CFU-S,[246,247] but the stroma was considered to be of donor origin.[247] Thus implantation subcutaneously of femurs and spleens has been considered to provide an assay for assessment of hematopoietic stromal cell influences.[241] Exposure to split dosages of irradiation[242] or to 950 rad X-irradiation impairs the function of the implanted stroma cells,[244,247,248] and no detectable recovery is seen for at least 6 weeks after the irradiation.[241,249] However, the number of CFU-S recovers to normal within 6 weeks. It was suggested that a submaximal stromal defect reduced the accumulation rate or proliferation of CFU-S in the site, but not necessarily the number that could be supported. Radiation sensitivity studies on cells which transfer the hematopoietic microenvironment were performed in mice in which femoral bone marrow was transplanted under the renal capsule of a mouse.[250] The D_o for in vitro gamma irradiation of these transferring units was 444 ± 5 rad and a quasi-threshold dose was approximately 500 rad which suggested a high capacity for repair of sublethal injury. The D_o for in vivo exposure was 325 ± 25 with a quasi-threshold dose of 635 rad. It was calculated that one femoral marrow plug contained about 50 hematopoietic microenvironment transferring units. Both cyclosphamide and busulphan have been shown also to damage the function of hematopoietic stroma cells.[251]

The livers of adult mice have been shown to contain CFU-S after repeated irradiation,[252] but it has been suggested that while CFU-S are found in livers of mice whose marrow cells have been oblated by ^{89}strontium these CFU-S do not proliferate.[253]

3. *Transient Receptor Theory*

Another concept of the regulation of stem cells involves stem cell differentiation based on inducers of differentiation which act on the same population of cells, but which demonstrate selectivity dependent on the time of synthesis of specific receptors for the inducers.[254] Support for this theory derives from the noted effects of erythropoietin on CFU-S.[255] Preincubation of bone marrow cells with erythropoietin prior to inoculation of the cells into irradiated mice resulted in an increase in the number of

CFU-S, which was dependent on the amount of erythropoietin added. This increase was due entirely to an increase in erythroid colonies.

B. Cell and Cell-Free Stimulatory and Inhibitory Feedback Mechanisms

Since the inital experiments which suggested that stem cell proliferation was controlled by stochastic[235] and/or hematopoietic inductive microenvironmental influences,[26] there has been a substantial literature developing around cell and cell-derived regulators. In essence, both stimulatory and inhibitory activities have been implicated.

The consideration that there are self-contained stem cell regulatory volumes or domains in mouse bone marrow led to a study of the kinetics of bone marrow replacement in W/W^v mice given stem cells from bg^J/bg^J (beige) mice.[256] Dose response curves suggested random seeding of stem cells in the host marrow and a decrease in the efficiency of secondary colonization by local migration. It was estimated that the W/W^v marrow contained approximately 2600 stem cell regulatory units with an average volume of 10^8 μm^3 which was considered to be consistent with the role of short range cell interactions in the regulation of stem cells.

Lymphoid cells have been implicated in the regulatory interactions.[257] It had been shown that when thymus cells which were syngeneic to marrow cells injected, but allogeneic to the recipient, were added there was an enhancement in spleen colony formation.[258] In a completely syngeneic system no enhancement was seen. In a different and probably unrelated experimental procedure it was noted that live thymus cells were necessary for spleen colony formation enhancement when the injected bone marrow cells were previously irradiated or when endogenous spleen colony formation in sublethally irradiated mice was assessed.[259] The influence of the thymus cells was apparent if they were given simultaneously with or 1 day after the injection of irradiated marrow cells, but not if they were given 2 days before the marrow cells. The effectiveness of the thymus cells was reduced even if given 1 day prior to the marrow cells. Optimal effectiveness was accomplished with 10^6 thymus cells, but if the thymus cells were killed they were not effective. Moreover, live thymus cells had no influence on spleen colony formation of nonirradiated donor marrow cells.

Although seeding efficiency was not calculated for the injected cells, changes in seeding efficiency were ruled out as a cause of the effects noticed. It had been suggested that a rabbit antimouse brain antiserum cross-reacted with antigenic determinants on pluripotential stem cells (CFU-S), and in the presence of complement the antisera could kill CFU-S as detected by a decrease in the number of spleen colonies seen.[89] However, it was suggested that, in fact, the antiserum was probably acting on an accessory cell necessary for the proliferation of cells derived from CFU-S.[98] The numbers of spleen colonies derived from bone marrow cells previously treated with the antiserum and complement could be restored to control values if the treated inoculum of bone marrow cells was injected into recipient mice with live thymus cells or if live thymus cells were injected within 1 day of the bone marrow suspension. Thymus cells irradiated with 1600 rad of gamma irradiation could not mimic this action. The live thymus cells had no effect on spleen colony formation by untreated donor bone marrow cells. Subdivision of donor bone marrow cells by density gradient separation demonstrated that the influence of the thymus cells was confined to CFU-S with a density greater than 1.075 g/cm^3. Thymus cell addition did not effect the seeding efficiency of CFU-S and preliminary experiments suggested that the enhancing activity of thymus cells was not due to a Thy-1 positive cell.

Interestingly, at least two populations of accessory cells for rat bone marrow CFU-S have been distinguished. These include putative helper cells which were strongly Thy-1 positive and cortisone sensitive and putative suppressor cells which were weakly Thy-

1 positive and cortisone resistant.[110] Further evidence for the role of thymus derived cells on this type of system came from studies on thymectomized mice which had decreased spleen colony forming cell capacity and whose CFU-S were cycling at a slower rate.[260] An increase in spleen colonies and cycling status of CFU-S was noted after implantation, into thymectomized mice, of thymus lobes in diffusion chambers or after addition of a thymus derived substance. The actions were restricted to thymectomized mice. Other T-cell derived substances have been implicated in stem cell regulation.[261–263] These mediators included a stem-cell activating material in the supernatant from lymphocytes stimulated by phytohemagglutinin and a material obtained in partially purified form from the supernatant of lymphocytes which were stimulated antigenically.[261,262] Both substances increased numbers of spleen colony forming cells, but only the former one stimulated DNA synthesis in the total population of bone marrow cells. This substance appeared to activate CFU-S in vitro rather than merely increasing the survival of these cells. The biological activity did not appear to be restricted by the K and Ia regions of the mouse histocompatibility complex (H_2).

The need for the presence of a theta-sensitive cell in normal bone marrow, thymus, and spleen for the promotion of differentiation of CFU-S along the erythroid pathway has been suggested.[264,265] These studies were performed in W/W^v mice which have a macrocytic anemia and defective CFU-S and the interpretation based on the fact that normal littermate thymocytes, when added to normal littermate bone marrow cells which had been first treated with antisera to Thy-1.2 plus complement, restored the ability of these bone marrow cells to cure the anemia in W/W^v mice.[10] These antitheta sensitive ''helper'' cells were deficient in W/W^v mice. The ''helper'' cells survived 1050 rad in vitro, the numbers needed were small (10^3 to 10^4), and the cells had to be injected at the same time as the marrow cells suggesting the need for close cell contact between these cells and the stem cells.[265] The anti theta-sensitive regulatory cell was found to bear the surface phenotype, anti-thymocyte globulin$^-$, mouse T-lymphocyte-specific antigen$^-$, Thy 1.2$^+$, Ly 1$^+$, 2$^-$, 3$^-$, and Ia$^-$.[266]

Other reports have indicated the presence of stem cell stimulatory activities.[267–273] Proliferation of stem cells was shown to be dependent on a fibroblast-derived factor which was apparently different from the factors necessary for stimulation of granulocyte-macrophage progenitor cells.[267] However, the actual cell of derivation of this substance may be open to further investigation as it has now become clear that very rigorous tests are needed to confirm that a cell can indeed be classified as a fibroblast.[274] Medium conditioned by human peripheral blood leukocytes has been reported to contain an initiator of DNA synthesis in CFU-S, which corresponds to increased maintenance of CFU-S and which increases numbers of granulocyte-macrophage progenitor cells.[268] Medium conditioned by mouse marrow adherent cells has been shown to increase the 24 hr survival of CFU-S in vitro.[269] Interestingly, medium conditioned by cells from Sl/Sl^d and W/W^v mice was as effective as medium conditioned by marrow cells from normal mice suggesting that the defective microenvironment of Sl/Sl^d mice was not due to a deficiency in production of this factor.

Studies on irradiated mice have allowed the suggestion that irradiation damage might cause the release of a humoral substance which stimulates proliferation of CFU-S surviving the irradiation[270] and pretreatment of mice with cyclophosphamide enhances stem cell recovery in mice subsequently subjected to irradiation.[271,272] Maximum enhancement occurred when cyclophosphamide was given 2 to 3 days before irradiation and marrow transplantation and was observed even at dosages of cyclophosphamide which were relatively toxic to the stem cells.[272] It was suggested that these effects might have been mediated by cell-cell interactions or by the release of humoral regulators,[271] and more recent evidence suggests a humorally mediated effect.[273] Similar studies have been reported by others.[275] Strontium-89 (^{89}Sr) is a beta-emitting, bone seeking radionuclide with a 55 day halflife and has been used to ablate the marrows of 12 to 16 week old CAF_1 mice. It was suggested that the spleen, after ^{89}Sr-irradiation to the mice, became a prime supplier of stem cells and that the spleen might suppress marrow stem cell proliferation in normal mice.[276] It was suggested that the granulocytic pool might regulate this proliferation. When bone marrow cells placed in diffusion chambers were implanted into ^{89}Sr-treated mice there was an enhancement in stem cell numbers above those in diffusion chambers inplanted into mice treated with cold-^{89}Sr.[277] A humoral stimulus was postulated for this effect.

Inhibitors of stem cell proliferation have also been detected. In has been suggested that cells in S-phase might inhibit the entry of noncycling cells into cycle,[278,279] and a substance extracted from the marrow of fetal calves was able to inhibit cycling of CFU-S induced by prior low dose irradiation (150 rad) of the animal.[280] This effect was not seen with extracts derived from thymic or liver cells. The dialysate of fetal bone marrow extracts was capable, when injected simultaneously with the drug Ara-C, of protecting a certain proportion of CFU-S against drug killing without a protective effect on nucleated cells or granulocyte-macrophage progenitor cells.[280] The use of a double diffusion chamber system implanted into mice has noted the elaboration of a diffusible material from both regenerating and steady state bone marrow cells which prevented CFU-S from entering cell cycle. Mature granulocytes and macrophages did not appear to be the source of these substances.[281]

The roles of stimulatory and inhibitory substances have been discussed,[282–285] and elaborate studies have defined more precisely the role of stimulatory and inhibitory factors in regulation of stem cell proliferation.[286–292] An extract of bone marrow cells from untreated mice contained an activity resident in the molecular weight range of 50,000 to 100,000 daltons which protected rapidly proliferating CFU-S from the lethal effects of tritiated thymidine.[286] This substance was not detected in bone marrow cells which were in active regeneration and was not toxic as it had no direct effect on numbers of CFU-S or on the granulocyte-macrophage progenitor cells. It was suggested that the active fraction might be a protein as it was inactivated by treatment with trypsin. A stimulator of CFU-S was detected in the molecular weight range of 30,000 to 50,000 daltons.[287] Further studies demonstrated that both stimulatory and inhibitory factors could be detected from bone marrow cells undergoing normal and regenerative proliferation, but high stimulatory activity was seen in cell suspensions with rapidly proliferating CFU-S and inhibitory activity was seen in those suspensions with slowly proliferating CFU-S.[288] Inhibitory activity was elaborated from bone marrow cells with a density of 1.052 to 1.060 g/cm^3 and stimulatory activity derived from cells with a density of 1.064 to 1.072 g/cm^3.[289] It has also been found that medium conditioned by normal human bone marrow cells contains an inhibitor of mouse CFU-S proliferation[290] similar in molecular ultrafiltration and dose response analysis to that isolated from freshly isolated mouse bone marrow cells.[286]

Studies on proliferation kinetics of CFU-S in long-term mouse bone marrow cultures[291] led to a study of proliferation inhibitors and stimulators in these cultures.[292] CFU-S have been detected in both the adherent and nonadherent layers in long-term cultures and CFU-S in the adherent layer were able to regenerate themselves and the nonadherent cells. It had been noted that one day after refeeding the cultures by removal of half the growth medium and addition of fresh culture medium both adherent and nonadherent CFU-S were actively cycling, whereas 5 to 7 days after refeeding most of the CFU-S were in slower cycle.[291] The mechanisms of this phenomenon were investigated.[292] It was noted that shortly after refeeding of the cultures, when CFU-S were in cycle, there were high levels of stimulator and later, when more slowly cycling CFU-S were detected, high levels of an inhibitor could be seen. The stimulatory and inhibitory substances appeared similar to those previously reported from freshly isolated marrow.[286,287] It was shown that the inhibitor could suppress proliferation of rapidly cycling CFU-S and the stimulator could enhance proliferation of the slowly cycling CFU-S within the culture.

The results presented in this section suggest that pluripotential hematopoietic stem cell proliferation both in vitro and in vivo may be regulated by opposing stimulatory and inhibitory activities. Future studies will no doubt define better the biochemistry of these molecules as well as the stimulus for their production and any molecules which may modulate this production.

VIII. APPLICATION OF STEM CELL KNOWLEDGE

A. Human Bone Marow Transplantation, Cryopreservation of Bone Marrow Cells and Animal Models of Disease Involving Defects in Stem Cells

Some select patients with severe combined immunodeficiency disease, aplastic anemia, and acute and chronic leukemia are considered candidates for treatment by bone marrrow transplantation. Four types of grafts are distinguishable between the host and donor.[293] These include, autologous bone marrow grafts in which the marrow to be grafted is placed back into the same donor from which it was removed, isogeneic grafts in which the host and donor are identical genetically and marrow is collected from an identical twin or in the case of animals from those of the same inbred strain, allogeneic grafts in which genetic differences exist between the donor and recipient but are from the same species, and xenogeneic grafts in which donor and host are from different species. Treatment by bone marrow transplantation was at the beginning reserved for those donors who had what was considered to be an end stage disease for which the currently available treatment protocols were no longer of use. The most successful transplants have been those from siblings matched with the patients at the major histocompatibility complex. It is beyond the scope of this chapter to discuss the genetics of transplantation but there are useful reviews on this for man[294] and mouse.[295,296]

Reviews of bone marrow transplantation are prevalent[297–300] and updated continuously. Information is now available on many clinical trials and this has suggested that treatment of patients who are not at the terminal stage of disease might profit better from bone marrow transplantation, and such treatments have now been extended to patients with acute leukemia during remission[301,302] and with chronic leukemia during the nonterminal phase.[303–305] Cures of leukemia have been reported after transplantation procedures,[306] but relapses are still frequent and there are reports of leukemia occurring in the cells originally derived from the normal donor.[307–311] The critical issues[312] and factors influencing the success and failure[313] of clinical bone marrow transplantation have been discussed. Among these issues are complications associated with high-dose chemotherapy or irradiation, the failure of the tissue to graft, graft-vs.-host disease, severe infections due to bacteria, fungus and viruses, immunoincompetence, and other late developments.[297] Experimental studies to evaluate some of these conditions have been described.[314]

In addition to transplantation with bone marrow cells, the combined use of fetal liver and thymus for immunological reconstitution in patients with variants of severe combined immunodeficiency has been considered.[315] To overcome many of the complications associated with allogeneic transplantation, the transplantation of autologous marrow has been considered and tried.[316–318] Two rationales are involved in autologous marrow transplantation. In nonleukemic patients with cancer it would be possible to place these patients under more intensive chemotherapeutic regimens and then rescue them from bone marrow and hematological failure by giving them back their own marrow cells.[316] In patients with leukemia it is hoped that marrow could be taken from patients during the remission phase of acute leukemia or the chronic phase of chronic leukemia, when the load of leukemia cells would be considered to be very low, and then frozen and returned to the same patients during the acute phase of their diseases and after intensive chemotherapy.[316–318] One of the crucial points in bone marrow transplantation, especially in the situation of autologous transplantation, is the cryopreservation and subsequent retrieval of viable and functional stem, progenitor, and perhaps even more mature cells. Techniques of cryopreservation have been refined[319,319–322] and various means of studying the functional capacities of these cells have been suggested.[323–325] The newer technologies discussed in Sections VI B and VI C of this chapter will also be valuable procedures for monitoring patients before and after bone marrow transplantation.

The phenomenon of hybrid, allogeneic, and xenogeneic resistance to marrow grafting has been observed in animal models.[326–329] One of these situations in paticular has been studied and revolves around the fact that bone marrow cells from parental mice would not grow in F_1 hybrids. Several names, including "hybrid resistance", "colony forming unit repression" and "poor growth phenomenon" have been used to describe this phenomenon.[330–332] This resistance did not fit into the then classical laws of genetics and was described as follows. It was mediated by an antigraft reaction that was immunologically specific, insensitive to a single exposure to whole body irradiation, was thymus-independent, suppressible by antimacrophage agents, and was genetically determined by a number of distinct noncodominant Hh (hemopoietic histocompatibility) genes, the strongest one (Hh-1) mapping in or near the D region.[326–329] An in vitro assay to study this has been described[333,334] as have various cells and agents which abrogate the manifestations of the phenomenon.[335–338]

Other animal models exist which have been useful in the study of stem cell proliferation and disease progression. The use of mice with genetic anemias has been valuable in dissecting out the influence of the stem cells themselves and factors which modulate their growth[339–341] and background information on these mice has been reviewed.[339] Two strains of mice of particular usefulness have been the W/W^v and Sl^d. It has been shown that the Sl/Sl^d anemia is intrinsic to the cells which constitute the environment influencing the stem cells. Studies on mice with autoimmune hemolytic anemia have demonstrated that NZB mice showed normal CFU-S activity when transplanted, but elevated levels of endogenous CFU-S. NZC mice which had elevated levels of endogenous CFU-S demonstrated defect when CFU-S were exogenously transplanted into them. It was suggested that NZC mice had a defect in the microenvironment of the spleen which did not allow them to nuture transplanted CFU-S.[324] In addition, an experimental model of chronic hypoplastic marrow failure has been induced in mice with a short course of busulphan.[343,344] The drug produced residual marrow damage characterized by mild or moderate marrow failure with defects in stem and progenitor cells. It was suggested in later works that unrecognized marrow damage could be an etiological factor in marrow failure due to drug idiosyncrasy.[345] Aplasia in mice has also been investigated in mice so induced by immunological methods and stem and progenitor cells were also decreased.[346] It was considered that this model would be useful in investigating the pathogenesis of aplastic anemia.

Studies with animal model systems such as those listed above will most likely yield valuable information to help us to understand better the genetic and cellular processes involved in human bone marrow transplantation.

B. Molecular Modification

The ability to transfer genes to cells which can repopulate the hematopoietic system of a recipient and then maintain a selective proliferative advantage is of clinical importance. Such applications have been suggested[346] and include: the transfer of drug-resistance genes which might help patients with cancer tolerate higher dosages of chemotherapeutic agents and insertion of these drug resistance genes attached to other genes which might modify certain human genetic diseases such as sickle cell disease and thalassemia. Recently,[346] the insertion and selection for genes conferring resistance to methotrexate in bone marrow cells of intact mice has been described. This procedure followed up on successes for inserting DNA into cells in culture.

Mouse bone marrow cells with a distinctive chromosome marker (T6T6) from CBA/T6T6 mice were obtained from intact mice treated previously with vinblastine in order to enrich the number of proliferating and hematopoietic stem and progenitor cells. The isolated marrow cells were treated in culture with a calcium microprecipate of DNA from a mouse cell line selected for resistance to methotrexate and containing reiterated sequences of genes coding for dihydrofolate reductase. Methotrexate is a drug with antiproliferative capacity and acts as a folic acid antagonist by inhibiting dihydrofolate reductase. Mouse bone marrow cells from the syngeneic mouse strain CBA/Ca were similarly removed but subjected to mock transformation procedures with control DNA lacking methotrexate resistence sequences. A 1:1 mixture of T6T6 and Ca cells were injected into genetically compatible animals that had been irradiated to reduce endogenous hematopoiesis. During the period of cellular regeneration the mice were treated with methotrexate to allow for a proliferative advantage for those cells which had taken in a functional gene for dehydrofolate reductase. The hematological status of mice receiving the "transformed" bone marrow treated with the resistance-conferring DNA in vitro returned to normal despite persistent treatment with methotrexate. No micro- or macro-scopic abnormalities were detected in sections of visceral organs upon autopsy at intervals of up to 150 days after transformation, and the mice were clinically well before death. It was found also that dehydrofolate reductase-specific activity was two to four times greater in the spleen cell extracts from mice receiving the "transformed" bone marrow than in controls, and the T6T6 karyotype was shown to predominate in the pluripotential hematopoietic stem cell, or progenitor cell compartments. It has not been determined yet if the inserted genes had become integrated into the nuclear or cytoplasmic DNA. It has been demonstrated by similar means that the gene for the herpes simplex virus thymidine kinase could be inserted into the DNA of marrow cells which could then repopulate the marrow of irradiated recipients.[348] At first DNA containing the herpes simplex virus thymidine kinase gene was used to transform wild type tK^+ mouse L cells to a tK^{++} state in culture using methotrexate as a selective agent. In vitro transformed marrow cells when then injected into the irradiated mice. The methotrexate-treated recipient mice allowed the proliferation predominately of the population of cells containing the appropriate gene sequences.

Several questions have been proposed regarding the above studies.[349] It must be determined if the resistant genes will remain with the cells, if correct control can be restored over the introduced genes, and if the required genes can be inserted into the appropriate position on the chromosome. Methods must be available to balance the expression of the newly introduced genes.

REFERENCES

1. **Lajtha, L. G.** (Rapporteur), Haemopoietic stem cells: concepts and definitions, *Blood Cells*, 5, 447, 1979.
2. **Yoffey, J. M.,** Stem cell role of the lymphocyte-transitional cell (LT) compartment, in *Haemopoietic Stem Cells*, North-Holland, New York, 1973, 5.
3. **Dicke, K. A., van Noord, M. J., Maat, B., Schaeffer, U. W., and van Bekkum, D. W.,** Attempts at morphological identification of haemopoietic stem cells in primates and rodents, in *Haemopoietic Stem Cells*, North-Holland, New York, 1973, 47.
4. **Moore, M. A. S.,** In vitro studies in the myeloid leukemias, in *Advances in Acute Leukemia*, Clefton, F. J., Crowther, D., and Malpas, J. S., Eds., North-Holland, New York, 1974, 161.
5. **McCulloch, E. A.,** Control of hematopoiesis at the cellular level, in *Regulation of Hematopoiesis*, Vol. 1, Gordon, A. S., Ed., Appleton-Century-Crofts, New York, 1970, 133.
6. **Metcalf, D. and Moore, M. A. S.,** *Haemopoietic Cells*, North-Holland, New York, 1971.
7. **Schofield, R.,** The pluripotential stem cell, in *Clinics in Haematology*, Vol. 8, W. B. Saunders, London, 1979, 221.
8. **Lorenz, E., Uphoff, D., Reid, T. R., and Shelton, E.,** Modification of irradiation injury in mice and guinea pigs by bone marrow injections, *J. Natl. Cancer Inst.*, 12, 197, 1951.
9. **Jacobson, L. O., Marks, E. K., and Gaston, E. O.,** Observations on the effect of spleen-shielding and the injection of cell suspensions on survival following irradiation, in *Radiobiology Symposium*, Bacq, Z. M. and Alexander, P., Eds., Butterworths, London, 1954, 122.
10. **Lindsley, D. L., Odell, T. T., Jr., and Tausche, F. G.,** Implantation of functional erythropoietic elements following whole body irradiation, *Proc. Soc. Exp. Biol. Med.*, 90, 512, 1955.
11. **Ford, C. E., Hamerton, J. L., Barnes, D. W. H., and Loutit, J. F.,** Cytological identification of radiation chimaeras, *Nature*, 177, 452, 1956.
12. **Nowell, P. C., Cole, L. J., Habermeyer, J. G., and Roan, P. L.,** Growth and continued function of rat marrow cells in X-radiated mice, *Cancer Res.*, 16, 258, 1956.
13. **Urso, P. and Congdon, C. C.,** The effect of the amount of isologous bone marrow injected after lethal irradiation injury in mice, *Blood*, 12, 251, 1957.
14. **McCulloch, E. A. and Till, J. E.,** The radiation sensitivity of normal mouse bone marrow cells, determined by quantitative marrow transplantation into irradiated mice, *Radiat. Res.*, 13, 115, 1960.
15. **Smith, L. H. and Vos, O.,** Sensitivity and protection of bone marrow cells X-irradiated *in vitro, Int. J. Radiat. Biol.*, 5, 461, 1962.
16. **Till, J. E. and McCulloch, E. A.,** A direct measurement of the radiation sensitivity of normal mouse bone marrow cells, *Radiat. Res.*, 14, 213, 1961.
17. **McCulloch, E. A. and Till, J. E.,** The sensitivity of cells from normal mouse bone to gamma radiation *in vitro* and *in vivo*, *Radiat. Res.*, 16, 822, 1962.
18. **Becker, A. J., McCulloch, E. A., and Till, J. E.,** Cytological demonstration of the clonal nature of spleen colonies derived from transplanted mouse marrow cells, *Nature*, 197, 452, 1963.
19. **Becker, A. J., McCulloch, E. A., Siminovitch, L., and Till, J. E.,** The effect of differing demands for blood cell production in DNA synthesis by hemopoietic colony forming cells of mice, *Blood*, 26, 296, 1965.
20. **McCulloch, E. A. and Till, J. E.,** Proliferation of hemopoietic colony-forming cells transplanted into irradiated mice, *Radiat. Res.*, 22, 383, 1964.
21. **Till, J. E. and McCulloch, E. A.,** The f-factor of the spleen-colony assay for hemopoietic stem cells, *Ser. Haematol.*, 5, 15, 1972.
22. **Fred, S. S. and Smith, W. W.,** Induced changes in transplantability of hemopoietic colony-forming cells, *Proc. Soc. Exp. Biol. Med.*, 128, 364, 1968.
23. **Lord, B. I. and Hendry, J. H.,** Observations on the settling and recoverability of transplanted hemopoietic colony-forming units in the mouse spleen, *Blood*, 41, 409, 1973.
24. **Monette, F. C. and deMello, J. B.,** The relationship between stem cell seeding efficiency and position in cell cycle, *Cell Tissue Kinet.*, 12, 161, 1979.
25. **Siminovitch, L., McCulloch, E. A., and Till, J. E.,** The distribution of colony-forming cells among spleen colonies, *J. Cell. Comp. Physiol.*, 62, 327, 1963.
26. **Trentin, J. J.,** Influence of hematopoietic organ stroma (hematopoietic inductive microenvironments) on stem cell differentiation, in *Regulation of Hematopoiesis*, Vol. 1, Gordon, A. S., Ed., Appleton-Century-Crofts, New York, 1970, 161.
27. **Jenkins, V. K., Trentin, J. J., Speirs, R. S., and McGarry, M. P.,** Hemopoietic colony studies. VI. Increased eosinophil-containing colonies obtained by antigen pre-treatment of irradiated mice reconstituted with bone marrow cells, *J. Cell. Physiol.*, 79, 413, 1972.

28. **Till, J. E.,** Overlap error in counts of splenic colonies, *Ser. Haematol.*, 5, 5, 1972.
29. **Blackett, N. M.,** Statistical accuracy to be expected from cell colony assays; with special reference to the spleen colony assay, *Cell Tissue Kinet.*, 7, 407, 1974.
30. **Hodgson, G. S. and Bradley, T. R.,** Properties of haemopoietic stem cells surviving 5-fluorouracil treatment: evidence for a pre-CFU-S cell?, *Nature,* 281, 381, 1979.
31. **Kitamura, Y., Tamai, M., Miyano, Y., and Shimada, M.,** Development of hematopoietic spleen colonies in nonirradiated genetically normal mice, *Blood,* 50, 1121, 1977.
32. **Davis, W. E., Jr., Cole, L. J., and Shaffer, W. I.,** Graft-versus-host reactions in nonirradiated mice. Early suppression of Jerne plaque and hemopoietic colony-forming units, *Transplantation,* 9, 529, 1970.
33. **Brecher, G., Tjio, J. H., Haley, J. E., Narla, J., and Beal, S. L.,** Transplantation of murine bone marrow without prior host irradiation, *Blood Cells,* 5, 237, 1979.
34. **Smith, W. W., Bud, R. A., and Cornfield, J.,** Estimation of radiation dose-reduction factor for β-mercaptoethylamine by endogenous spleen colony counts, *Radiat. Res.*, 27, 363, 1966.
35. **Boggs, S. S., Chervenick, P. A., and Boggs, D. R.,** The effect of postirradiation bleeding or endotoxin on proliferation and differentiation of hematopoietic stem cells, *Blood,* 40, 375, 1972.
36. **Chervenick, P. A. and Boggs, D. R.,** Patterns of proliferation and differentiation of hemopoietic stem cells after compartment depletion, *Blood,* 37, 568, 1971.
37. **Boggs, S. S., Boggs, D. R., Neil, G. L., and Sartiano, G.,** Cycling characteristics of endogenous spleen colony forming cells as measured with cytosine arabinoside and methotrexate, *J. Lab. Clin. Med.*, 82, 727, 1973.
38. **Wolf, N. S. and Trentin, J. J.,** Linearity of counts of endogenous and exogenous colonies in mouse bone marrow, *Exp. Hematol.*, 3, 54, 1975.
39. **Broxmeyer, H. E. and Moore, M. A. S.,** Communication between white cells and the abnormalities of this in leukemia, *Biochem. Biophys. Acta, Reviews on Cancer,* 516, 129, 1978.
40. **Metcalf, D.,** *Hemopoietic Colonies,* Springer-Verlag, Berlin, 1977.
41. **McLeod, D. L., Shreeve, M. M., and Axelrad, A. A.,** Induction of megakaryocytic colonies with platelet formation in vitro, *Nature,* 261, 492, 1976.
42. **Hara, J. and Ogawa, M.,** Murine hemopoietic colonies in culture containing normablasts, macrophages and megakaryocytes, *Am. J. Hematol.*, 4, 23, 1978.
43. **Johnson, G. R. and Metcalf, D.,** Pure and mixed erythroid colony formation in vitro stimulated by spleen conditioned medium with no detectable erythropoietin, *Proc. Natl. Acad. Sci. U.S.A.*, 74, 3879, 1977.
44. **Zucali, J. R., Stevens, V., and Mirand, E. A.,** In vitro production of erythropoietin by mouse fetal liver, *Blood,* 46, 85, 1975.
45. **Johnson, G. R. and Metcalf, D.,** Nature of cells forming erythroid colonies in agar after stimulation by spleen conditioned medium, *J. Cell. Physiol.*, 94, 243, 1978.
46. **Metcalf, D., Johnson, G. R., and Mandel, T. E.,** Colony formation in agar by multipotential hemopoietic cells, *J. Cell. Physiol.*, 98, 401, 1979.
47. **Johnson, G. R.,** Colony formation in agar by adult bone marrow multipotential hemopoietic cells, *J. Cell. Physiol.*, 103, 371, 1980.
48. **Metcalf, D. and Johnson, G. R.,** Production by spleen and lymph node cells of conditioned medium with erythroid and other hemopoietic colony-stimulating activity, *J. Cell. Physiol.*, 96, 31, 1978.
49. **Metcalf, D. and Johnson, G. R.,** Interactions between purified GM-CSF, purified erythropoietin and spleen conditioned medium on hemopoietic colony formation in vitro, *J. Cell. Physiol.*, 99, 159, 1979.
50. **Metcalf, D., Johnson, G. R., and Burgess, A. W.,** Direct stimulation by purified GM-CSF of the proliferation of multi-potential and erythroid precursor cells, *Blood,* 55, 138, 1980.
51. **Nowell, P. C. and Wilson, D. B.,** Lymphocytes and hemic stem cells, *Am. J. Pathol.*, 65, 641, 1971.
52. **Phillips R. A.,** Stem cell heterogeneity: pluripotent and committed stem cells of the myeloid and lymphoid systems, in *Differentiation of Normal and Neoplastic Hematopoietic Cells,* Book A, Clarkson, B., Marks, P. A., and Till, J. E., Eds., Cold Spring Harbor Laboratory, 1978, 109.
53. **Barnes, D. W. H., Ford, C. E., Gray, S. M., and Loutit, J. F.,** Spontaneous and induced changes in cell populations in heavily irradiated mice, *Prog. Nucl. Energy Ser. 6,* 2, 1, 1959.
54. **Micklem, H. S., Ford, C. E., Evans, E. P., and Gray, J.,** Interrelationships of myeloid and lymphoid cells: studies with chromosome-marked cells transfused into lethally irradiated mice, *Proc. R. Soc. Lond. Ser. B.*, 165, 78, 1966.
55. **Trentin, J., Wolf, N., Cheng, V., Fahlberg, W., Weiss, D., and Bonhag, R.,** Antibody production by mice repopulated with limited numbers of clones of lymphoid cell precursors, *J. Immunol.*, 98, 1326, 1967.

56. **Yung, L. L. L., Wyn-Evans, T. C., and Diener, E.,** Ontogeny of the murine immune system: development of antigen recognition and immune responsiveness, *Eur. J. Immunol.*, 3, 224, 1973.
57. **Wu, A. M., Till, J. E., Siminovitch, L., and McCulloch, E. A.,** Cytological evidence for a relationship between normal hemopoietic colony-forming cells and cells of the lymphoid system, *J. Exp. Med.*, 127, 455, 1968.
58. **Nowell, P. C., Hirsch, B. E., Fox, D. H., and Wilson, D. B.,** Evidence for the existence of multipotential lympho-hematopoietic stem cells in the adult rat, *J. Cell. Physiol.*, 75, 151, 1970.
59. **Edwards, G. E., Miller, R. G., and Phillips, R. A.,** Differentiation of rosette-forming cells from myeloid stem cells, *J. Immunol.*, 105, 719, 1970.
60. **Abramson, S., Miller, R. G., and Phillips, R. A.,** The identification in adult bone marrow of pluripotential and restricted stem cells of the myeloid and lymphoid systems, *J. Exp. Med.*, 145, 1567, 1977.
61. **Phillips, R. A., Jones, E. V., and Miller, R. G.,** Differentiative potential of hemopoietic stem cells, in *Hematopoietic Cell Differentiation*, Golde, D. W., Cline, M. J., Metcalf, D., and Fox, C. F., Eds., Academic Press, New York, 1978, 129.
62. **El-Arini, M. O. and Osoba, D.,** Differentiation of thymus-derived cells from precursors in mouse bone marrow, *J. Exp. Med.*, 137, 821, 1973.
63. **Paige, C. J., Kincade, P. W., Moore, M. A. S., and Lee, G.,** The fate of fetal and adult B-cell progenitors grafted into immunodeficient CBA/N mice, *J. Exp. Med.*, 150, 548, 1979.
64. **Paige, C. J., Kincade, P. W., Shinefeld, L. A., and Sata, V. L.,** Precursors of murine B lymphocytes. Physical and functional characterization, and distinctions from myeloid stem cells, *J. Exp. Med.*, 152, 458, 1980.
65. **Kincade, P. W.,** Defective colony formation by B lymphocytes from CBA/N and C3H/HeJ mice, *J. Exp. Med.*, 145, 249, 1977.
66. **Kincade, P. W., Moore, M. A. S., Lee, G., and Paige, C. J.,** Colony-forming B cells in F1 hybrid and transplanted CBA/N mice, *Cell. Immunol.*, 40, 294, 1978.
67. **Worton, R. G., McCulloch, E. A., and Till, J. E.,** Physical separation of hemopoietic stem cells from cells forming colonies in cultures, *J. Cell. Physiol.*, 74, 171, 1969.
68. **Haskill, J. S., McNeill, T. A., and Moore, M. A. S.,** Density distribution analysis of *in vivo* and *in vitro* colony forming cells in bone marrow, *J. Cell. Physiol.*, 75, 167, 1970.
69. **Messner, H., Till, J. E., and McCulloch, E. A.,** Density distributions of marrow cells from mouse and man, *Ser. Haematol.*, 5, 22, 1972.
70. **Worton, R. G., McCulloch, E. A., and Till, J. E.,** Physical separation of hemopoietic stem cells differing in their capacity for self-renewal, *J. Exp. Med.*, 130, 91, 1969.
71. **Metcalf, D. and Moore, M. A. S.,** *Haemopoietic Cells*, North-Holland, New York, 1971, 98.
72. **Monette, F. C., Gilio, M. J., and Chalifoux, P.,** Separation of proliferating CFU from Go cells of murine bone marrow, *Cell Tissue Kinet.*, 7, 443, 1974.
73. **Visser, J., van den Engh, G., Williams, N., and Mulder, D.,** Physical separation of the cycling and non-cycling compartments of murine hemopoietic stem cells, in *Experimental Hematology Today*, Baum, S. J. and Ledney, G. D., Eds., Springer-Verlag, New York, 1977, 21.
74. **Haskill, J. S. and Moore, M. A. S.,** Two dimensional cell separation: comparison of embryonic and adult haemopoietic stem cells, *Nature*, 226, 853, 1970.
75. **Moore, M. A. S., McNeill, T. A., and Haskill, J. S.,** Density distribution analysis of *in vivo* and *in vitro* colony forming cells in developing fetal liver, *J. Cell. Physiol.*, 75, 181, 1970.
76. **Metcalf, D., Moore, M. A. S., and Shortman, K.,** Adherence column and buoyant density separation of bone marrow stem cells and more differentiated cells, *J. Cell. Physiol.*, 78, 441, 1971.
77. **Pretlow, T. G., Williams, E. E., Davis, M. L., and Zettergren, J. G.,** Separation of spleen colony forming units (CFU-s) from mouse bone marrow cells using velocity sedimentation in an isokinetic gradient of ficoll in tissue culture medium, *Am. J. Pathol.*, 72, 201, 1973.
78. **Stephenson, J. R. and Axelrad, A. A.,** Separation of erythropoietin-sensitive cells from hemopoietic spleen colony-forming stem cells of mouse fetal liver by unit gravity sedimentation, *Blood*, 37, 417, 1971.
79. **Blazi-Poljak, M. and Boranic, M.,** The ability of cell fractions of mouse spleen to repopulate the hemopoietic tissue and to mount graft-versus-host reaction, *Exp. Hematol.*, 3, 85, 1975.
80. **Williams, N., Jackson, H., and Meyers, P.,** Isolation of pluripotential hemopoietic stem cells and clonable precursor cells of erythrocytes, granulocytes, macrophages and megakaryocytes from mouse bone marrow, *Exp. Hematol.*, 7, 524, 1979.
81. **van den Engh, G., Visser, J., and Trask, B.,** Identification CFU-s by scatter measurements on a light activated cell sorter, in *Experimental Hematology Today 1979*, Baum, S. J. and Ledney, G. D., Eds., Springer-Verlag, New York, 1979, 19.

82. **van den Engh, G. and Visser, J.,** Light scattering properties of pluripotential and committed haemopoietic stem cells, *Acta Haematol.,* 62, 289, 1979.
83. **Boyse, E. A. and Old, L. J.,** The immunogenetics of differentiation in the mouse, *Harvey Lect.,* 71, 23, 1978.
84. **Ross, D. R.,** Identification of human lymphocyte subpopulations by surface marker analysis, *Blood,* 53, 799, 1979.
85. **Till, J. E.,** Regulation of hemopoietic stem cells, in *Stem Cells of Renewing Cell Populations,* Cairnie, A. B., Lala, P. K., and Osmond, D. G., Eds. Academic Press, New York, 1976, 143.
86. **Kohler, G. and Milstein, C.,** Continuous cultures of fused cells secreting antibody of predefined specificity, *Nature,* 256, 495, 1975.
87. Workshop on lymphocyte hybridomas, *Curr. Top. Microbiol. Immunol.,* 81, 16, 1978.
88. **Kennett, R. H., McKern, T. J., and Bechtol, K. B.,** *Monoclonal Antibodies; Hybridomas: A New Dimension in Biological Analyses,* Plenum Press, New York, 1980.
89. **Golub, E. S.,** Brain-associated stem cell antigen. An antigen shared by brain and hemopoietic stem cells, *J. Exp. Med.,* 142, 1200, 1972.
90. **Golub, E. S.,** Brain-associated Θ antigen: reactivity of rabbit anti mouse brain with mouse lymphoid cells, *Cell. Immunol.,* 2, 353, 1971.
91. **Golub, E. S.,** Brain associated erythrocyte antigen: an antigen shared by brain and erythrocytes, *Exp. Hematol.,* 1, 105, 1973.
92. **Van den Engh, G. and Golub, E. S.,** Antigenic differences between hemopoietic stem cells and myeloid progenitors, *J. Exp. Med.,* 139, 1621, 1974.
93. **Monette, F. C., Eichacker, P. Q., Byrt, W., Garver, R. I., Gilio, M. J., and deMello, J. B.,** An immunologic approach to cell cycle analysis of the stem cell, in *Experimental Hematology Today,* Baum, S. J. and Ledney, G. D., Eds., Springer-Verlag, New York, 1977, 11.
94. **Adler, S. S., Kuznetsky, R. D., and Trobaugh, F. E., Jr.,** Rabbit antimouse brain serum (RAMBS): lack of specific inhibition of late committed erythroid stem cells in culture (CFU-E), *Blut,* 37, 211, 1978.
95. **Kuznetsky, R. D., Trobaugh, F. E., and Adler, S. S.,** Antiserum to mouse hematopoietic pluripotent stem cells (CFU-s): further investigation of its functional properties, *Exp. Hematol.,* 7, 369, 1979.
96. **Adler, S. S., Kuznetsky, R. D., and Trobaugh, F. E., Jr.,** Anti-CFU-s activity of rabbit antimouse brain serum: mechanisms of action in *Experimental Hematology Today 1978,* Baum, S. J. and Ledney, G. D., Eds., Springer-Verlag, New York, 1978, 23.
97. **Van den Engh, G. and Platenburg, M.,** Suppression of CFU-s activity by rabbit anti-mouse brain serum can be overcome by treatment with papain, *Exp. Hematol.,* 6, 627, 1978.
98. **Testa, N. G., Schofield, R., and Eliason, J. F.,** Enhancement of spleen colony formation by live syngeneic thymus cells: effects on subpopulations of CFU-s, in *Experimental Hematology Today, 1980,* Baum, S. J., Ledney, G. D., van Bekkum, D., Eds., S. Karger, Basel, 1980, 103.
99. **Krogsrud, R. L., Bain, J., and Price, G. B.,** Serological identification of hemopoietic progenitor cell antigens common to mouse and man, *J. Immunol.,* 119, 1486, 1977.
100. **Rosendaal, M.,** Age-dependent surface marker on haemopoietic stem cells, *Nature,* 265, 147, 1977.
101. **Van den Engh, G., Russel, J., and de Cicco, D.,** Surface antigens of hemopoietic stem cells: the expression of BAS, Thy-1, and H-2 antigens on CFU-s, in *Experimental Hematology Today 1978,* Baum, S. J. and Ledney, G. D., Eds., Springer-Verlag, New York, 1978, 9.
102. **Basch, R. S., Janossy, G., and Greaves, M. F.,** Murine pluripotential stem cells lack Ia antigen, *Nature,* 270, 520, 1977.
103. **Kincade, P. W., Paige, C. J., Parkhouse, R. M. E., and Lee, G.,** Characterization of murine colony-forming B cells. I. Distribution, resistance to antiimmunoglobulin antibodies, and expression of Ia antigens, *J. Immunol.,* 120, 1289, 1978.
104. **Krogsrud, R. L. and Price, G. B.,** Hemopoietic stem cells bear sperm-associated antigens, *Exp. Hematol.,* 7, 377, 1979.
105. **Moore, M. A. S., Broxmeyer, H. E., Sheridan, A. P. C., Meyers, P. A., Jacobsen, N., and Winchester, R. J.,** Continuous human bone marrow culture: Ia antigen characterization of probable pluripotential stem cells, *Blood,* 55, 682, 1980.
106. **Kincade, P. W., Flaherty, L., Lee, G., Wantanabe, T., and Michaelson, J.,** Qa antigen expression on functional lymphoid, myeloid, and stem cells in adult mice, *J. Immunol.,* 124, 2879, 1980.
107. **Berridge, M. V.,** A new class of cell surface antigens, quantitative absorption studies defining cell-lineage-specific antigens on hemopoietic cells, *J. Exp. Med.,* 150, 977, 1979.
108. **Berridge, M. V. and Okeck, N.,** Surface antigens of murine hemopoietic stem cells, I. Cross reactivity of antisera against differentiated hemopoietic cells with bone marrow stem cells, *Exp. Hematol.,* 7, 452, 1979.

109. **Goldschneider, I., Gordon, L. K., and Morris, R. J.,** Demonstration of Thy-1 antigen on pluripotential hemopoietic stem cells in the rat, *J. Exp. Med.*, 148, 1351, 1978.
110. **Goldschneider, I., Metcalf, D., Battye, F., and Mandel, T.,** Analysis of rat hemopoietic cells on the fluorescence-activated cell sorter. I. Isolation of pluripotential hemopoietic stem cells and granulocyte-macrophage progenitor cells, *J. Exp. Med.*, 152, 419, 1980.
111. **Reisner, Y., Itzicovitch, L., Meshorer, A., and Sharon, N.,** Hemopoietic stem cell transplantation using mouse bone marrow and spleen cells fractionated by lectins, *Proc. Natl. Acad. Sci. U.S.A.*, 75, 2933, 1978.
112. **Reisner, Y., Ikehara, S., Hodes, M. Z., and Good, R. A.,** Allogeneic hemopoietic stem cell transplantation using mouse spleen cells fractionated by lectins: *in vitro* study of cell fractions, *Proc. Natl. Acad. Sci. U.S.A.*, 77, 1164, 1980.
113. **Byron, J. W.,** Manipulation of the cell cycle of the hemopoietic stem cell, *Exp. Hematol.*, 3, 44, 1975.
114. **Byron, J. W.,** Cell mechanisms influencing the transition of hemopoietic stem cells from Go into S, in *Cell Cycle Controls*, Padilla, G. M., Cameron, I. L., and Zimmerman, A., Eds., Academic Press, New York, 1974, 87.
115. **Byron, J. W.,** Effects of steroids on the cycling of haemopoietic stem cells, *Nature*, 228, 1204, 1970.
116. **Byron, J. W.,** Comparison of the action of ^{3}H-thymidine and hydroxyurea on testosterone-treated hemopoietic stem cells, *Blood*, 40, 198, 1972.
117. **Byron, J. W.,** Effect of steroids and dibutyryl cyclic AMP on the sensitivity of haemopoietic stem cells to ^{3}H-thymidine in vitro, *Nature*, 234, 39, 1971.
118. **Byron, J. W.,** Evidence for a β-adrenergic receptor initiating DNA synthesis in haemopoietic stem cells, *Exp. Cell Res.*, 71, 228, 1972.
119. **Byron, J. W.,** Drug receptors and the haemopoietic stem cell, *Nature*, 241, 152, 1973.
120. **Byron, J. W.,** Cholinergic mechanisms and the hemopoietic stem cell, in *Erythropoiesis*, Nakao, K., Fisher, J. W., and TaKaKu, F., Eds., University Park Press, Baltimore, 1975, 141.
121. **Byron, J. W.,** Histamine H_2-receptor and the hematopoietic stem cell (CFU-s), in *Differentiation of Normal and Neoplastic Hematopoietic Cells*, Book A, Clarkson, B., Marks, P. A., and Till, J. E., Eds., Cold Spring Harbor Laboratory, New York, 1978, 121.
122. **Byron, J. W.,** Pharmacodynamic basis for the interaction of cimetidine with the bone marrow stem cells (CFU-s), *Exp. Hematol.*, 8, 256, 1980.
123. **Feher, I. and Gidali, J.,** Prostaglandin E_2 as stimulator of haemopoietic stem cell proliferation, *Nature*, 274, 550, 1974.
124. **Gidali, J. and Feher, I.,** The effect of E type prostaglandins on the proliferation of haemopoietic stem cells *in vivo*, *Cell Tissue Kinet.*, 10, 365, 1977.
125. **Spivak, J., Misiti, J., Stuart, R., Sharkis, S. S., and Sensenbrenner, L. L.,** Suppression and potentiation of mouse hematopoietic progenitor cell proliferation by Ouabain, *Blood*, 56, 315, 1980.
126. **Marsh, J. C.,** The effects of cancer chemotherapeutic agents on normal hematopoietic precursor cells: a review, *Cancer Res.*, 36, 1853, 1976.
127. **Delmonte, L., Williams, N., and Moore, M. A. S.,** Effect of myleran on murine hemopoiesis. III. Changes in the density distribution of spleen colony forming (CFU-s) and agar gel colony forming cells (CFU-c), *Cell Tissue Kinet.*, 11, 369, 1978.
128. **Delmonte, L.,** Effect of myleran on murine hemopoiesis. II. Direct and host mediated action on proliferative capacity and differentiation bias of spleen colony forming units (CFU-s), *Cell Tissue Kinet.*, 11, 359, 1978.
129. **Moore, M. A. S. and Owen, J. J. T.,** Chromosome marker studies on the development of the haemopoietic system of the chick embryo, *Nature*, 208, 956, 1965.
130. **Moore, M. A. S. and Owen, J. J. T.,** Stem cell migration in the developing myeloid and lymphoid systems, *Lancet*, 1, 658, 1967.
131. **Moore, M. A. S. and Johnson, G. R.,** Hemopoietic stem cells during embryonic development and growth, in *Stem Cells of Renewing Cell Populations*, Cairnie, A. B., Lala, P. K., and Osmond, D. G., Eds., Academic Press, New York, 1976, 323.
132. **Perah, G. and Feldman, M.,** In vitro activation of the *in vivo* colony-forming units of the mouse yolk sac, *J. Cell. Physiol.*, 91, 193, 1977.
133. **Micklem, H. S., Ford, C. E., Evans, E. P., Ogden, D. A., and Papworth, D. S.,** Competitive *in vivo* proliferation of foetel and adult haematopoietic cells in lethally irradiated mice, *J. Cell. Physiol.*, 79, 293, 1972.
134. **Rosendaal, M., Hodgson, G. S., and Bradley, T. R.,** Haemopoietic stem cells are organized for use on the basis of their generation-age, *Nature*, 264, 68, 1976.

135. **Rosendaal, M., Hodgson, G. S., and Bradley, T. R.,** Organization of haemopoietic stem cells: the generation-age hypothesis, *Cell Tissue Kinet.,* 12, 17, 1979.
136. **Hellman, S., Botnick, L. E., Hannon, E. C., and Vignuelle, R. M.,** Proliferative capacity of murine hematopoietic stem cells, *Proc. Natl. Acad. Sci. U.S.A.,* 75, 490, 1978.
137. **Schofield, R., Lord, B. I., Kyffin, S., and Gilbert, C. W.,** Self-maintenance capacity of CFU-s, *J. Cell. Physiol.,* 103, 355, 1980.
138. **Lajtha, L. G.,** Stem cell concepts, *Differentiation,* 14, 23, 1979.
139. **Boggs, S. S. and Boggs, D. R.,** Earlier onset of hematopoietic differentiation after expansion of the endogenous stem cell pool, *Radiat. Res.,* 63, 165, 1975.
140. **Harrison, D. E.,** Competitive repopulation: a new assay for long term stem cell functional capacity, *Blood,* 55, 77, 1980.
141. **Lord, B. I., Testa, N. G., and Hendry, J. H.,** The relative spatial distributions of CFUs and CFUc in the normal mouse femur, *Blood,* 46, 65, 1975.
142. **Lord, B. I.,** Cellular and architectural factors influencing the proliferation hematopoietic stem cells, in *Differentiation of Normal and Neoplastic Hematopoietic Cells,* Book B, Clarkson, B., Marks, P. A., and Till, J. E., Eds., Cold Spring Harbor Laboratory, New York, 1978, 775.
143. **Shackney, S. E.,** The orderliness of cell proliferation and cell differentiation in relation to kinetic heterogeneity in mouse bone marrow, in *Differentiation of Normal and Neoplastic Hematopoietic Cells,* Book B, Clarkson, B., Marks, P. A., and Till, J. E., Eds., Cold Spring Harbor Laboratory, New York, 1978, 789.
144. **Maloney, M. A., Lamela, R. A., Dorie, J. J., and Patt, H. M.,** Concentration gradient of blood stem cells in mouse bone marrow—an open question, *Blood,* 51, 521, 1978.
145. **Maloney, M. A. and Patt, H. M.,** Migration of cells from shielded to irradiated marrow, *Blood,* 39, 804, 1972.
146. **Micklem, H. S., Ogden, D. A., Evans, E. P., Ford, C. E., and Gray, J. G.,** Compartments and cell flows within the mouse haemopoietic system. II. Estimated rates of interchange, *Cell Tissue Kinet.,* 8, 233, 1975.
147. **Maloney, M. A. and Patt, A. M.,** Marrow stem cell release in the autorepopulation assay, *Exp. Hematol.,* 6, 227, 1978.
148. **Gidali, J., Feher, I., and Antal, S.,** Some properties of the circulating hemopoietic stem cells, *Blood,* 43, 573 ,1974.
149. **Dorie, M. J., Maloney, M. A., and Patt, H. M.,** Turnover of circulating hematopoietic stem cells, *Exp. Hematol.,* 7, 483, 1979.
150. **Micklem, H. S., Anderson, N., and Ross, E.,** Limited potential of circulating haemopoietic stem cells, *Nature,* 256, 41, 1975.
151. **Lajtha, L. G. and Schofield, R.,** Regulation of stem cell renewal and differentiation: possible significance in aging, in *Advances in Gerentological Research,* Strehler, B. L., Ed., Academic Press, New York, 1971, 3.
152. **Micklem, H. S. and Ogden, D. A.,** Ageing of haemopoietic stem cell populations in the mouse, in *Stem Cells of Renewing Cell Populations,* Cairnie, A. B., Lala, P. K., and Osmond, D. G., Eds., Academic Press, New York, 1976, 331.
153. **Harrison, D. E., Astle, C. M., and Delaittre, J. A.,** Loss of proliferative capacity in immunohemopoietic stem cells caused by serial transplantation rather than aging, *J. Exp. Med.,* 147, 1526, 1978.
154. **McCulloch, E. A., Thompson, M. W., Siminovitch, L., and Till, J. E.,** Effects of bacterial endotoxin on hemopoietic colony-forming cells in the spleens of normal mice and mice of genotype Sl/ Sl^d, *Cell Tissue Kinet.,* 3, 47, 1970.
155. **Reissmann, K. R., Udupa, K. B., and Okamura, H.,** Effect of endotoxin on normal and 5-fluorouracil suppressed hematopoietic stem cells, *J. Lab. Clin. Med.,* 76, 652, 1970.
156. **Vos, O.,** Effect of bacterial lipopolysaccharide on proliferation of CFU-s, *Exp. Hematol.,* 6, 688, 1978.
157. **Monette, F. C., Morse, B. S., Howard, D., Niskanen, E., and Stohlman, F., Jr.,** Hemopoietic stem cell proliferation and migration following Bordetella pertussis vaccine, *Cell Tissue Kinet.,* 5, 121, 1972.
158. **Vos, O., Buurman, W. A., and Ploemacher, R. E.,** Mobilization of haemopoietic stem cells (CFU) into the peripheral blood of the mouse; effects of endotoxin and other compounds, *Cell Tissue Kinet.,* 5, 467, 1972.
159. **Wilschut, I. J. C. and Vos, O.,** Further studies on mobilization of CFUs, *Cell Tissue Kinet.,* 12, 257, 1979.
160. **Zander, A. R., Spitzer, G., Verma, D. S., Beran, M., and Dicke, K. A.,** Effect of pyran copolymer on murine hemopoiesis, *Exp. Hematol.,* 8, 521, 1980.

161. **Wilschut, I. J. C., Erkens-Versluis, M. E., Ploemacher, R. E., Benner, R., and Vos, O.,** Studies on the mechanism of haemopoietic stem cell (CFUs) mobilization, a role of the complement system, *Cell Tissue Kinet.*, 12, 299, 1979.
162. **Quesenberry, P., Levin, J., Zuckerman, K., Rencricca, N., Sullivan, R., and Tyler, W.,** Stem cell migration by erythropoietin or haemolytic anaemia: the effects of actinomycin and endotoxin contamination of erythropoietin preparations, *Br. J. Haematol.*, 41, 253, 1979.
163. **Dexter, T. M., Allen, T. D., Lajtha, L. G., Schofield, R., and Lord, B. I.,** Stimulation of differentiation and proliferation of haemopoietic cells in vitro, *J. Cell. Physiol.*, 82, 461, 1973.
164. **Shulman, L. N. and Robinson, S. H.,** Maintenance of hemopoietic stem cells in diffusion chamber cultures, *J. Lab. Clin. Med.*, 90, 581, 1977.
165. **Dexter, T. M. and Lajtha, L. G.,** Proliferation of Haemopoietic stem cells in vitro, *Br. J. Haematol.*, 28, 525, 1974.
166. **Dexter, T. M., Allen, T. D., and Lajtha, L. G.,** Conditions controlling the proliferation of haemopoietic stem cells in vitro, *J. Cell. Physiol.*, 91, 335, 1977.
167. **Allen, T. D. and Dexter, T. M.,** Cellular interrelationships during in vitro granulopoiesis, *Differentiation,* 6, 191, 1976.
168. **Allen, T. D.,** Ultrastructural aspects of in vitro haemopoiesis, in *Stem Cells and Tissue Homeostasis,* Lord, B. I., Potten, C. S., and Cole, R. J., Eds., Cambridge University Press, London, 1978, 217.
169. **Mori, K. J., Fujitake, H., OKubo, H., Dexter, T. M., and Ito, Y.,** Quantitative development of adherent cell colonies in bone marrow cell culture *in vitro, Exp. Haematol.*, 7, 12, 1979.
170. **Bentlely, S. A. and Foidart, J. M.,** Some properties of marrow derived adherent cells in tissue culture, *Blood,* 56, 312, 1980.
171. **Dexter, T. M.,** Cell interactions in vitro, *Clin. Haematol.*, 8, 453, 1979.
172. **Williams, N., Jackson, H., and Rabellino, E. M.,** Proliferation and differentiation of normal granulopoietic cells in continuous bone marrow cultures, *J. Cell. Physiol.*, 93, 435, 1977.
173. **Greenberger, J. S.,** Sensitivity of corticosteroid-lipogenesis in marrow preadipocytes of obese-diabetic (db/db) mice, *Nature,* 275, 752, 1978.
174. **Potter, J. E. and Wright, E. G.,** Bone marrow lipids in normal and anemic mice, *Am. J. Hematol.*, 8, 361, 1980.
175. **Dexter, T. M. and Moore, M. A. S.,** *In vitro* duplication and "cure" of haemopoietic defects in genetically anaemic W/W^v and $S1/S1^d$ mice, *Nature,* 269, 412, 1977.
176. **Moore, M. A. S. and Dexter, T. M.,** Stem cell regulation in continuous hematopoietic cell culture, *Transplant. Proc.*, 10, 83, 1978.
177. **Dexter, T. M., Moore, M. A. S., and Sheridan, A. P. C.,** Maintenance of hemopoietic stem cells and production of differentiated progency in allogeneic bone marrow chimeras *in vitro, J. Exp. Med.*, 145, 1612, 1977.
178. **Dexter, T. M. and Spooncer, E.,** Loss of immunoreactivity in long-term bone marrow culture, *Nature,* 275, 135, 1978.
179. **Reimann, J. and Burger, H.,** *In Vitro* proliferation of haemopoietic cells in the presence of adherent cell layers. I. Culture conditions and strain dependence, *Exp. Hematol.*, 7, 45, 1979.
180. **Dexter, T. M., Allen, T. D., and Lajtha, L. G.,** Factors controlling the proliferation of haemopoietic stem cells in vitro, in *Molecular Control of Proliferation and Differentiation,* Papaconstantinou, J. and Rutler, W. J., Eds., Academic Press, New York, 1978, 149.
181. **Reimann, J. and Burger, H.,** *In vitro* proliferation of haemopoietic cells in the presence of adherent cell layers. II. Differential effect of adherent cell layers derived from various organs, *Exp. Hematol.*, 7, 52, 1979.
182. **Dexter, T. M. and Shadduck, R. K.,** The regulation of haemopoiesis in long term bone marrow cultures. I. Role of L-cell CSF, *J. Cell. Physiol.*, 102, 279, 1980.
183. **Williams, N. and Burgess, A. W.,** The effect of mouse lung granulocyte-macrophage colony stimulatory factor and other colony-stimulating activities on the proliferation and differentiation of murine bone marrow cells in long-term cultures, *J. Cell. Physiol.*, 102, 287, 1980.
184. **Williams, N., Jackson, H., Sheridan, A. P. C., Murphy, M. J., Elste, A., and Moore, M. A. S.,** Regulation of megakaryopoiesis in long-term murine bone marrow cultures, *Blood,* 51, 245, 1978.
185. **Testa, N. G. and Dexter, T. M.,** Long term production of erythroid precursor cells (BFU) in bone marrow cultures, *Differentiation,* 9, 193, 1977.
186. **Humphries, R. K., Eaves, A. C., and Eaves, C. J.,** Characterization of a primitive erythropoietic progenitor found in mouse marrow before and after several weeks in culture, *Blood,* 53, 746, 1979.
187. **Eliason, J. F., Testa, N. G., and Dexter, T. M.,** Erythropoietin-stimulated erythropoiesis in long-term bone marrow culture, *Nature,* 281, 382, 1979.
188. **Ralph, P., Williams, N., Cronin-Sheridan, A. P., Nakoinz, I., Jackson, H., and Moore, M. A. S.,** Effector cell functions in long term culture of murine, prosimian, and human bone marrow, in *Mononuclear Phagocytes,* Part 1, Van Furth, R., Ed., Martinus Nijhoff, The Hague, 1980, 13.

189. **Schrader, J. W. and Schrader, S.,** In vitro studies on lymphocyte differentiation. I. Long term *in vitro* culture of cells giving rise to functional lymphocytes in irradiated mice, *J. Exp. Med.*, 148, 823, 1978.
190. **Jones-Villeneuve, E. V., Rusthoven, J. J., Miller, R. G., and Phillips, R. A.,** Differentiation of Thy 1-bearing cells from progenitors in long-term bone marrow cultures, *J. Immunol.*, 124, 597, 1980.
191. **Mauch, P., Greenberger, J. S., Botnick, L., Hannon, E., and Hellman, S.,** Evidence for structured variation in self-renewal capacity within long-term bone marrow cultures, *Proc. Natl. Acad. Sci. U.S.A.*, 77, 2927, 1980.
192. **Levitt, L. J. and Quesenberry, P. J.,** The effect of lithium on murine hematopoiesis in a liquid culture system, *N. Engl. J. Med.*, 302, 713, 1980.
193. **Broxmeyer, H. E., deSousa, M., Smithyman, A., Ralph, P., Hamilton, J., Kurland, J. I., and Bognacki, J.,** Specificity and modulation of the action of lactoferrin, a negative feedback regulator of myelopoiesis, *Blood,* 55, 324, 1980.
194. **Dexter, T. M., Scott, D., and Teich, N. M.,** Infection of bone marrow cells *in vitro* with FLV: effects on stem cell proliferation, differentiation and leukemogenic capacity, *Cell,* 12, 355, 1977.
195. **Moore, M. A. S. and Sheridan, A. P.,** Pluripotential stem cell replication in continuous human, prosimian, and murine bone marrow culture, *Blood Cells,* 5, 297, 1979.
196. **Testa, N. G., Dexter, T. M., and Teich, N. M.,** Characterization of myelomonocytic leukemia cells induced by *in vitro* infection of bone marrow with FLV, in *Modern Trends in Human Leukemia III,* Neth, R., Gallo, R. C., Hofschneider, P.-H., and Mannweiler, K., Eds., Springer-Verlag, Berlin, 1979, 231.
197. **Teich, N., Boss, M., and Dexter, T. M.,** Infection of mouse bone marrow cells with abelson murine leukemia virus and establishment of producer cell lines, in *Modern Trends in Human Leukemia III,* Neth, R., Gallo, R. C., Hofschneider, P. H., and Mannweiler, K., Eds., Springer-Verlag, Berlin, 1979, 488.
198. **Greenberger, J. S., Davisson, P. B., Gans, P. J., and Maloney, W. C.,** *In vitro* induction of continuous acute promyelocytic leukemia cell lines by Friend or Abelson murine leukemia virus, *Blood,* 53, 987, 1979.
199. **Dexter, T. M. and Teich, N. M.,** Modification of the proliferative and differentiation capacity of stem cells following treatment with chemical and viral leukemogens, in *Modern Trends in Human Leukemia III,* Neth, R., Gallo, R. C., Hofschneider, P.-H., and Mannweiler, K., Eds., Springer-Verlag, Berlin, 1979, 223.
200. **Dexter, T. M., Allen, T. D., Scott, D., and Teich, N. M.,** Isolation characterization of a bipotential haematopoietic cell line, *Nature,* 277, 471, 1979.
201. **Boggs, D. R.,** Clonal diseases of the myeloid stem cell systems, in *Modern Trends in Human Leukemia III,* Neth, R., Gallo, R. C., Hofschneider, P.-H., and Mannweiler, K., Eds., Springer-Verlag, Berlin, 1979, 191.
202. **Whang, T., Frei, E., III, Tjio, J. H., Carbone, P. P., and Brecher, G.,** The distribution of the Philadelphia chromosome in patients with chronic myelogenous leukemia, *Blood,* 22, 664, 1963.
203. **Tough, I. M., Jacobs, P. A., Court-Brown, W. M., Baikie, A. G., and Williamson, E. R. D.,** Cytogenetic studies on bone marrow in chronic myeloid leukemia, *Lancet,* 1, 844, 1963.
204. **Nowell, P. C. and Hungerford, D. A.,** Chromosome studies on normal and leukemic human leukocytes, *J. Natl. Cancer Inst.*, 25, 85, 1960.
205. **Rowley, J. D.,** A new consistent chromosomal abnormality in chronic myelogneous leukemia identified by quinacrine fluorescence and giemsa staining, *Nature,* 243, 299, 1973.
206. **Rowley, J. D.,** Chromosomes in leukemia and lymphona, *Semin. Hematol.*, 15, 301, 1978.
207. **Cunningham, I., Gee, T., Dowling, M., Chaganti, T., Bailey, T., Hopfan, S., Bowden, L., Turnbull, A., Knapper, W., and Clarkson, B.,** Results of treatment of PH^1 + chronic myelogenous leukemia with an intensive treatment regimen (L-5 Protocol), *Blood,* 53, 375.
208. **Fialkow, P. J.,** Clonal origin of human tumors, *Biochim. Biophys. Acta,* 458, 283, 1976.
209. **Fialkow, P. J., Denman, A. M., Singer, J., Jacobson, R. J., and Lowenthal, M. N.,** Human myeloproliferative disorders: clonal origin in pluripotential stem cells, in *Differentiation of Normal and Neoplastic Hematopoietic Cells,* Book A, Clarkson, B., Marks, P. A., and Till, J. E., Eds., Cold Spring Harbor Laboratory, New York, 1978, 131.
210. **Fialkow, P. J., Gartler, S. M., and Yoshida, A.,** Clonal origin of chronic myelocytic leukemia in man, *Proc. Natl. Acad. Sci. U.S.A.*, 58, 1469, 1967.
211. **Fialkow, P. J., Jacobson, R. J., and Papayannopoulou, T.,** Chronic myelocytic leukemia: clonal origin in a stem cell common to the granulocyte, erythrocyte, platelet and macrocyte/macrophage, *Am. J. Med.*, 63, 125, 1977.
212. **Fialkow, P. J., Denman, A. M., Jacobson, R. J., and Lowenthal, M. N.,** Chronic leukemia. Origin of some lymphocytes from leukemic stem cells, *J. Clin. Invest.*, 62, 815, 1978.

213. **Prchal, J. T., Throchmorton, D. W., Carroll, A. J., Fuson, E. W., Gams, R. A., and Prchal, J. F.,** A common progenitor for human myeloid and lymphoid cells, *Nature,* 274, 590, 1978.
214. **Greaves, M. F., Verbi, W., Reeves, B. R., Hoffbrand, A. V., Drysdale, H. C., Jones, L., Sacker, L. S., and Samaratunga, I.,** "Pre-B" phenotypes in blast crisis of PH[1] positive CML: evidence for a pluripotential stem cell "target", *Leukemia Res.,* 3, 181, 1979.
215. **Fialkow, P. J.,** Use of glucose-6-phosphate dehydrogenase markers to study human myeloproliferative disorders, in *Modern Trends in Human Leukemia III,* Neth, R., Gallo, R. C., Hofschneider, P.-H., and Mannweiler, K., Eds., Springer-Verlag, Berlin, 1979, 53.
216. **Fialkow, P. J., Jacobson, R. J., Singer, J. W., Sacher, R. A., McGuffin, R. W., and Neefe, J. R.,** Philadphia chromosome (Ph[1])-negative chronic myelogenous leukemia (CML): a clonal disease with origin in a multipotent stem cell, *Blood,* 56, 70, 1980.
217. **Prchal, J. F., Adamson, J. W., Murphy, S., Steinman, L., and Fialkow, P. J.,** Polycythemia vera: the *in vitro* response of normal and abnormal stem cell lines to erythropoietin, *J. Clin. Invest.,* 61, 1044, 1978.
218. **Singer, J. W., Fialkow, P. J., Steinman, L., Najfeld, V., Stein, S. J., and Robinson, W. A.,** Chronic myelocytic leukemia: failure to detect residual normal committed stem cells *in vitro, Blood,* 53, 264, 1979.
219. **Singer, J. W., Arlin, Z. A., Najfeld, V., Adamson, J. W., Kempin, S. J., Clarkson, B. D., and Failkow, P. J.,** Restoration of nonclonal hematopoiesis in chronic myelogenous leukemia (CML) following a chemotherapy-induced loss of the PH[1] chromosome, *Blood,* 56, 356, 1980.
220. **Moore, M. A. S., Sheridan, A. P. C., Allen, T. D., and Dexter, T. M.,** Prolonged hematopoiesis in a primate bone marrow culture system: characteristics of stem cell production and the hematopoietic microenvironment, *Blood,* 54, 775, 1979.
221. **Hocking, W. G. and Golde, D. W.,** Long-term human bone marrow cultures, *Blood,* 56, 118, 1980.
222. **Gartner, S. and Kaplan, H. S.,** Long-term culture of human bone marrow cells, *Proc. Natl. Acad. Sci. U.S.A.,* 77, 4756, 1980.
223. **Greenberg, H. M., Parker, L. M., Newburger, P. E., Said, J., Cohen, G. I., and Greenberger, J. S.,** Corticosteroid dependence of continuous hemopoiesis *in vitro* with murine or human bone marrow, in *Modern Trends in Human Leukemia IV,* Neth, R., Gallo, R. C., Graf, T., Mannweiler, K., and Winkler, K., Eds., Springer-Verlag, Berlin, 1980.
224. **Winchester, R. J., Fu, S. M., Wernet, P., Kunkel, H. G., Dupont, B., and Jersild, C.,** Recognition of non HLA alloantigens selectively expressed on B lymphocytes, *J. Exp. Med.,* 141, 924, 1975.
225. **Winchester, R. J., Ross, G. D., Jarowski, C. I., Wang, C. Y., Halper, J., and Broxmeyer, H. E.,** Expression of Ia-like antigen molecules on human granulocytes during early phases of differentiation, *Proc. Natl. Acad. Sci. U.S.A.,* 74, 4012, 1977.
226. **Broxmeyer, H. E.,** Lactroferrin acts on Ia-like antigen positive subpopulations of human monocytes to inhibit production of colony stimulatory activity *in vitro, J. Clin. Invest.,* 64, 1717, 1979.
227. **Broxmeyer, H. E., Pelus, L. M., Gillis, S., Kincade, P., deSousa, M., and Moore, M. A. S.,** Heterogeneity in responsiveness of mononuclear phagocytes to receptor-binding of lactoferrin and to inhibition of the production of granulocyte-macrophage colony stimulatory factors by lactoferrin, in *Heterogeneity of Mononuclear Phagocytes,* Landy, M. and Forester, O., Eds., Academic Press, New York, 1980.
228. **Fauser, A. A. and Messner, H. A.,** Granuloerythropoietic colonies in human bone marrow, peripheral blood, and cord blood, 52, 1243, 1978.
229. **Fauser, A. A. and Messner, H. A.,** Identification of megakaryocytes, macrophages, and eosinophils in colonies of human bone marrow containing neutrophilic granulocytes and erythroblasts, *Blood,* 53, 1023, 1979.
230. **Fauser, A. A. and Messner, H. A.,** Proliferative state of human pluripotential hemopoietic progenitors (CFU-GEMM) in normal individuals and under regenerative conditions after bone marrow transplantation, *Blood,* 54, 1197, 1979.
231. **Messner, H. A. and Fauser, A. A.,** Human pluripotential hemopoietic progenitors (CFU-GEMM) in culture, in NIH Conference on Aplastic Anemia, San Francisco, 1979.
232. **Gregory, C. J. and Henkelman, R. M.,** Relationship between early hemopoietic progenitor cells determined by correlation analysis of their numbers in individual spleen colonies, in *Experimental Hematology Today,* Baum, S. J. and Ledney, G. D., Eds., Springer-Verlag, New York, 1977, 93.
233. **Adamson, J. W., Fialkow, P. J., Murphy, S., Prchal, J. F., and Steinmann, L.,** Polycythemia vera: stem cell and probable clonal origin of the disease, *N. Engl. J. Med.,* 295, 913, 1976.
234. **Messner, H. A. and Fauser, A. A.,** Culture studies of human pluripotential hemopoietic progenitors, in *Modern Trends in Human Leukemia IV,* Neth, R., Gallo, R. C., Graf, T., Mannweiler, K., and Winkler, K., Eds., Springer-Verlag, Berlin, 1980.

235. **Till, J. E., McCulloch, E. A., and Siminovitch, L.,** A stochastic, model of stem cell proliferation, based on the growth of spleen colony forming cells, *Proc. Natl. Acad. Sci. U.S.A.*, 51, 29, 1964.
236. **Korn, A. P., HenKelman, R. M., Ottensmeyer, F. P., and Till, J. E.,** Investigations of a stochastic model of haemopoiesis, *Exp. Hematol.*, 1, 362, 1973.
237. **Trentin, J. J.,** Hemopoietic inductive microenvironments, in *Stem Cells, of Renewing Cell Populations,* Cairnie, A. B., Lala, P. K., and Osmond, D. G., Eds., Academic Press, New York, 1976, 255.
238. **Trentin, J. J.,** Hemopoietic microenvironments, *Transplant. Proc.*, 10, 77, 1978.
239. **Wolf, N. S.,** The haemopoietic microenvironment, *Clin. Haematol.*, 8, 469, 1979.
240. **Tavassoli, M.,** Studies on hemopoietic microenvironments, report of a workshop, *Exp. Hematol.*, 3, 213, 1975.
241. **Chamberlin, W., Barone, J., Kedo, A., and Fried, W.,** Lack of recovery of murine hematopoietic stromal cells after irradiation-induced damage, *Blood,* 44, 385, 1974.
242. **Hendry, J. H. and Lajtha, L. G.,** The response of hemopoietic colony-forming units to repeated doses of X-rays, *Radiat. Res.*, 52, 309, 1972.
243. **Tavassoli, M. and Crosby, W. H.,** Transplantation of marrow to extramedullary sites, *Science,* 161, 54, 1968.
244. **Maniatis, A., Tavassoli, M., and Crosby, W. H.,** Origin of osteogenic precursor cells in extra medullary marrow grafts, *Blood,* 38, 569, 1971.
245. **Amsel, S. and Dell, E. S.,** Bone marrow repopulation of subcutaneously grafted mouse femurs, *Proc. Soc. Exp. Biol. Med.*, 138, 555, 1971.
246. **Friedenstein, A. Y., Petrakova, K. V., Kurolejova, A. I., and Frolova, G. P.,** Heterotropic transplants of bone marrow. Analysis of precursor cells for osteogenic and hematopoietic tissues, *Transplantation,* 6, 230, 1968.
247. **Fried, W., Husseini, S., Knospe, W., and Trobaugh, F. E., Jr.,** Studies on the source of hematopoietic tissue in the marrow of subcutaneously implanted femurs, *Exp. Hematol.*, 1, 29, 1973.
248. **Fried, W., Chamberlin, W., Knospe, W. H., Hussenini, S., and Trobaugh, F. E., Jr.,** Studies on the defective haematopoietic microenvironment of $S1/S1^d$ mice, *Br. J. Haematol.*, 24, 643, 1973.
249. **Fried, W., Chamberlain, W., Kedo, A., and Barone, J.,** Effects of radiation on hematopoietic stroma, *Exp. Hematol.*, 4, 310, 1976.
250. **Chertkov, J. L. and Gurevitch, O. A.,** Radiosensitivity of progenitor cells of the hematopoietic microenvironment, *Radiat. Res.*, 79, 177, 1979.
251. **Fried, W., Kedo, A., and Barone, J.,** Effects of cyclophosphamide and of busulfan on spleen colony-forming units and on hematopoietic stroma, *Cancer Res.*, 37, 1205, 1977.
252. **Testa, N. G. and Hendry, J. H.,** Radiation induced hemopoiesis in adult mouse liver, *Exp. Hematol.*, 5, 136, 1977.
253. **Adler, S. S. and Trobaugh, F. E., Jr.,** Hemopoietic support capacity of adult mouse liver. Studies in ^{89}Sr marrow-ablated mice, *Blood,* 52, 293, 1978.
254. **Goldwasser, E.,** Erythropoietin and the differentiation of red blood cells, *Fed. Proc.*, 34, 2285, 1975.
255. **Van Zant, G. and Goldwasser, E.,** The effects of erythropoietin *in vitro* on spleen colony-forming cells, *J. Cell. Physiol.*, 90, 241, 1977.
256. **Maloney, M. A., Dorie, M. J., Lamela, R. A., Rogers, Z. R., and Patt, H. M.,** Hematopoietic stem cell regulatory volumes as revealed in studies of the bg^J/bg^J:W/W^v Chimera, *J. Exp. Med.*, 147, 1189, 1978.
257. **Schofield, R.,** Lymphocyte co-operation in haemopoiesis, in *International Conference of Leukemia and Aplastic anemia,* Metcalf, D., Condorelli, M. and Peschle, C., Eds., Il Pensiero Scientifico, Italy, 1976, 392.
258. **Goodman, J. W. and Grubbs, G. G.,** The relationship of the thymus to erythropoiesis, in *Hemopoietic Cellular Proliferation,* Stohlman, F., Jr., Ed., Grune & Stratton, 1970, 26.
259. **Lord, B. I. and Schofield, R.,** Influence of thymus cells in hemopoiesis: stimulation of hemopoietic stem cells in a syngeneic, *in vivo,* situation, *Blood,* 42, 395, 1973.
260. **Zipori, D. and Tranin, N.,** The role of a thymus humoral factor in the proliferation of bone marrow CFU-s from thymectomized mice, *Exp. Hematol.*, 3, 389, 1975.
261. **Cerny, J.,** Stimulation of bone marrow haemopoietic stem cells by a factor from activated T cells, *Nature,* 249, 63, 1974.
262. **Cerny, J., Warner, E. B., and Rubin, A. S.,** T cell studies on the origin and action of the factor (s), *J. Immunol.*, 115, 513, 1975.
263. **Hamano, T. and Nagai, K.,** Effects of allogeneic stimulations on the proliferation and differentiation of the hemopoietic stem cell, *Transplantation,* 25, 23, 1978.
264. **Wiktor-Jedrzejczak, W., Sharkis, S., Ahmed, A., and Sell, K. W.,** Theta-sensitive cell and erythropoisis: identification of a defect in W/W^v anemic mice, *Science,* 196, 313, 1977.

265. **Sharkis, S. J., Wiktor-Jedrzejczak, W., Ahmed, A., Santos, G. W., McKnee, A., and Sell, K. W.,** Antitheta-sensitive regulatory cell (TSRc) and hematopoiesis: regulation of differentiation of transplanted stem cells in W/W^v anemic and normal mice, *Blood,* 52, 802, 1978.
266. **Wiktor-Jedrzejczak, W., Ahmed, A., Sharkis, S. J., Cahill, R. A., and Sell, K. W.,** Ly phenotype and other T-cell antisera sensitivity of an anti-theta sensitive cell that regulates hematopoiesis, in *Experimental Hematology Today 1979,* Baum, S. J. and Ledney, G. D., Eds., Springer-Verlag, New York, 1979, 33.
267. **Lowenberg, B. and Dicke, K. A.,** Induction of proliferation of haemopoietic stem cells in culture, *Exp. Hematol.,* 5, 319, 1977.
268. **Wagemaker, G. and Peters, M. F.,** Effects of human leukocyte conditioned medium on mouse haemopoietic progenitor cells, *Cell Tissue Kinet.,* 11, 45, 1978.
269. **Patt, H. M. and Blackburn, M.,** Increased survival of CBA pluripotential haemopoietic stem cells in vitro induced by a marrow stromal factor in $S1/S1^d$ mice, *Exp. Hematol.,* 7, 325, 1979.
270. **Fried, W., Knospe, W. H., Gregory, S. A., and Trobaugh, F. E., Jr.,** Factors regulating the proliferation and migration of hematopoietic stem cells, *J. Lab. Clin. Med.,* 77, 239, 1971.
271. **Gregory, S. A., Fried, W., Knospe, W. H., and Trobaugh, F. E., Jr.,** Accelerated regeneration of transplanted hematopoietic stem cells in irradiated mice pretreated with cyclophosphamide, *Blood,* 37, 196, 1971.
272. **Blackett, N. M. and Aguado, M.,** The enhancement of haemopoietic stem cell recovery in irradiated mice by prior treatment with cyclophosphamide, *Cell Tissue Kinet.,* 12, 291, 1979.
273. **Fried, W., Barone-Varelas, J., Helfgott, M., and Berman, M.,** Effect of plasma from cyclophosphamide treated mice on CFU-s in an *in vivo* culture system, *Blood,* 56, 940, 1980.
274. **Castro-Malaspina, H., Gay, R., Resnick, G., Kapoor, N., Meyers, P., Chiarieri, D., McKenzie, S., Broxmeyer, H. E., and Moore, M. A. S.,** Characterization of human bone marrow fibroblast colony forming cells (CFU-F) and their progeny, *Blood,* 56, 289, 1980.
275. **Croizat, H. and Frindel, E.,** Study of a CFUs stimulating factor liberated by bone marrow cells after total and partial body irradiation, *Exp. Hematol.,* 8, 185, 1980.
276. **Adler, S. S., Trobaugh, F. E., and Knospe, W. H.,** Hemopoietic stem cell dynamics in ^{89}Sr marrow-ablated mice, *J. Lab. Clin. Med.,* 89, 592, 1977.
277. **Adler, S. S. and Trobaugh, F. E., Jr.,** Hemopoiesis in diffusion chambers in strontium-89 marrow-ablated mice, *Proc. Soc. Exp. Biol. Med.,* 159, 260, 1978.
278. **Necas, E. and Neuwirt, J.,** Control of haemopoietic stem cell proliferation by cells in DNA synthesis, *Br. J. Haematol.,* 33, 395, 1976.
279. **Necas, E. and Newirt, J.,** Proliferation rate of haemopoietic stem cells after damage by several cytostatic agents, *Cell Tissue Kinet.,* 9, 479, 1976.
280. **Guigon, M., Enouf, J., and Frindel, E.,** Effects of CFU-s inhibitors on murine bone marrow during ara-c treatment. I. Effects on stem cells, *Leukemia Res.,* 4, 385, 1980.
281. **Benestad, H. B., Testa, N. G., and Lajtha, L. G.,** Inhibition of haemopoietic stem cell proliferation by a diffusible product of bone marrow cells, *Scand. J. Haematol.,* 20, 18, 1978.
282. **Lord, B. I., Wright, E. G., and Mori, K. J.,** The role of proliferation inhibitors in the regulation of haemopoiesis, in *Stem Cells and Tissue Homeostasis,* Lord, B. I., Potten, C. S., and Cole, R. J., Eds., Cambridge University Press, New York, 1978, 203.
283. **Lord, B. I.,** The assay of cell proliferation inhibitors, in *Chalones,* Houck, J. C., Ed., North-Holland, New York, 1976, 97.
284. **Lajtha, L. G., Lord, B. I., Dexter, T. M., Wright, E. G., and Allen, T. D.,** Inter-relationship of differentiation and proliferation control in hemopoietic stem cells, in *Cell Differentiation and Neoplasia,* Saunders, G. F., Ed., Raven Press, New York, 1978, 179.
285. **Lord, B. I.,** Proliferation regulators in haemopoiesis, *Clin. Haematol.,* 8, 435, 1979.
286. **Lord, B. I., Mori, K. J., Wright, E. G., and Lajtha, L. G.,** An inhibitor of stem cell proliferation in normal bone marrow, *Br. J. Haematol.,* 34, 441, 1976.
287. **Lord, B. I., Mori, K., and Wright, E. G.,** A stimulator of stem cell proliferation in regenerating bone marrow, *Biomedicine,* 27, 223, 1977.
288. **Wright, E. G. and Lord, B. I.,** Production of stem cell proliferation stimulators and inhibitors by haemopoietic cell suspensions, *Biomedicine,* 28, 156, 1978.
289. **Wright, E. G. and Lord, B. I.,** Production of stem cell proliferation regulators by fractionated haemopoietic cell suspensions, *Leukemia Res.,* 3, 15, 1979.
290. **Wright, E. G., Sheridan, P., and Moore, M. A. S.,** An inhibitor of murine stem cell proliferation produced by normal human bone marrow, *Leukemia Res.,* 4, 309, 1980.
291. **Dexter, T. M., Wright, E. G., Krizsa, F., and Lajtha, L. G.,** Regulation of haemopoietic stem cell proliferation in long term bone marrow cultures, *Biomedicine,* 27, 344, 1977.

292. **Toksoz, D., Dexter, T. M., Lord, B. I., Wright, E. G., and Lajtha, L. G.,** The regulation of hemopoiesis in long-term bone marrow cultures. II. Stimulation and inhibition of stem cell proliferation, *Blood,* 55, 931, 1980.
293. **Dicke, K. A., Lotzova, E., Spitzer, G., and McCredie, K. B.,** Immunobiology, *Semin. Hematol.,* 15, 263, 1978.
294. **Gotze, D. and Albert, E.,** The major histocompatibility system in man, in *The Major Histocompatibility System in Man and Animals,* Gotze, D., Ed., Springer-Verlag, Berlin, 1977, 7.
295. **Klein, J.,** *Biology of the Mouse histocompatibility—2 complex,* Springer-Verlag, New York, 1975.
296. **David, C. S.,** The major histocompatibility system of the mouse, in *The Major Histocompatibility System in Man and Animals,* Gotze, D., Ed., Springer-Verlag, Berlin, 1977, 255.
297. **Thomas, E. D., Storb, R., Cliff, R. A., Fefer, A., Johnson, L., Neiman, P. E., Lerner, K. G., Glucksberg, H., and Buckner, C. D.,** Bone marrow transplantation. I, *N. Engl. J. Med.,* 292, 832, 1975.
298. **Thomas, E. D., Storb, R., Clift, R. A., Fefer, A., Johnson, L., Neiman, P. E., Lerner, K. G., Glucksberg, H., and Buckner, C. D.,** II, *N. Engl. J. Med.,* 292, 895, 1975.
299. **Storb, R., Prentice, R. L., and Thomas, E. D.,** Marrow transplantation for treatment of aplastic anemia, *N. Engl. J. Med.,* 296, 61, 1977.
300. **Storb, R. and Thomas, E. D.,** Marrow transplantation for treatment of aplastic anemia, *Clin. Haematol.,* 7, 597, 1978.
301. **Thomas, E. D., Buckner, C. D., Clift, R. A., Fefer, A., Johnson, F. L., Neiman, P. E., Sale, G. E., Sanders, J. E., Singer, J. W., Shulman, H., Storb, R., and Weiden, P. L.,** Marrow transplantation for acute nonlymphoblastic leukemia in first remission, *N. Engl. J. Med.,* 301, 597, 1978.
302. **Thomas, E. D., Sanders, J. E., Flournoy, N., Johnson, F. L., Buckner, C. D., Clift, R. A., Fefer, A., Goodell, B. W., Storb, R., and Weiden, P. L.,** Marrow transplantation for patients with acute lymphoblastic leukemia in remission, *Blood,* 54, 468, 1979.
303. **Doney, K., Buckner, C. D., Sale, G. E., Ramberg, R., Boyd, C., and Thomas, E. D.,** Treatment of chronic granulocytic leukemia by chemotherapy, total body irradiation and allogeneic bone marrow transplantation, *Exp. Hematol.,* 6, 738, 1978.
304. **Fefer, A., Cheever, M. A., Thomas, E. D., Boyd, C., and Ramberg, R.,** Disappearance of Ph^1-positive cells in four patients with chronic granulocytic leukemia after chemotherapy, irradiation and marrow transplantation from an identical twin, *N. Eng. J. Med.,* 300, 333, 1979.
305. **Canellos, G. P.,** Reconstitution or resurrection of normal stem cells in chronic granulocytic leukemia, *N. Engl. J. Med.,* 300, 360, 1979.
306. **Thomas, E. D., Flournoy, N., Buckner, C. D., Clift, R. A., Fefer, A., Neiman, P. E., and Storb, R.,** Cure of leukemia by marrow transplantation, *Leukemia Res.,* 1, 67, 1977.
307. **Fialkow, P. J., Thomas, E. D., Bryant, J. I., and Neiman, P. E.,** Leukaemic transformation of engrafted human cells in vivo, *Lancet,* 1, 251, 1971.
308. **Thomas, E. D., Bryant, J. I., Buckner, C. D., Clift, R. A., Fefer, A., Johnson, F. L., Neiman, P., Ramberg, R. E., and Storb, R.,** Leukaemic transformation of engrafted human cells in vivo, *Lancet,* 1, 1310, 1972.
309. **Goh, K.,** Cytogenetic evidence of *in vivo* leukaemic transformation of engrafted marrow cells, *Lancet,* 1, 1338, 1975.
310. **Goh, K. and Klemperer, M. R.,** *In vivo* leukemic transformation: cytogenetic evidence of *in vivo* leukemic transformation of engrafted marrow cells, *Am. J. Hematol.,* 2, 283, 1977.
311. **Elfenbein, G. J., Brogaonkar, D. S., Bias, W. B., Burns, W. H., Saral, R., Sensenbrenner, L. L., Tutschka, P. J., Zaczek, B. S., Zander, A. R., Epstein, R. B., Rowley, J. D., and Santos, G. W.,** Cytogenetic evidence for recurrence of acute myelogenous leukemia after allogeneic bone marrow transplantation in donor hematopoietic cells, *Blood,* 52, 627, 1978.
312. **Storb, R.,** Critical issues in clinical bone marrow transplantation, in *Natural Resistance Systems Against Foreign Cells, Tumors, and Microbes,* Cudkowicz, G., Landy, M., and Shearer, G. M., Eds., Academic Press, New York, 1978, 49.
313. **Bortin, M. M. and Rimm, A. A.,** Factors influencing success and failure of human marrow transplantation: a review from the international bone marrow transplant registry, in *Experimental Hematology Today, 1979,* Baum, S. J., and Ledney, G. D., Eds., Springer-Verlag, New York, 1979, 173.
314. **Vitale, B. and Boranic, M.,** Clinical and theoretical implications of experimental bone marrow transplantation, *Br. J. Haematol.,* 42, 1, 1979.
315. **Pahwa, R., Pahwa, S., Good, R. A., Incefy, G. S., and O'Reilly, R. J.,** Rationale for combined use of fetal liver and thymus for immunological reconstitution in patients with variants of severe combined immunodeficiency, *Proc. Natl. Acad. Sci. U.S.A.,* 74, 3002, 1977.

316. **Tobias, J. S. and Tattersall, M. H. N.,** Prospectives in cancer research. Autologous marrow support and intensive chemotherapy in cancer patients, *Eur. J. Cancer,* 12, 1, 197.
317. **Heim, L. E.,** Ed., *Autologous bone marrow transplantation, Exp. Hematol.,* 7(Suppl. 5), 1979.
318. **Dicke, K. A., Spitzer, G., Peters, L., McCredie, K. B., Zander, A., Verma, D. S., Vellekoop, L., and Hester, J.,** Autologous bone-marrow transplantation in relapsed adult acute leukemia, *Lancet,* 514, 1979.
319. **Dicke, K. A. and Van Bekkum, D. W.,** Preparation and use of stem cell concentrates for restoration of immune deficiency diseases and bone marrow aplasia, *Rev. Eur. Etudes Clin. Biol.,* 17, 645, 1972.
320. **Lowenthal, R. M., Park, D. S., Goldman, J. M., Th'ng, K. H., Hill, R. S., and Whyte, G.,** The cryopreservation of leukaemia cells: morphological and functional changes, *Br. J. Haematol.,* 34, 105, 1976.
321. **Gorin, N. C., Herzig, G., Bull, M. I., and Graw, R. G., Jr.,** Long-term preservation of bone marrow and stem cell pool in dogs, *Blood,* 51, 257, 1978.
322. **Sarpel, S. C., Zander, A. R., Harvath, L., and Epstein, R. B.,** The collection preservation and function of peripheral blood hematopoietic cells in dogs, *Exp. Hematol.,* 7, 111, 1979.
323. **Moore, M. A. S., Hansen, J. A., Everson, L. K., O'Reilly, R. O., and Good, R. A.,** Hematological analysis of clinical bone marrow grafting evaluated by *in vitro* cultures, *Transplant. Proc.,* 8, 647, 1976.
324. **Broxmeyer, H. E.,** Culture characteristics of human granulocyte-macrophage progenitor celis and their regulation in the context of bone marrow transplantation, *Exp. Hematol.,* 7 (Suppl. 5), 149, 1979.
325. **Niskanen, E., Wells, J. R., Quesenberry, P. J., and Cline, M. J.,** Differential effect of cryopreservation on human and murine hematopoietic stem cells, *Exp. Hematol.,* 8 (Suppl. 7), 29, 1980.
326. **Cudkowicz, G.,** Genetic control of resistance to allogeneic and xenogeneic bone-marrow grafts in mice, *Transplant. Proc.,* 7, 155, 1975.
327. **Cudkowicz, G.,** Natural resistance to foreign hemopoietic and leukemia grafts, in *Natural Resistance Systems Against Foreign Cells, Tumors, and Microbes,* Cudkowicz, G., Landy, M., and Shearer, G. M., Eds., Academic Press, New York, 1978, 1.
328. **Lotzova, E.,** Resistance to parental, allogeneic and xenogeneic hemopoietic grafts in irradiated mice, *Exp. Hematol.,* 5, 215, 1977.
329. **Trentin, J. J., Gallagher, M. T., and Lotzova, E.,** Xenogeneic and genetic resistance to bone marrow transplantation: relationship to leukemia surveillance, *Transplant. Proc.,* 8, 463, 1976.
330. **Cudkowicz, G. and Stimpfling, J. H.,** Deficient growth of C57B1 marrow cells transplanted in F1 hybrid mice. Association with the histocompatibility-2 locus, *Immunology,* 7, 291, 1964.
331. **McCulloch, E. A. and Till, J. E.,** Repression of colony forming ability of C57B1 hematopoietic cells transplanted into non-isologous hosts, *J. Cell. Physiol.,* 61, 301, 1963.
332. **Goodman, J. W. and Wheeler, H. B.,** Factors that modify poor growth of parental marrow cells in F_1 hybrid mice, in *Advances in Transplantation,* Hamburger, J. and Mathe, G., Eds., Munksgaard, Copenhagen, 1968, 427.
333. **Shearer, G. M. and Cudkowicz, G.,** Induction of F_1 hybrid antiparent cytotoxic effector cells: an in vitro model for hemopoietic histoincompatibility, *Science,* 190, 890, 1975.
334. **Shearer, G. M., Waksal, H., and Cudkowicz, G.,** An in vitro model of hybrid resistance to bone marrow grafts, *Transplant. Proc.,* 8, 469, 1976.
335. **Buurman, W. A., Van Bruggen, I., and Vos, O.,** The influence of genetic resistance on CFU growth kinetics in spleen and femur, *Cell Tissue Kinet.,* 8, 111, 1975.
336. **Buurman, W. A., and Van Brugeen, I.,** Weakening of genetic resistance. II. The effect of injection of the macrophage toxic agents sibica and carragheenan and the cytostatic drugs cyclophasphamide, busulphan and vinblastin, *Exp. Hematol.,* 4, 382, 1976.
337. **Lemeneva, L. N. and Chertkov, J. L.,** Effect of hemic cells on hybrid resistance, *Exp. Hematol.,* 4, 209, 1976.
338. **Lotzova, E., Gallagher, M. T., and Trentin, J. J.,** Macrophage involvement in genetic resistance to bone marrow transplantation, *Transplant. Proc.,* 8, 477, 1976.
339. **Harrison, D. E.,** Use of genetic anaemias in mice as tools for haematological research, *Clin. Haematol.,* 8, 239, 1979.
340. **McCulloch, E. A., Siminovitch, L., and Till, J. E.,** Spleen-colony formation in anemic mice of genotype WW^v, *Science,* 144, 844, 1964.
341. **Sutherland, D. J. A., Till, J. E., and McCulloch, E. A.,** A kinetic study of the genetic control of hemopoietic progenitor cells assayed in culture and *in vivo, J. Cell. Physiol.,* 75, 267, 1970.
342. **Warner, N. L. and Moore, M. A. S.,** Defects in hematopoietic differentiation in NZB and NZC mice, *J. Exp. Med.,* 134, 313, 1971.

343. **Morley, A. and Blake, J.,** Haemopoietic precursor cells in experimental hypoplastic marrow failure, *Aust. J. Exp. Biol. Med. Sci.,* 52, 904, 1974.
344. **Morley, A., Trainor, K., and Blake, J.,** A primary stem cell lesion in experimental chronic hypoplastic marrow failure, *Blood,* 45, 681, 1975.
345. **Morley, A., Trainor, K., and Remes, J.,** Residual marrow damage: possible explanation for idiosyncrosy to chloramphenical, *Br. J. Haematol.,* 32, 525, 1976.
346. **Kubota, K., Mizoguchi, H., Miura, Y., Kano, S., and Takaku, F.,** Experimental hypoplastic marrow failure in the mouse, *Exp. Hematol.,* 6, 791, 1978.
347. **Cline, M. J., Strong, H., Mercola, K., Morse, L., Ruprecht, R., Browne, J., and Salser, W.,** Gene transfer in intact animals, *Nature,* 284, 422, 1980.
348. **Mercola, K. E., Stang, H. D., Browne, J., Salser, W., and Cline, M. J.,** Insertion of a new gene of viral origin into bone marrow cells of mice, *Science,* 208, 1033, 1980.
349. **Williamson, B.,** Reintroduction of genetically transformed bone marrow cells into mice, *Nature,* 284, 397, 1980.

Chapter 5

THE ERYTHROID SYSTEM AT THE LEVEL OF PROGENITOR CELLS—STRUCTURE AND REGULATION

Nydia G. Testa

TABLE OF CONTENTS

I. INTRODUCTION

The processes of differentiation and maturation which lead to the formation of functional red cells presumably require an orderly sequence of events which influence different stages of the progression of early committed erythroid cells towards mature erythrocytes. Considerable advances have been made towards achieving a working understanding of such progression. Distinct populations of erythroid progenitor cells may be characterized using assays which depend on the capacity of these cells to proliferate in vitro, forming clonal colonies of hemoglobinized cells. The influence of humoral factors, which may act as hormonal regulators of erythropoiesis, and of cell populations which may also play a regulatory role in erythroid colony formation, is actually being investigated in several laboratories. Furthermore, progress towards the understanding of the structure of the bone marrow and its likely influence in the regulation of hemopoiesis by providing permissive or inductive microenvironments, has been made recently. This chapter describes the assays available to study erythroid progenitor cells, and analyzes their usefulness for the study of normal erythropoiesis, its kinetics, and its regulation.

II. ERYTHROID COLONY FORMATION

A. General Remarks

Colony growth of erythroid cells in cultures of mouse fetal liver was first reported in 1971.[1] Reports of colonies derived from adult tissue of mouse[2,3] as well as of other species, followed to date from man,[3] and dog,[4] sheep,[5] rabbit,[6] and cat.[7] The first colonies reported achieved only a small size of up to about 60 hemoglobinized cells after an optimum period of incubation of only 2 days in the presence of erythropoietin (Epo).[1] The cells forming these colonies are usually called CFU-E, or colony-forming units-erythroid. As will be seen below, they have been characterized as relatively mature erythroid progenitor cells, probably very close to the earliest proerythroblasts recognizable under light microscopy.[8–9]

Perhaps more interesting from the point of view of understanding the erythroid system is the possibility of growing in culture colonies derived from earlier erythroid precursor cells.[2,10] These colonies, or bursts, which may contain thousands of hemoglobinized cells,[10] are derived from the BFU-E, or burst-forming units-erythroid.[2] The BFU-E are very heterogeneous with regard to proliferation and differentiation capacity. At present, cells which are very close or even overlap the compartment of multipotential cells and are therefore not yet restricted to the erythroid pathway of differentiation, to cells which are the immediate precursors of CFU-E are considered part of the BFU-E population. As their physical and functional characteristics change as they advance towards maturity, their progression through the erythroid compartment may be inferred from experimental observations. This, as will be seen below, allows the construction of schemes of the erythroid system which may be tested experimentally.

B. Colony Forming Cells

1. CFU-E

When hemopoietic cells are cultured in plasma clot[1] or methylcellulose[2] with adequate nutrients, and in the presence of Epo, the CFU-E give rise to colonies which contain up to about 60 late normoblasts and nonnucleated erythrocytes. The clonal nature of these colonies, inferred from the linear relationship between cell inoculum and colony numbers, has been documented using time-lapse photography.[8]

Both the limited size of the colonies (Figure 1) and the short incubation time required

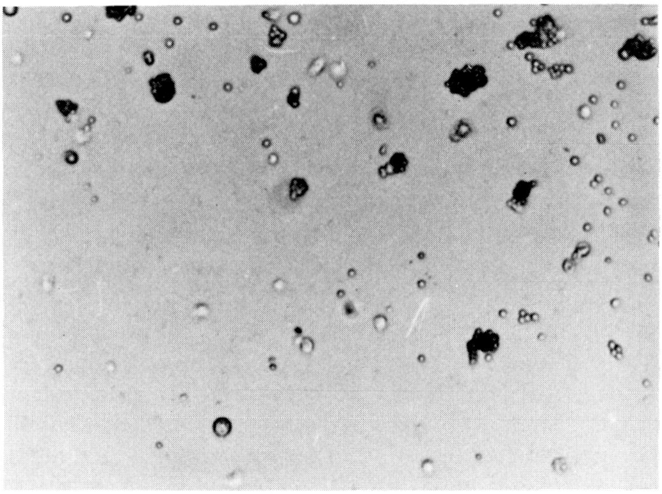

FIGURE 1. CFU-E derived colonies from normal mouse marrow grown in methylcellulose. Darker colonies show better hemoglobinization.

before the colony cells become hemoglobinized, of only 2 days in the case of mouse cells[1] and up to 7 for man,[3,11] indicates that CFU-E are relatively late progenitor cells. This is strengthened by their high incidence in normal bone marrow up to 600/per 10^5 nucleated mouse marrow cells,[12] which suggests that they are close to the recognizable proerythroblasts. This was confirmed by direct observation using time-lapse photography[8] which showed that only two or three cell divisions separate the CFU-E from hemoglobin-synthesizing cells.

CFU-E not only require Epo to proliferate in vitro, but their own survival is Epo dependent. In cultures initiated with Epo, more than 80% of the CFU-E die if Epo is not added before 24 hr.[13] This suggests that the CFU-E population itself may be regulated by this hormone.[4] In fact, the size of the CFU-E population in vivo is Epo dependent: when the levels of Epo are lowered by hypertransfusion, the numbers of CFU-E decrease markedly, by about 90%, and they increase two or threefold when Epo levels are increased by bleeding or by exogeneous administration.[2,14]

The CFU-E population proliferates actively during normal steady-state. A short exposure to high doses of tritiated thymidine, which regularly kill cells undergoing DNA synthesis, results in the elimination of 70 to 80% of the CFU-E.[15,16] It is of interest to note that in hypertransfused mice, the proportion killed remains high, at about 60%, in spite of the fact that there is no physiological need for red cell production.[15] In these polycythemic mice, no recognizable erythroid cells are found in the marrow and only insignificant amounts of injected radioactive iron are incorporated into red cells, showing that erythroid cell production has been arrested. The implications of the continued cycling of the CFU-E population for the regulation of red cell production under those circumstances are not known. The high level of cycling may be an equivalent, at the CFU-E level, of the normal degree of ineffective erythropoiesis which is found at later stages of erythroid cell maturation in man.[18] However, this ineffective erythropoiesis in the population of hemoglobin-synthesizing cells is small. Whether the high level suggested by the 60% cycling of the CFU-E is only a result of differences between man and mouse, is not known. It is of interest that no signs of ineffective erythropoiesis have been found in the population of recognizable erythroid cells in mouse.[19]

2. BFU-E

The BFU-E give rise to colonies which contain from several hundred up to about 10^4 cells, mainly late normoblasts and some nonnucleated red cells, in plasma clot[2] or methylcellulose[10] cultures in the presence of Epo. Not only is the colony size considerably larger than in CFU-E derived colonies, but the incubation time required to reach full development is longer. Colonies composed of several thousand cells (Figure 2), sometimes arranged in several tight clusters for any single burst, may require 8 to 14 days of incubation for mouse bone marrow cultures and about 14 to 20 days for human cells.[20,21] Their incidence at 50 to 100 bursts per 10^5 bone marrow cells is lower than that of CFU-E,[20-22] and is similar for human and mouse cells.[20-23] Although the presence of Epo is essential for the full differentiation of the BFU-E progeny, and therefore, for the visualization and recognition of the bursts, the first divisions (and perhaps some differentiation steps) of the BFU-E in vitro depend on the presence in the cultures of another factor(s): BPA, or burst-promoting activity,[12] which will be discussed below.

The multicentric appearance of some bursts, especially in cultures of human cells, made it important to establish beyond doubt the clonal nature of these colonies. This was elegantly demonstrated using the naturally occurring mosaic, the X-chromosome linked glucose-6-phosphate dehydrogenase (G-6-PD) isoenzyme system.[23] Bursts arising from hemopoietic cells of individuals heterozygous for G-6-PD contain only one type of the enzyme, and the ratio of colonies with each isoenzyme is similar to that found in circulating blood cells[23] and in nonhemopoietic mesenchymal cells.[24]

The wide spectrum of cells which belong to the BFU-E compartment encompasses all cells beginning with those close to the multipotential cell population, down to the immediate precursors of the CFU-E. By varying the length of the incubation time, subpopulations of BFU-E of different degrees of maturity may be detected.[21] They are usually identified by a prefix denoting the length of incubation (i.e., Day 3 BFU-E, Day 8 BFU-E, etc.) and may be scored sequentially in the same cultures. The most immature BFU-E originate the largest bursts which require longer periods of incubation. It is important to notice that in a proportion of these, multipotential cells, CFU-S (colony forming units-spleen) which give rise to spleen colonies in irradiated mice, are still found after several days of incubation.[25] This indicates that those BFU-E must be multipotential, and suggests that the concept of the early BFU-E being already committed to erythropoiesis may have to be revised. Furthermore, some bursts contain megakaryocytes[22,26,27] and one example is illustrated in Figure 3. The proportion of bursts derived from fresh marrow, which contain megakaryocytes in addition to erythroid cells may be as high as 40%.[27] Studies in cultures of mixed male and female bone marrow indicate that these bursts are of clonal origin, since both tetraploid and diploid metaphases forming individual bursts were found to belong to either male or female cells, for each burst studied.[27] As will be discussed below, the colony cells in culture may only express incompletely their potential for proliferation and differentiation, which is governed in vitro by the conditions provided by the culture. In that respect, the addition of the necessary stimulus for differentiation together with permissive culture conditions is all important.

The BFU-E population shares some characteristics with the CFU-S of mice. They have a similar size, as determined by their velocity of sedimentation at unit gravity[28] and a similar buoyant density in bovine serum albumin gradients.[22] Furthermore, the proportion of the population undergoing DNA synthesis, determined by exposure to high doses of tritiated thymidine, is only slightly higher (30%) than that reported for CFU-S (10%).[16] However, some kinetic parameters differ; after repeated doses of irradiation which result in residual damage to the bone marrow and reduced numbers of CFU-S in femur,[29] the BFU-E, although subnormal, reach a higher level than the CFU-

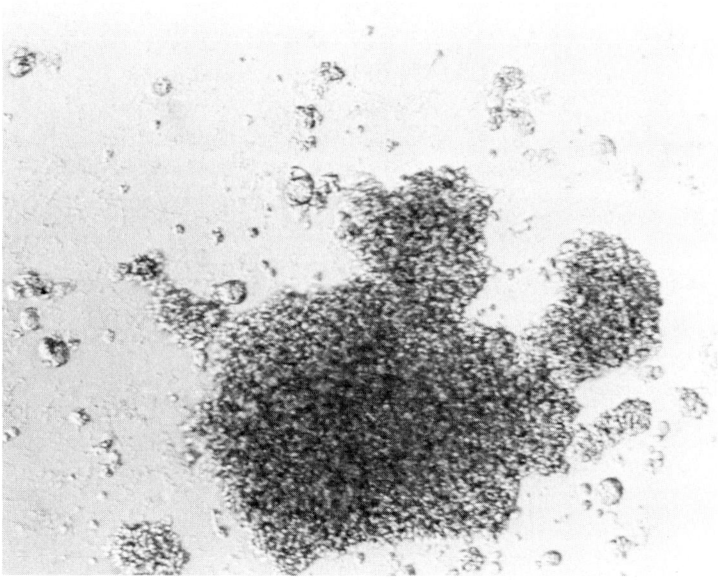

FIGURE 2. Large BFU-E derived colony with homogeneous hemoglobinization after 14 days of culture. Normal human marrow grown in methylcellulose.

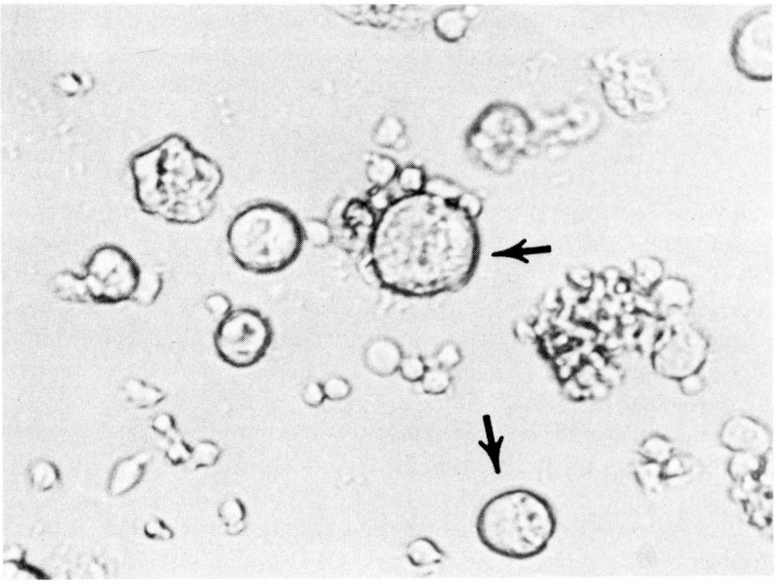

FIGURE 3. Section of a large burst showing megakaryocytes (arrows) and a cluster of erythroid cells.

S,[9] possibly reflecting some amplification within the erythroid compartment. Some kinetic differences are also apparent during regeneration following multiple injections of hydroxyurea. Although the pattern of regeneration of CFU-S and Day 10 BFU-E is similar, the exponential phase of growth appears to be initiated earlier for Day 10 BFU-E than for CFU-S.[30] The differences are more pronounced for Day 3 BFU-E: they reach

Table 1
SOME CHARACTERISTICS OF PROGENITOR CELLS IN HUMAN BONE MARROW

Progenitor	Potential for differentiation	Incidence per 10^5 bone marrow cells	Incubation time (days)	Cycling status (% kill by ^{3}HTdR)	Regulation	Ref.
Mix-CFU	Multipotential	5	≥20	Low (~20)	Factor (s) in CM (BPA-like?)	33 to 35
Early BFU-E	Bi- or unipotential	5—10	18—20	Low (~30)	BPA	12,20,21,23
Late BFU-E	Unipotential	40	7—12	Intermediate (~40)	BPA, Epo	11,20,21
CFU-E	Unipotential	100	6—8	High (~80)	Epo	3,11,21

control values faster than the other two cell populations.[30] The intermediate Day 3 BFU-E show more differences than the more immature BFU-E when compared to CFU-S; their turnover, with about 40 to 50% killed by tritiated thymidine, and their incidence in normal bone marrow, are intermediate between those of the earlier BFU-E and the CFU-E.[21] A summary of several parameters measured in the different populations of erythroid progenitors is shown in Table 1. It should be noted that Day 3 BFU-E of mice and Day 7 BFU-E of human are probably equivalent in terms of maturation, the difference in time of incubation reflecting the longer time human cells require to reach full maturity in culture.[20,21]

3. *Mix-CFU*

Mixed colonies that contain in addition to erythroblasts and megakaryocytes, granulocytes (neutrophils and/or eosinophils), and macrophages, can be grown from mouse[31,32] and human cells[33-35] in cultures which contain medium conditioned by mitogen stimulated cells. The cells giving rise to those colonies, will be called here Mix-CFU, or colony forming units which can give rise to a mixed progeny. As in all colony assays, strict proof of clonality is important to establish. This allows us to analyze the capacity of individual cells to respond to regulators and to divide and differentiate, ultimately placing them within a functional scheme in the hemopoietic system.

The single cell origin of mixed colonies was established beyond doubt by replating experiments using single cells and following the growth of the new mixed colonies they originated[32] and by co-cultivation of male and female cells, which yielded mixed colonies of male or female type.[33] Like the early BFU-E, the Mix-CFU share some physical and functional characteristics with the CFU-S, and a proportion of mixed colonies contains CFU-S.[32] However, both their proliferative capacity and their potential for differentiation appear to be more restricted,[31–35] at least as determined by the in vitro colony assay; the colonies are smaller than those produced in vivo by CFU-S, and, unlike them, appear to lack the capacity to originate lymphoid progeny. However, it should be borne in mind that these measurements are performed in vitro which may allow only partial expression of the true capacities of the colony forming cells. As these cell populations have not yet been isolated as pure populations, the criteria established by the experimental colony assays are the only ones available at present. On this basis, a maturation sequence CFU-S, Mix-CFU, BFU-E, CFU-E erythroblasts, may be postulated from the earliest cell which can be assayed functionally to the earliest erythroid cell recognizable under optical microscopy.

III. REGULATION OF COLONY FORMATION

A. Humoral Factors

1. Erythropoietin

The classic role of Epo is to induce the differentiation of erythroid precursor cells to hemoglobin synthesizing cells, an effect well documented in several experimental systems.[36] Using colony assays, the apparent requirements of Epo are lowest at the CFU-E level, with maximum colony formation observed after 0.1 to 0.2 U of exogenous Epo per milliliter of culture,[1] and highest at the more immature BFU-E level, with reports of maximum burst formation in the presence of 1 U Epo to more than 10 U/mℓ.[1,13,21,22] An important factor to be considered is the presence of both Epo and BPA in the serum used in most culture systems, which may be present at different levels in different batches of serum. The determination of the sensitivity of CFU-E to Epo done in serum-free cultures, gives values of 0.15 U/mℓ for maximum CFU-E growth,[37] and it seems likely that CFU-E are, as has been postulated,[13,21] more sensitive to Epo than BFU-E.

Erythropoietin is produced mainly in the kidney as a response to low O_2 content in the blood relative to demand. Its production, physiology, and metabolism have been expertly reviewed.[36] A great deal of effort has been devoted to the purification of this hormone and preparations of up to 70,000 units per milligram have been reported.[38] Availability of such preparations will be very useful to design experiments in which the role of Epo may be defined in a more exacting way than has been possible in the past. Some of the effects attributed to Epo may have been due to contaminants such as endotoxin or to other biologically active molecules, like colony stimulating factor (CSF),[3,39] which induce the growth of colonies of granulocytes and macrophages in vitro, and perhaps also megakaryocyte CSF. It is also possible that some Epo preparations currently in use may contain BPA.[9] This is suggested by the observation that an adequate supply of BPA added to cultures may reduce the requirement of Epo tenfold, without any effect in the number, size, or degree of hemoglobinization of the bursts produced.[13,22] The presence of BPA in Epo preparations may also explain the reported discrepancies in the dose of Epo required for maximum burst formation.

Relatively mature cells, defined in vivo as erythropoietin responsive cells (ERC),[40] assayed in polycythemic mice by their capacity to originate a wave of erythropoiesis in response to administered Epo,[17] respond to this hormone by acquiring the capacity to synthesize Hb.[36] Earlier cells, called pre-ERC[41,42] respond to Epo by increasing proliferation, which in time and if the erythropoietic stimulus is maintained, results in a bigger wave of mature RBC. Myleran®-treated mice, in which CFU-S and early BFU-E are only about 1 to 2% of control values, can respond to Epo in the way described,[43] indicating that the increased amplification takes place at the level of the intermediate BFU-E and perhaps a minority of the CFU-E.[44] As these results are also obtained using highly purified, endotoxin-free Epo[45] there appears to be little doubt about this dual role of Epo in the regulation of erythropoiesis.

An intriguing report of CFU-E growth in a serum-free, erythropoietin-free system suggests that Epo may not be the only stimulator of erythroid differentiation at the level of the late progenitor cells (CFU-E) and can be replaced by a factor contained in conditioned medium produced by mitogen stimulated cells.[37] As will be discussed below, several stimulators of hemopoiesis are found in that type of conditioned medium. If these results are confirmed and their physiological significance is established they will lead to a revision of our current concepts of regulation of erythropoiesis.

2. Burst-Promoting Activity

The early observations that BFU-E may be maintained in culture, and undergo substantial proliferation in the absence of exogenous Epo,[13] suggested that, although Epo is needed to achieve full maturation of the BFU-E progeny, early events in erythropoiesis may be regulated by a different factor, BPA.[13] BPA has been found in medium conditioned by lectin stimulated spleen cells,[13] and in the serum of man,[46] horse, and mice,[23] as well as in human urine. In profound perturbations of hemopoiesis like in aplastic anemia in humans,[47] or those resulting from the induction of hemolytic anemia in mice,[22] the levels of BPA are increased, a situation similar to that found for Epo. However, after cessation of exposure to hypoxia, increased levels of BPA together with decreased Epo are found,[22] suggesting that the production of each factor is regulated by different mechanisms.

Biochemical characterization of BPA is underway in several laboratories.[13,48,49] Although considerable progress has been made, it is not yet possible to establish whether BPA can be ascribed to a single molecule, or it is part of a family of molecules of similar nature, which may act at slightly different levels along the differentiation pathway. No clear information has yet emerged on whether this molecule(s) is active in a pathway-specific way (i.e., influencing only erythroid progenitor cells) or is a stimulator of divisions in more than one cell line.[13] In that respect, it is of interest to note that highly purified colony stimulating factor which induces the formation of colonies of granulocytes and macrophages (GM-CSF) may stimulate up to five cell divisions of Mix-CFU of mouse, but could not support subsequent proliferation to produce a fully developed mixed colony.[50] This latter step required the addition of cell line specific factors (eosinophil CSF, megakaryocytic CSF, and Epo), which probably act at later stages of maturation and/or differentiation. It will be of great interest to elucidate the window of action, and the effect of purified BPA, not only from the point of view of possible pathway specificity but in order to clarify its relationship to factors which stimulate the formation of mixed colonies.[48,49] Partially purified BPA has been obtained from mitogen stimulated spleen cell conditioned medium,[13] and has characteristics which are similar to those described for the factor which stimulates Mix-CFU: both are stable glycoproteins, of an apparent molecular weight of 35,000 to 45,000.[13,49,51]

In contrast with Epo, which has a well-established role in vivo in the regulation of erythropoiesis, no firm evidence of such a role for BPA has yet been obtained. However, suggestive evidence exists and some of it has already been discussed. The observation that normal cells, as will be seen below, produce BPA or similar activities emphasizes the possibility of a role in vivo. Although there is an urgent need to perform experiments designed to determine such role, the usefulness of BPA for the analysis of populations of erythroid progenitor cells is already apparent.

3. Others

Both Epo and BPA are absolute requirements for erythroid growth in vitro and have been discussed above with regard to their role in the regulation of erythropoiesis. There are other molecules which may stimulate the growth of erythroid cells in vitro by exerting the effect on the modulation of erythropoiesis which they show in vivo, or which may supplement the culture medium and favor growth by improving the general conditions in vitro.

Among the latter, the freshness of the culture medium, and an adequate source of serum or of the serum components shown to be essential for cell growth, like albumin, transferrin, selenium, and phospholipids, are important considerations. Alpha-thyoglycerol, or beta-mercaptoethanol may improve CFU-E as well as BFU-E growth.[52]

Hormones which enhance erythropoiesis in vivo, like thyroxine and other thyroid analogs, enhance erythroid growth in vitro, an action not related to their calorigenic effect.[53] This stimulation, shown by an increase in plating efficiency, is comparable in degree to that exerted by growth hormone[54] and appears to be more selective than the effect of some steroids with a 5β structure, which in addition to improving erythroid growth in vitro, also stimulate granulocyte-macrophage colony formation.[15] There may be species differences in the action of some pharmacological agents on erythroid growth.[54] For example, addition of prostaglandins of the E series results in a dose-dependent inhibition of BFU-E, but not CFU-E growth in cultures of mouse bone marrow, an effect also seen after the addition of theophylline (an inhibitor of phosphodiesterase). In contrast, comparable levels added to human bone marrow cultures enhance both BFU-E and CFU-E growth.[55]

B. Associated Cell Populations

1. Burst Feeder Activity

The first report that the growth of bursts could be modified by cells normally present in the hemopoietic tissue originated in experiments which showed that if bone marrow cells were cultured after separating the cells adhering to polyester fibers, erythroid growth could be enhanced by medium conditioned by human leukocytes.[11] The observation that CFU-E growth was not enhanced by leukocyte-conditioned medium[21] made feasible the suggestion that the stimulating factor involved might be BPA.

Activities provided by cells added directly to cultures have been called BFA, or burst feeder activity.[22] It is possible, although not proven, that BFA may be very similar, or indeed identical to BPA. However, there may be conditions associated to their production or release in culture which could result in different behavior of BFA and BPA in vitro in some circumstances.[56] But until the BFA-associated cells become fully characterized, and purified BPA becomes available, their relationship will remain uncertain.

The cells associated with BFA in marrow have high density (>1.08 g/mℓ^{-3}) in bovine serum albumin gradients.[22] They still produce and/or release normal levels of BFA after doses of irradiation up to 20 Gy,[57] which indicates that either they are very radioresistant, or that BFA release does not depend on cell proliferation.

Although a recent report suggests that human bone marrow may produce BPA, the specific population(s) responsible for its production has not yet been characterized.[58]

2. T Cells

Burst growth from circulating BFU-E may improve in terms of plating efficiency, colony size, and hemoglobinization if relatively large numbers of T cells are added to the cultures.[58] This, however, is a result that has not been obtained consistently, and similar growth of bursts in the presence or in the absence of T cells has also been reported.[59] These discrepancies may only be due to differences in culture and cell separation techniques which should be solved in the near future. Information reviewed recently indicates that the role of cell-cell interactions is important not only in the regulation of erythropoiesis, but also of multipotential cells and granulocytic-macrophage progenitors.[60-63] There are indications of a possible role of T cells in the regulation of erythropoiesis in vivo,[64] and evidence of production of erythroid potentiating activity (EPA) by a human T-lymphoblastic cell line in vitro.[49] EPA enhances the growth of BFU-E and also of human, but not mouse, CFU-E.[49] Its partial biochemical characterization shows that it is an acidic glycoprotein with an apparent molecular weight of 45,000 which is similar to BPA.[13] This cell line also produces a factor that stimulates Mix-CFU; whether the latter is equivalent to EPA (or BPA?) remains to be determined.

3. Monocytes, Macrophages

As in the case of T cells, conflicting reports in the literature make it difficult to establish with certainty the role of monocytes and macrophages in erythropoiesis. It is likely, however, that in the case of granulopoiesis[65] these cells are part of complicated feedback rings which will require extensive experimental work for their analysis and understanding.

Classically, the macrophage has been considered a cell that is involved in the transfer of iron to erythroblasts.[66] More recently it has been shown that macrophages potentiate the effect of Epo in vitro by the release of diffusible substances.[59] In contrast to their reported role in iron transfer, the latter effect does not require cell contact and results in increased plating efficiency of CFU-E and BFU-E. However, there is no indication that the presence of macrophages is an absolute requirement for erythroid growth, although the presence of a macrophage in the center of an erythroblastic island is frequently observed both in vivo and in vitro.[66,67]

The macrophage products responsible for the increased plating efficiency have not yet been identified, although it is likely that BFA may be involved.[59] However, the role of macrophages in erythropoiesis may be more extensive than just as providers of BFA and iron; indeed, the increase in plating efficiency of the CFU-E, a cell not considered to be influenced by BPA, which macrophages induced, supports that suggestion.[59] The stimulatory or inhibitory effect of monocytes-macrophages on erythroid colony growth may be dose dependent, with high numbers tending to be inhibitory,[68] perhaps by release of PGE which may be inhibitory of murine BFU-E growth.[55] In man, removal of monocytes resulted in a significant stimulation of CFU-E growth.[68] Furthermore, when increasing numbers of purified monocytes were added to peripheral blood BFU-E, growth was inhibited in a dose-dependent fashion. The mechanism of such inhibition does not appear to be related to inactivation of Epo or to nutritional depletion of the cultures.[68]

At present, it seems reasonable to postulate that monocytes-macrophages may contribute to the regulation of erythropoiesis not only by their involvement in the production and/or release of BFA-BPA, but possibly by their relationship to other active molecules, like prostaglandins.[55] Whether the effects described in vitro are of importance physiologically in vivo remains to be determined.

IV. STRUCTURE AND REGULATION OF THE ERYTHROID COMPARTMENT

The erythroid compartment starts at the level of the earliest cells committed to erythroid differentiation. From studies on the multipotential cells which originate mixed colonies, it is apparent that the separation into compartments is not clear-cut, and that a certain degree of overlap can be expected in the cell populations detected by the Mix-CFU and the early BFU-E assays. As described above, not only do these cells have some similar physical and functional characteristics, but both require products of lectin-stimulated cells to proliferate and/or differentiate in culture. Current investigation of the molecules, or families of molecules which act at this level is aimed at establishing whether there are active moieties exerting their effect on cells at different levels of maturation.[48-51] Another problem, highly relevant for our understanding of differentiation, is to establish whether they act as pathway indifferent stem cell-like regulators,[13]

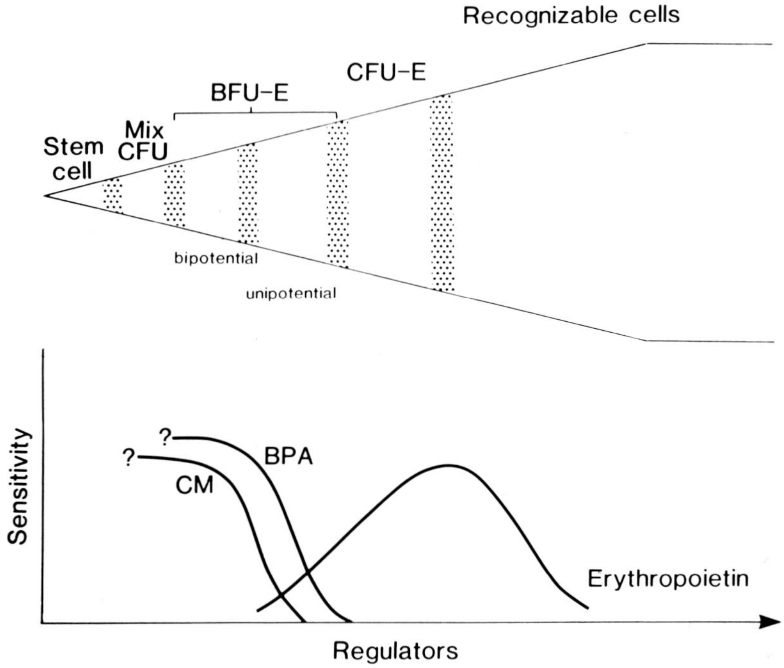

FIGURE 4. Diagram of the erythroid compartment. The erythroid system is considered to start at the level of the earliest unipotential BFU-E, which will undergo maturation and proliferation to originate, in time, intermediate and late BFU-E and CFU-E. The latter will originate recognizable erythroblasts and eventually mature, nondividing red blood cells. The grey areas indicate overlap in the cell populations detected by the different assays. Sensitivity to humoral regulators is plotted in the lower part of the diagram. Cell populations sensitive to each regulator are those above the curves shown. Factors in conditioned medium (CM) may be similar or identical to BPA. The question marks indicate that the earliest target cells for these factors may be at the Mix-CFU or even at the stem cell level.

to be followed at later stages by pathway specific molecules like erythropoietin for red blood cell production, or some types of CSF for granulocytes and macrophages.[48] The early regulators may act as humoral regulators, like BPA or BPA-like molecules, or through cell-cell interactions. Less is known about the latter, but studies on the structure of the bone marrow suggest, as will be discussed below, that cell-cell interactions, or short range mechanisms may be important in erythropoiesis. However, the concept that regulation at the Mix-CFU, early BFU-E level may be pathway indifferent suggests that the mechanisms by which the line of differentiation is determined, remain unknown.

Once the pathway has been established, and the committed cells progress toward maturation, they become less sensitive to the lectin-stimulated cell products, or BPA type molecules, and become responsive to specific pathway regulators, in this case Epo.[13] In the scheme shown in Figure 4, the most immature BFU-E (bi- and unipotential) are sensitive only to the former type of regulators, while the intermediate also became sensitive to Epo. These may respond, according to the circumstances and to the dose of Epo, with increased proliferation, therefore amplifying the erythroid compartment, or by acquiring the capacity to synthesize Hb.[42-45] It may be postulated that the probability of the latter effect is higher for the more mature BFU-E and the CFU-

E. Sensitivity to Epo is probably maximal at the CFU-E level,[13,39] although it is known that recognizable erythroblasts are also sensitive to it.

The possible role of putative regulatory cells has not been illustrated in Figure 4, as it is apparent from the conflicting reports in the literature that the cell types involved have not yet been identified, and their action has not yet been clarified. As discussed above, the main cell types likely to be involved belong to the monocyte-macrophage and the T-cell populations, both of which are notoriously heterogeneous. Further characterization of the cells involved may allow the definition of the relevant cells and their possible roles. In fact two subpopulations of T cells, one stimulatory and one inhibitory of BFU-E growth, have been identified recently by the use of monoclonal antibodies.[69]

As erythroid precursor cells advance along the maturation pathway, they undergo multiplication and change some physical characteristics; their size increases,[28] the proportion of the population undergoing DNA synthesis becomes higher,[16] their incidence in bone marrow increases,[12] and the proliferation capacity of individual cells diminishes.[2] Discrete steps in this progression will probably be defined in the near future using long-term bone marrow cultures. In these cultures, multipotential cells and extensive granulopoiesis are maintained for several weeks, depending on the presence of an adherent layer of bone marrow derived cells, which contains macrophages, fat cells, and endothelial cells, and which is thought to have a regulatory role.[61] In the basic culture conditions, the erythroid lineage is blocked at the early BFU-E stage.[70] By adding purified Epo, progression up to the CFU-E stage can be achieved;[71] further progression to nonnucleated hemoglobinized red cells is seen in conditions that do not favor cell attachment to the culture dishes,[71] or by the addition of serum from anemic irradiated and phenyl-hydrazine-treated mice to standard cultures.[67] Although the anemic mouse serum is rich in Epo, and probably in BPA, some factors other than these may also influence erythropoiesis under these conditions since (1) addition of purified Epo alone does not suffice,[70,71] and (2) the adherent cell layer has high levels of BFA.[56] If BPA present in the serum is the factor responsible, it has to be postulated that BFA in the cultures is not readily released into the culture medium, and therefore local conditions in the adherent layer (cell-cell interactions or short-range factors?) are important for erythropoiesis. It is also worthy of notice that in these cultures, T cells have not been detected.[61]

V. DISTRIBUTION OF ERYTHROID PRECURSOR CELLS IN THE BONE MARROW

There are several indications that the distribution of different cell types within the bone marrow is not random. Labeling studies using tritiated thymidine established a gradient between the subendosteal and the central, capillary rich regions of the marrow, which suggests migration of mature cells towards the capillaries.[72] At the level of the precursor cells, it has been shown that, at least in mouse femur, the multipotential cells and the precursors of granulocytes and macrophages conform to a well defined, nonrandom, spacial distribution characteristic of each population.[73] Recent work indicates that the granulocytic-macrophage precursors, as well as the cells which produce CSF, also show a nonrandom spacial distribution in human sternum and rib with a lower incidence in regions associated with the bone trabeculae than in the rest of the marrow.[74] Although experiments to establish the distribution of human erythroid precursor cells are still in progress it has already been established that, in the mouse femur, erythroid precursor cells are not randomly distributed, and precursors of different degree of maturity follow different patterns.[75] Figure 5 shows a diagramatic representation of the relative incidence of CFU-E and BFU-E in mouse femur. It shows that BFU-E has a

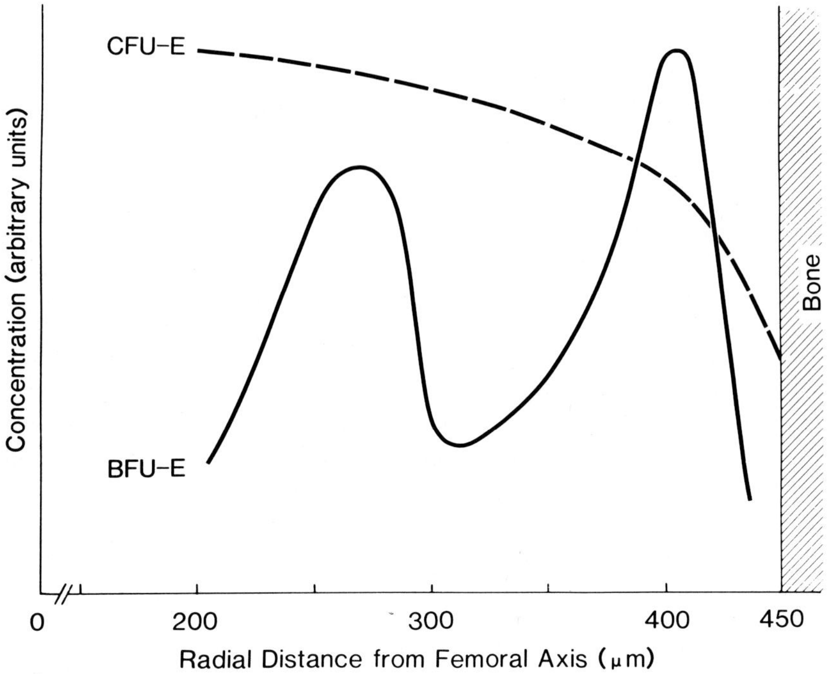

FIGURE 5. Spatial distribution of BFU-E and CFU-E in mouse femur.

bimodal distribution with a peak close to, but not in contact with, the bone surface and a second peak in an intermediate position between the femoral bone and the axis of the cavity. There are indications that the first peak contains a higher proportion of the more immature BFU-E, some of which may be bipotential. In the same region, CFU-S are also found in high concentrations, although unlike the BFU-E, they do not decrease close to the bone surface.[73] The second peak has a longer proportion of relatively more mature BFU-E while the CFU-E show a broad distribution with the highest incidence towards the axis of the femur, and the lowest close to the endosteal surface. Although no definitive data are yet available, preliminary results suggest that BFA-associated cells also follow a nonrandom distribution.[75]

It is likely, and indeed experiments in progress support this concept, that erythroid progenitor cells also may conform to a well-defined distribution in the human bone marrow. The implications of these observations for the understanding of the regulation of differentiation and proliferation of hemopoietic cells, and especially for the role of cell-cell interactions, may be important.

VI. ERYTHROID COLONIES IN HEMOPOIETIC DISORDERS

A. Anemia

1. Aplastic Anemia

As can be expected, the incidence of mixed and erythroid colonies is very low, reflecting the low proliferative activity of the hemopoietic tissue.[76,77] Perhaps a more interesting aspect of colony studies in aplastic anemia is the possibility of investigating imbalances of environmental regulation of erythropoiesis. This is illustrated by a recent case report of a patient with long-standing hypoplastic anemia, whose marrow showed a florid growth of BFU-E and CFU-E, with good cellular maturation and synthesis of heme. As material from a nondispersed marrow biopsy failed to show heme synthesis, and no cellular or humoral inhibitors of erythropoiesis could be demonstrated in the patient's cells or serum, it was concluded that the anemia was due to a defect in the bone marrow environment.[78] Although the possibility of a defective environment as a cause of aplasia had been postulated before,[79-81] this is the first clinical report which substantiates that hypothesis. It is worth mentioning that an apparent similar case, but involving normal granulocyte-macrophage colony growth in vitro with no detectable inhibitors of granulopoiesis, has also been reported.[82]

The possibility that some cases of aplastic anemia may be of immunological origin has been revived recently.[80-83] Bone marrow culture studies provide a useful tool to investigate this problem.

2. Congenital Hypoplastic Anemia

Patients with Diamond-Blackfan syndrome have been studied using marrow culture techniques with a view to determine whether putative regulatory cell populations are involved in the pathogenesis of the disease. Inhibition of CFU-E from normal allogeneic bone marrow by patient's lymphoid cells has been reported,[84] although this has not been a consistent finding.[85] The possibility of inhibition being related to the history of the patients has to be considered from the point of view of possible sensitization induced by blood transfusions[9] which may account for the inhibitory effect reported. In this context, it is of interest that no inhibition has been found in nontransfused patients.[85] Another possibility is that steroid treatment may change the sensitivity of erythroid progenitors to possible suppression effects of regulatory cells. The reported stimulatory role of T cells on BFU-E appears to be conserved in these patients.[86]

B. Myeloproliferative Syndromes

1. Preleukemia

Only limited information is available in the literature about erythroid colony growth in this syndrome. The characteristic refractory cytopenia may be accompanied by normal or even increased incidence of CFU-E in the bone marrow.[87,88] This increase is probably related to the high degree of ineffective erythropoiesis these patients may present, since there is no correlation between CFU-E numbers and Hb levels.[9]

2. Polycythemia Vera

A high level of CFU-E growth in the absence of exogenous Epo is a consistent finding in this disease.[89-91] However, a large proportion of the colonies would only grow in cultures with added Epo. This finding, together with the observation that CFU-E in polycythemia vera responds to steroids in a manner comparable to normal cells,[89] confirms earlier in vivo observations that the erythroid compartment is influenced by normal regulatory factors [92,93] and validates in vitro studies in hematological patients.

The clonal nature of the disease was established in patients heterozygous for G-6-PD.[94] Using the same marker, it has been shown that some of the bursts which appeared in cultures with large doses of Epo were derived from cells which contained the other isoenzyme, and were, therefore, presumably remaining normal BFU-E.[95] Investigation of the factors that allow the expression of normal erythropoiesis in vitro, but not in vivo may throw light on the pathophysiology of polycythemia vera.

3. Chronic Myeloid Leukemia

Although the main manifestation of chronic myeloid leukemia is an overproduction of granulocytic cells and of their precursors,[96] it has been demonstrated recently that there is also considerable expansion at the level of the erythroid progenitor cells. Both

BFU-E and CFU-E numbers are increased in the bone marrow[97] and still more strikingly in the peripheral blood,[98] where the BFU-E may be up to 180 times the normal value. These findings indicate that the amplification of early cells is not an exclusive phenomenon of the granulocytic series. There was also considerable colony growth in cultures containing only minimum amounts of Epo,[97] a phenomenom also seen consistently in polycythemia vera.[89,90] However, in chronic myeloid leukemia this pattern of growth was associated with anemia,[97] suggesting a block in erythroid cell production at or after the CFU-E level.

Another similarity may be the conservation of some normal regulatory mechanisms in both diseases: in a case of juvenile chronic myeloid leukemia undergoing an erythroblastic phase, the numbers of erythroid colonies in the marrow decreased after transfusion, as did Epo level in serum.[99] However, the situation may be different in the adult type of the disease.

VII. GENERAL CONCLUSIONS

Considerable ground has been covered since the first clonal assays for hemopoietic cells were described.[100,101] The possibility of studying populations of progenitor cells, and putative regulatory factors which influence them has already thrown considerable light on our understanding of the structure and physiology of the normal erythroid system, and of their alterations in disease. The relative importance of humoral and short-range factors and of possible cell to cell interactions in the regulation of proliferation and differentiation in the erythroid cell lineage is now being studied actively in several laboratories. The possibility of analyzing possible regulatory networks involving such highly reactive cells as lymphocytes and monocytes-macrophages in defined in vitro conditions now exists. As these studies are being extended to the diseased state, concepts related to alterations in regulatory mechanisms in syndromes with abnormal cell proliferation, can be tested.

REFERENCES

1. **Stephenson, J. R., Axelrad, A. A., McLeod, D. L., and Shreeve, M. M.,** Induction of colonies of hemoglobin-synthesizing cells by erythropoietin in vitro, *Proc. Natl. Acad. Sci. U.S.A.*, 68, 1542, 1971.
2. **Axelrad, A. A., McLeod, D. L., Shreeve, H. M., and Heath, D. A.,** Properties of cells that produce erythrocytic colonies in vitro, in *Hemopoiesis in Culture*, Robinson, W., Ed., U.S. Government Printing Office, Washington, D.C., 1974, 226.
3. **Iscove, N. N., Sieber, F., and Winterhalter, K. H.,** Erythroid colony formation in cultures of mouse and human bone marrow: analysis of the requirement for erythropoietin by gel filtration and affinity chromatography on agarose-concavalin A, *J. Cell. Physiol.*, 83, 309, 1974.
4. **Adamson, J. W. and Brown, J. E.,** Aspects of erythroid differentiation and proliferation, in *Molecular Control of Proliferation and Differentiation*, Papaconstantinou, J. and Rutter, W. J., Eds., Academic Press, London, 1978, 161.
5. **Darbre, P. D., Adamson, J. W., Wood, W. G., Weatherall, D. J., and Robinson, J. S.,** Patterns of globin chain synthesis in erythroid colonies grown from sheep marrow of different developmental stages, *Brit. J. Haematol.* 41, 459, 1979.
6. **Ohno, Y. and Fisher, J. W.,** Inhibition of bone marrow erythroid colony forming cells (CFU-E) by serum from chronic anemic uremic rabbits, *Proc. Soc. Exp. Biol. Med.*, 156, 56, 1977.
7. **Testa, N. G., Eliason, J. F., Onions, P., and Harrett, O.,** In vitro growth of colonies derived from cat marrow, *Annu. Rep. Paterson Labs and Med. Oncol.*, Manchester, 1978, 142.

8. **Cormack, D.,** Time-lapse characterization of erythrocyte colony-forming cells in plasma cultures, *Exp. Hematol.,* 14, 319, 1976.
9. **Testa, N. G.,** Erythroid progenitor cells: their relevance for the study of haematological disease, *Clin. Haematol.,* 8, 311, 1979.
10. **Iscove, N. N. and Sieber, F.,** Erythroid progenitors in mouse bone marrow detected by macroscopic colony formation in culture, *Exp. Hematol.,* 3, 32, 1975.
11. **Aye, M. T.,** Erythroid colony formation in cultures of human marrow: effect of leukocyte conditioned medium, *J. Cell. Physiol.,* 91, 69, 1977.
12. **Isocove, N. N.,** Regulation of proliferation and maturation at early and late ages of erythroid differentiation, in *Cell Differentiation and Neoplasia,* Sanders, G. F., Ed., Raven Press, New York, 1972, 195.
13. **Iscove, N. N.,** Erythropoietin independent stimulation of early erythropoiesis in adult marrow cultures by conditioned media from lectin-stimulated spleen cells, in *Hemopoietic Cell Differentiation,* Golde, D. W., Cline, M. J., Metcalf, D., and Fox, C. F., Eds., Academic Press, New York, 1978, 37.
14. **Gregory, C. J., McCullough, E. A., and Till, J. E.,** Erythropoietic progenitors capable of colony formation in culture: state of differentiation, *J. Cell. Physiol.,* 81, 411, 1973.
15. **Singer, J. W. and Adamson, J. W.,** Steroids and hematopoiesis. II. The effect of steroids on in vitro erythroid colony growth: evidence for different target cells for different classes of steroids, *J. Cell. Physiol.,* 88, 135, 1976.
16. **Iscove, N. N.,** The role of erythropoietin in regulation of population size and cell cycling of early and late erythroid precursors in mouse bone marrow, *Cell Tissue Kinet.,* 10, 323, 1977.
17. **Filmanovicz, E. and Gurney, C. W.,** Studies on erythropoiesis. XVI. Response to a single dose of erythropoietin in polycythemic mouse, *J. Lab. Clin. Med.,* 57, 65, 1961.
18. **Stohlman, F., Breaker, G., and Moores, R. R.,** Humoral regulation of erythropoiesis. VIII. The kinetics of red cell production and the effect of erythropoietin, in *Erythropoiesis,* Jacobson, L. O. and Doyle, M., Ed., Grune & Stratton, New York, 1962.
19. **Bond, V. P., Fliedner, T. M., Cronkite, E. P., Rubini, G. R., and Robertson, G. S.,** Cell turnover in blood and blood forming tissues studied by tritiated thymidine, in *The Kinetics of Cellular Proliferation,* Stohlman, F., Ed., Grunne & Stratton, New York, 1959, 188.
20. **Ogawa, M., Parmley, R. T., Bank, H. L., and Spicer, S. S.,** Human marrow erythropoiesis in culture. I. Characterization of methylcellulose colony assay, *Blood,* 48, 407, 1976.
21. **Gregory, C. J. and Eaves, A. C.,** Three stages of erythropoietic progenitor cell differentiation distinguished by a number of physical and biologic properties, *Blood,* 51, 527, 1978.
22. **Wagemaker, G.,** Cellular and soluble factors influencing the differentiation of primitive erythroid progenitor cells (BFU-E) in vitro, in *In Vitro Aspects of Erythropoiesis,* Murphy, M. J., Ed., Springer-Verlag, New York, 1978, 44.
23. **Prchal, J. F., Adamson, J. W., Steinman, L., and Fialkow, P. J.,** Human erythroid colony formation in vitro: evidence for clonal origin, *J. Cell. Physiol.,* 89, 489, 1976.
24. **Fialkow, P. J.,** Primordial cell pool size and lineage relationships of five human cell types, *Ann. Hum. Genet.,* 37, 39, 1973.
25. **Humphries, R. K., Jacky, P. B., Dill, F. J., Eaves, A. C., and Eaves, C. J.,** CFU-S in individual erythroid colonies derived in vitro from adult mouse marrow, *Nature,* 279, 718, 1979.
26. **McLeod, D. L., Shreeve, M. M., and Axelrad, A. A.,** Induction of megakaryocyte colonies with platelet formation in vitro, *Nature,* 261, 462, 1976.
27. **McLeod, D. L., Shreeve, M. M., and Axelrad, A. A.,** Chromosome marker evidence for the bipotentiality of BFU-E, *Blood,* 56, 318, 1980.
28. **Heath, D. S., Axelrad, A. A., McLeod, D. L., and Shreeve, M. M.,** Separation of the erythropoietin responsive progenitors BFU-E and CFU-E in mouse bone marrow by unit gravity sedimentation, *Blood,* 47, 777, 1976.
29. **Hendry, J. H. and Lajtha, L. G.,** The response of haemopoietic colony-forming units to repeated doses of X-rays, *Radiat. Res.,* 52, 309, 1972.
30. **Wagemaker, G. and Visser, T. P.,** Erythropoietin-independent regeneration of erythroid progenitor cells following multiple injections of hydroxyurea, *Cell Tissue Kinet.,* 13, 505, 1980.
31. **Johnson, G. R. and Metcalf, D.,** Pure and mixed erythroid colony formation in vitro stimulated by spleen conditioned medium with no detectable erythropoietin, *Proc. Natl. Acad. Sci. U.S.A.,* 74, 3879, 1977.
32. **Metcalf, D., Johnson, G. R., and Mandel, T. E.,** Colony formation in agar by multipotential hemopoietic cells, *J. Cell. Physiol.* 98, 401, 1979.
33. **Fauser, A. A. and Messner, H. A.,** Granuloerythropoietic colonies in human bone marrow, peripheral blood and cord blood, *Blood,* 52, 1243, 1978.

34. **Fauser, A. A. and Messner, H. A.,** Proliferative state of human pluripotent hemopoietic progenitors (CFU-GEMM) in normal individuals and under regenerative conditions after bone marrow transplantation, *Blood,* 54, 1197, 1979.
35. **Messner, H. A. and Fauser, A. A.,** Culture studies of human pluripotent hemopoietic progenitors, *Blut.* 41, 327, 1980.
36. **Gordon, A. S.,** Erythropoietin, in *Vitamins and Hormones,* Vol. 31, Academic Press, New York 1973, 105.
37. **Fagg, B.,** Is erythropoietin the only factor which regulates late erythroid differentiation?, *Nature,* 289, 184, 1981.
38. **Miyake, T., Jung, C. K. H., and Goldwasser, E.,** Purification of human erythropoietin, *J. Biol. Chem.,* 252, 5558, 1977.
39. **Gregory, C.,** Erythropoietin sensitivity as a differentiation marker in the hemopoietic system: studies of three erythropoietic colony responses in culture, *J. Cell Physiol.,* 89, 289, 1976.
40. **Bruce, W. R. and McCulloch, E. A.,** The effect of erythropoietic stimulation on the hemopoietic colony forming cells of mice, *Blood,* 23, 216, 1964.
41. **Schofield, R. and Lajtha, L. G.,** Erythropoietic effects on stem cell population, in *Kidney Hormones,* Fisher, S. W., Ed., Academic Press, London, 1977, 283.
42. **Lajtha, L. G., Gilbert, C. W., and Guzman, E.,** Kinetics of haemopoietic colony growth, *Br. J. Haematol.,* 20, 343, 1971.
43. **Reissmann, K. R. and Udupa, K. B.,** Effect of erythropoietin on proliferation of erythropoietin responsive cells, *Cell Tissue Kinet.,* 5, 481, 1972.
44. **Udupa, K. B. and Reissmann, K. R.,** In vivo erythropoietin requirements of regenerating erythroid progenitors (BFU-E, CFU-E) in bone marrow of mice, *Blood,* 53, 1164, 1979.
45. **Testa, N. G., Eliason, J. F., and Frassoni, F.,** Role of purified erythropoietin in the amplification of the erythroid compartment, *Exp. Hematol.,* Suppl., 8, 144, 1980.
46. **Dukes, P. P., Meytes, D., Ma, A., Di Rocco, G., Ortega, J. A., and Shore, N. A.,** A urinary factor which stimulates erythroid burst formation more effectively than erythropoietin, in *Hematopoietic Cell Differentiation,* Golde, D. W., Cline, M. J., Metcalf, D., and Fox, C. D., Eds., Academic Press, New York, 1978, 119.
47. **Nissen, C., Iscove, N. N., and Speck, B.,** High burst-promoting activity (BPA) in serum of patients with acquired aplastic anemia, in *Experimental Hematology Today,* Baum, S. J. and Ledney, G. D., Eds., Springer-Verlag, Berlin, 1979, 79.
48. **Burgess, A. W. and Metcalf, D.,** The nature and action of granulocyte-macrophage colony stimulating factors, *Blood,* 56, 947, 1980.
49. **Golde, D. W., Bersch, N., Quan, S. G., and Lusis, A. J.,** Production of erythroid potentiating activity by a human T-lymphoblast cell line, *Proc. Natl. Acad. Sci. U.S.A.,* 77, 593, 1980.
50. **Metcalf, D., Johnson, G. R., and Burgess, A. W.,** Direct stimulation by purified GM-CSF of the proliferation of multipotential and erythroid precursor cells, *Blood,* 55, 138, 1980.
51. **Burgess, A. W., Metcalf, D., Russell, S. H. M., and Nicola, N. A.,** Granulocyte-macrophage-megakaryocyte-eosynophil and erythroid colony stimulating factors produced by mouse spleen cells, *Biochem. J.,* 185, 301, 1980.
52. **Guilbert, L. J. and Iscove, N. N.,** Partial replacement of serum by selenite, transferrin, albumin and lecithin in haemopoietic cell cultures, *Nature,* 263, 594, 1976.
53. **Golde, D. W., Bersch, N., Chopra, I. J., and Cline, M. J.,** Thyroid hormones stimulate erythropoiesis in vitro, *Br. J. Haematol.,* 37, 173, 1977.
54. **Golde, D. W., Bersch, N., and Li, C. H.,** Growth hormone: species specific stimulation of erythropoiesis in vitro, *Science,* 196, 1112, 1977.
55. **Rossi, G. B., Migliaccio, A. R., Migliaccio, G., Lettieri, F., Di Rosa, M., Mastroberardino, G., and Pesche, C.,** In vitro interactions of PGE and cAMP with murine and human erythroid precursors, *Blood,* 56, 74, 1980.
56. **Eliason, J. F., Dexter, T. M., and Testa, N. G.,** The regulation of hemopoiesis in long-term bone marrow culture. III. The roles of Epo and BFA, *Exp. Hematol.,* in press.
57. **Wagemaker, G., Peters, M. F., and Bol, S. J. L.,** Induction of erythropoietin responsiveness in vitro by a distinct population of bone marrow cells, *Cell Tissue Kinet.,* 12, 521, 1979.
58. **Nathan, D. G., Ches, L., Hillman, D. G., Clarke, B., Breard, J., Merler, E., and Housman, D. E.,** Human erythroid burst-forming unit: T-cell requirement for proliferation in vitro, *J. Exp. Med.,* 147, 324, 1978.
59. **Kurland, J. I., Meyers, P. A., and Moore, M. A. S.,** Synthesis and release of erythroid colony and burst potentiating activities by purified populations of murine peritoneal macrophages, *J. Exp. Med.,* 151, 839, 1980.

60. **Wolf, N. S.,** The haemopoietic microenvironment, *Clin. Haematol.,* 8, 469, 1979.
61. **Dexter, T. M.,** Cell interactions in vitro, *Clin. Haematol.,* 8, 453, 1979.
62. **Harrison, D. E.,** Use of genetic anaemias in mice as tools for haematological research, *Clin. Haematol.,* 8, 239, 1979.
63. **Testa, N. G., Schofield, R., and Eliason, J. F.,** Enhancement of spleen colony formation by live syngeneic thymus cells: effects on subpopulations of CFU-S, in *Experimental Hematology Today,* Baum, S. J., Ed., Springer-Verlag, New York, 1979.
64. **Jedrzejczak, W. W., Sharkis, S., Ahmed, A., Sell, K. W., and Santor, W. S.,** Theta, sensitive cell and erythropoiesis: identification of a defect in W/W^v anemic mice, *Science,* 196, 313, 1977.
65. **Moore, M. A. S.,** Humoral regulation of granulopoiesis, *Clin. Haematol.,* 9, 297, 1979.
66. **Bessis, M.,** in *Living Blood Cells and Their Ultrastructure,* Springer-Verlag, Berlin, 1973, 87.
67. **Dexter, T. M., Testa, N. G., Allen, T. D., Rutherford, T., and Scolnick, E.,** Molecular and cell biological aspects of erythropoiesis in long-term bone marrow cultures, *Blood,* 58, 699, 1981.
68. **Zanjani, E. D., and Kaplan, M. E.,** Cell-cell interaction in erythropoiesis, in *Progress in Hematology,* Vol. II, Brown, E. B., Ed., Grune & Stratton, New York, 1979, 173.
69. **Torok-Storb, B. and Hausen, J.,** Differential effects of T-cell subpopulations in the regulation of in vitro erythropoiesis identified using 2 monoclonal antibodies, presented at the 2nd Conf. Hemoglobin Switching, Airlie House, Virginia, June 22—26, 1980.
70. **Testa, N. G. and Dexter, T. M.,** Long-term production of erythroid precursor cells (BFU) in bone marrow culture, *Differentiation,* 9, 193, 1977.
71. **Eliason, J. F., Testa, N. G., and Dexter, T. M.,** Erythropoietin-stimulated erythropoiesis in long-term bone marrow culture, *Nature,* 281, 382, 1979.
72. **Shackny, S. E., Ford, S. S., and Witting, A. B.,** Kinetics microarchitecture correlations in the bone marrow of the mouse, *Cell Tissue Kinet.,* 8, 505, 1975.
73. **Lord, B. I., Testa, N. G., and Hendry, J. H.,** The relative spatial distribution of CFU-S and CFU-C in the mouse femur, *Blood,* 46, 65, 1975.
74. **Trivissone, R., Testa, N. G., and Lord, B. I.,** Non-random distribution of CFU-C in human sternum and rib, submitted for publication, 1982.
75. **Frassoni, F., Testa, N. G., and Lord, B. I.,** The relative spatial distribution of erythroid progenitor cell (BFU-E and CFU-E) in the normal mouse femur, *Cell Tissue Kinet.,* in press.
76. **Hara, H., Kai, S., Fushimi, M., Taniwaki, S., Okamoto, T., Ohe, Y., Fujita, S., Noguchi, K., Senba, M., Hamano, T., Kanamaru, A., and Nagai, K.,** Pluripotent hemopoietic precursors in vitro (CFU-E Mix) in aplastic anemia, *Exp. Hematol.,* 8, 1165, 1980.
77. **Hausi, W., Rich, I., Heimpel, H., Hert, W., and Kubanek, B.,** Erythroid colony forming cells in aplastic anemia, *Br. J. Hematol.,* 37, 483, 1977.
78. **Ershler, W. B., Ross, J., Finlay, J. L., and Shahidi, N. T.,** Bone marrow microenvironment defect in congenital hypoplastic anemia, *N. Engl. J. Med.,* 302, 1321, 1980.
79. **Boggs, D. R. and Boggs, S. S.,** The pathogenesis of aplastic anemia: a defective pluripotent hematopoietic stem cell with inappropriate balance of differentiation and self-replication, *Blood,* 48, 71, 1976.
80. **Geary, C. G. and Testa, N. G.,** Pathophysiology of marrow hypoplasia, in *Aplastic Anaemia,* Geary, C. G., Ed., Baillieu-Tindall, London, 1978.
81. **Fitchen, J. H. and Cline, M. J.,** Recent developments in understanding the pathogenesis of aplastic anemia, *Am. J. Hematol.,* 5, 365, 1978.
82. **Kagan, W. A., Ascensao, J. L., Fialk, M. A., Coleman, M., Valera, E. B., and Good, R. A.,** Studies on the pathogenesis of aplastic anemia, *Am. J. Med.,* 66, 444, 1979.
83. **Cline, M. J. and Golde, D. W.,** Immune suppression of hematopoiesis, *Am. J. Med.,* 64, 301, 1979.
84. **Hoffman, R., Zanjani, E. D., Vila, J., Zalusky, R., and Wasserman, L. R.,** Diamond-Blackfan syndrome: lymphocyte-mediated suppression of erythropoiesis, *Science,* 193, 899, 1966.
85. **Friedman, M. H. and Saunders, E. F.,** Diamond-Blackfan syndrome—evidence against cell-mediated erythropoietic suppression, *Blood,* 51, 1125, 1978.
86. **Nathan, D. G., Hillman, D. G., Chess, L., Alter, B. P., Clarke, B. J., Breard, J., and Housman, D. E.,** Normal erythropoietic helper T-cells in congenital hypoplastic (Diamond-Blackfan) anemia, *N. Engl. J. Med.,* 298, 1049, 1978.
87. **Milner, G. R., Testa, N. G., Geary, C. G., Dexter, T. M., Muldal, S., MacIver, J. E., and Lajtha, L. G.,** Bone marrow culture studies in refractory cytopenia and smouldering leukaemia, *Br. J. Haematol.,* 35, 251, 1977.
88. **Koeffler, H. P., Cline, M. J., and Golde, D. W.,** Erythropoiesis in preleukaemia, *Blood,* 51, 1013, 1978.
89. **Golde, D. W., Bersch, N., and Cline, M. S.,** Polycythemia vera: hormonal modulation of erythropoiesis in vitro, *Blood,* 49, 399, 1977.

90. **Eaves, C. J. and Eaves, A. C.,** Erythropoietin (Ep) dose-response curves for three classes of erythroid progenitors in normal human marrow and in patients with polycythemia vera, *Blood,* 52, 1196, 1978.
91. **Lacombe, C., Casadevall, N., and Varet, B.,** Polycythemia vera: in vitro studies of circulating erythroid progenitors, *Br. J. Haematol.,* 44, 189, 1980.
92. **Bomchil, G., Carmena, A. O., Segade, A., Cavagnaro, F., and Testa, N. G.,** Studies on the response to hypoxia and relative hyperoxia in two polycythemia vera patients, *Indian J. Med. Res.,* 55, 543, 1967.
93. **Adamson, J. W.,** The erythropoietin-hematocrit relationship in normal and polycythemia man: implications of marrow regulation, *Blood,* 32, 597, 1968.
94. **Adamson, J. W., Fialknow, P. J., Murphy, S., Prchal, J. F., and Steinman, L.,** Polycythemia vera: stem-cell and probable clonal origin of the disease, *N. Engl. J. Med.,* 295, 913, 1976.
95. **Prchal, J. F., Adamson, J. W., Murphy, S., Steinman, L., and Fialkow, P. J.,** Polycythemia vera: the in vitro response of normal and abnormal stem cell lines to erythropoietin, *J. Clin. Invest.,* 61, 1044, 1978.
96. **Moore, M. A. S., Williams, N., and Metcalf, D.,** In vitro colony formation by normal and leukaemic human hematopoietic cells. Characterisation of colony-forming cells, *J. Natl. Cancer Inst.,* 50, 603, 1973.
97. **Eaves, A. C. and Eaves, C. J.,** Abnormalities in the erythroid progenitor compartments in patients with chronic myelogenous leukaemia (CML), *Exp. Hematol,* 7 (Suppl.), 65, 1979.
98. **Goldman, J. M., Shiota, F., Th'ng, K. H., and Orchard, K. H.,** Circulating granulocytic and erythroid progenitor cells in chronic granulocytic leukaemia, *Br. J. Haematol.,* 46, 7, 1980.
99. **Hoffman, R. and Zanjani, E. D.,** Erythropoietin dependent erythropoiesis during the erythroblastic phase of juvenile chronic granulocytic leukaemia, *Br. J. Haematol.,* 38, 511, 1978.
100. **Till, J. E. and McCulloch, E. A.,** A direct measurement of the radiation sensitivity of normal mouse bone marrow cells, *Radiat. Res.,* 14, 213, 1961.
101. **Bradley, T. R. and Metcalf, D.,** The growth of mouse bone marrow cells in vitro, *Aust. J. Exp. Biol. Med. Sci.,* 44, 287, 1966.

Chapter 6

GRANULOPOIESIS*

Hal E. Broxmeyer

TABLE OF CONTENTS

*Supported by Public Health Service Grant CA-23528 from the National Cancer Institute, grant CH-138 from the American Cancer Society, the Gar Reichman Foundation, and a Scholar award from the Leukemia Society of America.

I. INTRODUCTION AND CHARACTERIZATION OF GRANULOCYTES

The granulocytic series contains neutrophils, eosinophils, and basophils. The largest amount of data, however, are available for the neutrophilic granulocytes which are considered to be one of the body's first lines of defense against microbial infection. This chapter will discuss the intricacies involved in granulopoiesis from the viewpoint of the kinetics and the regulation of the production of granulocytes. The main focus of this chapter will be on cells of the neutrophilic lineage. The production of granulocytes is a dynamic and rapidly expanding process which is nevertheless under precise and stringent control via stimulatory and inhibitory feedback systems. These feedback mechanisms, which we are just beginning to understand through the use of in vitro culture systems, form the basis of this chapter. Before discussing the regulation of the production of granulocytes, information will be presented, briefly, on the morphological, biochemical, and functional aspects of granulocytes. This information is of importance for better understanding the control of granulopoiesis.

Granulocytes derive originally from totipotent or pluripotent hematopoietic stem cells which have the capacity for differentiation along the various hematopoietic lineages, but which as a pool of cells also retain the capacity for extensive cell renewal. This pool of cells has been described in depth in the chapter in this volume on hematopoietic stem cells. A catenated system of movement from hematopoietic stem cells to the end stage granulocytes is apparent with various compartments of cells noted in between. Hematopoietic stem cells give rise to progenitor cells committed to the granulocytic and/or monocytic lineages which then give rise to the first set of cells which can be recognized morphologically with some degree of certainty, the precursor cells. The precursor cell compartment includes the immature and dividing myeloblasts, promyelocytes, and then myelocytes. Following these precursor cells are the nondividing but transitory maturation cell compartments, the metamyelocytes and bands. Further differentiation of these cells yields the more functional end stage cells, the polymorphonuclear neutrophils. Approximately 1 of 1000 nucleated cells in the bone marrow are considered to be granulocyte and/or macrophage progenitor cells, and myeloblasts are less than 1 to 5% of marrow cells under normal conditions.

Morphological characterization of immature and mature granulocytes has been accomplished by light microscopy using various procedures to stain the nucleus and cytoplasmic constituents and by electron microscopy.[1,2] Myeloblasts are approximately 15 to 20 μm in diameter, and have a large round nucleus with a small amount of chromatin. The nuclear chromatin is finely dispersed; there are usually two or more nucleoli and the cytoplasm usually has no clear zone around the nucleus. Promyelocytes are distinguishable by coarse blue or violet granules in the cytoplasm. Azurophilic granules represent the prominent granule in this cell. Fewer mitochondria are seen than in myeloblasts, but the endoplasmic reticulum is more fully developed. Clumping of nuclear chromatin becomes evident at first during the myelocyte stage. Two distinct patterns of granules are noted now and include the primary azurophilic granules detected in the promyelocyte and the secondary or specific granules. The constituents of azurophil and specific granules from human polymorphonuclear neutrophils have been described.[3] The azurophil granules contain the following acid hydrolases: β-glycerophosphate, *N*-acetyl-β-glucosaminidase, β-glucuronidase β-mannosidase, cathepsin D, and cathepsin B. Acid hydrolases were not detected in the specific granules. Azurophil granules contained the neutral proteinases, elastase, cathepsin G, and proteinase 3, while specific granules contained the neutral proteinases, collagenase and second collagenolytic metalloproteinase. Lysozyme was found in both the azurophil and specific granules while myeloperoxidase was localized in the azurophil granules, and lactoferrin and vitamin B_{12}-binding protein were detected only in the specific granules.

Lactoferrin will be described below as a regulator of granulocyte production. A monograph on neutral proteases describing the more recent work in this area has been published.[4] Enriched fractions of mature and immature guinea pig neutrophilic granulocytes were isolated and assessed for ornithine decarboxylase activity and polyamine content.[5] This study was initiated because of the finding that the content and rate of synthesis of polyamines was greater in tissues with high growth rates than in nongrowing tissue.[6] Immature granulocytes contained at least ten times more ornithine decarboxylase activity and two times more spermidine than mature granulocytes.[5] It was suggested that polyamine synthesis in the granulocytic pool of cells was mainly associated with immature proliferating cells and that this synthesis preceded increased granulocyte proliferation in the bone marrow following an inflammatory stimulus.[5] It has been noted also that polymorphonuclear neutrophils secrete plasminogen activator.[7] Secretion was stimulated by concanavalin A and low concentrations of phorbol myristate acetate and was inhibited by low concentrations of glucocorticoids and by cyclic AMP, actinomycin D, and cycloheximide. The release kinetics of plasminogen activatior were different from granule-bound enzymes such as elastase.

It is at the myelocyte stage that neurophilic, basophilic, and eosinophilic granules are first prominent and distinguishable. Metamyelocytes, the first in the series of nondividing cells, have the cytoplasmic features of mature granulocytes with the most notable changes from this stage onward being changes in nuclear morphology which eventually result in segmentation of the nucleus. The ultrastructural characteristics of neutrophilils,[8–10] basophils,[11] and eosinophils[9,10,12] have been described.

Various surface markers have been analyzed on neutrophilic granulocytes, and heterogeneity among even the polymorphonuclear neutrophils has been detected. A distinct sequence of marker appearance during the terminal phases of granulocyte differentiation was noted on mouse bone marrow cells grown in culture.[13] The order of appearance of markers was considered to be first the presence of receptors for the Fc portion of immunoglobulin G (FcR), then in addition complement receptor type two (C 3d receptor), then also the capacity for ingestion of particles, and finally the acquisition also of complement receptor type one (C 3b receptor). Although 95% of blood polymorphonuclear neutrophils contained the four markers, only half of the spleen—and 20% of bone marrow—polymorphonuclear neutrophils contained all four markers. Ia (immune-associated)-antigenic determinants were found on human progenitor cells for granulocytes, on myeloblasts, and on a few promyelocytes, but were not detected on more mature neutrophils.[14]

However, two different complement receptors are found later on during maturation and by the polymorphonuclear neutrophilic stage the complement 2-receptors have been lost and only complement 1-receptors retained.[15] The detection of receptors on human polymorphonuclear neutrophils and evidence for subpopulations of these cells, which were previously considered to be a homogeneous population of cells, are available. The receptors noted include Fc receptors, complement receptors, and receptors for IgA.[16–23]

Polymorphonuclear neutrophils separated by rosetting with IgG-coated human erythrocytes differed in functional capacity from nonrosetting neutrophils with regard to adherence to nylon wool, phagocytosis of *Staphylococcus aureus,* killing of *Staphylococcus aureus,* and responsiveness to endotoxin-activated human serum in a ^{51}Cr chemotaxis assay.[18] Polymorphonuclear neutrophils separated by rosetting with rabbit IgG antibody-coated sheep erythrocytes were found to differ in the functional activity, but not in the actual content, of lactoferrin, a negative feedback regulator of granulopoiesis.[19] Those neutrophils containing Fc receptors were the more adherent neutrophils,[18] and studies in rats have shown that the adherent neutrophils were the older cells that had been in the circulation the longest.[24] Thus, if extrapolation between human and rat neutrophils can be made, then those neutrophils with detectable Fc receptors may be the older circulating neutrophils. When the membrane receptor for the Fc portions of IgG were examined on the cell surface of human neutrophils by electron microscopy, it was suggested that the clustering of Fc receptors seen was a natural surface representation on these cells rather than an initial redistribution induced by the ligands used.[25]

Subpopulations of polymorphonuclear neutrophils have been detected during disease states.[26,27] Immunoglobulin (Ig)G receptors were analyzed by rosette formations in suspension with human Rh-positive erythryocytes sensitized with high-titer Rh antiserum.[26] IgG receptors were detected on 19% of neutrophils from normal subjects, but in polycythemia vera and myeloid metaplasia the percentage increased to 70. Normal values were detected in polycythemic states not due to myeloproliferative disease and in chronic myeloid leukemia, but the percent of rosette-forming neutrophils increased to 52 in infection and inflammation. Two populations of granulocytes differing in susceptibility to lysis by complement were detected in five of six patients with paroxysmal nocturnal hemoglobinuria.[27] It was suggested that the binding of complement 3 and the efficiency of the terminal stages of complement lysis were increased in a portion of the granulocytes.

Surface labeling was performed on mouse polymorphonuclear neutrophils isolated from peritoneal cells and purified on the basis of light scattering using a cell sorter or by density gradient centrifugation.[28] Electrophoretic studies of the proteins from this population of cells demonstrated an abundance of lactoferrin and actin and other proteins. Surface iodination indicated six tyrosine-containing proteins present on the external cell membranes. The apparent molecular weights of these proteins ranged from 90,000 to 185,000 with the major protein at 90,000. Interestingly, neither actin nor lactoferrin were labeled with ^{125}I, and using biosynthetic labeling with ^{35}S-methionine some of the granule storage proteins, such as lactoferrin, were not labeled within 3 hr. These results suggested that lactoferrin might not be synthesized in the polymorphonuclear neutrophils but might be carried over during the maturation of these cells from the myelocyte or metamyelocyte stages.

It has been suggested that neutrophils could act as exocrine cells.[29] Polymorphonuclear neutrophils were stained simultaneously with fluorescein and rhodamine-labeled monospecific antisera to myeloperoxidase (found in azurophil granules) and lactoferrin (found in specific granules) to identify the granules within single cells and the degranulation of these granules after phagocytic challenge with *Escherichia coli.*[30] The results suggested that bacteria made contact with granule-associated antimicrobial substances within 5 sec after the initiation of phagocytosis, and that free communication of granule constituents occurred between the newly formed phagolysosome and the extracellular space. Phagocytosis itself is not necessarily a prerequisite for degranulation by human neutrophils.[31] Kinetic studies have shown that the extracellular release of specific and azurophil granules occur sequentially in human neutrophils with both soluble and particulate stimuli.[32] Release of lactoferrin was noted first, followed by myeloperoxidase and then β-glucuronidase. It was suggested that the two types of granules were subjected to separate controlling factors for the release of their constituents. This has been noted by others also.[33] The spontaneous release of lysozyme, found in both the azurophil and specific granules, reflected a selected mobilization and exocytosis of the specific granules, since it occured without the release of products from the azurophil granulocytes.[33]

During exposure of neutrophils to various stimuli, changes in oxygen metabolism occur and are manifested as increases in oxygen consumption, superoxide and hydrogen peroxide production, and hexose monophosphate shunt activity.[34–38] These activities are releated to the functional capacities of the neutrophils in their role of protection of the body against invading microorganisms. It is clear that these metabolic events can be stimulated in the absence of phagocytosis.[35,39–41]

Various abnormalities in neutrophil functions have been described and are related to alcohol,[42] collection procedures using continuous flow filtration leukopheresis,[43] and to various disease states such as cyclic neutropenia in dogs,[44] Chediak-Higashi syndrome,[45,46] and chronic granulomatous disease in man,[47] iron deficiency in children,[48] acute and chronic leukemia[49–55] and ''preleukemia.''[56] In many of these studies the defects have correlated with the susceptibility of the host to infection. Neutrophil replacement therapy has been considered[57] and newer methods that preserve neutrophils and their functional capacity better have been described.[58]

Studies on eosinophils[59] have shown that they have receptors for complement and for aggregated immunoglobulin G. Eosinophils differed from mature neutrophils since eosinophils had receptors for complement 3d and relatively weak immune adherence receptors (complement 4 or 3b). Neutrophils did not have complement 3d receptors but had strong immune adherence receptors. No surface immunoglobulin or spontaneous erythrocyte rosette formation was observed with eosinophils. Eosinophils isolated from the peritoneal capacity of Balb/c mice infected with the parasite *Mesocestoides corti* were purified further to greater than 95% and the proteins of these cells analyzed.[60] Using SDS-polyacrylamide gel electrophoresis a group of high molecular weight proteins were detected between 160 to 250,000 which were not as evident in the profile of neutrophil proteins. Using ^{125}I-labeled proteins, four of the eosinophil surface labeled proteins (>50,000) corresponded to those on neutrophils, but the major surface component of eosinphils (79,000) appear to be smaller than the major neutrophil protein (90,000).

Eosinophils have been shown to contain a similar but in some ways more potent oxidative burst than neutrophils with a role for NADPH oxidase suggested in the initiation of the burst.[61] In spite of comparable rates of phagocytosis between eosinophils from a patient with hyperosinophilia and neutrophils from a normal donor, the eosinophils were less able to kill bacteria. This correlated with an inability of eosinophil peroxidase to catalyze the peroxidase-H_2O_2-Cl^--mediated decarboxylation of amino acids.[62,63]

Due to the small number of eosinophils in the blood of normal individuals and the difficulty of isolating these cells, most studies on eosinophils have been done on cells procured from patients with eosinophilia. A comparison of eosinophils of greater than 95% purity from normal donors and patients with eosinophilia of varying etiologies was made.[64] Using the criteria of surface change, activation of lysosomal acid phosphatase, membrane hexose transport, and hexose monophosphate shunt activities, it was shown that eosinophils obtained from patients with eosinophilia were significantly activated when compared with normal eosinophils.

Basophils are also present in low numbers in the peripheral blood of normal donors.

Isolation procedures using unoccupied IgE-Fc receptors have yielded populations of basophils which are 65 to 85% pure,[65] and this should allow more precise biochemical and functional analysis of these cells. Evidence has now been given, through ultrastructural analysis of an intermediary cell, that basophils and mast cells which have many things in common may actually be derived from the same precursor cell.[66]

II. KINETICS OF THE PRODUCTION OF MORPHOLOGICALLY IDENTIFIABLE GRANULOCYTES

A. Bone Marrow Production and Release to the Blood

The use of radioactive tracers such as tritiated thymidine (TdR-^{3}H), diisopropylfluorophosphate (DF^{32}P), and carbon (^{14}C) compounds have allowed the elucidation of the cell parameters of immature dividing granulocytic precursor cells and the characteristics of the flow of populations of these cells from an immature cell compartment to another more mature compartment of cells, and ultimately also the flow from marrow to blood and then to the tissue areas. Many fine reviews are available describing the mathematics and theory behind calculations involved in these kinetic parameters for human and murine cells and the areas in which caution in interpretation must be exercised.[67–79]

The cell cycle is considered to be composed of four or more compartments.[67,68] These include S-phase, or the time spent in the synthesis of DNA, G_2, or the postsynthetic-premitotic period, M, or the period of cell division or mitosis, and G_1, or the post-mitotic-presynthetic period. There have also been suggestions for the existence of a G_0 phase for some cells which are not actively participating in the cell cycle but which can be triggered to enter cell cycle and divide. G_0 has been considered by some to be actually a very extended G_1 phase.[67] It has been suggested that there is one mitotic division at the myeloblast and promyelocyte stages and two or more sequential divisions at the myelocyte stage.[79] The rate of cell production in man varies from 3.5×10^7 to 6.8×10^7 cells per kilogram per hour depending on the methods used to assess the production rate. Estimates of the transit time through the nonproliferating compartment range from 130 to 158 hr. The total time from stem cell to mature blood neutrophil in man has been estimated to be in the range of 11 to 12 days,[76] but this will have to be considered a very crude estimate as it is not clear yet how many cell cycles are involved in movement from a toti- or pluripotential stem cell to that of a morphologically recognizable precursor cell.

There appears to be a marrow granulocyte reserve which is capable of acting as a buffer system which can release large numbers of granulocytes upon demand without need for immediate recruitment from the more immature cell compartments. Evidence is strong that the bone marrow granulocytes that enter the nondividing maturation compartment first are first out to the circulation.[24,67,80,81] An evaluation of the release of blood granulocytes from the isolated perfused hind legs of rats pretreated with vinblastine-sulfate showed that even after depletion of the marrow granulocyte reserve to 15% of normal values normal circulating numbers of neutrophils were sustained.[82] The calculations given above for man are assumed to be normal steady-state values but the transit time to blood is shortened substantially under certain conditions such as during infection and disease. The total blood granulocyte compartment is composed of both circulating and marginated pools of cells and the proportions of these pools of cells vary during different clinical situations.[69,76] It is apparent that determination of cell kinetics during leukemia has been helpful in designing more effective treatment protocols[83,84] that more efficiently utilize the cycle-specific and cycle-nonspecific drugs.

The capacity of eosinophils to influence cytotoxic reactions against nonphagocytosable targets is believed to be of major importance in defense reactions against invasion by some parasites.[85] The cycle compartment flow characteristics of esonophils in rats have been evaluated, and a marrow reserve of eosinophils is apparent in rats and guinea pigs.[86–91]

B. Neutrophil-Releasing Factors

Various agents are known to cause the release of granulocytes from the bone marrow to the blood and from the blood to the tissue areas.[92] Bacterial products can act as such agents,[93–95] and it is through the use of these products that a humoral mechanism mediating the release of granulocytes to the blood has been evaluated. Several lines of evidence suggested initially the presence of releasing factors, termed leukocytosis-inducing factors or neutrophil releasing factors, in mice, rats, dogs, and man. These included studies employing parabiosis of rats,[96,97] perfusion of the isolated hind legs or femurs of rats,[98–100] and serum or plasma transfers from animals previously injected with bacterial products and/or from whom leukocytes had been removed from the peritoneal cavity.[96,101–108] Repeated leukocytapheresis of one of the members of parabiotic pairs of rats resulted in an increase in blood leukocyte levels in the nonleukocytapheresed mate.[96]

Perfusion of isolated hind legs or femurs with blood maintained these organs in good conditions, and perfusion of leukocyte depleted blood caused the release of blood leukocytes from the organs; perfusion of leukocyte-rich blood suppressed the release phenomenon.[98–100] Animals from whom leukocytes had been removed were able to elaborate into the serum factors which upon injection into normal intact animals or upon perfusion of isolated hind legs or femurs caused the release of leukocytes. It was demonstrated that the releasing factors, while being induced by bacterial products, were not themselves bacterial products.[107–109] Several observations confirmed this: bacterial products did not cause release of neutrophils from isolated hind legs of rats, intravenous injections of plasma from leukocytapheresed rats did not induce a febrile reaction in rabbits, leukocyte-inducing activity of plasma from rats was destroyed by heating to 100°C while exogenous endotoxins required higher temperatures for biological inactivation, sham leukocytapheresed rats did not contain the activity, plasma harvested shortly after endotoxin injection into dogs was usually inactive, there were qualitative differences in the characteristics of the curve of developing neutrophilia in response to active plasma, compared to the curve after endotoxin injection, and the neutrophil response to postendotoxin plasma was not changed in animals in which tolerance to endotoxin was induced. Preliminary characterization of the neutrophil releasing factor in rats demonstrated that it was thermolabile, nondialyzable, and insoluble in 1.4 to 2.4 *M* ammonium sulfate.[109] The active factor appeared to be associated with weakly anionic alphaglobulins. The neutrophil-releasing factor was shown to be biologically separable from the colony stimulatory factors necessary for the production in vitro of colonies of granulocytes and macrophages,[101,110,111] and the mechanisms regulating release of granulocytes and granulocyte-macrophage progenitor cells from the bone marrow appeared to be different.[112]

In studies on the marrow granulocyte reserve in man the factor which predicted best for the endotoxin response was the percent of marrow band and segmented neutrophils.[113] The responders to endotoxin had more than 25% neutrophils in the bone marrow samples. Characterization of the surface qualities of human granulocytes during maturation demonstrated functionally useful changes in these cells as they differentiated into mature forms.[114] Immature granulocytes were characterized by a high neuraminadase-susceptible negative surface charge density, a high degree of cellular rigidity, low adhesiveness to glass and plastic, low propensity to aggregate, a slow rate of cell spreading, pseudopod extension and motility, and a low rate of phagocytosis. In contrast, polymorphonuclear neutrophils had a lower negative surface charge density, a higher degree of surface deformability, higher adhesiveness, a higher propensity to aggregate, a higher rate of cell spreading, pseudopod formation and motility, and a higher rate of phagocytosis. Studies have given support for a preferential migration site for cells at the parajunctional zone of the endothelial cell rather than through intercellular junctions and for the concept that pores are made at the time of egress.[115]

A soluble plasma factor inducing the release of eosinophils from rat bone marrow has also been suggested.[116]

C. Mobilization to Tissues—Chemotaxis

Responding cells can be induced towards directed motility by various chemoattractants. An historical overview of the chemotaxis of leukocytes has been written,[117] and evidence is accumulating rapidly that many of these factors and their modifiers may play a role in vivo.[117–120] Some of the factors known to be chemotactic for neutrophils have been reviewed[118,121] and include complement-related C3 fragment, C5 fragment and C567, endogenous enzymes, such as kallikrein and plasminogen activator, coagulation-related products such as fibrinopeptide B and fibrin degradation products, bacterial factors including *N*-formyl-methionyl-oligopeptides, oxidized lipids and other uncharacterized agents, products of the granules of mature granulocytes, lymphokines, monokines, transfer factor and supernatants of cells infected with viruses, some denatured proteins and agents such as casein, gluten, and starch granules. As is apparent from this list, many substances exist in a precursor form and need activation by enzymes prior to the acquisition of chemotactic activity.[118] It appears as if neutrophil granules themselves can interact with complement to generate and also to inactivate complement-derived factors.[119] Thus exudate neutrophils can increase and localize an inflammatory reaction and also limit the response. It has also been shown that cationic polyelectrolytes and inflammatory exudates influence the surfaces of mature granulocytes and modify their interaction with chemoattractants.[120]

Specific membrane binding sites for certain peptides with chemoattractant activity have been demonstrated on polymorphonuclear neutrophils.[122–125] Such binding sites were studied with synthetic *N*-formylmethionyl peptides.[123] Binding was rapid with a halftime of less than 2 min and was reversible. The value at which half the receptors were saturated at 37°C was 12 to 14 m*M* and there were approximately 2000 receptors per cell although only 100 to 200 sites had to be occupied for a maximal migratory response. The specificity of the binding sites for a series of these peptides reflected the correlation between binding and initiation of chemotaxis. It was suggested that the binding sites initiated the specific response of the motile cells to the peptides. Incubation of human polymorphonuclear neutrophils with concentrations of degranulating stimuli which caused limited release of granule constituents increased receptor availability for f-met-leu-phe and decreased the apparent affinity of binding.[124]

It had been suggested that equine polymorphonuclear neutrophils could be used as a model for the study of events which lead to a biological response after occupation of the receptors as the equine cells had a high-affinity receptor for *N*-formylated peptides and secreted lysozyme as a response, but did not exhibit chemotaxis.[125] Chemotactic factors have various influences on mature granulocytes. These have been summarized[118] and include increased transmembrane fluxes of Na^+, K^+, and Ca^{++}, increased intracellular pool of exchangeable Ca^{++}, induced release of membrane-bound Ca^{++}, activation of Na^+ K^+ ATPase, increased surface membrane ruffling and pseudopoda formation, depolarized surface membranes, induced cellular swelling, activation of proesterase I, enhanced microtubule assembly, enhanced glycolysis and superoxide anion production, increased adhesiveness of surface membranes, induced cellular aggregation, endothelial margination, neutropenia and neutrophilia, enhanced random or directed movement, enhanced accumulation at tissue sites, inhibition or enhancement of phagocytosis and induction of degranulation. Many of the effects of these chemotactic factors appear to better equip the polymorphonuclear neutrophil for functional activity inducing enhanced adhesiveness, neutrophil oxidative metabolism, chemiluminescence and bactericidal activity.[126–130] There is evidence that the formylmethionyl peptides stimulate neutrophil locomotion, granule enzyme secretion, aggregation and initiation of the respiratory burst by interacting with a single population of receptors.[131]

Maintenance of the chemotactic response of cryopreserved human granulocytes has been demonstrated,[132] but defects in chemotactic migration in vitro of neutrophils from patients with chronic myelogenous leukemia have been observed.[133]

Monocyte and macrophage-derived chemotactic factors for polymorphonuclear neutrophils have been described[134–136] and may play a role in the interaction of cells of the mononuclear phagocytic series with mature granulocytes. After in vitro culture of normal human alveolar macrophages two chemotactic substances were released into the culture supernatant.[134] The release of these substances was stimulated maximally by aggregated human immunoglobulin G or zymosan, but adhesion of the cells to plastic surfaces also caused the release of these substances. The larger substance was 10,000 daltons, immunologically distinct from complement 5a and interacted with different receptors than formyl-methionyl-leucyl-phenylalanine. Its activity was inactivated by trypsin and localized to a pI value of 5.0. Production of a chemotactic factor from human blood monocytes stimulated by bacterial lipopolysaccharide or anti-β_2 microglobulin has been reported.[135] Phytohemagglutinin, concanavalin A, and sepharose-protein A did not induce the production of significant amounts of this chemotactic factor. These chemotactic factors[134,135] had no influence on the migration of cells of the mononuclear phagocytic system. It has been suggested also that the peritoneal chemotactic signal for mature granulocytes in vivo is triggered after the interaction of bacterial lipopolysaccharide with cells of the adherent mononuclear cell lineage.[136]

Chemotactic factors have also been isolated for eosinophils and have been characterized partially.[137] An eosinophil chemotactic factor of the parasite in extracts from the body cavity fluid of the Ascares species was isolated, found to be active in vivo and in vitro, was heat labile, nondialyzable, stable to lyophilization, had an approximate molecular weight of 30,000 daltons and an isoelectric point of 8.5.[137]

III. REGULATION OF THE PRODUCTION OF NORMAL GRANULOCYTES AND MACROPHAGES

Regulation of the production of granulocytes and cells of the monocyte-macrophage lineage are connected intimately and it is necessary to discuss each in order to understand the other. The dual involvement of these cells originates in what is apparently a bipotent progenitor cell committed to both lineages and extends to the cell-derived regulatory substances elaborated from the end stage cells of these lineages. It is becoming increasingly clear that the progeny of the progenitor cells have the capacity to regulate the production of more of their own kind of cells. These intricate feedback systems form the basis of the next few sections of this chapter.

Several assay systems are available for studying the production and regulation of granulocytes and macrophages. These include systems in which hematopoietic cells are grown in liquid suspension cultures in vitro,[138,139] in liquid suspension within diffusion chambers implanted into host animals,[140–154] on macrophage coated membranes within the peritoneal cavity of mice,[155,156] in semisolid culture systems in vitro,[157] and in semisolid cultures within diffusion chambers implanted into host animals.[158–165] The suspension culture assays allow calculations on the kinetics of proliferation of cells and when studied in diffusion chambers offer a combination of *in vitro* and *in vivo* methodologies. Semisolid medium cultures allow studies on production of cells from a single progenitor cell and diffusion chamber studies have combined the in vitro and in vivo approach. A recent monograph traces the history of the use of diffusion chambers as well as offering a view of more recent studies and the pros and cons of using this assay.[166] Technologies involved in the use of semisolid clonal assays have been modified by many authors but the basic principles and culture ingredients used have been summarized.[157,167] Some of these assay systems have been used in combination and have allowed the elucidation of heterogeneity within populations of progenitor cells.[168,169] The characteristics of progenitor cells and the stimulatory and inhibitory interactions regulating their proliferation and differentiation will be discussed below in the context of normal as well as abnormal situations.

A. Characteristics of Progenitor Cells

1. Information on Culture Systems

The analysis of a set of progenitor cells committed to the granulocyte-macrophage lineage was first approached for mouse cells using semisolid culture medium support systems,[170–176] but now encompasses cells from rats,[177,178] dogs,[179,180] chicks,[181] and humans.[182–184] Granulocyte-macrophage progenitor cells have been studied in humans from bone marrow,[182–184] blood,[185–187] spleen, and cord blood.[188] The counting of colonies is a time-consuming affair and some attempts have been made to automate the counting procedure for murine and human colonies.[189–192] The accuracy of the currently used automated counters has not yet, however, been found to be as good or better than the human eye. This is especially true with regards to scoring colonies of more than 40 cells vs. clusters of 3 to 40 cells from human bone marrow which in many cases are not found as tight aggregates of cells. Rather they are found as loose aggregates, especially in the case of macrophages and cells from patients with leukemia. The scoring of colonies and clusters from murine cells can be expressed not only as per the number of cells plated but as the number of cells per organ. This latter expression of results is most important when discussing events occuring within an animal as it takes into account the expansion and decrease of the total nucleated cell profile within an organ and allows one to describe the absolute number of colony forming or progenitor cells per organ. Unfortunately, studies on human progenitor cells can at the present be discussed only in terms of the number of cells plated as it is not possible to determine the actual number of cells per organ unless the entire organ, such as a spleen, is removed. Withdrawing marrow from human donors carries with it the problem of variable blood dilution within the samples as well as differing distributions of progenitor cells within different areas of the skeleton.

Several attempts have been made to express the results of human studies in a more meaningful fashion rather than as the number of nucleated cells plated. It has been found helpful to describe the ratio of colonies to clusters especially when comparing results from patients with leukemia to those of normal donors.[193] For studies on normal marrow it has been suggested that results be expressed per milliliter of aspirate[194] or per number of metamyelocytes plated.[195] Each had its pitfalls and the situation has not been resolved satisfactorily.[196,197] It has been suggested that lowering the oxygen tension will increase the cloning efficiency of murine progenitor cells[198] and it is now possible to study progenitor cell growth in a system almost completely free of unknown serum factors.[199] The single cell origin of colonies and clusters has been demonstrated by a variety of procedures including documenting the linear relationships between the number of cells plated and the number of colonies formed, karyotypic analysis of the progeny of progenitor cells, single cell manipulations and, more recently, analysis of the glucose-6-phosphate dehydrogenase isoenzyme patterns of the progeny.[157,167,200] Using the latter method it has been shown that the single cell origin of colonies in semisolid medium is best seen when the density of colonies on a plate is low.[200]

Neutrophils, eosinophils, and basophils have been found in colonies[157,201] and the mitotic rate of promyelocytes and myelocytes is higher than that reported in vivo.[202] With mouse cells within colonies it was determined that the G_1, S, G_2, and M cycle phases were respectively 6.3 ± 1.6 hr, 5.8 ± 1.4 hr., 1.7 ± 0.1 hr, and 0.7 ± 0.1 hr (42 ± 8 min).[203] An analysis of surface receptors on the cells within colonies from mouse bone marrow cells has shown that neutrophils and macrophages possessed complement 3 and IgG-receptors, whereas eosinophil colony cells contained only IgG-receptors.[204] The neutrophils did not appear actively phagocytic under the conditions used[204] which may reflect their lack of terminal differentiation. Mature polymorphonuclear neutrophils are only found rarely in colonies. Results have suggested that pluripotential stem cells are contained within or in close proximity to developing in vitro colonies from mouse cells[205] and natural killer cells have been found in such colonies.[206] Variations and oscillations in the numbers of progenitor cells circulating in human blood have been seen[207–209] with evidence of diurnal variations being detected.[210,211] The mean half-life of circulating progenitor cells in man was found to be 4.6 hr after bone marrow transplantation, and no correlation was seen between the maximum number of circulating progenitor cells and the disappearance from the blood.[212]

Radiation sensitivity[213,214] and cycling status have been used to characterize the granulocyte-macrophage progenitor cells. The radiation sensitivity for human progenitor cells was similar to that of a comparable class of mouse marrow cells,[213] but it was found that the apparent kill of human colony forming cells by irradiation was dependent on the relative levels of colony stimulatory activities supplied to the culture system after irradiation of target marrow cells.[214] Thus the D_0 value (the dose of irradiation required to reduce survival to 37% of control) increased from 40 to 160 rad as the net level of colony stimulatory activity increased.[214] This suggested that other factors besides the actual kill of the colony forming cells were involved in the survival of these cells and illuminated the complexities of cellular interactions occuring in the culture dish. It was suggested that high levels of stimulation might be necessary to overcome the effects of noted inhibitory substances released from irradiated cells and that colony forming cells at different phases of the cell cycle might have different thresholds for damage by irradiation and stimulation by various factors. The data could also be explained if radiation-injured colony forming cells needed higher levels of stimulation to proliferate. The proliferative capacity of progenitor cells at the time of study has been evaluated by means of cell kill with pulse exposures of cells to high specific activity tritiated thymidine or hydroxyurea. The proliferative capacity, expressed as the percentage of colony forming cells in DNA synthesis has been evaluated for murine, monkey, canine, and human cells.[214–223] Variations in the cycling status of granulocyte-macrophage progenitor cells have been reported and a statistical analysis of these studies with murine cells performed.[224] In a study evaluating the cycle status of human colony forming cells it was found that this also was dependent on the stimulus applied to the cells after treatment by hydroxyurea.[214] The apparent percent of cells in cycle increased as the net level of colony stimulatory activity increased, and it was suggested that the range of estimates of kill reported in the literature could be due to differences in the level of factors used to stimulate cultures.[214] These studies were confirmed by others,[225] and it now appears as if these results may be due not only to the actual level of stimulatory factors but also to the presence of inhibitory factors within the conditioned medium used to stimulate colony formation.[801] Regardless of the reasons for these results, it is apparent that some studies may be underestimating the actual number of progenitor cells cycling at any point in time.

The study of eosinophil colonies has been made easier by the use of specific staining procedures utilizing either Dominici's stain containing phloxine or Luxol-fast-blue stain.[226–229] The eosinophil colony forming cell probably derives from a progenitor cell distinct from the neutrophil-macrophage progenitor cell as eosinophil colonies and clusters always contained pure populations of eosinophils, and no mixed colonies of eosinophils with other cells were observed.[226] A minor population of basophil colonies has been detected in semisolid cultures.[201] Basophils and mast cells may be derived from the same precursor cell,[66] and using specific stains and electron microscopy a small number of mast cells were detected in human but not mouse bone marrow cultures.[230] Long term in vitro cultures of murine mast cells have been described.[231,232] The cells were identified by their morphology, characteristic ultrastructure of granules, positive reaction with toluidine blue and alcian blue, presence of receptors for IgG and IgE, as well as the presence of histamine, serotonin, L-Dopa, 5-hydroxytryptophan and sulfated products within the cytoplasm.[231] The source of stimulation derived from concanavalin A activated murine spleen leukocytes and mast cell lines were established from the spleen and bone marrow of athymic nude mice, long-term cultured marrow cells, and T-cell depleted normal marrow.[230] The cultured mast cells were absolutely dependent on the growth factors in the conditioned medium for their growth and viability.[231] The mast cell growth factor could be separated biochemically from a T-cell growth factor present in the same conditioned medium.[232] A continuously growing mast cell line has also been isolated which depends on a factor in pokeweed mitogen spleen cell conditioned medium.[233] The production of basophils from guinea pigs in suspension culture has been shown to depend on a conditioned medium prepared from T cells within the spleen.[234]

A primitive macrophage progenitor cell with high proliferative potential has been detected in mouse bone marrow after treatment with fluorouracil and/or endotoxin, using a combination of colony stimulatory factors from pregnant uterus extract and human spleen cell conditioned medium.[235] Colonies of macrophages have also been described which appear to originate from a more mature cell than a progenitor cell. These macrophage colony forming cells have been characterized in liquid and in semisolid culture medium systems.[236–241]

2. *Heterogeneity of Granulocyte-Macrophage Progenitor Cell Populations*

Physical, immunological, and biochemical procedures have been used to isolate and characterize granulocyte-macrophage progenitor cells from humans,[168,169,242–247] mice,[248–264] and monkeys.[265] Separation of human bone marrow cells has detected heterogeneity in progenitor cell populations.[168,169,245–247] Cells which form granulocytic colonies in fibrin clot diffusion chambers implanted intraperitoneally in sublethally irradiated mice and cells cultured in suspension culture in vitro have a similar slow sedimentation rate after separation by velocity sedimentation in the range of 5 mm/hr.[168,169] These cells appear to generate progenitor cells in the range of 6 mm/hr which form colonies in agar after 14 days of incubation. These progenitor cells appear to further mature into progenitor cells seen in the range of 7.3 mm/hr which are detected as colonies in agar after 7 days of incubation. While evidence is not yet available that a single cell actually matures from one progenitor cell to the next, the population kinetics do suggest such a movement with increased cycling status apparent as a progression to the more mature population occurs.[168,169] Differential responsiveness of these progenitor cell populations to stimulation by various factors[168,169,245–247] has provided further evidence for heterogeneity. Rapidly sedimenting and probably more mature cells appeared to be more responsive to stimulation than the slowly sedimenting cells.[245] The more quickly sedimenting cells responded to a stimulus in culture supernatants from an established human fibroblast cell line, while the more slowly sedimenting, and presumably more immature cells, responded to a stimulus from medium conditioned by peripheral blood leukocytes in the presence of phytohemagglutin.[246]

Variations in responsiveness were also detected with factors separated electrophoretically from human lung conditioned medium.[247] Other evidence for heterogeneity was based on oscillations of progenitor cells noted in cyclic neutropenia in man.[248] An inverse relationship was observed between cells forming colonies in diffusion chambers and cells forming colonies in agar culture in vitro, which cycled out of phase with the diffusion chamber colony forming cells. A similar maturation sequence has been postulated for mouse marrow cells separated by velocity sedimentation[249] and density-gradient centrifugation.[250] A combination of techniques involving drug treatment, cell separation procedures, and culture in diffusion chambers demonstrated the existence of colonies of granulocytes from mouse containing more than 1×10^6 cells.[251] It would be of interest to determine where this cell belongs in the hierarchy of progenitor cells. Granulocyte-macrophage progenitor cells are essentially nonadherent and nonphagocytic cells[252–267] which has allowed a simple procedure for removing the progenitor cells from cells endogenous to the sample which elaborate constitutively factors which can stimulate colony and cluster formation. These studies have shown that the proliferation and differentiation of progenitor cells is absolutely dependent on a source of such stimulatory factors under normal conditions and during leukemia.[268]

3. *Surface Characteristics of Granulocyte-Macrophage Progenitor Cells*

Granulocyte-macrophage progenitor cells lack detectable T-cell antigens, Fc receptors, and complement receptors.[265,269–271] The use of hypotonic lysis has allowed the isolation of granulocyte-macrophage progenitor cells from other cell types,[272,273] and various lectins have been used to separate bone marrow cells[274] and, more recently, mouse[275] and human[276] granulocyte-macrophage progenitor cells. The differential expression of surface carbohydrate residues and lectin probes were analyzed. The use of pokeweed mitogen, *Helix pomatia* agglutinin, soybean agglutinin, and peanut agglutinin preferentially bound to the mouse colony forming cells and enriched their numbers by four- to tenfold using fluorescence activated cell sorting.[275] The best enrichment was obtained with pokeweed mitogen. Sorting of cells using low angle scatter, high angle scatter, and pokeweed mitogen fluorescence enriched numbers of colony forming cells by 16- to 50-fold.[275] The fucose-binding lectin from *Lotus tetragonolobus* in combination with cell sorting procedures yielded a fraction containing 23% progenitor cells with a 36% yield.[276] The more mature day 7 colony forming cells appeared to contain more receptors for the fucose binding lectin than the more immature day 14 colony forming cells. An interesting sequence was thus apparent since granulocytes and marrow monocytes also contained this receptor, suggesting the possibility of functional significance.

Membrane sialoglycolipids have also been implicated as a structural component of progenitor cells involved in the functional interrelationship with stimulatory factors.[277] This was based on the following observations: (1) cholera toxin, which bound strongly to membrane gangiosides, inhibited colony formation; (2) different sources of stimulatory factors were sensitive similarly to the cholera toxin effect; (3) choleragenoid, a structural analogue of cholera toxin, was as effective as the parent toxin; (4) the cholera toxin inhibitory action was not observed in other clonal assays not mediated by binding of stimulatory factors, (5) other competitive substances, such as human chorionic gonadotropin and serotonin inhibited the action of the stimulatory factors; (6) the addition of exogenous gangliosides inactivated the stimulatory factors; and (7) the sialic acid on the cell membrane was essential for the responsiveness of the colony forming cells to the stimulatory factors.

Of the antigenic determinants found on granulocyte-macrophage progenitor cells, the most complete studies thus far have been done on the Ia-antigenic system.[14,278–284] Ia antigens are products of genes of the major histocompatibility complex which can be recognized by alloantibodies, heteroantisera, and monoclonal antibodies. A comprehensive review of the human Ia system is available.[285] It appears that the Ia antigens are absent on the pluripotential stem cells analyzed in continuous marrow cultures[280] (described in Chapter 4 on hematopoietic stem cells), but are gained when commitment to the various progenitor cell types occurs and are subsequently lost as these cells undergo differentiation within the marrow. Ia-antigenic determinants have been detected on colony forming cells in diffusion chambers, the equivalent of these cells in liquid suspension culture as well as on the day 14 and 7 colony forming cells.[278–284] Ia antigenic determinants have been detected on these cells using heteroantisera, alloantisera, and monoclonal antibodies. It is now becoming apparent, however, that different monoclonal antibodies to Ia antigens may be recognizing different portions of the determinants or epitomes of the Ia antigen.[286] Monoclonal antibodies to Ia antigens have now been obtained which may preferentially recognize to a greater extent Ia antigenic determinants on one vs. another human granulocyte-macrophage progenitor cell population.[802]

The identity of Ia-antigenic determinants on human progenitor cells was first assessed by complement-dependent cytotoxicity assays and subsequently confirmed by cell sorter analysis which was able to separate progenitor cells with varying densities of determinants from those cells which did not contain Ia-antigenic determinants. It has been suggested that the Ia determinants may play a role in the regulation of myelopoiesis,[14] and evidence for this is beginning to accumulate and will be described later in this chapter. Ia antigens have also been shown to be differentiation markers on human eosinophils.[287] Interestingly, and as yet unexplained, is the finding that Ia antigens have not been detected on mouse granulocyte-macrophage progenitor cells.[288] Heteroantisera[289] and monoclonal antibodies[284] have detected HLA-A and -B antigens of human progenitor cells, and heteroantisera to the i red blood cell antigen has demonstrated i-antigen on granulocyte, as well as on erythroid, progenitor cells.[290] Interestingly, the i-antigen was only detected on the cycling population of cells, or those cells which were synthesizing DNA.[290] Monoclonal antibodies to T cell antigens have substantiated the absence of T-cell antigens on granulocyte-macrophage progenitor cells from human bone marrow.[291] Antibodies against a series of serologically defined cell surface antigens, termed Qa, which were encoded by genes in the Tla region which is distal to the H-2D end of the major histocompatibility complex of the mouse, has demonstrated the presence of Qa antigens on a subpopulation of mouse granulocyte-macrophage progenitor cells.[292] It is apparent that the surface topography of the progenitor cells is just beginning to be elucidated and advances will no doubt be rapid in this area with the advent of monoclonal antibodies which are already being used to help determine the surface characteristics of these cells.[283–286,291,293]

B. Stimulatory Interactions

1. Source of Granulocyte-Macrophage Colony Stimulatory Factors

Many tissues contain and appear to synthesize colony stimulatory factors for granulocytes and macrophages. These factors appear to be released constitutively from cells of the monocyte-macrophage lineage, but these cells can be induced to release greater quantities of factors after antigenic stimulation. The production of these factors also derives from lymphocytes after activation, from endothelial cells, and after interactions between monocytes-macrophages and lymphocytes.

Monocytes and macrophages constitute the mononuclear phagocytic series. These cells are multifaceted in function and release a diverse group of substances,[294–296] and it is becoming apparent that they constitute a heterogenous population cells.[297,298] Among the substances released from these cells are factors which sustain and trigger granulocyte-macrophage progenitor cells to proliferate and differentiate.[299–307] The cells from human blood elaborating the stimulating factors were adherent and phagocytic mononuclear cells.[299–307] It has been noted that the percentage of monocytes in normal blood is at least twice as high as is commonly recognized on routine smears,[308] suggesting that morphology alone would not have been adequate to demonstrate the monocyte origin of these factors. Separation of mouse peritoneal macrophages by velocity sedimentation demonstrated two peaks of nucleated cells which corresponded to a profile of two peaks of colony stimulatory factor producing cells.[297] Both peaks were composed of cells of the mononuclear phagocytic lineage, but the more slowly sedimenting or smaller cells appeared to be more immature as they were mainly cells which were nonadherent, nonphagocytic, stained poorly for nonspecific esterase, produced low levels of lysozyme, had low levels of the ectoenzyme 5′-nucleotidase, but they did contain Fc receptors. The more rapidly sedimenting or larger cells appeared to be more mature cells of the mononuclear phagocytic lineage as they were adherent, phagocytic, stained heavily for nonspecific esterase, produced large quantities of lysozyme, had high levels of 5′-nucleotidase, and contained Fc receptors.

These results demonstrated that both the immature and mature cells of the mononuclear phagocyte series could release the colony stimulatory factors, but as will be described later in this chapter it was only the apparently mature population of cells which was under feedback regulation. It is generally assumed that monocytes and macrophages release colony stimulatory factors constitutively; however, it cannot be ruled out definitively that this release is induced by extremely low levels of bacterial endotoxin or some other activating agents. The mouse monocyte cell line Pu5-1.8 does not produce these factors constitutively, but will respond to nanogram levels of endotoxin and release these factors,[309] and it may be that normal monocytes and macrophages are exquisitively sensitive to low levels of endotoxin which are already present in the culture medium to which the cells are added. Alternatively the cells may already have been activated in vivo before removal from the host environment. Interestingly, corticosteroids will block the newly induced but not constitutive production of colony stimulatory factors from PU5 1.8 cells.[310]

Lymphocytes also have been shown to release granulocyte-macrophage colony stimulatory factors but only after activation by such agents as phytohemagglutinin or concanavalin A.[307,311–315] It is generally assumed that the source of these factors is T lymphocytes. A mouse T-cell line, EL4, will produce these factors when cultured in the presence of Con A but not PHA,[316] and human T lymphocytes growing continuously in culture in the presence of media obtained from mitogen-stimulated peripheral blood lymphocytes will in the presence of mitogens release colony stimulatory factors.[313] A permanent human T-lymphocyte line established from the spleen cells of a patient with a T-lymphocyte variant of hairy cell leukemia can also elaborate colony stimulatory factors.[317] This elaboration appeared to be constitutive although augmented release of factors was detected when the cells were cultured in the presence of phytohemagglutinin. The granulocyte-macrophage colony stimulatory factors from lymphocytes have been separated from other lymphokines such as migration inhibition factor and lymphotoxin[315] and purified T-cell growth factors.[318,319] The production of stimulatory factors by lymphoid tissues has been reviewed.[320]

Subpopulations of lymphocytes are now distinguishable and rapid advances in the characterization of T lymphocytes is being accomplished with the use of monoclonal antibodies directed against surface components of T lymphocytes.[321–325] It should not be long before the subpopulations of lymphocytes which produce the stimulatory factors are defined more precisely. In fact, the hybridoma technology used to make monoclonal antibodies has been used to make cell lines with "infinite" proliferative capacity which can produce granulocyte-macrophage colony stimulatory factors.[326,327] Mouse spleen cells stimulated in vitro with pokeweed mitogen were fused with a thymoma, and a stable cloned T-cell hybridoma was isolated which expressed the H-2 antigens of both fusion parents and the thy 1.1 associated with the parent tumor.[326] The production of factors could be enhanced from this cell line by lipopolysaccharide or if the cells were held at high density in a serum-free medium.[326] Another cloned T-cell hybridoma in the presence of concanavalin A also released colony stimulatory factors.[327] Such activities from both hybridoma cell lines[326,327] were not produced when the parental tumors were exposed to the respective mitogens.

Colony stimulatory factors for granulocytes and macrophages have been produced in mixed leukocyte cultures although the actual cellular source of these factors could not be established firmly.[328,329] It is known that a cooperation exists between mononuclear phagocytes and lymphocytes in immune reactions,[330] and it now appears that these cell populations can collaborate to produce colony stimulatory factors.[331–334] The effect of coincubation of human monocytes and macrophages with autologous lymphocytes in the presence of the methanol extraction residue of Bacillus Calmette Guerin (BCG) was investigated, and it was determined that T lymphocytes could augment as well as suppress the elaboration of the colony stimulatory factors.[331] The kinetics of this response were reported elsewhere.[332] Helper T cells in the form of pure clonal populations of known physiological function and antigenic specificity were used, and the colony stimulatory factors were released when the helper T cells were cultured with specific antigen.[334] The release of factors depended on an H-2 (I-A region) restricted interaction with accessory cells present in the spleen or normal peritoneal cavity.[334]

Vascular endothelial cells were purported to produce granulocyte-macrophage colony stimulatory factors.[335] This was confirmed by the use of extremely well characterized populations of endothelial cells.[336] The release of factors was enhanced from endothelial cells by *S. typhosa* endotoxin as well as by lysates of human blood granulocytes. It was determined that the effective substance in the lysates was not lactoferrin,[336] a metal-binding glycoprotein shown to inhibit the production and/or release of the colony stimulatory factors from monocytes and macrophages.[337]

Two other human cell lines have been shown to elaborate granulocyte-macrophage colony stimulatory factors,[338] and such factors are released by human placental cells,[339] human lung,[340,341] and mouse fetal tissues.[342,343] A list of the mouse and human monocyte and macrophage lines releasing these factors has been published.[344]

It has been suggested that fibroblasts may be a source of these stimulatory factors; however, colony stimulatory factors were not produced by well-defined human bone marrow fibroblasts,[345] suggesting that extensive characterization of cells are necessary before assuming that fibroblast-like cells are fibroblasts. The growth stimulus for fibroblasts derived from megakaryocytes and platelets.[346]

Eosinophilic stimulatory factors have also been isolated and were mainly from populations of lymphocytes.[347–353]

Regardless of the source of the stimulatory factors, local production is believed to be of most relevance in terms of regulation,[354,355] and the relevance of circulating levels of these factors is open to question.[356]

2. *Role of Endotoxin and Other Agents in Granulopoiesis*

Bacteria and their products are efficient stimulators of the release of granulocyte-macrophage colony stimulatory factors both in vitro and in vivo and enhance granulopoiesis in vivo in animals and in man.[24,357–371] It has been suggested that intermittent endotoxemia may play a role in regulating granulopoiesis.[358]

Bacterial endotoxins elicit many host responses and these have been discussed in an extensive review article.[372] The active fraction of bacterial endotoxin has been considered to be the lipid A component of bacterial lipopolysaccharide;[373,374] however, the non lipid component has been shown to be active[375–380] and in fact the lipid A-associated protein may be even more active than the lipid A component,[803] at least in terms of activity in vitro. The action of bacterial products may be under genetic control[381–383] and injections in vivo have been shown to change the size[384] and density[385] distributions of granulocyte and macrophage progenitor cells. Glycoprotein lectin-like receptors have been demonstrated on mouse peritoneal macrophages which bind to the cell wall sugars of various Gram-negative and Gram-positive bacteria.[386–388] Interestingly, the receptor activity may be associated with the Ia region of the mouse histocompatibility complex.[388] These receptors may play a role in the recognition of bacteria or their cell wall products. Different types of colony-stimulatory factors released from adherent blood cells by endotoxin in the presence of fresh and heat-inactivated autologous serum have been reported.[389]

Due to the potent effects of endotoxin, which appear to mediate their effects through the intermediary action of granulocyte-macrophage colony stimulatory factors or other regulators of granulopoiesis, it is important to make sure that endotoxin is removed from test samples and a report is available on the removal of endotoxin from purified colony stimulatory factors.[390]

An intriguing and as yet not fully explained phenomenon is the tolerance of GM-CSF release to endotoxin which occurs after a threshold amount of endotoxin is administered to mice.[391–395] This tolerance phenomenon is most likely intimately associated with the regulation of granulopoiesis and has been used by some to suggest that the granulocyte-macrophage colony stimulating factors may not be the only regulators of granulopoiesis.[394]

Various other agents are known to enhance granulopoiesis in vitro and/or in vivo and these include glucan,[396] *C. parvum,*[397] BCG,[398] lithium,[399–401] and some tumor promotors such as the phorbol esters.[309,402–405] Lithium enhances the release of granulocyte-macrophage colony stimulatory factors from monocytes and macrophages[399,400] as well as counteracting the inhibitory influence of lactoferrin on stimulatory factor production from these cells. It has been shown that lithium also enhances the proliferation of murine pluripotential stem cells,[407,408] but this also may be mediated by stimulatory factors. Purified granulocyte-macrophage stimulatory factors have been shown to stimulate the growth in vitro of colony forming cells with multipotentialities.[409] (See Chapter 4.) It is not clear whether the phorbol esters work by means of the production of stimulatory factors, by increasing the sensitivity of the progenitor cells to stimulation, and/or by stimulating the proliferation of the progenitor cells directly.

3. *Colony Stimulatory Factors—Isolation and Characterization*

It has been suggested that these factors may derive from the cell membrane[410] although work with a human monocyte cell line suggests that there are pools of preformed factors associated mainly with the cell cytosol which have apparent molecular weights similar to their secreted counterparts.[411]

The isolation and purity of various colony stimulatory factors have been discussed in two recent review articles.[412,413] At least four subclasses of these molecules have been reported[413] and include those that stimulate the production of macrophages exclusively,[414–416] those which stimulate granulocytes and macrophages,[417–424] those which stimulate neutrophils,[425,426] and those which stimulate eosinophil production.[427]

Not all colony stimulatory factors act on all cell types, and in general those factors derived from mouse tissue will not directly stimulate human progenitor cells.[428] In addition some factors derived from human cells will only stimulate mouse progenitor cells.[307] Thus it is obvious that the assay system used is of great importance for interpretation of the results. Two human active granulocyte-macrophage colony stimulatory factors have been isolated from human placental cell-conditioned medium.[427] One preferentially stimulates colony formation by day 14 of culture, with increased proportions of macrophages and decreased proportions of neutrophil colonies as the strength of the stimulus is decreased. The other acts more specifically on colony formation noted after 7 days, with approximately 80% of the colonies being neutrophilic. Eosinophilic activity was found in the first fraction. Human active stimulatory factors are not as well isolated as the mouse derived, mouse active factors. An analysis of mouse active factors from serum and medium conditioned by various organs has suggested that many factors are glycoproteins with apparent molecular weights of 23,000.[429] A radioimmunoassay[416] and a radioreceptor assay[430] have been reported that detect a subclass of colony stimulatory factors stimulating only macrophage production. Another radioimmunoassay may also detect other subclasses of factors.[431]

It has been suggested that one form of human stimulatory factor bears microglobulin determinants,[432,433] and that a form of mouse factor interacts with anti-I^k serum.[434] It has been suggested that this effect may be due however to anti-β_2 microglobulin determinants on the progenitor cells.[435]

At one time it was considered that the same molecule could regulate both granulocyte and macrophage differentiation,[436] but it then became apparent that separate molecules for both could be found.[413–427] More recent efforts with clonal analysis of the proliferation of paired daughter cells has demonstrated that granulocyte-macrophage colony stimulating factor can influence not only the cell cycle time but also the pathway of differentiation entered by bipotential granulocyte-macrophage progenitor cells.[437]

Serum halflives for human urine containing mouse active stimulatory factors[438] and mouse lung, mouse active factors[439] in intact mice were calculated at 2.9 hr and 7.3 hr, respectively. The serum half-life for mouse L-cell, mouse active factors[440] were biphasic and were 24 to 40 min in the first phase and 2 to 2.5 hr in the second phase. The organ distribution for the latter two radiolabeled compounds[439,440] were described.

A subclass of mouse stimulatory factors interacts with mononuclear phagocytic cells,[441] and it is now apparent that the granulocyte-macrophage colony stimulatory activities have functions in addition to stimulation of the proliferation and differentiation of granulocyte-macrophage progenitor cells. These other activities include stimulation of the release of E type prostaglandins from mouse macrophages,[442,443] specifically by a macrophage type stimulatory factor,[444] stimulation of RNA synthesis by mouse bone marrow cells,[445] stimulation of the release of plasminogen activator by mouse macrophages,[446,447] stimulation of the killing of *Leishmania tropica* by macrophages,[448] and stimulation of interleukin 1 from mouse macrophages.[449]

Various substances have been shown to potentiate the release of granulocyte-macrophage colony stimulatory factors and/or the action of these factors on the progenitor cells. These substances themselves have no direct effect on the progenitor cells when care is taken to remove endogenous stimulatory-factor-producing cells from the target assay system and when no stimulatory factors are added exogenously. These enhancing agents include serum and red blood cells or their lysates.[450–461] It has been suggested that granulocyte-macrophage colony stimulatory factors are not present in human sera.[462] However, a biological assay has been described which uses analysis of dose-response curves of colony formation in vitro and allows the simultaneous assay of serum factors which stimulate progenitor cells directly and those serum factors which act indirectly on bone marrow adherent factor producing cells.[463]

Other stimulatory agents which work on a pregranulocyte macrophage progenitor cell have been noted,[297,406,464] and these factors have been biochemically separated from those activities acting on the progenitor cells.[465]

A workshop to standardize culture procedures has been held,[466] but it is clear that much has to be learned before all culture systems can be totally standardized. This includes elucidation of the mechanisms by which factor production and factor action occur.

4. In Vivo Relevance of Granulocyte-Macrophage Colony Stimulating Factors

It is most likely that these factors will be demonstrated to be physiologically relevant, but as of now this has not been demonstrated definitively. Studies which suggest an in vivo role for these factors are available. Injections of partially purified human urine preparations enriched with stimulatory factors stimulated a monocytosis and a polymorphonuclear leukocytosis or increased granulopoiesis in neonatal and adult mice with increases of granulocyte progenitor cells and early granulocytes.[467] However, the effects of contaminating proteins or nonspecific stimulators of granulopoiesis could not be eliminated, and multiple injections of this preparation did not result in sustained leukocytosis. Reports on cyclical fluctuation in urine stimulator levels in cyclic neutropenia[468,469] and in chronic myelogenous leukemia with cyclic features[470] suggest an in vivo role, and measurement of plasma stimulator levels in a child with familial cyclic neutropenia demonstrated regular cycles with peak stimulator levels coincident with peaks of monocytes and nadirs of neutrophils.[305] Also, a human lung cancer, which was coincident with neutrophilia in the patient when serially transplanted to nude mice, caused a neutrophilia with increases in progenitor cells.[471] The plasma of nude mice bearing this tumor contained human active as well as mouse active stimulatory factors, and removal of the tumors was followed by the return to normal levels of stimulatory factors and granulopoiesis. A similar study has been reported by others.[472]

Antibodies to a subclass of stimulatory factors have been made,[473] fractionated,[474] and analyzed in an in vivo diffusion chamber assay.[475] Total cellularity and proliferating and nonproliferating granulocytes were markedly suppressed after 4 days of injection of antiserum, and granulocyte progenitor cells were markedly decreased. However, granulopoiesis was not totally suppressed, which may be due to the use of antibodies against only subclasses of stimulatory molecules, and it was not demonstrated that granulopoiesis once suppressed could be reactivated with purified sources of stimulatory factors. Proving the in vivo relevance of stimulatory factors is obviously a complicated matter as other stimulatory activities and cell interactions may be involved. Perhaps the best evidence for an in vivo role for granulocyte-macrophage colony stimulatory factors derives from experiments in which lactoferrin, an in vitro and in vivo suppressor of the production and/or release of stimulatory factors, suppressed granulopoiesis within mice.[337,476] This action occurred in vivo with μg quantities of lactoferrin and was reversed by μg quantities of bacterial lipopolysaccharide. The evidence from these studies was also indirect. Moreover, the production of stimulatory factors was not totally decreased and purified samples of stimulatory factors not added back. However, approaches such as this in which production of stimulatory factors is suppressed, may ultimately yield the definitive proof on whether these stimulatory factors are indeed physiological regulators.

C. Inhibitory Interactions

Myelopoiesis is a dynamic process regulated by inhibitory as well as stimulatory feedback mechanisms. Various inhibitors of myelopoiesis have been described and some are better characterized in terms of biochemistry, site of production, and site of action than others. Those inhibitory substances that will be discussed include lactoferrin, acidic isoferritins, E-type prostaglandins, interferon, chalones and other factors found in serum, including immunoglobulins. This section will be devoted to normal regulatory feedback systems and will not discuss inhibitory activities acting on pluripotential stem cells since these were covered in the chapter on hematopoietic stem cells.

1. Lactoferrin

The existence of a negative feedback control mechanism mediated by a glycoprotein inhibitory factor derived from mature granulocytes was described. It limited colony formation in vitro and myelopoiesis in vivo by decreasing the production and/or release of granulocyte-macrophage colony stimulatory factors from normal and leukemic monocytes and macrophages.[476–480] These studies were based on prior work that demonstrated the inhibitory capacity of intact granulocytes.[481–483]

This factor was similar in many respects to lactoferrin, a metal binding protein first isolated from milk and also present in epithelial secretions and mature granulocytes.[337] This included a similar biochemistry, a similar site of production, and a similar site of action. Three experimental approaches were used to identify lactoferrin as the granulocyte inhibitory factor. The first showed that both acted in vitro and in vivo in a similar manner, the second demonstrated that the inhibitory activity was localized in the same region after separation by isoelectric focusing, and the third demonstrated that antibodies to lactoferrin could inactivate the action of both molecules. The functional capacity of lactoferrin to act as a negative feedback regulator was then shown to depend on the structure of the molecule itself and on the presence and absence of agents that could modulate its activity.[406]

Lactoferrin had a specific requirement for iron in terms of its functional capacity. Each molecule of lactoferrin could bind two molecules of iron.[484] The physical chemistry of lactoferrin has been reported[485] as has a comparative study with transferrin, a biochemically similar but antigenically distinct molecule.[486] Lactoferrin was most effective in inhibiting the production of granulocyte-macrophage colony stimulatory factors from monocytes and macrophages when it was fully saturated with iron. In this condition it was active to concentrations as low as 10^{-17} *M*. In this context it is of interest that increased levels of stimulatory factors have been noted in iron deficiency anemia.[487] Lactoferrin inhibited production of stimulatory factors necessary for neutrophil, eosinophil, and macrophage colony formation.[444,488] Lactoferrin saturated with copper or zinc was functionally ineffective; moreover copper and zinc actually interfered with the inhibitory properties of partially iron saturated lactoferrin. It is known that the conformation of lactoferrin changes depending on its metal saturation,[485] suggesting that fully iron saturated lactoferrin is in a conformational form necessary for activity. Transferrin, even in its fully iron saturated form was relatively inactive in this assay and only acted at concentrations greater than 10^{-6} *M*.[337,406] A radioimmunoassay for lactoferrin did not distinguish between the functionally active and inactive samples of metal-unsaturated and metal-saturated lactoferrin, demonstrating that the detection of a molecule does not necessarily imply the functional activity of the molecule.[406] Bacterial lipopolysaccharide, lithium, testosterone, and estradiol abrogated lactoferrin action in vitro, but the mechanisms were probably different since lithium but not lipopolysaccharide could equally reverse lactoferrin inhibition of C3H/HeJ (poor lipopolysaccharide responder) and C3HeB/FeJ (normal responder) macrophages. Bacterial lipopolysaccharide could also reverse the in vivo action of lactoferrin.[337,476] While the corticosteroids, hydrocortisone, and dexamethasone, did not influence the production of stimulatory factors or the action of lactoferrin, they did block the lipopolysaccharide abrogation of lactoferrin action in vitro.

An hypothesis for the diverse actions of one molecule which focus ultimately on a similar means of regulation has been postulated for lactoferrin.[489] Iron-depleted (Apo-) lactoferrin is considered to be a bacteriostatic or bactericidal agent, presumably through its capacity to remove iron, which bacteria need in order to proliferate, from the milieu. This role, however, need not be mutually exclusive of the action of iron-saturated lactoferrin as a myelopoietic inhibitor. Bacteria and their products are known to enhance myelopoiesis, most probably through their action in enhancing the production of the stimulatory factors for granulocyte and macrophage colony formation. It has been suggested that neutrophils reduce this factor production by removing the positive stimulus, bacteria.[490] This may be mediated by lactoferrin which is present in a relatively iron-unsaturated form in neutrophils.[491,492] Lactoferrin is released from neutrophils in response to phagocytic challenge[493] or in response to a specific stimulus such as endogenous pyrogen.[494] With an iron association constant of 3×10^{38}, which is 300 times greater than that of transferrin,[484] lactoferrin would bind iron from the serum, and bacteria would no longer have access to the free iron needed for growth. This would reduce enhanced stimulatory factor production attributed to bacterial product activation of the mononuclear phagocytes and leave the iron-saturated lactoferrin to bind to the mononuclear phagocytes,[19,297,406] thereby decreasing constitutive production of stimulatory factors. Lactoferrin has been shown to bind to specific receptors on mononuclear phagocytes,[495,496] but it is not clear how lactoferrin can act at concentrations as low as 10^{-17} *M;* activity at this low concentration has been substantiated by others.[497] An unproven but possible explanation is a chemotactic response between lactoferrin and mononuclear phagocytes since it is known that monocytes and macrophages have receptors for certain chemotactic agents.[498,499]

Subpopulations of polymorphonuclear neutrophils containing an active form of lactoferrin[19] as well as subpopulations of mononuclear phagocytes responding to lactoferrin[297,496,500] have been detected. As pointed out earlier in this chapter, evidence is available that subpopulations of polymorphonuclear neutrophils can be distinguished on the basis of membrane characteristics. Subpopulations of these cells from human peripheral blood differing in functional capacity were separated by a rosetting procedure by using rabbit IgG antibody coated sheep erythrocytes.[19] Both Fc receptor positive and negative cells contained lactoferrin. However, only lactoferrin (10^{-16} to 10^{-6} *M*) obtained from the Fc receptor positive cells was able to bind to blood monocytes and to inhibit stimulator production and/or release from these cells. Lactoferrin from the Fc receptor negative cells did not bind to blood monocytes and was inactive as an inhibitor at concentrations as high as 10^{-5} *M*. As suggested earlier in this chapter, the Fc receptor positive cells may be the more mature cells in the blood having been in the circulation longest. Extracts of Fc receptor negative cells contained proteolytic enzymes, not apparent in Fc receptor positive cells, that inactivated the capacity of active lactoferrin to bind to blood monocytes and to inhibit factor production from these cells.

Titration of the activity of lactoferrin has revealed a wide plateau of maximum inhibition,[337,406] but total inhibition of the production of granulocyte-macrophage colony stimulatory factors has not been observed. This suggested that the effects of lactoferrin could be specific for a subpopulation of factor producing cells. Subpopulations of human monocytes and mouse peritoneal macrophages express Ia-antigenic determinants.[278,501–503] Using heteroantisera and more recently monoclonal antibodies to human and mouse Ia antigens, it has been shown that lactoferrin inhibits factor production from an Ia antigen-positive subpopulation of human blood monocytes and mouse peritoneal macrophages.[496,500] Lactoferrin also works on a subpopulation of mouse macrophages which contain $Qa_{2,3}$-antigenic determinants.[496] The blocking of lactoferrin action by anti-Ia and anti-$Qa_{2,3}$ suggests an intimate association between Ia antigens, $Qa_{2,3}$ antigens, and lactoferrin receptors. These antigenic determinants may be of significance to regulation, and the interaction could depend on the heterogeneity of Ia-antigen expression, shedding and replacement of Ia-antigens, and the presence of substances that might be able to modulate the numbers or distribution of Ia antigens on the cell surface. Various agents have been shown to modulate Ia expression on mouse macrophages,[504–506] and it has been demonstrated that the synthesis and expression of Ia antigens on these cells are transient events.[505] Lactoferrin acts on a subpopulation of mouse macrophages separated by velocity sedimentation, which appear to be the more mature macrophages, and using radiolabeled lactoferrin, the population of mouse macrophages which sedimented in the range of 5.3 to 8.5 mm/hr had up to 280,000 lactoferrin receptors per cell.[297,496] Thus it appears as if the interactions involved in lactoferrin action may involve the more mature polymorphonuclear neutrophils as well as the more mature mononuclear phagocytes.

A technique used to localize antigens within a cell immunologically with the electron microscope has been used to study terminal transferase[507] and more recently to trace lactoferrin into human blood monocytes after a pulse exposure of the cells to lactoferrin.[508] Lactoferrin was found in the cytoplasm as well as in the nucleus where it was associated only with the euchromatin. Lactoferrin was found only in 5 to 20% of the monocyte population, but could be detected within these cells after pulse exposure to concentrations as low as 10^{-14} *M*. These results suggest that lactoferrin may exert its effect in the nucleus.

The specificity of action of lactoferrin has been explored. Lactoferrin had no effect on B-lymphocyte colony stimulating activity production by mouse macrophages,[406] erythropoietin production by fetal mouse liver cells,[509] or on the pregranulocyte macrophage progenitor cell stimulatory activity production by adherent mononuclear blood or bone marrow cells,[406] although it did inhibit granulocyte-macrophage colony stimulatory factor production from these same populations of cells. Lactoferrin had no direct effect on the progenitor cells for granulocytes, macrophages, erythroid cells, or B lymphocytes,[337,406] and did not influence the release of lysozyme from human monocytes and mouse macrophages, the release of β-glucuronidase from J774 cells, and the production of plasminogen activator by mouse macrophages.[406] Moreover, lactoferrin did not bind to or inhibit granulocyte-macrophage colony stimulating factor production from human lymphocytes.

It has been suggested that lactoferrin could be a physiological regulator.[337] This was based on the low concentrations needed for activity in vitro, on its specificity of action, and on its action in vivo in a mouse model of rebound myelopoiesis. It is now apparent that lactoferrin will also work in untreated mice where the actual number of granulocyte-macrophage progenitor cells per femur was decreased and the cycling status of these cells curtailed.[804] The fact that lactoferrin decreases the absolute number of granulocyte-macrophage progenitor cells in vivo when it has no direct effect on these cells in vitro suggests that lactoferrin may also be inhibiting the production of stimulatory factors necessary for stem cells or earlier progenitor cells. It has been shown that granulocyte-macrophage colony stimulatory factors act on multipotential hematopoietic colony forming cells in vitro.[409]

Lactoferrin has been shown to act on the production and/or release of two other regulatory factors from cells of the mononuclear phagocytic series. These are the E-type prostaglandins[442,444] and acidic isoferritins.[801] These two factors are discussed below.

2. Acidic Isoferritins

The absence of normal hematopoiesis during acute leukemia not in remission and the recovery of apparently normal blood cells during chemotherapy induced remission suggest that suppressive cell interactions may be involved in the pathogenesis of acute leukemia. It had been shown that there was inhibition of normal progenitor cell proliferation and differentiation by cells from patients with leukemia, but little or no information was provided regarding the actual characterization of the inhibitory cells or the mechanisms of action.[510–522] The existence of an S-phase specific inhibitory activity, leukemia associated inhibitory activity (LIA), against normal granulocyte-macrophage progenitor cells which was produced by bone marrow, spleen, and blood cells from patients with acute and chronic myeloid and lymphoid leukemia and "preleukemia" was demonstrated.[523–527] Greater concentrations of LIA were found during acute leukemia (newly disgnosed and untreated, or on therapy but not in remission) than during chronic leukemia.[523,524] Remission of acute leukemia was associated with low levels of LIA,[524,525] and LIA at that time was not found in hemopoietic cells from normal donors.[523–527] In contrast to its action on normal progenitor cells, LIA was not effective in suppressing the growth of progenitor cells from patients with acute leukemia who were not in remission and from many patients with acute leukemia during remission and with chronic leukemia.[524–527] It was postulated that LIA might confer a proliferative advantage to abnormally responsive cells.[524]

These inhibitory interactions have been documented in neonatal and adult Balb/c mice infected with Abelson virus.[528] Within 2 to 4 days after virus infection, the progenitor cells from bone marrow and spleen became insensitive to inhibition by human LIA and by mouse LIA-like material, even though colony morphology appeared normal. Shortly after, or simultaneously with, the detection of the colony forming cell resistance phenomenon LIA was found in bone marrow, spleen, and thymus cells. The abnormal interactions appeared to be related to induction of lymphoma in Balb/c neonates and to a lymphoproliferative disease in adult Balb/c mice. In contrast, normal cellular interactions were noted in adult C57B1/6 mice which were not susceptible to Abelson disease after virus inoculation and in untreated neonatal and adult Balb/c and adult C57B1/6 mice. Their progenitor cells were sensitive to inhibition by LIA and no LIA-like material was detected in their bone marrow, spleen, and thymus cells. LIA interactions have also been noted in mice given Friend virus (SFFV plus helper) or helper virus,[805] and others have developed a model for LIA based on induction of leukemia in mice with the RFV strain of Friend virus, the spontaneous regression of the disease and its recurrance.[529–531]

After isolating and characterizing LIA[532] it was noted that it was similar to a subclass of isoferritins. Ferritin is considered to be the main storage form for iron in mammalian cells and to play a role in iron metabolism.[533–535] Ferritin is separable by isoelectric focusing into isoforms,[536] and interest had been generated for acidic (low pH) isoferritins as tumor associated substances which might be of value in the diagnosis and prognosis of cancer.[536–543] Relatively little evidence had been presented which suggested that ferritin might have a role other than as a storage molecule for iron.[544–546] The demonstration that LIA was actually acidic isoferritins[547,548] indicated that it was a normally occurring substance, and was the first clear demonstration that the acidic and basic isoferritins could be distinguished in terms of biological function. Evidence has been presented by others that they could be distinguished by the kinetics of iron uptake.[549]

The LIA to be purified was pooled from more than 5000 samples of extracts from bone marrow, spleen, and blood cells collected over a 5-year period from more than 1000 different patients with all types of acute and chronic leukemia and at all stages of disease progression. LIA was isolated by a combination of procedures including ultracentrifugation, Sephadex ® G-200, carboxymethyl cellulose, SDS-polyacrylamide gel electrophoresis, analytical and preparative isoelectric focusing, and concanavalin A Sepharose ®.[532] LIA had an apparent molecular weight of ~550,000 and a pI of 4.7 and copurified with the acidic isoferritins. LIA was detected in all the ferritin preparations tested.[547] Additionally, purified preparations of LIA were composed almost entirely (>90%) of acidic isoferritins, as determined by immunoassay, radioimmunoassay, and isoelectric focusing, and the inhibitory activity in the LIA and ferritin samples was inactivated by a battery of antisera specific for ferritins, including those prepared against acidic isoferritins from normal heart and spleen tissues from patients with Hodgkin's disease.[547] LIA and the acidic isoferritin-inhibitory activity had similar physicochemical characteristics as treatment with trypsin, chymotrypsin, pronase, and periodate and breakdown of the ferritin into subunits by reduction inactivated the inhibitory activity. DNase, RNase, neuraminidase, lipase, phospholipase C, iron depletion, and heat treatment (75°C for 20 min) did not inactivate the activity.[547] Inhibitory activity was detected at concentrations as low as 10^{-17} to 10^{-19} *M* even with completely iron-depleted molecules, and all samples were inactive against progenitor cells from patients with nonremission acute leukemia.[547] A similar curve of inhibition was noted when mouse ferritin was assayed against mouse progenitor cells. The human and mouse acidic isoferritin inhibitory activity suppressed colony formation of cells giving rise to colonies containing purely granulocytes, macrophages, or eosinophils or mixtures of granulocytes and macrophages. Evidence now suggests inhibitory activity against cycling populations of colony forming cells for early erythroid burst formation and for mixed colonies of erythroid cells, granulocytes, and macrophages.[805]

LIA was not detected previously in bone marrow and blood cells from normal donors, but it was found in heart, spleen, placentae, and liver ferritin isolated from normal individuals[547] and mice. This was considered to be due to a combination of factors.[548] Acidic isoferritins are elevated in leukemia and lymphoma, but are in very low concentrations in bone marrow and blood cells and in serum from normal donors. Additionally, evidence demonstrated that medium conditioned by normal human bone marrow and blood monocytes, placental cells, mouse macrophages and WEHI-3 cells, which were used to stimulate colony formation, contained acidic isoferritins. Removal of the ferritins by preincubation with antisera to acidic isoferritins, or by passing the material over Sepharose® 6B columns or over columns to which ferritin antibodies had been fixed to Sephadex® beads by CNBr enhanced the stimulatory capacity of the conditioned medium by 50 to 100%. Not surprisingly, acidic isoferritins (LIA) demonstrated greater inhibition of colony and cluster formation (e.g., 60% inhibition vs. 40%) when the preparations free of ferritin were used to stimulate colony and cluster formation.

The relevance in vivo of acidic isoferritins as regulators of myelopoiesis is still to be determined, but low concentrations needed for activity on the progenitor cells in vitro (10^{-17} to $10^{-19}M$) suggest that they may be of importance as physiological regulators, a role postulated previously for lactoferrin. It remains to be determined if the final effect of acidic isoferritins is due to a direct action on the progenitor cells, a single molecule multiple target hit situation or a cascading set of events set off by one or more acidic isoferritin molecules. Additionally, it is not yet clear if all acidic isoferritin molecules can act as inhibitors or if this activity is confined to a subset of these molecules. At the present time the acidic isoferritin-inhibitory activity appears to derive only from cells of the mononuclear phagocytic lineage.[801]

Using a monoclonal antibody against human Ia-antigens it has been found that the Ia antigens detected by this antibody are either only expressed while the granulocyte-macrophage progenitor cells are cycling (during DNA synthesis) or are at a much greater density on the cell surface of these cells at this time. Acidic isoferritins act on the progenitor cells during S phase, but only on those cells in cycle that also express Ia-antigenic determinants.[801] These studies plus those described above for lactoferrin suggest a role for metal-binding glycoproteins and Ia antigenic determinants in the regulation of myelopoiesis.

Another leukemia associated inhibitor, termed LAI, has been isolated.[550,551] LAI shares many characteristics with acidic isoferritins as well as some perhaps superficial differences. It remains to be determined whether LAI is or is not part of the acidic isoferritin population of molecules.

3. E-type Prostaglandins

The prostaglandins are a large family of compounds with similar structures but diverse functions,[552–554] but it is the E-type prostaglandins (PGE) which play a role in the regulation of macrophage production.[444,555] PGE_1 and PGE_2 are produced by human monocytes and mouse macrophages[442,556,557] and directly affect bone marrow target cell proliferation[442,558–563] by selectively inhibiting human and murine progenitor cells committed to monocyte-macrophage differentiation.[444,488,555,562] Fifty percent inhibition of murine macrophage colony formation occurs with 10^{-8} to 10^{-9} *M* PGE and significant inhibition is noted with 10^{-10} to 10^{-11} *M* PGE.[444] The growth of mixed colonies containing both macrophages and neutrophils is less sensitive to the inhibitory effects of PGE, but the macrophage component of these colonies is reduced. Neutrophil colony formation is not influenced by PGE concentrations below 10^{-6} *M*.[444]

A number of prostaglandins were evaluated for their capacity to inhibit human marrow macrophage progenitor cell proliferation.[488] Both day 7 and day 14 progenitor cells were most sensitive to the effects of the E series prostaglandins. Little difference was observed between PGE_1 and PGE_2 in their ability to inhibit either day 7 (ID_{50}: PGE_1 4×10^{-9} *M*, PGE_2 7×10^{-9} *M*), or day 14 colony forming cells (ID_{50}: PGE_1 2.2×10^{-8} *M*, PGE_2 1.2×10^{-8} *M*. Prostaglandins of the A series were more effective than the E series PGs in inhibiting colony forming cell proliferation at 10^{-5} *M* concentrations; however, below 10^{-6} *M* they were markedly less effective, requiring more than 50 to 140-fold higher concentration for equivalent 50% inhibition of day 7 cells and 40 to 46-fold greater concentrations for day 14 cells. Similar results were observed with the D series prostaglandins; however, day 7 cells were sensitive to the effects of PGD_2 between 10^{-5} *M* and 10^{-8} *M*. The synthetic endoperoxide PGH_2 analogs inhibited macrophage progenitor cell proliferation only at the highest concentrations tested. Thromboxane B_2, 6-keto $PGF_{1\alpha}$ (the stable metabolite of PGI_2), $PGF_{1\alpha}$ and $PGF_{2\alpha}$ had no effect on either day 7 or day 14 colony forming cell proliferation. The facts that circulating levels of PGE of 10^{-10} to 10^{-11} *M* can routinely be demonstrated in human plasma[564] and that during trauma, inflammation, or infection, PGE levels can approach 10^{-7} *M*,[565] place the in vitro sensitivity of the mononuclear phagocyte, but not granulocyte, progenitor cells within physiologically demonstrable prostaglandin limits. This suggests that PGE might serve as an in vivo regulator of monocytopoiesis. Some evidence for in vivo action has been presented.[566]

In comparison to the effect of PGE_1 and PGE_2 on human macrophage progenitor cells, two log greater concentrations of prostaglandins of the A series were required for 50% inhibition. Since PGA has not been detected in human plasma and there is evidence that it results from chemical dehydration of PGE, it is possible that as PGE continually degrades to the more stable PGA, its inhibitory effects can still be exerted.[488] The role of PGD in physiological functions is largely unknown since few tissues produce this prostaglandin and those that do, produce very small quantities of it.[488] Further feedback loops are apparent in macrophage proliferation since various agents activate prostaglandin synthesis.[567–571] The common theme in this activation may be the release of stimulatory factors first since mouse macrophage PGE synthesis is induced by mouse colony stimulatory factor preparations with the selective capacity to stimulate macrophage proliferation differentially, but not by those which preferentially stimulate neutrophil colony formation.[444] It has been suggested that prostaglandins can decrease the release of colony stimulatory factors induced by bacterial lipopolysaccharide;[572] however, prostaglandins have had no influence on constitutive production of colony stimulatory factors from noninduced monocytes and macrophages.[442] Prostaglandins of the E series have been shown to be produced by subpopulations of mouse peritoneal macrophages,[443] and human blood monocytes,[573] and increased prostaglandin synthesis by mouse macrophages has been detected in tumor bearing mice.[574]

4. Interferon, Chalones, and Serum Activities

Interferons are a family of inducible secretory glycoproteins produced by cells in response to infection by viruses or other stimuli. Tumor therapy using interferon has been considered, clinical trials begun, and the production, properties and in vivo effects of interferon have been discussed.[575–577] Progress in the area of characterization of interferons has moved rapidly, and new suggestions for interferon nomenclature have been given.[578] Preparations of interferon have been shown to inhibit human and murine granulocyte-macrophage progenitor cells as well as erythroid progenitor cells.[579–586] It has been suggested by one group that interferon actually blocks differentiation of marrow myeloid precursors,[587] and interferon has been shown to inhibit both the primary and self-renewal capacity of blast cell progenitors.[588] While it appears as if the inhibitory effects are due to interferon, definitive evidence for this awaits the use of pure preparations of interferon. It is likely that the new techniques for gene cloning may show more heterogeneity in action of various interferon preparations as this heterogeneity is already apparent in the samples prepared by standard procedures.

Chalones are considered to be tissue specific, species nonspecific regulator substances produced in the same tissue on which they act with inhibition of cell proliferation being reversible. Several review on granulocytic chalones are available.[589–593] The concept of chalones is not totally accepted, and most reports on chalones have not demonstrated adequately the specificity of the source or the site of action of the material. One problem is perhaps the attempts by the authors to fit their substances into a category associated with a man-made definition of what it is believed such molecules should do, rather than what they can actually do.

Various serum inhibitory activities have been reported and include those of lipoprotein nature, immunoglobulins, and those of an undefined nature.[594–606] The serum inhibitory activities may include some of the defined factors discussed above, but until the factors have been isolated from the serum and characterized it will be difficult to compare them to other inhibitory activities.

IV. ABNORMAL REGULATION OF GRANULOCYTE-MACROPHAGE PRODUCTION DURING LEUKEMIA AND OTHER DISORDERS

A. Progenitor Cells and Stimulatory Interactions

Leukemia cells can form colonies in semisolid medium and in diffusion chambers implanted into mice and can grow in suspension culture in vitro and in diffusion chambers.[268] The leukemic origin of these cells is substantiated by morphology, karyotypic analysis of cells,[607–610] glucose 6-phosphate dehydrogenase isoenzyme analysis of cells (see Chapter 4), biophysical characteristics,[242,611] in vitro clonal growth patterns of bone marrow and blood cells,[612–627] and abnormal responsiveness to bioregulatory molecules.[268] Growth patterns are abnormal during leukemia,[612–627] but the progenitor cells retain some capacity to respond to normal regulators and human leukemia cells do not proliferate autonomously.[268]

Leukemia cells in semisolid agar give rise to abnormal numbers of colonies and manifest heterogeneity in growth patterns among patients with the same morphological disease. Colony formation is usually absent or outside the normal range, but of more importance to disease diagnosis and prognosis is the growth pattern or colony to cluster ratio.[612]

Four main growth patterns were recognized originally.[612] These were colony forming (40 cells or greater per aggregate), large cluster forming (20 to 39 cells per aggregate), small cluster forming (3 to 19 cells per aggregate) and nongrowing. Highly significant differences in remission rate were observed in the different groups. These studies were based on untreated marrow samples and scoring for colonies and clusters were done after cultures were incubated for 7 days. Assays using methylcellulose as the semisolid supporting medium have not detected these differences.[628] The possible reasons for this have been discussed.[268,617]

In a recent updated study 98 consecutive patients with acute nonlymphoblastic leukemia entering the Memorial Sloan Kettering Cancer Center were studied at diagnosis.[616] The microcluster (<20 cells per aggregate) growth pattern indicative of acute myelogenous leukemia was found in 57% of the patients, and this was associated with higher remission rates on two treatment protocols. However, no relationship was seen between the growth pattern at presentation and the duration of remission. The ''acute myelogenous leukemia-''growth pattern was most frequently found to be associated with leukemias exhibiting morphological evidence for partial myeloid or monocytic differentiation. The favorable prognostic significance of Auer rods was recognized in all growth pattern categories. Patients demonstrating the microcluster growth pattern and Auer rods obtained complete remissions in 89% of cases compared to 38% in the Auer rod negative group showing other growth patterns.

The demonstration of a group of patients with poor prognosis characteristics may suggest alternate means of therapy. These growth pattern assays were performed on 354 samples of 48 different patients with acute nonlymphoblastic leukemia and marked spontaneous as well as chemotherapy related fluctuations of aggregate incidence and growth patterns were seen.[616] These fluctuations have been noted by others and are probably of relevance to the pathophysiological condition.[622–624] The growth pattern assay has allowed a diagnostic distinction between acute myeloid and acute lymphoid leukemia and has helped especially in placing those patients with acute undifferentiated leukemia into one of the two categories.[612,616] It has also been helpful in categorizing patients into or out of the acute monocytic group.[627] Patients with acute lymphoblastic leukemia usually form very low numbers of colonies and clusters with a normal colony to cluster ratio, and it had been considered that these were derived from residual normal progenitor cells and that the lymphoblastic clone would not grow under these circumstances.[612,616] A report of the clonal growth of lymphoblastic leukemia cells has appeared.[629]

The colony and cluster assay has also been used to study bone marrow and blood cells from patients with myeloproliferative as well as myelodysplastic syndromes,[630–642] including the selective neutropenias[643] of varying etiologies.[644–654] Alterations of colony formation have been studied after chemotherapy[655] and prior to and after bone marrow transplantion.[656,657] Plating of bone marrow cells in agar after a period of growth in suspension culture gives a measure of a pregranulocyte-macrophage compartment[169] and has been used also as a correlation to clinical status.[658] The normally observed increase in progenitor cells during liquid culture was absent in most marrow samples from patients with leukemia, and persistent low recovery of progenitor cells during remission of acute myelogenous leukemia was associated in three patients with a short duration of remission.[658] A different method of feeding the culture plates has been reported in which increased plating efficiency of cells from patients with leukemia was noted,[659] and this assay was deemed useful in predicting the response of patients to chemotherapy and in chosing the more effective drugs.[660] A relationship between in vitro drug sensitivity and in vivo response to drugs has been noted.[661]

The responsiveness in vitro of granulocyte-macrophage progenitor cells to stimulation by colony stimulatory factors has been studied.[662,663] In the first report[662] it was noted that cells from patients with acute leukemia were slightly more responsive than normal at low concentrations of conditioned medium, but cells from patients with chronic myeloid leukemia were slightly less responsive at all concentrations.[662] These studies did not use nonadherent target marrows and thus endogenous cells producing stimulatory activities were not removed from the target marrow population. In a later study by others the mean threshold of stimulation was estimated by analysis of dose response curves of colony and cluster growth against concentrations of stimulatory activities.[663] Nonadherent cells were not used in this study either but it was claimed that this method of assessment had the advantage that contaminating populations of stimulator-factor producing cells did not affect the results. In this study the marrow cells from patients with acute myeloid leukemia were less sensitive to stimulation than cells from normal donors, and the sensitivities of cells from patients with chronic myeloid leukemia were within the normal range, but this group also tended to require more stimulation. The sensitivity to stimulation was related to the probability of remission.[663] The concept of increased or decreased sensitivity to stimulation is an important one in terms of disease progression, and studies on repetitive samples during disease progression using nonadherent target marrows in the presence of enhancing agents as well as in the presence of varying dilutions of stimulatory factors needs to be done.

The production and/or release of stimulatory factors from marrow cells of patients with leukemia[664] have been reported. Reduced release has been detected in some patients. Chemotherapy induced complete remission in 7 of 8 patients with leukemia who had normal levels whereas remission was only detected in 4 of 13 patients with low levels.[664] Remission was associated with normal or increased levels in 42 of 46 studies in nine patients. Decreased levels of stimulatory activity production has been detected after stimulation of peripheral blood mononuclear cells from patients with aplastic anemia by phytohemagglutinin.[665] Interestingly, the progenitor cells from mice of the autoimmune NZB strain were normally sensitive to stimulation by factors in L-cell conditioned medium or endotoxin serum, but were poor responders in cultures stimulated by WEHI-3 cell conditioned medium.[666] The reasons for the differential sensitivity were not clear but did suggest heterogeneity in response patterns.

Cycling status of granulocyte-macrophage progenitors has been studied in many disease states,[242,268,617] and it has been noted that cycling increases after surgical trauma.[667]

The colony assay has also been used to evaluate those patients with aplastic anemia who might be responsive to treatment with prednisone. A correlation was noted between prednisone-responsiveness in vivo and the inactivation of suppressor T lymphocytes by cortisol in vitro.[668]

An assay for a rapidly proliferating subpopulation of clonogenic blood myeloblasts with self renewal capacity has been developed which requires stimulation by a medium conditioned by human blood leukocytes in the presence of phytohemagglutinin.[669–672]

Using a procedure to remove T cells from the nonrosetting fraction of cells has allowed detection of this clonogenic population of cells even when myeloblasts on a smear were low or absent.[673] This assay has been used to study drug sensitivity[674] and sensitivity to inhibition by interferon.[588] Self-renewal or recloning capacity of granulocyte-macrophage progenitor cells has been identified as a unique feature of some patients with chronic myelogenous leukemia.[675]

Other methods have been used to distinguish abnormal from normal cells. These include the use of premature chromosome condensation[676,677] which has been used to detect residual abnormal cells and to monitor for patient responsiveness to treatment[678–680] and merocyanine 540 which is used as a fluorescent probe of membranes[681] and which has demonstrated selective staining of immature hematopoietic cells from normal donors and patients with leukemia.[682]

B. Inhibitory Interactions

1. The Role of Feedback Regulators and Ia-Antigenic Determinants in the Proliferative Advantage of Abnormally Responsive Cells

Various inhibitory interactions have been described in Section III C, and abnormalities in these interactions have been noted during leukemia and related disorders. Inhibitory activities deriving from cells of patients with leukemia have been reported,[510–522,550,551] But it is not clear if these activities derived from leukemia or residual normal cells. In many cases these activities were not detected from the bone marrow or blood cells of normal donors. This might only mean that the activities were present normally but below the detection sensitivity of the assay systems used. An example of this is the leukemia associated inhibitory activity (LIA)[523–528,532] which was subsequently identified as an acidic isoferritin and later found in normal cells.[547,548] Thus, while this material is most likely a normal regulator,[547,548] it is found in much greater quantity during leukemia and along with other inhibitors such as another leukemia-associated inhibitor (LAI),[550,551] and E-type prostaglandins[444,555] may be involved in the growth advantage of leukemia colony forming cells. Acidic isoferritins (LIA),[547,548] LAI,[550,551] and E type prostaglandins[444,555,558–563] inhibit, respectively, granulocyte and macrophage colony forming cells, the cycling of granulocyte colony forming cells, and macrophage colony forming cells from normal donors, but do not influence the colony forming cells from most patients with leukemia. Therefore, abnormally responsive ''leukemia'' progenitor cells would be able to proliferate while the normal progenitor cells were supressed.

Evidence for the progression of abnormal clones during leukemia has been substantiated by chromosomal[607–610] as well as glucose 6-phosphate dehydrogenase isoenzyme analysis (see Chapter 4).[683] Interestingly, another normal feedback regulator, lactoferrin, is quantitatively and qualitatively deficient during leukemia.[476–478,481] Lactoferrin suppresses the production of granulocyte-macrophage colony stimulatory factors from normal and leukemic mononuclear phagocytes. However, the levels of active lactoferrin are decreased during leukemia, and the factor-producing cells from patients with leukemia are less sensitive to feedback inhibition by lactoferrin. The increased presence of acidic isoferritin inhibitory activity and the decreased presence of active lactoferrin during leukemia suggested that a compensatory system was in effect and that the production and/or release of acidic isoferritin inhibitory activity might be regulated by lactoferrin. This appears to be the case since it is now apparent that lactoferrin can inhibit the production and/or release of acidic isoferritin inhibitory activity as well as E-type prostaglandins from cells of the mononuclear phagocytic lineage.[442,444,801] An important question was why these feedback regulators did not act against the cells from patients with leukemia. Acidic isoferritin-inhibitory activity acts on normal colony forming cells during S phase but not on patient colony forming cells even though they are in cycle at the time the acidic isoferritin is added. A possible explanation is now apparent. Ia antigenic determinants are present on granulocyte-macrophage progenitor cells,[14,278–284] and information now suggests that these determinants are either only expressed during S phase or their expression is much greater during S phase. Acidic isoferritin inhibitory activity only works on Ia-antigen positive cells.[801] Ia antigens are nondetectable on the colony forming cells from many patients[684,806] suggesting that the absence of Ia antigens is responsible for the inactivity of acidic isoferritins. E type prostaglandins also act on Ia-antigen positive cells, although they appear to work on a minor population of Ia negative cells.[807] Lack of Ia antigenic determinants on patient progenitor cells may also explain the inability of E type prostaglandins to act on the patient cells. Furthermore, lactoferrin acts on an Ia-antigen positive population of human monocytes and mouse peritoneal macrophages[496,500] and the decreased sensitivity of patient cells to feedback regulation with lactoferrin also may be manifested because of a lack of Ia-antigen positive target cells. The exact relationship of Ia-antigens on the surface of cells to the action of acidic isoferritins, E-type prostaglandins, and lactoferrin remains to be determined but the results do suggest that the Ia antigens are of importance for the action of these regulatory molecules.

2. *Inhibitory Interactions during Neutropenia and Aplastic Anemia*

Lymphocytes and lymphocyte-derived factors have been implicated in the neutropenic states associated with the selective neutropenias as well as in aplastic anemia.[685–698] In some of the studies it had not been definitively proved that lymphocytes were the source of the inhibition, and the inhibitory activity associated with aplastic anemia has not been noted with all patients[699,700] or by all authors.[701,702]

An immunological mechanism has been suggested in many of these studies, but a hematological mechanism can be considered also.[703] Bone marrow and peripheral blood cells of patients with nonleukemic neutropenia contained and elaborated a granulocyte-progenitor cell inhibitory activity.[703] This inhibitory activity was common to the neutropenias of the various etiologies studied, which included congenital, idiopathic, autoimmune, cyclical, common variable immunodeficiency with hypogammaglobulinemia, and drug induced states. It came from nonadherent, low density, slowly sedimenting, and non-E-rosetting cells, suggesting a non-T-lymphocyte origin for the factors. RNA and protein synthesis, but not cell division, were required for its production. The material was not species specific, inhibited autologous as well as allogeneic normal, and leukemia granulocyte colony forming cells. It was most effective against granulocyte-, less effective against granulocyte-macrophage-, and least or noneffective against macrophage progenitor cells. This inhibitory activity had no influence on pregranulocyte-progenitor cells or on erythroid progenitor cells. It was different from other known inhibitory activities such as lactoferrin, acidic isoferritin, E-type prostaglandins, interferon, and immunoglobulins and could not be detected in normal bone marrow and blood cells. It was considered that this activity, while at present an in vitro phenomenon, might be produced as a secondary response within a compromised host.[703] This same inhibitory activity fluctuates drastically during cyclic neutropenia[703] and has been detected in the bone marrow cells of some patients with aplastic anemia.[801] It cannot be ruled out that this inhibitory activity, under more sensitive assay conditions, will be found in normal bone marrow and blood cells and this may be a missing link in normal feedback regulation. E-type prostaglandins act on macrophage colony forming cells.[444,555] acidic isoferritins act on granulocyte and macrophage colony forming cells,[805] and lactoferrin inhibits the production and/or release of stimulatory factors for granulocyte and macrophage colony forming cells.[444,488] The neutropenia-associated inhibitory activity in comparison acts mainly on granulocyte colony forming cells.[703]

V. DIFFERENTIATION OF LEUKEMIA CELLS

Certain cellular functions are not entirely normal during the remission status of patients with acute leukemia,[268] and the possibility exists that at least some mature cells noted during remission derive from leukemia cells. Differentiation of cells from blast cells of patients with leukemia has been reported in suspension culture and in semisolid medium culture systems in vitro[268,704] as well as in diffusion chambers implanted into the peritoneum of host mice.[527,705–708] The most consistent results appear to involve those assays using diffusion chambers; cells which could not differentiate in vitro were able to differentiate in the diffusion chambers.[527] This suggests that certain differentiation factors, as yet not present in in vitro assays, can be produced in intact mice.[527] It cannot be definitively proved that the differentiation of primary cells from patients with leukemia derive from leukemia cells as there is no marker available yet that distinguishes the leukemic nature of mature cells. The possibility remains that differentiation proceeds from a residual but previously suppressed population of normal cells. Most likely, the differentiation noted does proceed from leukemia cells and the functionally mature nature of these morphologically-mature looking cells has been substantiated.[705,706] The differentiation of murine myelomonocytic leukemia cells in diffusion chambers was coincident with a large decrease in levels of acidic isoferritin-inhibitory activity suggesting that the removal of a suppressive influence may be associated with the phenomenon of differentiation. Lactoferrin, a marker of mature granulocytes,[337] has been found in the differentiated cells in diffusion chambers derived from cells of patients with leukemia[808] and may have been responsible for the decrease in acidic isoferritin inhibitory activity.

Another approach to studying the differentiation of leukemia cells involves the use of leukemia cell lines where the derivation of mature cells from leukemia cells is obvious.

Several human cell lines have been studied extensively and these will be discussed.

The HL-60 line is a promyelocytic cell line which shows some capacity to differentiate spontaneously to mature granulocytes and which can be induced to almost total differentiation by various agents including dimethylsulfoxide, hexamethylene, bisacetamide, certain purines, actinomycin D, retinoic acid, arginase, L-ethionine, and various tumor promoters.[709–721] Induction of differentiation along the macrophage, as well as the granulocyte pathway has been reported, and a subpopulation of HL60 can form colonies in semisolid medium spontaneously although increased colony formation is apparent when an exogenous source of colony stimulatory factors is supplied. There is also evidence of differentiation along the eosinophilic series as HL60 cells cloned in agar stain with Luxol-fast blue, a stain known to be specific for cells of the eosinophilic lineage.[809] Chemotaxis, development of complement receptors, phagocytosis, superoxide production, and nitroblue tetrazolium dye reduction were apparent after induction of differentiation of HL60 cells.[711,722] Two types of Fc receptors have been detected on HL60 cells[723] and specific changes in the surface glycoprotein pattern of these cells has been noted coincident with functional and morphological differentiation.[724,725] Also noted were changes in membrane fluidity[726] and lipid metabolism.[727] The isolation of a subpopulation of thioquanine resistent HL60 cells has been reported.[728] Serum-free cultures are available for the growth of many cells,[729] and the replacement of serum by insulin and transferrin supports growth and differentiation of HL60 cells.[730]

HL60 cells release two leukemia associated inhibitory activities, LAI[731] and acidic isoferritins,[801] but HL60 cells do not respond to inhibition by acidic isoferritins. This is interesting in view of the fact that Ia antigens have not been detected on HL60 cells.[725,732]

Another human myelogenous leukemia cell line, KG-1 has been shown to be responsive to stimulatory factors in vitro and in vivo.[733–735] Glucocorticoid receptors have been detected on these cells,[736] and both KG-1 and HL60 cells were responsive to inhibition by E-type prostaglandins.[734] KG-1 cells expressed Ia- and HLA-A and -B antigens.[732] A subclone (KG1a) did not respond to colony stimulatory factors and lacked Ia antigens.[737]

Two other human cell lines have been studied. One is K562 which was originally established from a pleural effusion of a patient with chronic myelogenous leukemia in terminal blastic crisis and which has been characterized as a highly undifferentiated cell of the granulocytic series, although some sublines manifesting erythroid differentiation have been reported.[738] The other is U937 which was derived from a patient with histiocytic lymphoma.[739] U937 cells synthesize lysozyme, lack immunoglobulin and Epstein-Barr virus genome, but bear receptors for immunoglobulin and complement and are considered to be cells of the monocytic lineage.[740] The subpopulation of U937 cells which forms colonies in semisolid culture medium expresses Ia antigens during S-phase and is responsive to inhibition by acidic isoferritins, lactoferrin, and E-type prostaglandins[806] which makes this a unique line for studying regulatory interactions.

Much information on the differentiation of leukemia cells has derived from established murine leukemia cell lines in which clones of cells capable of differentiating have been isolated from other clones in which differentiation cannot be induced.[741–784] Induction of differentiation in these cells is coincident with a decrease in leukemogenicity.[785–787] The use of these cell lines for screening of therapeutic agents has been considered[788] and studies with these lines have suggested the use of regulatory agents in the treatment of leukemia.[789,790] Differentiation inducing factors have been separated from growth inducing factors.[791] Cell lines have been produced from long-term cultures of mouse bone marrow cells.[792] The long-term cultures are described in Chapter 4 on hematopoietic stem cells. Some of these lines are dependent on a factor present in medium conditioned by WEHI-3 cells, a mouse myelomonocytic leukemia cell line,[740] or by normal spleen cells. The cell lines were obtained from nonvirus treated cultures, were not leukemogenic, maintained a normal karyotype, and formed colonies demonstrating maturation along the granulocytic series when plated in semisolid culture medium. The active moiety involved in the maintenance of these cells was distinct from the granulocyte-macrophage colony stimulating factors.

The use of cell lines offer many possibilities for understanding the regulation of the growth and differentiation of cells, but cell lines are usually far removed from the primary cells taken from the patients or animals with leukemia. The autonomous growth of cell lines has been reported. Such autonomous growth does not occur with primary cells taken from patients with leukemia, and the relevance of studies using autonomously growing cell lines might be questioned. However autonomous growth may be a misconception for many of the cell lines since these cells may still need growth factors and factors produced by the cells, whether or not released into the culture medium, may support the growth of these same cells. A few precedents for this are available. One involves growth factors from murine sarcoma virus-transformed cells which have receptors for these factors.[793–795] The sarcoma growth factor stimulates cell division, causes normal cells to grow in soft agar and produces rapid, reversible morphological transformation of cells in mononuclear culture. Sarcoma growth factor does not appear to produce permanent cell transformation. The phenotypic cell transformation by sarcoma growth factor can be blocked with retinoids.[796] Another example is the cell line WEHI-3 which was believed to be capable of autonomous proliferation. WEHI-3 cells were first obtained as a transplantable myelomonocytic leukemia in Balb/c mice after induction by mineral oil.[797] The cells secreted lysozyme and contained Fc receptors[797,798] and less than 1% of the cells functioned as leukemic stem cells. They had limited self-renewal capacity and formed colonies of neoplastic granulocytes and monocytes in semisolid culture medium.[799,800] They did not require colony stimulatory factor for their proliferation, but the cloning efficiency and size of colonies was increased in its presence.[167] The cells themselves elaborated large amounts of these stimulatory factors, and with the passaging of the cells they appeared to lose responsiveness to the factors completely.[167] These cells were adapted to culture[740] and while they produced the stimulatory factors they appeared to be insensitive to their action. However, lactoferrin could decrease the production and/or release of colony stimulatory factors from WEHI-3 cells, in culture,[337,479] and only then could it be demonstrated that the WEHI-3 cells were sensitive to stimulation by their own stimulatory factors.[479]

REFERENCES

1. **Laszlo, J. and Rundles, R. W.,** Morphology of granulocytes and their precursors, in *Hematology*, Williams, W. J., Beutler, E., Erslev, A. J., and Rundles, R. W., Eds., McGraw-Hill, New York, 1972, chap. 66.
2. **Wintrobe, M. M.,** *Clinical Hematology*, Lea & Febiger, Philadelphia, 1967, chap. 4.
3. **Baggiolini, M., Bretz, U., and Dewald, B.,** Subcellular localization of granulocyte enzymes, in *Neutral Proteases of Human Polymorphonuclear Leukocytes*, Haverman, K. and Janoff, A., Eds., Urban and Schwarzenberg, Baltimore, 1978, 3.
4. **Haverman, K. and Janoff, A.,** Eds., *Neutral Proteases of Human Polymorphonuclear Leukocytes*, Urban and Schwarzenberg, Baltimore, 1978.
5. **Evans, W. H., Grieshaber, C. K., Miller, W. C., Wilson, S. M., and Hoffman, H. A.,** Polyamine synthesis in bone marrow granulocytes: effect of cell maturity and early changes following an inflammatory stimulus, *Blood*, 51, 1021, 1978.
6. **Bachrack, U.,** *Function of Naturally Occurring Polyamines*, Academic Press, New York, 1973, 82.
7. **Granelli-Piperno, A., Vassalli, J.-D., and Reich, E.,** Secretion of plasminogen activator by human polymorphonuclear leukocytes, *J. Exp. Med.*, 146, 1693, 1977.
8. **Zucker-Franklin, D.,** Physiological and pathological variations in the ultrastructure of neutrophils and basophils, *Clin. Haematol.*, 4, 485, 1975.
9. **Wetzel, B. K.,** The comparative fine structure of normal and diseased mammalian granulocytes, in *Regulation of Hematopoiesis*, Gordon, A. S., Ed., Appleton-Century-Crofts, New York, 1970, 819.
10. **Sainte-Marie, G. and Sin, Y. M.,** Morphologic aspects and kinetics of the formation of neutrophils and eosinophils, in *Regulation of Hematopoiesis*, Gordon, A. S., Ed., Appleton-Century-Crofts, New York, 1970, 1109.
11. **Dvorak, H. F. and Dvorak, A. M.,** Basophilic leucocytes: structure, function and role in disease, *Clin. Haematol.*, 4, 651, 1975.
12. **Clark, R. A. F. and Kaplan, A. P.,** Eosinophil leucocytes: structure and function, *Clin. Haematol.*, 4, 635, 1975.
13. **Rabellino, E. M., Ross, G. D., Trang, H. T. G., Williams, N., and Metcalf, D.,** Membrane receptors of mouse leukocytes. II. Sequential expression of membrane receptors and phagocytic capacity during leukocyte differentiation, *J. Exp. Med.*, 147, 434, 1978.
14. **Winchester, R. J., Ross, G. D., Jarowski, C. I., Wang, C. Y., Halper, J., and Broxmeyer, H. E.,** Expression of Ia-like antigen molecules on human granulocytes during early phases of differentiation, *Proc. Natl. Acad. Sci. U.S.A.*, 74, 4012, 1977.
15. **Ross, G. D., Jarowski, C. I., Rabellino, E. M., and Winchester, R. J.,** The sequential appearance of Ia-like antigens and two different complement receptors during the maturation of human neutrophils, *J. Exp. Med.*, 147, 730, 1978.
16. **Messner, R. P. and Jelinek, J. A.,** Receptors for human γG globulin on human neutrophils, *J. Clin. Invest.*, 49, 2165, 1970.
17. **Wong, L. and Wilson, J. D.,** The identification of Fc and C3 receptors on human neutrophils, *J. Immunol. Methods*, 7, 69, 1975.

18. **Klempner, M. S. and Gallin, J. I.,** Separation and functional characterization of human neutrophil subpopulations, *Blood,* 51, 659, 1978.
19. **Broxmeyer, H. E., Ralph, P., Bognacki, J., Kincade, P. W., and DeSousa, M.,** A subpopulation of human polymorphonuclear neutrophils contains an active form of lactoferrin capable of binding to human monocytes and inhibiting production of granulocyte-macrophage colony stimulatory activities, *J. Immunol.,* 125, 903, 1980.
20. **Heborn, H. A., Valdimarsson, H., and Wickramasinghe, S. N.,** Development of human granulocyte and monocyte Fc receptors, *Scand. J. Haematol.,* 22, 364, 1979.
21. **Hensen, P. M.,** Membrane receptors on neutrophils, in *Immunology of Receptors,* Cinader, B., Ed., Marcel Dekker, New York, 1977, 131.
22. **Barrett, S., Garratty, E., and Garratty, G.,** Cell surface heterogeneity of human blood neutrophils and monocytes, *Br. J. Haematol.,* 43, 575, 1979.
23. **Fanger, M. W., Shen, L., Pugh, J., and Bernier, G. M.,** Subpopulations of human peripheral blood granulocytes and monocytes express receptors for IgA., *Proc. Natl. Acad. Sci. U.S.A.,* 77, 3640, 1980.
24. **Broxmeyer, H. E., Van Zant, G., Schultz, E. F., LoBue, J., and Gordon, A. S.,** Glass wool separation of rat PMNs according to adherence and maturity, *J. Reticuloendothel. Soc.,* 18, 118, 1975.
25. **An, T.,** Fc receptors on human neutrophils: electron microscopic study of natural surface distribution, *Immunology,* 40, 1, 1980.
26. **Gilbert, H. S., Goldberg, R., and Ward, L.,** Increased circulating neutrophils with surface receptor activity for immunoglobulin G in polycythemia vera and myeloid metaplasia, *Blood,* 53, 1106, 1979.
27. **Stern, M. and Rosse, W. F.,** Two populations of granulocytes in paroxysmal nocturnal hemoglobinuria, *Blood,* 53, 928, 1979.
28. **Watt, S. M., Burgess, A. W., and Metcalf, D.,** Isolation and surface labeling of murine polymorphonuclear neutrophils, *J. Cell. Physiol.,* 100, 1, 1979.
29. **Zucker-Franklin, D. and Hirsch, J. G.,** Electron microscope studies on the degranulation of rabbit peritoneal leukocytes during phagocytosis, *J. Exp. Med.,* 120, 569, 1964.
30. **Pryzwansky, K. B., MacRae, E. K., Spitznagel, J. K., and Cooney, M. H.,** Early degranulation of human neutrophils: immunocytochemical studies of surface and intracellular phagocytic events, *Cell,* 18, 1025, 1979.
31. **Goldstein, I. M. and Weissman, G.,** Non-phagocytic stimulation of human polymorphonuclear leukocytes: role of the plasma membrane, *Semin. Hematol.,* 16, 175, 1979.
32. **Bentwood, B. J. and Henson, P. M.,** The sequential release of granule constituents from human neutrophils, *J. Immunol.,* 124, 855, 1980.
33. **Wright, D. G. and Gallin, J. I.,** Secretary responses of human neutrophils: exocytosis of specific (secondary) granules by human neutrophils during adherence *in vitro, J. Immunol.,* 123, 285, 1979.
34. **Weissman, G., Korchak, H. M., Perez, H. D., Smolen, J. E., Goldstein, I. M., and Hoffstein, S. T.,** The secretary code of the neutrophil, *J. Ret. Soc.,* 26, 687, 1979.
35. **Baehner, R. L.,** Microbe ingestion and killing by neutrophils: normal mechanisms and abnormalities, *Clin. Haematol.,* 4, 609, 1975.
36. **Babior, B. M. and Kipnes, R. S.,** Superoxide-forming enzyme from human neutrophils: evidence for a flavin requirement, *Blood,* 50, 517, 1977.
37. **Tauber, A. I., Gabig, T. G., and Babior, B. M.,** Evidence for production of oxidizing radicals by the particulate O_2^--forming system from human neutrophils, *Blood,* 53, 666, 1979.
38. **Newburger, P. E., Chovaniec, M. E., and Cohen, H. J.,** Activity and activation of the granulocyte superoxide-generating system, *Blood,* 55, 85, 1980.
39. **Goldstein, I. M.,** Effects of phorbol esters on polymorphonuclear leukocyte functions *in vitro,* in *Carcinogenesis, Mechanisms of Tumor Promotion and Cocarcinogenesis,* Vol. 2, Slaga, T. S., Sivak, A., and Boutwell, R. K., Eds., Raven Press, New York, 1978, 389.
40. **DeChatelet, L. R., Shirley, P. S., and Johnston, R. B., Jr.,** Effect of phorbol myristate acetate on the oxidative metabolism of human polymorphonuclear leukocytes, *Blood,* 47, 545, 1976.
41. **Cohen, M. S., Metcalf, J. A., and Root, R. K.,** Regulation of oxygen metabolism in human granulocytes: relationship between stimulus binding and oxidative response using plant lectins as probes, *Blood,* 55, 1003, 1980.
42. **Liu, Y. K.,** Effects of alcohol on granulocytes and lymphocytes, *Semin. Hematol.,* 17, 130, 1980.
43. **Wright, D. G., Kauffmann, J. C., Chusid, M. J., Herzig, G. P., and Gallin, J. I.,** Functional abnormalities of human neutrophils collected by continuous flow filtration leukopheresis, *Blood,* 46, 901, 1975.
44. **Chusid, M. J., Bujak, J. S., and Dale, D. C.,** Defective polymorphonuclear leukocyte metabolism and function in canine cyclic neutropenia, *Blood,* 46, 921, 1975.

45. **Boxer, L. A., Albertini, D. F., Baehner, R. L., and Oliver, J. M.,** Impaired microtubule assembly and polymorphonuclear leucocytic function in the Chediak-Higashi syndrome correctable by ascorbic acid, *Br. J. Haematol.*, 43, 207, 1979.
46. **Baehner, R. L. and Boxer, L. A.,** Disorders of polymorphonuclear leukocyte function related to alterations in the integrated reactions of cytoplasmic constituents with the plasma membrane, *Semin. Hematol.*, 16, 148, 1979.
47. **Pinkerton, P. H. and Robinson, J. B.,** Granulocyte function in untreated acute and chronic granulocytic leukemia, *Acta Haematol.*, 56, 65, 1976.
48. **MacDougall, L. G., Anderson, R., McNab, G. M., and Katz, J.,** The immune response in iron-deficient children: impaired cellular defense mechanisms with altered humoral components, *J. Pediatr.*, 86, 833, 1975.
49. **Humbert, J. R., Hutter, J. J., Thoren, C. H., and DeArmy, P. A.,** Decreased neutrophil bactericidal activity in acute leukemia of childhood, *Cancer,* 37, 2194, 1976.
50. **Coiffier, B., Frobert, Y., and Revol, L.,** Polymorphonuclear function in acute myeloblastic leukemia, *Biomedicine,* 27, 94, 1977.
51. **Heilmann, C. and Pedersen, F. K.,** Granulocyte function in children with acute lymphoblastic leukaemia during remission, *Scand. J. Haematol.*, 25, 30, 1980.
52. **Olofsson, T., Odeberg, H., and Olsson, I.,** Granulocytic leukemia. II. Bactericidal capacity, phagocytic rate, oxygen consumption, and granule protein composition in isolated granulocytes, *Blood,* 48, 581, 1976.
53. **El-Maalem, H. and Fletcher, J.,** Defective neutrophil function in chronic granulocytic leukaemia, *Br. J. Haematol.*, 34, 95, 1976.
54. **El-Maalem, H. and Fletcher, J.,** Defective hydrogen peroxide production in chronic granulocytic leukaemia neutrophils, *Br. J. Haematol.*, 41, 49, 1979.
55. **Taub, R. N., Baker, M. A., and Madyastha, K. R.,** Masking of neutrophil surface lectin-binding sites in chronic myelogenous leukemia (CML), *Blood,* 55, 294, 1980.
56. **Ruutu, P., Ruutu, T., Vuopio, P., Kosunen, T. U., and de La Chapelle, A.,** Function of neutrophils in preleukaemia, *Scan. J. Haematol.*, 18, 317, 1977.
57. **Athens, J. W.,** An evaluation of the present status of neutrophil replacement therapy, in *Blood As a Tissue,* Holmes, W. L., Ed., Plenum Press, New York, 1970, 277.
58. **Boonlayangoor, P., Telischi, M., Boonlayangoor, S., Sinclair, T. F., and Millhouse, E. W.,** Cryopreservation of human granulocytes: study of granulocyte function and ultrastructure, *Blood,* 56, 237, 1980.
59. **Gupta, S., Ross, G. D., Good, R. A., and Siegal, F. P.,** Surface markers of human eosinophils, *Blood,* 48, 755, 1976.
60. **Burgess, A. W., Cruise, K. M., Mitchell, G. F., and Watt, S. M.,** Preparation and surface labeling of murine eosinophils, *Exp. Hematol.*, 8, 108, 1980.
61. **DeChatelet, L. R., Shirley, P. S., McPhail, L. C., Huntley, C. C., Muss, H. B., and Bass, D. A.,** Oxidative metabolism of the human eosinophil, *Blood,* 50, 525, 1977.
62. **DeChatelet, L. R., Migler, R. A., Shirley, P. S., Muss, H. B., Szejda, P., and Bass, D. A.,** Comparison of intracellular bactericidal activities of human neutrophils and eosinophils, *Blood,* 52, 609, 1978.
63. **Migler, R., DeChatelet, L. R., and Bass, D. A.,** Human eosinophilic peroxidase: role in bactericidal activity, *Blood,* 51, 445, 1978.
64. **Bass, D. A., Grover, W. H., Lewis, J. C., Szejda, P., DeChalelet, L. R., and McCall, C. E.,** Comparison of human eosinophils from normals and patients with eosinophila, *J. Clin. Invest.*, 66, 1265, 1980.
65. **Macglashan, D. W., Jr. and Lichtenstein, L. M.,** The purification of human basophils, *J. Immunol.*, 124, 2519, 1980.
66. **Zucker-Franklin, D.,** Ultrastructural evidence for the common origin of human mast cells and basophils, *Blood,* 56, 534, 1980.
67. **Cronkite, E. P. and Vincent, P. C.,** Granulocytopoiesis, *Ser. Haematol.*, 2, 3, 1969.
68. **LoBue, J.,** Analysis of normal granulocyte production and release, in *Regulation of Hematopoiesis,* Gordon, A. S., Ed., Appleton-Century-Crofts, New York, 1970, 1167.
69. **Athens, J. W.,** Neutrophilic granulocyte kinetics and granulocytopoiesis, in *Regulation of Hematopoiesis,* Gordon, A. S., Ed., Appleton-Century-Crofts, New York, 1970, 1143.
70. **Boggs, D. R.,** Homeostatic regulatory mechanisms of hematopoiesis, *Ann. Rev. Physiol.*, 28, 39, 1966.
71. **LoBue, J., Monette, F. C., Gordon, A. S., Chan, P-C., and Alexander, P., Jr.,** in Myeloproliferative Disorders of Animals and Man, Atomic Energy Commission Symposium Series 19, Clarke, W. J., Howard, E. B., and Hackett, P. L., Eds., Division of Technical Information, Atomic Energy Commission, Washington, D.C., 1970, 84.

72. **Cronkite, E. P. and Vincent, P. C.,** Granulocytopoiesis, in Myeloproliferative Disorders of Animals and Man, Atomic Energy Commission Symposium Series 19, Clarke, W. J., Howard, E. B., and Hackett, P. L., Eds., Division of Technical Information, Atomic Energy Commission, Washington, D.C., 1970, 3.
73. **Perry, S.,** Proliferation of myeloid cells, *Ann. Rev. Med.,* 22, 171, 1971.
74. **Constable, T. B. and Blackett, N. M.,** The cell population kinetics of neutrophilic cells, *Cell Tissue Kinet.,* 5, 289, 1972.
75. **LoBue, J.,** Stem cell and neutrophilic granulocyte kinetics, *Med. Clin. N. Am.,* 57, 265, 1973.
76. **Vincent, P. C.,** Granulocyte kinetics in health and disease, *Clin. Haematol.,* 6, 695, 1977.
77. **Vincent, P. C.,** The measurement of granulocyte kinetics, *Br. J. Haematol.,* 36, 1, 1977.
78. **Finch, C. A., Harker, L. A., and Cook, J. D.,** Kinetics of the formed elements of human blood, *Blood,* 50, 699, 1977.
79. **Cronkite, E. P.,** Kinetics of granulocytopoiesis, *Clin. Haematol.,* 8, 351, 1979.
80. **Boggs, D. R., Athens, J. W., Cartwright, G. E., and Wintrobe, M. M.,** Leukokinetic studies, IX. Experimental evaluation of a model of granulopoiesis, *J. Clin. Invest.,* 44, 643, 1965.
81. **Maloney, M. A. and Patt, H. M.,** Granulocyte transit from bone marrow to blood, *Blood,* 31, 195, 1968.
82. **Van Zant, G., Broxmeyer, H. E., LoBue, J., and Gordon, A. S.,** Rat hindleg perfusion: correlation of bone marrow leukocyte cellularity with release, *Am. J. Physiol.,* 225, 1327, 1973.
83. **Mauer, A. M. and Lampkin, B. C.,** Studies of leukemia cell proliferation, in *Advances in Acute Leukemia,* Cleton, F. J., Crowther, D., and Malpas, J. S., Eds., North-Holland, Amsterdam, 1974, 69.
84. **Arlin, Z. A., Fried, J., and Clarkson, B. D.,** Therapeutic role of cell kinetics in actue leukemia, *Clin. Haematol.,* 7, 339, 1978.
85. **Sullivan, T. J.,** The role of eosinophils in inflammatory reactions, *Prog. Hematol.,* 11, 65, 1979.
86. **Cohen, N. S., LoBue, J., and Gordon, A. S.,** Mechanisms of leukocyte production and release. VIII. Eosinophil and neutrophil kinetics in rats, *Scand. J. Haematol.,* 4, 339, 1967.
87. **Alexander, P., Monette, F. C., LoBue, J., Gordon, A. S., and Chan, P.-C.,** Mechanisms of leukocyte production and release. X. Eosinophil proliferation in rats of different ages, *Scand. J. Haematol.,* 6, 319, 1969.
88. **Hudson, G., Chin, K. N., and Moffatt, D. J.,** Changes in eosinophil granulocyte kinetics in severe hypoxia, *Acta Haematol.,* 48, 58, 1972.
89. **Hudson, G., Chin, K. N., and Moffatt, D. J.,** Marrow reserve of eosinophils: estimation of transit time in normal guinea-pigs, *Cell Tissue Kinet.,* 5, 191, 1972.
90. **Hudson, G.,** Quantitative study of the eosinophil granulocytes, *Semin. Hematol.,* 5, 166, 1968.
91. **Spry, C. J. F.,** Mechanisms of eosinophilia. V. Kinetics of normal and accelerated eosinopoiesis, *Cell Tissue Kinet.,* 4, 351, 1971.
92. **Fruhman, G. J.,** Factors influencing neutrophil mobilization, in *Regulation of Hematopoiesis,* Gordon, A. S., Ed., Appleton-Century-Crofts, New York, 1970, 873.
93. **Fruhman, G. J.,** Extravacular mobilzation of neutrophils, *Ann. N.Y. Acad. Sci.,* 113, 968, 1964.
94. **Fruhman, G. J.,** Endotoxins and leukocyte mobilization, *J. Ret. Soc.,* 12, 62, 1972.
95. **Chervenick, P. A., Boggs, D. R., Marsh, J. C., Cartwright, G. E., and Wintrobe, M. M.,** The blood and bone marrow neutrophil response to graded doses of endotoxin in mice, *Proc. Soc. Exp. Biol. Med.,* 126, 891, 1967.
96. **Gordon, A. S., Neri, R. O., Siegel, C. D., Dornfest, B. S., Handler, E. S., LoBue, J., and Eisler, M.,** Evidence for a circulating leukocytosis-inducing factor (LIF), *Acta Haematol.,* 23, 323, 1960.
97. **Ludwig, F. C., Smoke, M. E., and Wellington, J. S.,** Studies of the humoral regulation of leukocytes, *Ann. N.Y. Acad. Sci.,* 136, 784, 1964.
98. **Dornfest, B. S., LoBue, J., Handler, E. S., Gordon, A. S., and Quastler, H.,** Mechanisms of leukocyte production and release. II. Factors influencing leukocyte release from isolated perfused rat legs, *J. Lab. Clin. Med.,* 60, 777, 1962.
99. **Dornfest, B. S., LoBue, J., Handler, E. S., Gordon, A. S., and Quastler, H.,** Mechanisms of leukocyte production and release. I. Factors influencing leukocyte release from isolated perfused rat femora, *Acta Hematol.,* 28, 42, 1962.
100. **Dornfest, B. S.,** Perfusion techniques—a tool in elucidating blood cell release phenomena, in *Regulation of Hematopoiesis,* Gordon, A. S., Ed., Appleton-Century-Crofts, New York, 1970, 237.
101. **Broxmeyer, H., Van Zant, G., Zucali, J. R., LoBue, J., and Gordon, A. S.,** Mechanisms of leukocyte production and release. XII. A comparative assay of the leukocytosis-inducing factor (LIF) and the colony-stimulating factor (CSF), *Proc. Soc. Exp. Biol. Med.,* 145, 1262, 1974.

102. **Gordon, A. S., Handler, E. S., Siegel, C. D., Dornfest, B. S., and LoBue, J.,** Plasma factors influencing leukocyte release in rats, *Ann. N.Y. Acad. Sci.*, 113, 766, 1964.
103. **Handler, E. S., Varsa, E. E., and Gordon, A. S.,** Mechanisms of leukocyte production and release. V. Studies of leukocytosis-inducing factor in the plasma of rats treated with typhoid-paratyphoid vaccine, *J. Lab. Clin. Med.*, 67, 398, 1966.
104. **Lapin, D. M., LoBue, J., Gordon, A. S., Zanjani, E. D., and Schultz, E. F.,** Mechanisms of leukocyte production and release. IX. Kinetics of leukocyte release in leukocytapheresed rats, *Proc. Soc. Exp. Biol. Med.*, 131, 756, 1969.
105. **Schultz, E. F., Lapin, D. M., LoBue, J., Gordon, A. S., Siegel, C. D., and Rakowitz, F.,** Mechanisms of leukocyte production and release. XIII. Assay of plasma for marrow neutrophil-releasing activity, *J. Ret. Soc.*, 14, 287, 1973.
106. **Boggs, D. R., Cartwright, G. E., and Wintrobe, M. M.,** Neutrophilia-inducing activity in plasma of dogs recovering from drug-induced myelotoxicity, *Am. J. Physiol.*, 211, 51, 1966.
107. **Boggs, D. R., Chervenick, P. A., Marsh, J. C., Cartwright, G. E., and Wintrobe, M. M.,** Neutrophil-releasing activity in plasma of dogs injected with endotoxin, *J. Lab. Clin. Med.*, 72, 177, 1968.
108. **Chervenick, P. A. and Boggs, D. R.,** Granulocytic hyperplasia and induction of tolerance in response to chronic endotoxin administration, *J. Ret. Soc.*, 9, 288, 1971.
109. **Katz, R., Gordon, A. S., and Lapin, D. M.,** Mechanisms of leukocyte production and release. VI. Studies on the purification of the leukocytosis-inducing factor (LIF), *J. Ret. Soc.*, 3. 103, 1966.
110. **Quesenbery, P., Halperin, J., Ryan, M. and Stohlman, F., Jr.,** Tolerance to the granulocyte-releasing and colony-stimulating factor elevating effects of endotoxin, *Blood,* 45, 789, 1975.
111. **Chikkapa, G., Chanana, A. D., Chandra, P., Commerford, S. L., and Cronkite, E. P.,** Granulocytopoiesis: studies on leukocytosis-inducing and colony-stimulating factors, *Proc. Soc. Exp. Biol. Med.*, 154, 192, 1977.
112. **Quesenbery, P., Zuckerman, K., Ryan, M., and Stohlman, F., Jr.,** A dichotomy between the release of bone marrow granulocytes and stem cells, *Proc. Soc. Exp. Biol. Med.*, 154, 53, 1977.
113. **Joyce, R. A. and Boggs, D. R.,** Visualizing the marrow granulocyte reserve, *J. Lab. Clin. Med.*, 93, 101, 1979.
114. **Lichtman, M. A. and Weed, R. I.,** Alteration of the cell periphery during granulocyte maturation: relationship to cell function, *Blood,* 39, 301, 1972.
115. **Chamberlain, J. K. and Lichtman, M. A.,** Marrow cell egress: specificity of the site of penetration into the sinus, *Blood,* 52, 959, 1978.
116. **Spry, C. J. F.,** Mechanism of eosinophilia. VI. Eosinophil mobilization, *Cell Tissue Kinet.*, 4, 365, 1971.
117. **Ward, P. A.,** Overview, in *Leukocyte Chemotaxis,* Quie, P. G. and Gallin, J. I., Eds., Raven Press, New York, 1978, 405.
118. **O'Flaherty, J. T. and Ward, P. A.,** Chemotactic factors and the neutrophil, *Semin. Hematol.*, 16, 163, 1979.
119. **Wright, D. G. and Gallin, J. I.,** Mechanisms for modulation of the inflammatory response: generation and inactiviation of C5a by products stored in the granules of human neutrophils, in *Leukocyte Chemotaxis,* Gallin, J. I. and Quie, P. G., Eds., Raven Press, New York, 1978, 211.
120. **Ginsburg, I. and Quie, P. G.,** Modulation of human polymorphonuclear leukocyte chemotaxis by leukocyte extracts, bacterial products, inflammatory exudates, and polyelectrolytes, *Inflamation,* 4, 301, 1980.
121. **Becker, E. L. and Stossel, T. P.,** Chemotaxis, *Fed. Proc.*, 39, 2949, 1980.
122. **Snyderman, R. and Pike, M. C.,** Pathophysiologic aspects of leukocyte chemotaxis: identification of a specific chemotactic factor binding site on human granulocytes and defects of macrophage function associated with neoplasia, in *Leukocyte Chemotaxis,* Gallin, J. I. and Quie, P. G., Eds., Raven Press, New York, 1978, 357.
123. **Williams, L. T., Snyderman, R., Pike, M. C., and Lefkowitz, R. J.,** Specific receptor sites for chemotactic peptides on human polymorphonuclear leukocytes, *Proc. Natl. Acad. Sci. U.S.A.*, 74, 1204, 1977.
124. **Fletcher, M. P. and Gallin, J. I.,** Degranulating stimuli increase the availability of receptors on human neutrophils for the chemoattractant F-Met-Leu-Phe, *J. Immunol.*, 124, 1585, 1980.
125. **Snyderman, R. and Pike, M. C.,** *N*-Formylmethionyl peptide receptors on equine leukocytes initiate secretion but not chemotaxis, *Science,* 209, 493, 1980.
126. **Lehmeyer, J. E., Snyderman, R., and Johnston, R. B., Jr.,** Stimulation of neutrophil oxidative metabolism by chemotactic peptides: influence of calcium ion concentration and cytochalasin B and comparison with stimulation by phorbol myristate acetate, *Blood,* 54, 35, 1979.

127. **Van Epps, D. E. and Garcia, M. L.,** Enhancement of neutrophil function as a result of prior exposure to chemotactic factor, *J. Clin. Invest.*, 66, 167, 1980.
128. **Issekutz, A. C., Lee, K.-Y., and Biggar, W. D.,** Enhancement of human neutrophil bactericidal activity by chemotactic factors, *Infect. Immun.*, 24, 295, 1979.
129. **Boxer, L. A., Yoder, M., Bonsib, S., Schmidt, M., Ho, P., Jersild, R., and Baehner, R. L.,** Effects of a chemotactic factor, *N*-formylmethionyl peptide, on adherence, superoxide anion generation, phagocytosis, and microtubule assembly of human polymorphonuclear leukocytes, *J. Lab. Clin. Med.*, 93, 506, 1979.
130. **Gallin, J. I.,** Degranulating stimuli decrease the negative surface charge and increase the adhesiveness of human neutrophils, *J. Clin. Invest.*, 65, 298, 1980.
131. **Becker, E. L.,** A multifunctional receptor on the neutrophil for synthetic chemotactic oligopeptides, *J. Ret. Soc.*, 26, 701, 1979.
132. **Absolom, D. R. and Van Oss, C. J.,** Chemotactic response of cryopreserved human granulocytes, *J. Ret. Soc.*, 25, 231, 1979.
133. **Clawson, C. C., Nesbit, M. E., White, J. G., and Repine, J. E.,** Quantitation of chemotaxis and maximal bactericidal capacity of mature neutrophils in chronic myelogenous leukemia, *J. Ret. Soc.*, 26, 515, 1979.
134. **Merrill, W. W., Naegel, G. P., Matthay, R. A., and Reynolds, H. Y.,** Aveolar macrophage-derived chemotactic factor. Kinetics of *in vitro* production and partial characterization, *J. Clin. Invest.*, 65, 268, 1980.
135. **Tono-Oka, T., NaKayama, M., and Matsumoto, S.,** Human monocyte-derived chemotactic factor for granulocytes, *Immunology*, 39, 607, 1980.
136. **Russo, M.,** The role of macrophages in the chemotactic response of polymorphonuclear leukocytes to bacterial lipopolysaccharides, *Proc. Soc. Exp. Biol. Med.*, 164, 326, 1980.
137. **Tanaka, J., Baba, T., and Torisu, M.,** Ascaris and eosinophil. II. Isolation and characterization of eosinophil chemotactic factor and neutrophil chemotactic factor of parasite in ascaris antigen, *J. Immunol.*, 122, 302, 1979.
138. **Sumner, M. A., Bradley, T. R., Hodgson, G. S., Cline, M. J., Fry, P. A., and Sutherland, L.,** The growth of bone marrow cells in liquid culture, *Br. J. Haematol.*, 23, 221, 1972.
139. **Golde, D. W. and Cline, M. J.,** Growth of human bone marrow in liquid culture, *Blood*, 41, 45, 1973.
140. **Boyum, A. and Borgstrom, R.,** The concentration of granulocytic stem cells in mouse bone marrow, determined with diffusion chamber technique, *Scand. J. Haematol.*, 7, 294, 1970.
141. **Breivik, H.,** Haematopoietic stem cell content of murine bone marrow, spleen, and blood. Limiting dilution analysis of diffusion chamber cultures, *J. Cell. Physiol.*, 78, 73, 1971
142. **Breivik, H., Benestad, H. B., and Boyum, A.,** Diffusion chamber and spleen colony assay of murine haematopoietic stem cells, *J. Cell. physiol.*, 78, 65, 1971.
143. **Brevik, H. and Benestad, H. B.,** Regulation of granulocyte and macrophage formation in diffusion chamber cultures of mouse haematopoietic cells, *Exp. Cell Res.*, 70, 340, 1972.
144. **Benestad, H. B.,** Cell kinetics in diffusion chambers: survival, resumption of proliferation, and maturation rate of murine haemopoietic cells, *Cell Tissue Kinet.*, 5, 421, 1972.
145. **Boyum, A. and Breivik, H.,** Kinetics of murine haemopoietic cell proliferation in diffusion chambers, *Cell Tissue Kinet.*, 6, 101, 1973.
146. **Boyum, A., Carsten, A. L., and Laerum, O. D.,** Hematopoiesis measured by spleen colony and diffusion chamber techniques in mice treated with one or two injections of cyclophosphamide, *Br. J. Haematol.*, 26, 605, 1974.
147. **Quesenbery, P., Niskanen, E., Symann, M., Howard, D., Ryan, M., Halpern, J., and Stohlman, F., Jr.,** Growth of stem cell concentrates in diffusion chambers (DC), *Cell Tissue Kinet.*, 7, 337, 1974.
148. **Laissue, J. A., Chanana, A. D., Cronkite, E. P., Joel, D. D., and Pavelec, M.,** Culture of autologous bone marrow in diffusion chambers: effects of host irradiation, *Blood*, 45, 417, 1975.
149. **Marmor, J. B., Russel, J. L., Miller, A. M., and Robinson, S. H.,** Modulation of murine granulocyte proliferation in diffusion chamber cultures, *Blood*, 46, 39, 1975.
150. **Boyum, A., Carsten, A. L., Laerum, O. D., and Cronkite, E. P.,** Kinetics of cell proliferation of murine bone marrow cells cultured in diffusion chambers: effect of hypoxia, bleeding, erythropoietin injections, polycythemia, and irradiation of the host, *Blood*, 40, 174, 1972.
151. **Boyum, A., Boecker, W., Carsten, A. L., and Cronkite, E. P.,** Proliferation of human bone marrow cells in diffusion chambers implanted into normal or irradiated mice, *Blood*, 40, 163, 1972.
152. **Hoelzer, D., Harriss, E. B., Slade, M., and Kurrle, E.,** Growth of *in vitro* colony-forming cells from normal human peripheral blood leukocytes cultured in diffusion chambers, *J. Cell. Physiol.*, 89, 89, 1976.

153. **Chikkappa, G., Carsten, A. L., Chanana, A. D., and Cronkite, E. P.,** Culture of normal human blood cells in diffusion chamber systems. I. Granulocyte survival and proliferation, *Exp. Hematol.*, 6, 28, 1978.
154. **Niskanen, E. and Cline, M. J.,** Growth of mouse and human bone marrow in diffusion chambers in mice. Development of proliferation of myeloid stem cells in cyclophosphamide- and erythropoietin-treated mice, *Cell Tissue Kinet.*, 12, 59, 1979.
155. **Seki, M.,** Hematopoietic colony formation in a macrophage layer provided by intraperitoneal insertion of cellulose acetate membrane, *Transplantation,* 16, 544, 1973.
156. **Turner, A. R., Pfrimmer, W. J., Torok-Storb, B. J., and Boggs, D. R.,** Granulocytic colonies on macrophage-coated membranes, *Am. J. Hematol.*, 4, 105, 1978.
157. **Metcalf, D.,** *Hemopoietic Colonies,* Springer-Verlag, Berlin, 1977.
158. **Elmgreen, J., Jacobsen, N., and Knudtzon, S.,** The effect of syngeneic peripheral blood cells on the formation of colonies by normal human bone marrow cells in diffusion chambers in mice, *Scand. J. Haematol.*, 17, 379, 1976.
159. **Jacobsen, N. and Fauerholdt, L.,** Human granulocytopoietic colonies in diffusion chambers in mice: growth of colonies and the effect of host irradiation, *Scand. J. Haematol.*, 16, 101, 1976.
160. **Jacobsen, N. and Fauerholdt, L.,** Quantitative aspects of an *in vivo* diffusion chamber assay for normal human hemopoietic colony forming units, *Exp. Hematol.*, 5, 171, 1977.
161. **Jacobsen, N.,** Human granulopoietic progenitor cell diversity and regulation studied in diffusion chambers, *Diffusion Chamber Culture,* Cronkite, E. P. and Carsten, A. L., Eds., Springer-Verlag, Berlin, 1980, 28.
162. **Jacobsen, N.,** Proliferation of diffusion chamber colony-forming units (CFU-D) in cultures of normal human bone marrow in diffusion chambers in mice, *Blood,* 49, 415, 1977.
163. **Gordon, M. Y., Blackett, N. M., and Douglas, I. D. C.,** Colony formation by human haemopoietic precursor cells cultured in semi-solid agar in diffusion chambers, *Br. J. Haematol.*, 31, 103, 1975.
164. **Gordon, M. Y., Douglas, I. D. C., Clink, H. M., and Pickering, B. M. J.,** Distribution of granulopoietic activity in the human skeleton, studied by colony growth in agar diffusion chambers, *Br. J. Haematol.*, 32, 537, 1976.
165. **Steinberg, H. N., Handler, E. S., and Handler, E. E.,** Assessment of erythrocytic and granulocytic colony formation in an *in vivo* plasma clot diffusion chamber culture system, *Blood,* 47, 1041, 1976.
166. **Cronkite, E. P. and Carsten, A. L.,** Eds., *Diffusion Chamber Culture: Hemopoiesis Cloning of Tumors, Cytogenetic and Carcinogenic Assays,* Springer-Verlag, Berlin, 1980.
167. **Metcalf, D. and Moore, M. A. S.,** *Haemopoietic Cells,* North-Holland, Amsterdam, 1971.
168. **Jacobsen, N., Broxmeyer, H. E., Grossbard, E., and Moore, M. A. S.,** Diversity of human granulopoietic precursor cells: separation of cells that form colonies in diffusion chambers (CFU-d) from populations of colony-forming cells *in vitro* (CFU-c) by velocity sedimentation, *Blood,* 52, 221, 1978.
169. **Jacobsen, N., Broxmeyer, H. E., Grossbard, E., and Moore, M. A. S.,** Colony-forming units in diffusion chambers (CFU-d) and colony-forming units in agar culture (CFU-c) obtained from normal human bone marrow: a possible parent-progeny relationship, *Cell Tissue Kinet.*, 12, 213, 1979.
170. **Bradley, T. R. and Metcalf, D.,** The growth of mouse bone marrow cells *in vitro, Aust. J. Exp. Biol. Med.*, 44, 287, 1966.
171. **Pluznik, D. H. and Sachs, L.,** The cloning of normal "mast" cells in tissue culture, *J. Cell Comp. Physiol.*, 66, 319, 1965.
172. **Pluznik, D. H. and Sachs, L.,** The induction of clones of normal mast cells by a substance from conditioned medium, *Exp. Cell Res.*, 43, 553, 1966.
173. **Ichikawa, Y., Pluznik, D. H., and Sachs, L.,** In vitro control of the development of macrophage colonies, *Proc. Natl. Acad. Sci. U.S.A.*, 56, 488, 1966.
174. **Metcalf, D., Bradley, T. R., and Robinson, W. A.,** Analysis of colonies developing *in vitro* from mouse bone marrow cells stimulated by kidney "feeder layers" and leukemic serum, *J. Cell. Physiol.*, 69, 93, 1967.
175. **Bradley, T. R.,** Aspects of bone marrow colony growth *in vitro, Aust. J. Exp. Biol. Med. Sci.*, 46, 335, 1968.
176. **Bradley, T. R. and Sumner, M. A.,** Stimulation of bone marrow colony growth *in vitro, Aust. J. Exp. Biol. Med. Sci.*, 46, 607, 1968.
177. **Bradley, T. R. and Siemienowicz, R.,** Colony growth of rat bone marrow cells in vitro, *Aust. J. Exp. Biol. Med.*, 46, 595, 1968.
178. **Zucali, J. R., Rakowitz, F., Van Zant, G., and Gordon, A. S.,** Separation of agar colony forming cells from rat bone marrow, *Proc. Soc. Exp. Biol. Med.*, 145, 519, 1974.
179. **Marsh, J. C., Levitt, M., and Katzenstein, A.,** The growth of leukocyte colonies *in vitro* from dog bone marrow, *J. Lab. Clin. Med.*, 79, 1041, 1972.

180. **Levitt, M., Katzenstein, A., and Marsh, J. C.,** Kinetics of canine hematopoietic colonies grown *in vitro, Proc. Soc. Exp. Biol. Med.,* 141, 408, 1972.
181. **Dodge, W. H. and Moscovici, C.,** Colony formation by normal chick hematopoietic cells and leukemic myeloblasts, *J. Cell. Physiol.,* 81, 371, 1973.
182. **Senn, J. S., McCulloch, E. A., and Till, J. E.,** Comparison of colony-forming ability of normal and leukaemic human marrow in cell culture, *Lancet,* 2, 597, 1967.
183. **Pike, B. L. and Robinson, W. A.,** Human bone marrow colony formation in agar-gel, *J. Cell. Physiol.,* 76, 77, 1970.
184. **Iscove, N. N., Senn, J. G., Till, J. E., and McCulloch, E. A.,** Colony formation by normal and leukemic human marrow cells in culture: effect of conditioned medium from human leukocytes, *Blood,* 37, 1, 1971.
185. **Chervenick, P. A. and Boggs, D. R.,** In vitro growth of granulocytic and mononuclear cell colonies from blood of normal individuals, *Blood,* 37, 131, 1971.
186. **Kurnick, J. E. and Robinson, W. A.,** Colony growth of human peripheral white blood cells *in vitro, Blood,* 37, 136, 1971.
187. **McCredie, K. B., Hersh, E. M., and Freireich, E. J.,** Cells capable of colony formation in the peripheral blood of man, *Science,* 171, 293, 1971.
188. **Knudtzon, S.,** In vitro growth of granulocytic colonies from circulating cells in human cord blood, *Blood,* 43, 357, 1974.
189. **Maurer, H. R. and Henry, R.,** Automated scanning of bone marrow cell colonies growing in agar-containing glass capillaries, *Exp. Cell Res.,* 103, 271, 1976.
190. **Maurer, H. R. and Henry, R.,** Colony growth of mouse bone marrow cells in agar contained in glass capillaries, *Blut,* 33, 11, 1976.
191. **Maurer, H. R. and Henry, R.,** Growth kinetics by scanning of granulocytic cell colonies in glass capillaries, *Blut,* 34, 89, 1977.
192. **Maurer, H. R., Neumeier, R., and Bombik, B. M.,** A micromethod to culture granulocytic colonies from human bone marrow in agar-containing glass capillaries, *Exp. Hematol.,* 1981, in press.
193. **Moore, M. A. S., Spitzer, G., Williams, N., Metcalf, D., and Buckley, J.,** Agar culture studies in 127 cases of untreated acute leukemia: the prognostic value of reclassification of leukemia according to *in vitro* growth characteristics, *Blood,* 44, 1, 1974.
194. **Blackett, N. M. and Gordon, M. Y.,** Observations on the distribution of granulocytic progenitor cells (CFU-c) in human bone marrow: the importance of the manner in which the results of *in vitro* cultures are reported, *Br. J. Haematol.,* 40, 355, 1978.
195. **Parmentier, C., Maraninchi, D., Morardet, N., and Droz, J. P.,** Observations on the distribution of granulocytic progenitor cells (CFU-c) in human bone marrow: the importance of the manner in which the results of *in vitro* cultures are reported, *Br. J. Haematol.,* 40, 353, 1978.
196. **Coiffier, B., Sicard, B., Bryon, P. A., and Germain, D.,** Observations on human bone marrow granulocytic progenitor cell culture: a comparison of two ways to express results, *Br. J. Haematol.,* 44, 335, 1980.
197. **Blackett, N. M. and Gordon, M. Y.,** Correspondence, *Br. J. Haematol.,* 40, 355, 1978.
198. **Bradley, T. R., Hodgson, G. S., and Rosendaal, M.,** The effect of oxygen tension on haemopoietic and fibroblast cell proliferation *in vitro, J. Cell Physiol.,* 97, 517, 1978.
199. **Guilbert, L. J. and Iscove, N. N.,** Partial replacement of serum by selenite, transferrin, albumin, and lecithin in haemopoietic cell cultures, *Nature,* 263, 594, 1976.
200. **Singer, J. W., Fialkow, P. J., Dow, L. W., Ernst, C., and Steinmann, L.,** Unicellular or multicellular origin of human granulocyte-macrophage colonies *in vitro, Blood,* 54, 1395, 1979.
201. **Dao, C., Metcalf, D., Zittoun, R., and Bilski-pasquier, G.,** Normal human bone marrow cultures *in vitro:* cellular composition and maturation of the granulocytic colonies, *Br. J. Haematol.,* 37, 127, 1977.
202. **Baccarani, M., Ricci, P., Santucci, M. A., and Tura, S.,** Growth patterns, cell composition and mitotic activity of granulocytic aggregates developing in methyl cellulose from normal marrow cells, *Exp. Hematol.,* 7, 297, 1979.
203. **Testa, N. G. and Lord, B. I.,** Kinetics of growth of haemopoietic colony cells in agar, *Cell Tissue Kinet.,* 6, 425, 1973.
204. **Rabellino, E. and Metcalf, D.,** Receptors for C3 and IgG on macrophage, neutrophil and eosinophil colony cells grown *in vitro, J. Immunol.,* 115, 688, 1975.
205. **Chervenick, P. A.,** Spleen colonies produced by cells obtained from colonies grown *in vitro, Proc. Soc. Exp. Biol. Med.,* 138, 967, 1971.
206. **Claesson, M. H. and Olsson, L.,** Autoreactive natural killer-like cells from agar-cloned murine bone marrow cells, *Nature,* 283, 578, 1980.

207. **Kreutzmann, H. and Fliedner, T. M.,** Studies on the presence and possible oscillations of granulocytic progenitor cells (CFU-c) in human blood, *Scand. J. Haematol.,* 23, 360, 1979.
208. **Barrett, A. J., Faille, A., and Ketels, F.,** Variations in granulocyte colony forming cell numbers in adult blood, *Br. J. Haematol.,* 42, 337, 1979.
209. **Grilli, G., Carbonell, F., and Fliedner, T. M.,** Variations in erythroid and myeloid progenitor cell numbers in normal human peripheral blood, *Br. J. Haematol.,* 44, 679, 1980.
210. **Ross, D. D., Pollak, A., Akman, S. A., and Bachur, N. R.,** Diurnal variation of circulating human myeloid progenitor cells, *Exp. Hematol.,* 8, 954, 1980.
211. **Verma, D. S., Fisher, R., Spitzer, G., Zander, A. R., McCredie, K. B., and Dicke, K. A.,** Diurnal changes in circulating myeloid progenitor cells in man, *Am. J. Hematol.,* 9, 185, 1980.
212. **Koeffler, H. P., Gale, R. P., and Golde, D. W.,** Myeloid colony-forming cell kinetics in man, *Exp. Hematol.,* 8, 271, 1980.
213. **Senn, J. S. and McCulloch, E. A.,** Radiation sensitivity of human bone marrow cells measured by a cell culture method, *Blood,* 35, 56, 1970.
214. **Broxmeyer, H. E., Galbraith, P. R., and Baker, F. L.,** Relationships of colony-stimulating activity to apparent kill of human colony-forming cells by irradiation and hydroxyurea, *Blood,* 47, 403, 1976.
215. **Iscove, N. N., Till, J. E., and McCulloch, E. A.,** The proliferative states of mouse granulopoietic progenitor cells, *Proc. Soc. Exp. Biol. Med.,* 134, 33, 1970.
216. **Metcalf, D.,** Effect of thymidine suiciding on colony formation *in vitro* by mouse hematopoietic cells, *Proc. Soc. Exp. Biol. Med.,* 139, 511, 1972.
217. **Dresch, C., Faille, A., Poirier, O., Balitrand, N., and Najean, Y.,** Hydroxyurea suicide study of the kinetic heterogeneity of colony forming cells in human bone marrow, *Exp. Hematol.,* 7, 337, 1979.
218. **Richard, K. A., Brown, R. D., and Kronenberg, H.,** Studies on the proliferative capacity of the *in vitro* colony forming cell in normal human bone marrow, *Aust. N.Z.J. Med.,* 3, 361, 1973.
219. **Gerhartz, H. H. and Fliedner, T. M.,** Velocity sedimentation and cell cycle characteristics of granulopoietic progenitor cells (CFUc) in canine blood and bone marrow: influence of mobilization and CFUc depletion, *Exp. Hematol.,* 8, 209, 1980.
220. **Williams, N. and Moore, M.,** Sedimentation velocity characterisation of the cell cycle of granulocytic progenitor cells in monkey hemopoietic tissue, *J. Cell. Physiol.,* 82, 81, 1973.
221. **Liu, Y. K., Stallard, S. S., Koo, V., and Dannaher, C. L.,** The proliferative states of circulating granulopoietic stem cells in man, *Scand. J. Haematol.,* 22, 258, 1979.
222. **Moore, M. A. S. and Williams, N.,** Analysis of proliferation and differentiation of foetal granulocyte-macrophage progenitor cells in haemopoietic tissue, *Cell Tissue Kinet.,* 6, 461, 1973.
223. **Byrne, P. V., Heit, W., and Kubanek, B.,** The proliferative states of density subpopulations of granulocyte-macrophage progenitor cells, *Exp. Hematol.,* 7, 105, 1979.
224. **Quesenbery, P. J. and Stanley, K. A.,** Statistical analysis of murine stem cell suicide techniques, *Blood,* 56, 1000, 1980.
225. **Standen, G., Philip, M. A., and Fletcher, J.,** The proliferative state of granulocytic progenitor cells in human blood and marrow, *Cell Tissue Kinet.,* 13, 105, 1980.
226. **Dresch, C., Johnson, G. R., and Metcalf, D.,** Eosinophil colony formation in semi-solid cultures of human bone marrow cells, *Blood,* 49, 835, 1977.
227. **Dao, C., Metcalf, D., and Bilski-Pasquier, G.,** Eosinophil and neutrophil colony-forming cells in culture, *Blood,* 50, 833, 1977.
228. **Metcalf, D., Parker, J., Chester, H. M., and Kincade, P. W.,** Formation of eosinophilic-like granulocytic colonies by mouse bone marrow cells in vitro, *J. Cell. Physiol.,* 84, 275, 1974.
229. **Johnson, G. R. and Metcalf, D.,** Detection of a new type of mouse eosinophil colony by luxol-fast-blue staining, *Exp. Hematol.,* 8, 549, 1980.
230. **McCarthy, J. H., Mandel, T. E., Garson, O. M., and Metcalf, D.,** The presence of mast cells in agar cultures, *Exp. Hematol.,* 8, 562, 1980.
231. **Tertian, G., Yung, Y-P., Guy-Grand, D., and Moore, M. A. S.,** Long term *in vitro* culture of murine mast cells. I. Description of a growth factor culture technique, *J. Immun.,* 127, 788, 1981.
232. **Yung, Y-P., Eger, R., Tertian, G., and Moore, M. A. S.,** Long-term *in vitro* culture of murine mast cells. II. Purification of a mast cell growth factor and its dissociation from TCGF, *J. Immun.,* 127, 794, 1981.
233. **Hasthorpe, S.,** A hemopoietic cell line dependent upon a factor in pokeweed mitogen-stimulated spleen cell conditioning medium, *J. Cell. Physiol.,* 105, 379, 1980.
234. **Denburg, J. A., Davison, M., and Bienenstock, J.,** Basophil production, *J. Clin. Invest.,* 65, 390, 1980.
235. **Bradley, T. R. and Hodgson, G. S.,** Detection of primitive macrophage progenitor cells in mouse bone marrow, *Blood,* 54, 1446, 1979.

236. **Lin, H-S. and Stewart, C. C.,** Colony formation by mouse peritoneal exudate cells *in vitro, Nature,* 243, 176, 1973.
237. **Lin, H-S. and Stewart, C. C.,** Peritoneal exudate cells. I. Growth requirement of cells capable of forming colonies in soft agar, *J. Cell. Physiol.,* 83, 369, 1974.
238. **Stewart, C. C., Lin, H-S., and Adles, C.,** Proliferation and colony-forming ability of peritoneal exudate cells in liquid culture, *J. Exp. Med.,* 141, 1114, 1975.
239. **Lin, H-S.,** Peritoneal exudate cells. III. Effect of gamma irradiation on mouse peritoneal colony-forming cells, *Radiat. Res.,* 63, 560, 1975.
240. **Lin, H-S. and Freeman, P. G.,** Peritoneal exudate cells. IV. Characterization of colony forming cells, *J. Cell. Physiol.,* 90, 407, 1977.
241. **Reppun, T. S., Lin, H.-S., and Kuhn, C.,** III. Isokinetic separation and characterization of mouse pulmonary alveolar colony forming cells, *J. Ret. Soc.,* 25, 379, 1979.
242. **Moore, M. A. S., Williams, N., and Metcalf, D.,** *In vitro* colony formation by normal and leukemic human hematopoietic cells: characterization of the colony-forming cells, *J. Natl. Cancer. Inst.,* 50, 603, 1973.
243. **Zucker-Franklin, D., Grusky, G., and L'Esperance, P.,** Granulocyte colonies derived from lymphocyte fractions of normal human peripheral blood, *Proc. Natl. Acad. Sci. U.S.A.,* 71, 2711, 1974.
244. **Messner, H. A., Till, J. E., and McCulloch, E. A.,** Specificity of interacting populations affecting granulopoiesis in culture, *Blood,* 44, 671, 1974.
245. **Johnson, G. R., Dresch, C., and Metcalf, D.,** Heterogeneity in human neutrophil, macrophage, and eosinophil progenitor cells demonstrated by velocity sedimentation separation, *Blood,* 50, 823, 1977.
246. **Inoue, S. and Ottenbreit, M. J.,** Heterogeneity of human colony-forming cells, *Blood,* 51, 195, 1978.
247. **Miller, A. M., Gross, M. A., and Yunis, A. A.,** Heterogeneity of human colony-forming cells (CFU-c): differences in size, rate of colony formation and responsiveness to colony-stimulating factor, *J. Lab. Clin. Med.,* 92, 38, 1978.
248. **Jacobsen, N. and Broxmeyer, H. E.,** Oscillations of granulocytic and megakaryocytic progenitor cell populations in cyclic neutropenia in man, *Scand. J. Haematol.,* 23, 33, 1979.
249. **Bol, S., Visser, J., and van den Engh, G.,** The physical separation of three subpopulations of granulocyte/macrophage progenitor cells from mouse bone marrow, *Exp. Hematol.,* 7, 541, 1979.
250. **Bol, S. and Williams, N.,** The maturation state of three types of granulocyte/macrophage progenitor cells from mouse bone marrow, *J. Cell. Physiol.,* 102, 233, 1980.
251. **Cronkite, E. P., Carsten, A. L., Inoue, T., and Bullis, J.,** Colossal granulocytic and erythropoietic colonies and bursts formed by culture of regenerating bone marrow in plasma clot diffusion chambers (PCDC), in *Experimental Hematology Today 1980,* Baum, S. J., Ledney, G. D., and van Bekkum, D. W., Eds., S. Karger, Besel, 1980, 255.
252. **Janoshwitz, H., Moore, M. A. S., and Metcalf, D.,** Density gradient segregation of bone marrow cells with the capacity to form granulocytic and macrophage colonies *in vitro, Exp. Cell. Res.,* 68, 220, 1971.
253. **Haskil, J. S., McNeill, T. A., and Moore, M. A. S.,** Density distribution analyses of *in vivo* and *in vitro* colony forming cells in bone marrow, *J. Cell. Physiol.,* 75, 167, 1970.
254. **Iscove, N. N., Messner, H., Till, J. E., and McCulloch, E. A.,** Human marrow cells forming colonies in culture: analysis by velocity sedimentation and suspension culture, *Ser. Haematol.,* 5, 37, 1972.
255. **Sutherland, D. J. A., Till, J. E., and McCulloch, E. A.,** Short-term cultures of mouse marrow cells separated by velocity sedimentation, *Cell Tissue Kinet.,* 4, 479, 1971.
256. **Williams, N. and van den Engh, G. J.,** Separation of subpopulations of *in vitro* colony forming cells from mouse marrow by equilibrum density centrifugation, *J. Cell. Physiol.,* 86, 237, 1975.
257. **Metcalf, D. and MacDonald, H. R.,** Heterogeneity of *in vitro* colony-forming cells in mouse marrow: segregation by velocity sedimentation, *J. Cell. Physiol.,* 85, 643, 1975.
258. **Williams, N. and Jackson, H.,** Analysis of populations of macrophage-granulocyte progenitor cells stimulated by activities in mouse lung-conditioned medium, *Exp. Hematol.,* 5, 523, 1977.
259. **Byrne, P., Heit, W., and Kubanek, B.,** The *in vitro* differentiation of density sub-populations of colony-forming cells under the influence of different types of colony-stimulating factor, *Cell Tissue Kinet.,* 10, 341, 1977.
260. **Kolitsky, M. A. and Chervenick, P. A.,** Dissimilarity of *in vitro* colony-forming cells and erythrocyte-enhanced colony forming cells from mouse bone marrow, *J. Lab. Clin. Med.,* 89, 829, 1977.
261. **Johnson, G. R. and Metcalf, D.,** Characterization of mouse fetal liver granulocyte-macrophage colony-forming cells using velocity sedimentation, *Exp. Hematol.,* 6, 246, 1978.

262. **Williams, N. and Pluznik, D. H.,** Differences in the buoyant density characteristics of murine granulocyte-macrophage progenitor cells cloned in the presence of serum and/or hemolysate, *Exp. Hematol.,* 6, 383, 1978.

263. **Greenberg, P. L.,** Implications of *in vitro* marrow clonal growth studies for human disorders of granulopoietic regulation, in *Hematopoietic Cell Differentiation,* Golde, D. W., Cline, M. J., Metcalf, D., and Fox, C. F., Eds., Academic Press, New York, 1978, 295.

264. **Williams, N. and Eger, R. R.,** Purification and characterization of clonable murine granulocyte-macrophage precursor cell populations, in *Hematopoietic Cell Differentiation,* Golde, D. W., Cline, M. J., Metcalf, D., and Fox, C. F., Eds., Academic Press, New York, 1978, 385.

265. **Williams, N., Jackson, H., and Meyers, P.,** Isolation of pluripotential hemopoietic stem cells of erythrocytes, granulocytes, macrophages and megakaryocytes from mouse bone marrow, *Exp. Hematol.,* 7, 524, 1979.

266. **Byrne, P. V., Heit, H., and Heit, W.,** Buoyant density analysis of myeloid colony-forming cells in germfree and conventional mice, *Cell Tissue Kinet.,* 12, 635, 1979.

267. **Moore, M. A. S., Williams, N., and Metcalf, D.,** Purification and characterization of the *in vitro* clony forming cell in monkey hemopoietic tissue, *J. Cell Physiol.,* 79, 283, 1972.

268. **Broxmeyer, H. E. and Moore, M. A. S.,** Communication between white cells and the abnormalities of this in leukemia, *Biochem. Biophys. Acta,* 516, 129, 1978.

269. **Richman, C. M., Chess, L., and Yankee, R. A.,** Purification and characterization of granulocytic progenitor cells (CFU-c) from human peripheral blood using immunologic surface markers, *Blood,* 51, 1, 1978.

270. **Oehl, S., Schaefer, U. W., Boecker, W. R., Kalden, J. R., and Peter, H. H.,** Human peripheral blood "null lymphocytes", a highly enriched pool for granulocytic stem cells (CFU-c), *Z. Immunitaettsforsch. Exp. Ther.,* 152, 423, 1977.

271. **Goldberg, J., McGuire, L. A., Dock, N. L., Williams, W. J., and Davey, F. R.,** Purification of human peripheral blood colony forming cells (CFUc), *Exp. Hematol.,* 8, 1086, 1980.

272. **Lovhaug, D., Boyum, A., and Kristiansen, T.,** Culture of hemopoietic cells in diffusion chambers, in *Hemopoietic Cell Differentiation,* Golde, D. W., Cline, M. J., Metcalf, D., and Fox, C. F., Eds., Academic Press, New York, 1978, 175.

273. **Niskanen, E. and Cline, M. J.,** Differentiation of subpopulations of human and murine hemopoietic stem cells by hypotonic lysis, *J. Clin. Invest.,* 65, 285, 1980.

274. **Nicola, N. A., Burgess, A. W., Metcalf, D., and Battye, F. L.,** Separation of mouse bone marrow cells using wheat germ agglutinin affinity chromatography, *Aust. J. Exp. Biol. Med. Sci.,* 56, 663, 1978.

275. **Nicola, N. A., Burgess, A. W., Staber, F. G., Johnson, G. R., Metcalf, D., and Battye, F. L.,** Differential expression of lectin receptors during hemopoietic differentiation: enrichment for granulocyte-macrophage progenitor cells, *J. Cell. Physiol.,* 103, 217, 1980.

276. **Morstyn, G., Nicola, N. A., and Metcalf, D.,** Purification of hemopoietic progenitor cells from human marrow using a fucose-binding lectin and cell sorting, *Blood,* 56, 798, 1980.

277. **Lenz, R. and Pluznik, D. H.,** Membranal gangliosides present on committed hemopoietic stem cells (CFU-c): possible receptors for colony-stimulating factor (CSF), in *Experimental Hematology Today, 1980,* Baum, S. J., Ledney, G. D., and van Bekkum, D. W., Eds., S. Karger, Basel, 1980, 13.

278. **Broxmeyer, H. E.,** Culture characteristics of human granulocyte-macrophage progenitor cells and their regulation in the context of bone marrow transplantation, *Exp. Hematol.,* 7 (Suppl. 5), 149, 1979.

279. **Cline, M. J. and Billing, R.,** Antigens expressed by human B lymphocytes and myeloid stem cells, *J. Exp. Med.,* 146, 1143, 1977.

280. **Moore, M. A. S., Broxmeyer, H. E., Sheridan, A. P. C., Meyers, P. A., Jacobsen, N., and Winchester, R. J.,** Continuous human bone marrow culture: Ia antigen characterization of probable pluripotential stem cells, *Blood,* 55, 682, 1980.

281. **Jacobsen, N., Broxmeyer, H. E., Winchester, R. J., and Moore, M. A. S.,** Expression of DR antigens on early human progenitors of neutrophilic and eosinophilic colonies in diffusion chambers (CFUd), *Scand. J. Haematol.,* 24, 227, 1980.

282. **Koeffler, H. P., Niskanen, E., Cline, M., Billing, R., and Golde, D.,** Human myeloid precursors forming colonies in diffusion chambers express the Ia-like antigen, *Blood,* 54, 1188, 1979.

283. **Janossy, G., Francis, G. E., Capellaro, D., Goldstone, A. H., and Greaves, M. F.,** Cell sorter analysis of leukaemia-associated antigens on human myeloid precursors, *Nature,* 276, 176, 1978.

284. **Fitchen, J. H., Ferrone, S., Quaranta, V., Molinaro., G. A., and Cline, M. J.,** Monoclonal antibodies to HLA-A,B, and Ia-like antigens inhibit colony formation by human myeloid progenitor cells, *J. Immunol.,* 125, 2004, 1980.

285. **Winchester, R. J. and Kunkel, H. G.,** The human Ia system, *Adv. Immunol.,* 28, 221, 1979.
286. **Grumet, F. C., Charron, D. J., Fendly, B. M., Levy, R., and Ness, D. B.,** HLA-DR epitope region definition by use of monoclonal antibody probes, *J. Immunol.,* 125, 2785, 1980.
287. **Koeffler, H. P., Billing, R., Levine, A. M., and Golde, D. W.,** Ia antigen is a differentiation marker on human eosinophils, *Blood,* 56, 11, 1980.
288. **Kincade, P. W., Paige, C. J., Parkhouse, R. M. E., and Lee, G.,** Characterization of murine colony-forming B cells. I. Distribution, resistance to anti-immunoglobulin antibodies, and expression of Ia antigens, *J. Immunol.,* 120, 1289, 1978.
289. **Fitchen, J. H. and Cline, M. J.,** Human myeloid progenitor cells expressing HLA antigens, *Blood,* 53, 794, 1979.
290. **O'Hara, C. J., Shumak, K. H., and Price, G. B.,** The I antigen on human myeloid progenitors, *Clin. Immunol. Immunopathol.,* 10, 420, 1978.
291. **Taetle, R. and Royston, I.,** Human T-cell antigens defined by monoclonal antibodies. Absence of T65 on committed myeloid and erythroid progenitors, *Blood,* 56, 943, 1980.
292. **Kincade, P. W., Flaherty, L., Lee, G., Watanaber, T., and Michaelson, J.,** Qa antigen expression on functional, lymphoid, myeloid and stem cells in adult mice, *J. Immunol.,* 124, 2879, 1980.
293. **Beverly, P. C. L., Linch, D., and Delia, D.,** Isolation of human haemopoietic progenitor cells using monoclonal antibodies, *Nature,* 287, 332, 1980.
294. **Morahan, P. S.,** Macrophage nomenclature. Where are we going?, *J. Ret. Soc.,* 27, 223, 1980.
295. **Nathan, C. F., Murray, H. W., and Cohn, Z. A.,** The macrophage as an effector cell, *N. Engl. J. Med.,* 303, 622, 1980.
296. **Davies, P. and Bonney, R. J.,** Secretary products of mononuclear phagocytes: a brief review, *J. Ret. Soc.,* 26, 37, 1979.
297. **Pelus, L. M., Broxmeyer, H. E., DeSousa, M., and Moore, M. A. S.,** Heterogeneity among resident murine peritoneal macrophages: separation and functional characterization of monocytoid cells producing granulocyte-macrophage colony stimulating factor (GVCSF), and responding to regulation by lactoferrin, *J. Immunol.,* 126, 1016, 1981.
298. **Pelus, L. M. and Moore, M. A. S.,** Use of velocity sedimentation at unit gravity to separate mononuclear phagocytes, in *Methods for Studying Mononuclear Phagocytes,* Adams, D.O., Ed., Academic Press, New York, 1981, 207.
299. **Chervenick, P. A. and Boggs, D. R.,** Bone marrow colonies: stimulation *in vitro* by supernatant from incubated human blood cells, *Sceince,* 169, 691, 1970.
300. **Moore, M. A. S. and Williams, N.,** Physical separation of colony stimulating cells from *in vitro* colony forming cells in hemopoietic tissue, *J. Cell. Physiol.,* 80, 195, 1972.
301. **Chervenick, P. A. and LoBuglio, A. F.,** Human blood monocytes: stimulators of granulocyte and mononuclear colony formation *in vitro, Science,* 178, 164, 1972.
302. **Golde, D. W. and Cline, M. J.,** Identification of the colony-stimulating cell in human peripheral blood, *J. Clin. Invest.,* 51, 2981, 1972.
303. **Golde, D. W., Finley, T. N., and Cline, M. J.,** Production of colony-stimulating factor by human macrophages, *Lancet,* 2, 1397, 1972.
304. **Moore, M. A. S., Williams, N., and Metcalf, D.,** *In vitro* colony formation by normal and leukemic human hematopoietic cells: interaction between colony-forming and colony-stimulating cells, *J. Natl. Cancer Inst.,* 50, 591, 1973.
305. **Moore, M. A. S., Spitzer, G., Metcalf, D., and Penington, D. G.,** Monocyte production of colony stimulating factor in familial cyclic neutropenia, *Br. J. Haematol.,* 27, 47, 1974.
306. **Joyce, R. A. and Chervenick, P. A.,** Stimulation of granulopoiesis by liver macrophages, *J. Lab. Clin. Med.,* 86, 112, 1975.
307. **Shah, R. G., Caporale, L. H., and Moore, M. A. S.,** Characterization of colony-stimulating activity produced by human monocytes and phytohemagglutinin-stimulated lymphocytes, *Blood,* 50, 811, 1977.
308. **Zucker-Franklin, D.,** The percentage of monocytes among "mononuclear" cell functions obtained from normal human blood, *J. Immunol.,* 112, 234, 1974.
309. **Ralph, P., Broxmeyer, H. E., and Nakoinz, I.,** Immunostimulators induce granulocyte/macrophage colony-stimulating activity and block proliferation in a monocyte tumor cell line, *J. Exp. Med.,* 146, 611, 1977.
310. **Ralph, P., Ito, M., Broxmeyer, H. E., and Nakoinz, I.,** Corticosteroids block newly induced but not constitutive functions of macrophage lines: CSA production, latex phagocytosis, antibody-dependent lysis of rbc and tumor targets, *J. Immunol.,* 121, 300, 1978.
311. **Cline, M. J. and Golde, D. W.,** Production of colony-stimulating activity by human lymphocytes, *Nature,* 248, 703, 1974.
312. **Ruscetti, F. W. and Chervenick, P. A.,** Release of colony-stimulating activity from thymus-derived lymphocytes, *J. Clin. Invest.,* 55, 520, 1975.

313. **Ruscetti, F. W., Morgan, D. A., and Gallo, R. C.,** Functional and morphologic characterization of human T cells continuously grown *in vitro, J. Immunol.,* 119, 131, 1977.
314. **Ruscetti, F. W. and Chervenick, P. A.,** Regulation of the release of colony-stimulating activity from mitogen-stimulated lymphocytes, *J. Immunol.,* 114, 1513, 1975.
315. **Ruscetti, F. W., Allalunis, J., and Chervenick, P. A.,** Granulocyte colony stimulating activity from lymphocytes: separation from lymphokines by cytochalasin B, *Cell. Immunol.,* 36, 388, 1978.
316. **Ralph, P., Broxmeyer, H. E., Moore, M. A. S., and Nakoinz, I.,** Induction of myeloid colony stimulating activity (CSA) in murine monocyte tumor cell lines by macrophage activators, and in a T-cell line by Con A, *Cancer Res.,* 38, 1414, 1978.
317. **Golde, D., Quan, S. G., and Cline, M. J.,** Human T lymphocyte cell line producing colony-stimulating activity, *Blood,* 52, 1068, 1978.
318. **Mier, J. W. and Gallo, R. C.,** Purification and some characteristics of human T-cell growth factor from phytohemagglutinin-stimulated lymphocyte-conditioned medium, *Proc. Natl. Acad. Sci. U.S.A.,* 77, 6134, 1980.
319. **Wu, A. M.,** Properties and separation of T lymphocyte growth stimulatory activity (TL-GSA) produced separately from two human T lymphocyte subpopulations, *J. Cell. Physiol.,* 101, 237, 1979.
320. **Metcalf, D.,** Production of colony stimulating factors by lymphoid tissues, in *Biology of The Lymphokines,* Cohen, S, Pick, E., and Oppenheim, J. J., Eds., Academic Press, New York, 1979, 515.
321. **Ross, G. D.,** Identification of human lymphocyte subpopulations by surface marker analysis, *Blood,* 53, 799, 1979.
322. **Vogler, L. B., Grossi, C. E., and Cooper, M. D.,** Human lymphocyte subpopulations, *Prog. Hematol.,* 11, 1, 1979.
323. **Reinherz, E. L. and Schlossman, S. F.,** The differentiation and function of human T lymphocytes, *Cell,* 19, 821, 1980.
324. **Reinherz, E. L. and Schlossman, S. F.,** Regulation of the immune response-inducer and suppressor T-lymphocyte subsets in human beings, *N. Engl. J. Med.,* 303, 370, 1980.
325. **Hoffman, R. A., Kung, P. C., Hansen, W. P., and Goldstein, G.,** Simple and rapid measurement of human T lymphocytes and their subclasses in peripheral blood, *Proc. Natl. Acad. Sci., U.S.A.,* 77, 4914, 1980.
326. **Howard, M., Burgess, A., McPhee, D., and Metcalf, D.,** T-Cell hybridoma secreting hemopoietic regulatory molecules: granulocyte-macrophage and eosinophil colony-stimulating factors, *Cell,* 18, 993, 1979.
327. **Schrader, J. W., Arnold, B., and Clark-Lewis, I.,** A Con A-stimulated T-cell hybridoma releases factors affecting haematopoietic colony-forming cells and B-cell antibody responses, *Nature,* 283, 197, 1980.
328. **Parker, J. W. and Metcalf, D.,** Production of colony-stimulating factor in mixed leucocyte cultures, *Immunology,* 26, 1039, 1974.
329. **Hellmann, A., Th'ng, K. H., and Goldman, J. M.,** Production of colony stimulating activity in mixed mononuclear cell culture, *Br. J. Haematol.,* 45, 245, 1980.
330. **Unanue, E. R.,** Cooperation between mononuclear phagocytes and lymphocytes in immunity, *N. Engl. J. Med.,* 303, 977, 1980.
331. **Verma, D. S., Spitzer, E., Zander, A. R., Fisher, R., McCredie, K. B., and Dicke, K. A.,** T lymphocyte and monocyte-macrophate interaction in colony stimulating activity elaboration in man, *Blood,* 54, 1376, 1979.
332. **Verma, D. S., Spitzer, G., Zander, A. R., Beran, M., Dicke, K. A., and McCredie, K. B.,** The kinetics of colony-stimulating activity elaboration from human bone marrow cells by immunoadjuvants: interactions between light density adherent and nonadherent cells in vitro, *Leuk. Res.,* 4, 371, 1980.
333. **Apte, R. N., Hertogs, C. F., and Pluznik, D. H.,** Generation of colony stimulating factors by purified macrophages and lymphocytes, *J. Ret. Soc.,* 26, 491, 1979.
334. **Schreier, M. H. and Iscove, N. N.,** Haematopoietic growth factors are released in cultures of H-2-restricted helper T cells, accessory cells and specific antigen, *Nature,* 287, 226, 1980.
335. **Knudtzon, S. and Mortensen, B. T.,** Growth stimulation of human bone marrow cells in agar culture by vascular cells, *Blood,* 46, 937, 1975.
336. **Quesenbery, P. J. and Gimbrone, M. A., Jr.,** Vascular endothelium as a regulator of granulopoiesis: production of colony-stimulating activity by cultured human endothelial cells, *Blood,* 56, 1060, 1980.
337. **Broxmeyer, H. E., Smithyman, A., Eger, R. R., Meyers, P. A., and DeSousa, M.,** Identification of lactoferrin as the granulocyte-derived inhibitor of colony stimulating activity (CSA)-production, *J. Exp. Med.,* 148, 1052, 1978.

338. **DiPersio, J. F., Brennan, J. K., Lichtman, M. A. and Speiser, B. L.,** Human cell lines that elaborate colony-stimulating activity for the marrow cells of man and other species, *Blood,* 51, 507, 1978.
339. **Burgess, A. W., Wilson, E. M. A., and Metcalf, D.,** Stimulation by human placental conditioned medium of hemopoietic colony formation by human bone marrow cells, *Blood,* 49, 573, 1977.
340. **Fojo, S. S., Wu, M. C., Gross, M. A., and Yunis, A. A.,** The isolation and characterization of a colony-stimulating factor from human lung, *Biochem. Biophys. Acta,* 494, 92, 1977.
341. **Neumeier, R. and Maurer, H. R.,** Bovine lung conditioned medium as a source of both human and murine colony-stimulating factor, *Exp. Hematol.,* 8, 728, 1980.
342. **Zucali, J. R., McDonald, T. P., Gruber, D. F., and Mirand, E. A.,** Erythropoietin, thrombopoietin and colony stimulating factor in fetal mouse liver culture media, *Exp. Hematol.,* 5, 385, 1977.
343. **Johnson, G. R. and Metcalf, D.,** Sources and nature of granulocyte-macrophage colony stimulating factor in fetal mice, *Exp. Hematol.,* 6, 327, 1978.
344. **Ralph, P.,** Functions of macrophage cell lines, in *Mononuclear Phagocytes,* van Furth, R., Ed., Martinus Nijhoff, The Hague, 1980, 439.
345. **Castro-Malaspina, H., Gay, R., Resnick, G., Kapoor, N., Meyers, P., Chiarieri, D., McKenzie, S., Broxmeyer, H. E., and Moore, M. A. S.,** Characterization of human bone marrow fibroblast colony forming cells (CFU-F) and their progeny, *Blood,* 56, 289, 1980.
346. **Castro-Malaspina, H., Rabellino, E. M., Yen, A., Nachman, R. L., and Moore, M. A. S.,** Human megakaryocyte stimulation of proliferation of bone marrow fibroblasts, *Blood,* 57, 781, 1981.
347. **Ruscetti, F. W., Cypress, R. H., and Chervenick, P. A.,** Specific release of neutrophilic- and eosinophilic-stimulating factors from sensitized lymphocytes, *Blood,* 47, 757, 1976.
348. **McGarry, M. P. and Miller, A. M.,** Evidence for the humoral stimulation of eosinophil granulocytopoiesis in *in vivo* diffusion chambers, *Exp. Hematol.,* 2, 372, 1974.
349. **Miller, A. M., Colley, D. G., and McGarry, M. P.,** Spleen cells from Schistoma Mansoni-infected mice produce diffusible stimulator of eosinophilopoieis *in vivo, Nature,* 262, 586, 1976.
350. **Miller, A. M. and McGarry, M. P.,** A diffusible stimulator of eosinophilopoiesis produced by lymphoid cells as demonstrated with diffusion chambers, *Blood,* 48, 293, 1976.
351. **McGarry, M. P., Miller, A. M., and Colley, D. G.,** Eosinophil granulocytopoiesis: a model system, in *Experimental Hematology Today,* Baum, S. J. and Ledney, G. D., Eds., Springer-Verlag, New York, 1977, 63.
352. **Mahmoud, A. A. F., Stone, M. K., and Kellermeyer, R. W.,** Eosinophilopoietin, a circulating low molecular weight peptide-like substance which stimulates the production of eosinophils in mice, *J. Clin. Invest.,* 60, 675, 1977.
353. **Bartelmez, S. H., Dodge, W. H., Mahmoud, A. A. F., and Bass, D. A.,** Stimulation of eosinophil production *in vitro* by eosinophilopoietin and spleen-cell-derived eosinophil growth-stimulating factor, *Blood,* 56, 706, 1980.
354. **Chan, S. H. and Metcalf, D.,** Local production of colony-stimulating factor within the bone marrow: role of nonhematopoietic cells, *Blood,* 40, 646, 1972.
355. **Chan, S. H. and Metcalf, D.,** Local and systemic control of granulocytic and macrophage progenitor cell regeneration after irradiation, *Cell Tissue Kinet.,* 6, 185, 1973.
356. **Galbraith, P. R. and Broxmeyer, H. E.,** Studies on control of granulopoiesis in man. I. Relationship of leukocyte colony-stimulating activity *in vitro* to neutrophil count *in vivo, Can. Med. Assoc. J.,* 111, 141, 1974.
357. **Metcalf, D.,** Acute antigen-induced elevation of serum colony stimulating factor (CSF) levels, *Immunology,* 21, 427, 1971.
358. **Quesenbery, P., Morley, A., Stohlman, F., Jr., Rickard, K., Howard, D., and Smith M.,** Effect of endotoxin on granulopoiesis and colony stimulating factor., *N. Engl. J. Med.,* 286, 227, 1972.
359. **Metcalf, D. and Stevens, S.,** Influence of age and antigenic stimulation on granulocyte and macrophage progenitor cells in the mouse spleen, *Cell Tissue Kinet.,* 5, 433, 1972.
360. **NcNeill, T. A.,** Release of bone marrow colony stimulating activity during immunological reactions *in vitro, Nature,* 244, 175, 1973.
361. **Quesenberry, P. J., Morley, A., Ryan, M., Howard, D., and Stohlman, F., Jr.,** The effect of endotoxin on murine stem cells, *J. Cell. Physiol.,* 82, 239, 1973.
362. **Quesenbery, P. J., Morley, A., Miller, M., Rickard, K., Howard, D., and Stohlman, F., Jr.,** Effect of endotoxin on granulopoiesis and the *in vitro* colony-forming cell, *Blood,* 41, 391, 1973.
363. **Eaves, A. C. and Bruce, W. R.,** *In vitro* production of colony-stimulating activity. I. Exposure of mouse peritoneal cells to endotoxin, *Cell Tissue Kinet.,* 7, 19, 1974.
364. **Cline, M. J., Rothman, B., and Golde, D. W.,** Effect of endotoxin on the production of colony-stimulating factor by human monocytes and macrophages, *J. Cell. Physiol.,* 84, 193, 1974.
365. **Ruscetti, F. W. and Chervenick, P. A.,** Release of colony-stimulating factor from monocytes by endotoxin and polyinosinic-polycytidylic acid, *J. Lab. Clin. Med.,* 83, 64, 1974.

366. **Bolin, R. W. and Robinson, W. A.,** Bacterial, serum and cellular modulation of granulopoietic activity, *J. Cell. Physiol.*, 92, 145, 1977.
367. **Cline, M. J. and Golde, D. W.,** Mobilization of hematopoietic stem cells (CFU-c) into the peripheral blood of man by endotoxin, *Exp. Hematol.*, 5, 186, 1977.
368. **MacVittie, T. J. and Walker, R. I.,** Endotoxin-induced alterations in canine granulopoiesis: colony-stimulating factor, colony forming cells in culture, and growth of cells in diffusion chambers, *Exp. Hematol.*, 6, 613, 1978.
369. **Staber, F. G. and Metcalf, D.,** Cellular and molecular basis of the increased splenic hemopoiesis in mice treated with bacterial cell wall components, *Proc. Natl. Acad. Sci. U.S.A.*, 77, 4322, 1980.
370. **Golde, D. W. and Cline, M. J.,** Endotoxin-induced release of colony-stimulating activity in man, *Proc. Soc. Exp. Biol. Med.*, 149, 845, 1975.
371. **Hinterberger, W., Paukovits, W. R., and Mittermayer, K.,** Endotoxin-induced colony stimulating activity in normal and myeloid leukaemic subjects, *Scand. J. Haematol.*, 22, 280, 1979.
372. **Morrison, D. C. and Ryan, J. L.,** Bacterial endotoxins and host immune responses, *Adv. Immunol.*, 28, 293, 1979.
373. **Apte, R. N., Galanos, C., and Pluznik, D. H.,** Lipid A, the active part of bacterial endotoxins in inducing serum colony stimulating activity and proliferation of splenic granulocyte macrophage progenitor cells, *J. Cell. Physiol.*, 87, 71, 1975.
374. **Apte, R. N., Hertogs, C. F., and Pluznik, D. H.,** Regulation of lipopolysaccharide-induced granulopoieis and macrophage formation by spleen cells. I. Relationship between colony-stimulating factor release and lymphocyte activation in vitro, *J. Immunol.*, 118, 1435, 1977.
375. **Chang, H., Thompson, J. J., and Nowotny, A.,** Release of colony stimulatory factor (CSF) by non-endotoxic breakdown products of bacterial lipopolysaccharides, *Immunol. Commun.*, 3, 401, 1974.
376. **Butler, R. C., Abdelnoor, A. M., and Nowotny, A.,** Bone marrow colony-stimulating factor and tumor resistance-enhancing activity of postendotoxin mouse sera, *Proc. Natl. Acad. Sci. U.S.A.*, 75, 2896, 1978.
377. **Staber, F. G., Tarcsay, L., and Dukor, P.,** Modulation of myelopoiesis *in vivo* by chemically pure preparations of cell wall components from gram-negative bacteria: effects at different stages, *Infect. Immun.*, 20, 40, 1978.
378. **Staber, F. G., Gisler, R. H., Schuman, G., Tarcsay, L., Schlafli, E., and Dukor, P.,** Modulation of myelopoiesis by different bacterial cell-wall components: induction of colony-stimulating activity (by pure preparations, low molecular weight degradation products and a synthetic low molecular analog of bacterial cell-wall components) *in vitro, Cell Immunol.*, 37, 174, 1978.
379. **Staber, F. G.,** Comparative effects in mice of purified bacterial cell-wall components on granulocyte-macrophage progenitor cells and their regulators, *J. Immunol.*, 122, 1726, 1979.
380. **Staber, F. G. and Burgess, A. W.,** Serum of lipopolysaccharide-treated mice contains two types of colony-stimulating factor, separable by affinity chromatography, *J. Cell. Physiol.*, 102, 1, 1980.
381. **Apte, R. N. and Pluznik, D. H.,** Genetic control of lipopolysaccharide induced generation of serum colony stimulating factor and proliferation of splenic granulocyte/macrophage precursor cells, *J. Cell. Physiol.*, 89, 313, 1976.
382. **Apte, R. N. and Pluznik, D. H.,** Control of mechanisms of endotoxin and particulate material stimulation of hemopoietic colony forming cell differentiation, *Exp. Hematol.*, 4, 10, 1976.
383. **Russo, M. and Lutton, J. D.,** Decreased *in vitro* colony stimulating activity responses to bacterial lipopolysaccharide in C3H/HeJ mice, *J. Cell. Physiol.*, 92, 303, 1977.
384. **Metcalf, D. and Wilson, J. W.,** Endotoxin-induced size change in bone marrow progenitors of granulocytes and macrophages, *J. Cell. Physiol.*, 89, 381, 1976.
385. **Byrne, P. V., Heit, W., Heit, H., and Kubanek, B.,** Endotoxin-induced changes in the interrelationship of density subpopulations of granulocyte-macrophage progenitor cells, *J. Lab. Clin. Med.*, 96, 903, 1980.
386. **Ogmundsdottir, H. M., Weir, D. M., and Marmion, B. P.,** Binding of microorganisms to the macrophage plasma membrane; effects of enzymes and periodate, *Br. J. Exp. Pathol.*, 59, 1, 1978.
387. **Freimer, N. B., Ogmundsdottir, H. M., Blackwell, C. C., Sutherland, I. W., Graham, L., and Weir, D. M.,** The role of cell wall carbohydrates in binding of microorganisms to mouse peritoneal exudate macrophages, *Acta Pathol. Microbiol. Scand.*, 86, 53, 1978.
388. **Weir, D. M., Stewart, J., Glass, E. J., Oliver, A., Blackwell, C. C., and Doyle, J.,** Macrophage lectin receptors and bacterial recognition, in *Heterogeneity of Mononuclear Phagocytes*, Landy, M. and Forester, O., Eds., Academic Press, New York, 1981.
389. **Hinterberger, W., Mittermayer, K., Paukovits, W., and Singer, J.,** Different types of endotoxin-induced release of colony stimulating factors by adherent leukocytes in the presence of fresh and heat-inactivated autologous serum, *Scand. J. Haematol.*, 25, 221, 1980.

390. **Shadduck, R. K., Waheed, A., Porcellini, A., Rizzoli, V., and Levin, J.,** A method for removal of endotoxin from purified colony-stimulating factor, *Proc. Soc. Exp. Biol. Med.*, 164, 40, 1980.
391. **Metcalf, D.,** Depressed responses of the granulocyte-macrophage system to bacterial antigens following preimmunization, *Immunology*, 26, 1115, 1974.
392. **Quesenbery, P., Halperin, J., Ryan, M., and Stohlman, F., Jr.,** Tolerance to the granulocyte-releasing and colony stimulating factor elevating effects of endotoxin, *Blood*, 45, 789, 1975.
393. **Quesenbery, P., Cohen, H., Levin, J., Sullivan, R., Bealmear, P., and Ryan, M.,** Effects of bacterial infection and irradiation on serum colony-stimulating factor levels in tolerant and nontolerant CF, mice, *Blood*, 51, 229, 1978.
394. **Hartmann, D. W., Entringer, M. A., Vasil, M. L., and Robinson, W. A.,** Relationship between colony stimulating factor (CSF) and colony forming unit in culture (CFU-c) in nonimmunized and immunized C57/B1 mice infected with *Escherichia coli*, *Exp. Hematol.*, 8, 1222, 1980.
395. **Staber, F. G.,** Diminished response of granulocyte-macrophage colony stimulating factor (GM-CSF) in mice after sensitisation with bacterial cell-wall components, *Exp. Hematol.*, 8, 120, 1980.
396. **Burgaleta, C. and Golde, D. W.,** Effect of glucan on granulopoiesis and macrophage genesis in mice, *Cancer Res.*, 38, 1739, 1977.
397. **Foster, R. S., MacPherson, B. R., and Browdie, D. A.,** Effect of Cornynebacterium parvum on colony-stimulating factor and granulocyte-macrophage colony formation, *Cancer Res.*, 38, 1349, 1977.
398. **Singer, J. W. and Bernstein, I. D.,** Granulopoietic increase by BCG in mice, *Exp. Hematol.*, 6, 760, 1978.
399. **Harker, W. G., Rothstein, G., Clarkson, D., Athens, J. W., and MacFarlane, J. L.,** Enhancement of colony-stimulating activity production by lithium, *Blood*, 49, 263, 1977.
400. **Spitzer, G., Verma, D. S., Barlogie, B., Beran, M. A., and Dicke, K. A.,** Possible mechanisms of action of *in vitro* spontaneous myeloid colony formation, *Cancer Res.*, 39, 3215, 1979.
401. **Rossof, A. H. and Fehir, K. M.,** Lithium carbonate increases marrow granulocyte-committed colony forming units and periphral blood granulocytes in a canine model, *Exp. Hematol.*, 7, 255, 1979.
402. **Svet-Moldavskaya, I. A., Zinzar, S. N., Svet-Moldarsky, G. J., Mann, P. E., Bekesi, J. G., Holland, J. F., Clarkson, B. D., Arlin, Z., and Koziner, B.,** Macrophage-like cell transformation and CFU (C) flucuations in normal and leukemic human marrow cultures treated by phorbol diester, *Biomedicine*, 31, 252, 1979.
403. **Stuart, R. K. and Hamilton, J. A.,** Tumor-promoting phorbol esters stimulate hematopoietic colony formation *in vitro*, *Science*, 208, 402, 1980.
404. **Fibach, E., Marks, P. A., and Rifkind, R. A.,** Tumor promoters enhance myeloid and erythoid colony formation by normal mouse hemopoietic cells, *Proc. Natl. Acad. Sci. U.S.A.*, 77, 4152, 1980.
405. **Greenberger, J. S., Newburger, P. E., and Sakakeeny, M.,** Phorbol myristate acetate stimulates macrophage differentiation and replication and alters granulopoiesis and leukemogenesis in long-term bone marrow cultures, *Blood*, 56, 368, 1980.
406. **Broxmeyer, H. E., deSousa, M., Smithyman, A., Ralph, P., Hamilton, J., Kurland, J. I., and Bognacki, J.,** Specificity and modulation of the action of lactoferrin, a negative feedback regulator of myelopoiesis, *Blood*, 55, 324, 1980.
407. **Levitt, L. J. and Quesenbery, P. J.,** The effect of lithium on murine hematopoiesis in a liquid culture system, *N. Engl. J. Med.*, 302, 713, 1980.
408. **Gallicchio, V. S. and Chen, M. G.,** Modulation of murine pluripotential stem cell proliferation *in vivo* by lithium carbonate, *Blood*, 56, 1150, 1980.
409. **Metcalf, D., Johnson, G. R., and Burgess, A. W.,** Direct stimulation by purified GM-CSF of the proliferation of multipotential and erythroid precursor cells, *Blood*, 55, 138, 1980.
410. **Price, G. B., McCulloch, E. A., and Till, J. E.,** Cell membranes as sources of granulocyte colony stimulating activities, *Exp. Hematol.*, 3, 227, 1975.
411. **DiPersio, J. F., Brennan, J. K., Lichtman, M. A., Abboud, C. N., and Kirkpatrick, F. H.,** The fractionation, characterization, and subcellular localization of colony stimulating activities released by the human monocyte-like cell line, GCT, *Blood*, 56, 717, 1980.
412. **Burgess, A. W. and Metcalf, D.,** The nature and action of granulocyte-macrophage colony stimulating factors, *Blood*, 56, 947, 1980.
413. **Stanley, E. R.,** Colony stimulating factors, in *Molecular Mediators of Cellular Immunity: Characterization and Actions*, Hadden, J. W. and Stewart, W. E., II, Eds., Humana, New Jersey, 1980, chap. 3.
414. **Stanley, E. R., Cifone, M., Heard, P. M., and deFendi, V.,** Factors regulating macrophage production and growth: identity of colony-stimulating factor and macrophage growth factor, *J. Exp. Med.*, 143, 631, 1976.

415. **Stanley, E. R., Chen, D. M., and Lin, H.-S.,** Induction of macrophage production and proliferation by a purified colony stimulating factor, *Nature*, 274, 168, 1978.
416. **Stanley, E. R.,** Colony-stimulating factor (CSF) radioimmunoassay: detection of a CSF subclass stimulating macrophage production, *Proc. Natl. Acad. Sci. U.S.A.*, 76, 2969, 1979; see also erratum, **Stanley, E. R.,** *Proc. Natl. Acad. Sci. U.S.A.*, 76, 5411, 1979.
417. **Burgess, A. W., Camakaris, J., and Metcalf, D.,** Purification and properties of colony-stimulating factor from mouse lung-conditioned medium, *J. Biol. Chem.*, 242, 1998, 1977.
418. **Price, G. B., McCulloch, E. A., and Till, J. E.,** A new human low molecular weight granulocyte colony stimulating activity, *Blood*, 42, 341, 1973.
419. **Price, G. B., Senn, J. S., McCulloch, E. A., and Till, J. E.,** Heterogeneity of molecules with low molecular weight isolated from media conditioned by human leukocytes and capable of stimulating colony formation by human granulopoietic progenitor cells, *J. Cell. Physiol.*, 84, 385, 1974.
420. **Price, G. B., Senn, J. S., McCulloch, E. A., and Till, J. E.,** The isolation and properties of granulocytic colony-stimulating activities from medium conditioned by human peripheral leucocytes, *Biochem. J.*, 148, 209, 1975.
421. **Wu, M-C. and Yunis, A. A.,** Common pattern of two distinct types of colony stimulating factor in human tissues and cultured cells, *J. Clin. Invest.*, 65, 772, 1980.
422. **Nicola, N. A., Metcalf, D., Johnson, G. R., and Burgess, A. W.,** Preparation of colony stimulating factors from human placental conditioned medium, *Leuk. Res.*, 2, 313, 1978.
423. **Wu, M-C., Cini, J. K., and Yunis, A. A.,** Purification of a colony-stimulating factor from cultured pancreatic carcinoma cells, *J. Biol. Chem.*, 254, 6226, 1979.
424. **Waheed, A. and Shadduck, R. K.,** Purification of L cell-derived colony-stimulating factor, *J. Lab. Clin. Med.*, 94, 180, 1979.
425. **Williams, N., Eger, R. R., Moore, M. A. S., and Mendelsohn, N.,** Differentiation of mouse bone marrow precursor cells into neutrophil granulocytes by an activity separation from WEHI-3 cell conditioned medium, *Differentiation*, 11, 59, 1978.
426. **Horiuchi, M. and Ichikawa, Y.,** Control of macrophage and granulocyte colony formation by two different factors, *Exp. Cell Res.*, 110, 79, 1977.
427. **Nicola, N. A., Metcalf, D., Johnson, G. R., and Burgess, A. W.,** Separation of functionally distinct human granulocyte-macrophage colony-stimulating factors, *Blood*, 54, 614, 1979.
428. **Lind, D. E., Bradley, M. L., Gunz, F. W., and Vincent, P. C.,** The nonequivalence of mouse and human marrow culture in the assay of granulopoietic stimulatory factors, *J. Cell. Physiol.*, 83, 35, 1973.
429. **Nicola, N. A., Burgess, A. W., and Metcalf, D.,** Similar molecular properties of granulocyte-macrophage colony stimulating factors produced by different mouse organs *in vitro* and *in vivo*, *J. Biol. Chem.*, 254, 5290, 1979.
430. **Das, S. K., Stanley, E. R., Guilbert, L. J., and Forman, L. W.,** Discrimination of a colony stimulating factor subclass by a specific receptor on a macrophage cell line, *J. Cell. Physiol.*, 104, 359, 1980.
431. **Shadduck, R. K. and Waheed, A.,** Development of a radioimmuno-assay for colony stimulating factor, *Blood Cells*, 5, 421, 1979.
432. **Price, G. B., McCulloch, E. A., and Till, J. E.,** Cross reactivity of human β_2-microglobulin with human granulocyte colony-stimulating activity, *J. Immunol.*, 117, 416, 1976.
433. **Price, G. B. and Gorczynski, R. M.,** The role of macrophages in stimulation of immune induction and myelopoiesis. I. Comparison of activity of macrophage derived factors in granulopoiesis and immunostimulation, *Immunopharmacology*, 1, 175, 1979.
434. **Gorczynski, R. M. and Price, G. B.,** The role of macrophages in stimulation of immune induction and myelopoiesis. II. Analysis of genetic restriction involved in the stimulation of granulocyte colony precursors on mature lymphocytes using factors prepared from different recombinant inbred strains of mice, *Immunopharmacology*, 1, 187, 1979.
435. **Fitchen, J. H., Ferrone, S., Lusis, A. J., and Cline, M. J.,** Cytotoxicity of anti-β_2-microglobulin xenoantisera to human and murine myeloid progenitor cells and lack of cross-reactivity with colony stimulating activity, *J. Immunol.*, 124, 2906, 1980.
436. **Moore, M. A. S.,** In vitro studies in the myeloid leukaemias, in *Advances in Acute Leukemia*, Cleton, F. J., Crowther, D., and Malpas, J. S., Eds., North-Holland, Amsterdam, 1974, 169.
437. **Metcalf, D.,** Clonal analysis of proliferation and differentiation of paired daughter cells: action of granulocyte-macrophage colony-stimulating factor on granulocyte-macrophage progenitors, *Proc. Natl. Acad. Sci. U.S.A.*, 77, 5327, 1980.
438. **Metcalf, D. and Stanley, E. R.,** Serum half-life in mice of colony stimulating factor prepared from human urine, *Br. J. Haematol.*, 20, 549, 1971.

439. **Burgess, A. W. and Metcalf, D.,** Serum half-life and organ distribution of radiolabeled colony stimulating factor in mice, *Exp. Hematol.*, 5, 456, 1977.
440. **Shadduck, R. K., Waheed, A., Porcellini, A., Rizzoli, V., and Pigoli, G.,** Physiologic distribution of colony-stimulating factor *in vivo, Blood,* 54, 894, 1979.
441. **Guilbert, L. J. and Stanley, E. R.,** Specific interaction of murine colony-stimulating factor with mononuclear phagocytic cells, *J. Cell Biol.*, 85, 153, 1980.
442. **Kurland, J. I., Broxmeyer, H. E., Bockman, R. S., and Moore, M. A. S.,** Role for the monocyte-macrophage colony stimulating factor and prostaglandin E in the positive and negative feedback control of myeloid stem cell proliferation, *Blood,* 52, 388, 1978.
443. **Kurland, J. I., Pelus, L. M., Ralph, P., Bockman, R. S., and Moore, M. A. S.,** Induction of prostaglandin E synthesis in normal and neoplastic macrophages: role for colony-stimulating factor (S) distinct from effects on myeloid progenitor cell proliferation, *Proc. Natl. Acad. Sci. U.S.A.*, 76, 2326, 1979.
444. **Pelus, L. M., Broxmeyer, H. E., Kurland, J. I., and Moore, M. A. S.,** Regulation of macrophage and granulocyte proliferation: specificities of prostaglandin E and lactoferrin, *J. Exp. Med.*, 150, 277, 1979.
445. **Burgess, A. W. and Metcalf, D.,** The effect of colony stimulating factor on the synthesis of ribonucleic acid by mouse bone marrow cells *in vitro, J. Cell. Physiol.*, 90, 471, 1976.
446. **Lin, H-S. and Gordon, S.,** Secretion of plasminogen activator by bone marrow-derived mononuclear phagocytes and its enhancement by colony stimulating factor, *J. Exp. Med.*, 150, 231, 1979.
447. **Hamilton, J. A., Stanley, E. R., Burgess, A. W., and Shadduck, R. K.,** Stimulation of macrophage plasminogen activator activity by colony stimulating factors, *J. Cell. Physiol.*, 103, 435, 1980.
448. **Handman, E. and Burgess, A. W.,** Stimulation by granulocyte-macrophage colony-stimulating factor of *Leishmania tropica* killing by macrophages, *J. Immunol.*, 122, 1134, 1979.
449. **Moore, R. N., Oppenheim, J. J., Farrar, J. J., Carter, C. S., Jr., Waheed, A., and Shadduck, R. K.,** Production of lymphocyte activating factor (Interleukin 1) by macrophages activated with colony-stimulatory factors, *J. Immunol.*, 125, 1302, 1980.
450. **Bradley, T. R., Telfer, P. A., and Fry, P.,** The effect of erythrocytes on mouse bone marrow colony development *in vitro, Blood,* 38, 353, 1971.
451. **van den Engh, G. and Bol. S.,** The presence of a CSF enhancing activity in the serum of endotoxin-treated mice, *Cell Tissue Kinet.*, 8, 579, 1975.
452. **Marbry, J., Carbone, P. P., and Bull, J. M.,** Amplification of colony stimulating activity in human serum by interaction with CSA from other sources, *Exp. Hematol.*, 3, 354, 1975.
453. **Metcalf, D., MacDonald, H. R., and Chester, H. M.,** Serum potentiation of granulocyte and macrophage colony formation in vitro, *Exp. Haematol.*, 3, 261, 1975.
454. **Rothmann, J., Hertogs, C. F., and Pluznik, D. H.,** Replacement of serum by hemolysate as growth promotor for murine leukemic and normal hemopoietic progenitor cells in culture, *Exp. Hematol.*, 5, 117, 1977.
455. **Francis, G. E., Berney, J. J., and Hoffrand, A. V.,** Stimulation of human haemopoietic cells by colony stimulating factors: adherent cell dependent colony stimulating activity in human serum, *Br. J. Haematol.*, 35, 625, 1977.
456. **Furusawa, S., Komatsu, H., Saito, K., Enokihara, H., Hirose, K., and Shishido, H.,** Effect of normal human serum on granulocyte colony formation by human bone marrow cells, *J. Lab. Clin. Med.*, 91, 377, 1978.
457. **Tsuneoka, K., Takagi, Y., Hirashima, K., and Shikita, M.,** Enhancement of the action of colony stimulating factor (CSF) by soluble component (S) of erythrocytes in mouse bone marrow cell cultures, *Exp. Hematol.*, 6, 445, 1978.
458. **Rothmann, J., Hertogs, C. F., and Pluznik, D. H.,** Growth enhancement and serum replacement in cloning of murine mastocytoma and granulocyte/macrophage precursor cells: two distinct activities present in hemolysates, *Exp. Hematol.*, 7, 352, 1979.
459. **Aye, M. T., Sequin, J. A., and McBurney, J. P.,** Erythroid and granulocytic colony growth in cultures supplemented with human serum lipoproteins, *J. Cell. Physiol.*, 99, 233, 1979.
460. **Francis, G. E., Berney, J. J., Murray, V. S. G., Jackson, B., and Hoffbrand, A. V.,** Adherent cell dependent colony stimulating activity in human serum: a granulopoietic regulator, *Scand. J. Haematol.*, 24, 13, 1980.
461. **Boyum, A., Lovhaug, D., Viken, K. E., and Kristiansen, T.,** Medium conditioned for 24 hours by mononuclear human blood cells contains an inducer of granulopoiesis lacking colony stimulating activity, *Scand. J. Haematol.*, 25, 385, 1980.
462. **Baker, F. L. and Galbraith, P. R.,** Nutritional and regulatory roles of human serum in cultures of human granulopoietic cells, *Blood,* 52, 241, 1978.

463. **Francis, G. E.,** A bioassay system for two types of colony stimulating factor in human serum, *Exp. Hematol.*, 8, 749, 1980.
464. **Niho, Y., Till, J. E., and McCulloch, E. A.,** Granulopoietic progenitors in suspension culture: a comparison of stimulatory cells and conditioned media, *Blood,* 45, 811, 1975.
465. **Hoang, T.,** Generation of new CFU-C in liquid culture of human bone marrow cells depends on molecules different from G-CSA, *Exp. Hematol.*, 8 (Suppl. 7), 106, 1980.
466. **Moore, M. A. S., Burgess, A. W., Metcalf, D., McCulloch, E. A., Robinson, W. A., Dicke, K. A., Chervenick, P. A., Bull, J. M., Wu, A. M., Stanley, E. R., Goldman, J., and Testa, N.,** Report of a workshop on standardization of selective cultures for normal and leukaemic cells, *Br. J. Haematol.*, 35, 500, 1975.
467. **Metcalf, D. and Stanley, E. R.,** Haematological effects in mice of partially purified colony stimulating factor (CSF) prepared from human urine, *Br. J. Haematol.*, 21, 481, 1971.
468. **Dale, D. C., Brown, C. H., Carbone, P., and Wolff, S. M.,** Cyclic urinary leukopoietic activity in gray collie dogs, *Science,* 173, 152, 1971.
469. **Mangalik, A. and Robinson, W. A.,** Cyclic neutropenia: the relationship between urine granulocyte colony stimulating activity and neutrophil count, *Blood,* 41, 79, 1973.
470. **Gatti, R. A., Robinson, J. J., Deinard, A. S., Nesbit, M., McCullough, J. J., Ballois, M., and Good, R. A.,** Cyclic leukocytosis in chronic myelogenous leukemia: new perspectives on pathogenesis and therapy, *Blood,* 51, 771, 1973.
471. **Asano, S., Urabe, A., Okabe, T., Sato, N., Kondo, Y., Ueyama, Y., Chiba, S., Ohsawa, N., and Kosaka, K.,** Demonstration of a granulopoietic factor (s) in the plasma of nude mice transplanted with human lung cancer and in the tumor tissue, *Blood,* 49, 845, 1977.
472. **Suda, T., Miura, Y., Mizoguchi, H., Kubota, K., and Takaku, F.,** A case of lung cancer associated with granulocytosis and production of colony-stimulating activity by the tumour, *Br. J. Cancer,* 41, 980, 1980.
473. **Shadduck, R. K. and Metcalf, D.,** Preparation and neutralization characteristics of an anti-CSF antibody, *J. Cell. Physiol.*, 86, 247, 1975.
474. **Shadduck, R. W., Waheed, A., Pigoli, G., Boegel, F., and Higgens, L.,** Fractionation of antibodies to L-cell colony stimulating factor by affinity chromatography, *Blood,* 53, 1182, 1979.
475. **Shadduck, R. K., Carsten, A. L., Chikkappa, G., Cronkite, E., and Gerard, E.,** Inhibition of diffusion chamber (DC) granulopoiesis by anti-CSF serum, *Proc. Soc. Exp. Bio. Med.*, 158, 542, 1978.
476. **Broxmeyer, H. E.,** Inhibition *in vivo* of mouse granulopoiesis by cell-free activity derived from human polymorphonuclear neutrophils, *Blood,* 41, 889, 1978.
477. **Broxmeyer, H. E., Moore, M. A. S., and Ralph, P.,** Cell-free granulocyte colony inhibiting activity derived from human polymorphonuclear neutrophils, *Exp. Hematol.*, 5, 87, 1976.
478. **Broxmeyer, H. E., Mendelsohn, N., and Moore, M. A. S.,** Abnormal granulocyte feedback regulation of colony forming and stimulating activity-producing cells from patients with chronic myelogenous leukemia, *Leuk. Res.*, 1, 3, 1977.
479. **Broxmeyer, H. E. and Ralph, P.,** *In vitro* regulation of a mouse myelomonocytic leukemia cell line adapted to culture, *Cancer Res.*, 37, 3578, 1977.
480. **Mendelsohn, N., Eger, R. R., Broxmeyer, H. E., and Moore, M. A. S.,** Isolation of a granulocyte colony inhibitory factor derived from human polymorphonuclear neutrophils, *Biochim. Biophys. Acta,* 533, 238, 1978.
481. **Broxmeyer, H. E., Baker, F., and Galbraith, P. R.,** *In vitro* regulation of granulopoiesis in human leukemia: application of an assay for colony inhibiting cells, *Blood,* 47, 389, 1976.
482. **Baker, F., Broxmeyer, H. E., and Galbraith, P. R.,** Control of granulopoiesis in man. III. Inhibition of colony stimulating activity (CSF) by dense leukocytes, *J. Cell. Physiol.*, 86, 337, 1975.
483. **Haskill, J. S., McKnight, R. D., and Galbraith, P. R.,** Cell-cell interaction in vitro: studied by density separation of colony-forming, stimulating and inhibiting cells from human bone marrow, *Blood,* 40, 394, 1972.
484. **BezKorovainy, A. and Zschocke, R. H.,** Structure and function for transferrins. I. Physical, chemical and iron-binding properties, *Arzneim. Forsch.*, 24, 476, 1974.
485. **Ainscough, E. W., Brodie, A. M., Plowman, J. E., Bloor, S. J., Loehr, J., and Loehr, T. M.,** Studies on human lactoferrin by electron paramagnetic resonance, fluorescence, and resonance ramon spectroscopy, *Biochemistry,* 19, 4072, 1980.
486. **Aisen, P. and Leibman, A.,** Lactoferrin and transferrin: a comparative study, *Biochim. Biophys. Acta,* 257, 314, 1972.
487. **Mahmood, T., Robinson, W. A., Kurnick, J. E., and Vautrin, R.,** Granulopoietic and erythropoietic activity in patients with anemias of iron deficiency and chronic disease, *Blood,* 50, 449, 1977.

488. **Pelus, L. M., Broxmeyer, H. E., and Moore, M. A. S.,** Regulation of human myelopoiesis by prostaglandin E and lactoferrin, *Cell Tissue Kinet.*, 14, 515, 1981.
489. **Broxmeyer, H. E., Pelus, L. M., Ralph, P., Bognacki, J., Moore, M. A. S., and deSousa, M.,** Regulation of myelopoiesis: inhibitors of production and action of granulocyte and macrophage colony-stimulatory factors, in *Microbiology 1980*, American Society of Microbiology, Washington, D.C., 1980, 108.
490. **Robinson, W. A., Entringer, M. A., Bolin, R. W., and Stonington, O. G.,** Bacterial stimulation and granulocyte inhibition of granuloietic factor production, *N. Engl. J. Med.*, 297, 1129, 1977.
491. **Bullen, J. J. and Armstrong, J. A.,** The role of lactoferrin in the bactericidal function of polymorphonuclear leukocytes, *Immunology*, 36, 781, 1979.
492. **Van Snick, J. L., Masson, P. L., and Heremans, J. F.,** The involvement of lactoferrin in the hyposideremia of acute inflammation, *J. Exp. Med.*, 140, 1068, 1974.
493. **Leffell, M. S. and Spitznagel, J. K.,** Fate of human lactoferrin and myeloperoxidase in phagocytizing human neutrophils: effects of immunoglobulin G subclasses and immune complexes coated on latex beads, *Infect. Immun.*, 12, 813, 1975.
494. **Klempner, M. S., Dinarello, C. A., and Gallin, J. I.,** Human leukocyte pyrogen induces release of specific granule contents from human neutrophils, *J. Clin. Invest.*, 61, 1330, 1978.
495. **Van Snick, J. L. and Masson, P. L.,** The binding of human lactoferrin to mouse peritoneal cells, *J. Exp. Med.*, 144, 1568, 1976.
496. **Broxmeyer, H. E., Pelus, L. M., Gillis, S., Kincade, P., deSousa, M., and Moore, M. A. S.,** Heterogeneity in responsiveness of mononuclear phagocytes to receptor-binding of lactoferrin and to inhibition of the production of granulocyte-macrophage colony stimulating factors by lactoferrin, in *Heterogeneity of Mononuclear Phagocytes*, Landy, M. and Forester, O., Eds., Academic Press, New York, 1981.
497. **Bagby, G. C., Bennett, R. M., Stankova, L., Bigley, R., Davis, J., and Wilkinson, B.,** CSA production by mononuclear phagocytes: paradoxical effects of high and low dose lactoferrin (LF), *Exp. Hematol.*, 8 (Suppl 7), 75, 1980.
498. **Synderman, R. and Fudman, E. J.,** Demonstration of a chemotactic factor receptor on macrophages, *J. Immunol.*, 124, 2754, 1980.
499. **Falk, W. and Leonard, E. J.,** Human monocyte chemotaxis: migrating cells are subpopulation with multiple chemotaxin specificities on each cell, *Infect. Immun.*, 29, 953, 1980.
500. **Broxmeyer, H. E.,** Lactoferrin acts on Ia-like antigen positive subpopulations of human monocytes to inhibit production of colony stimulatory activity *in vitro*, *J. Clin. Invest.*, 64, 1717, 1979.
501. **McKinney, T. K., Boto, N. O., Spiro, R. C., and Humphreys, R. E.,** Membrane expression and synthesis of p. 23, 30 (HLA-DR antigen) by human peripheral blood monocytes, *Exp. Hematol.*, 8, 709, 1980.
502. **Beller, D. I., Kiely, J-M., and Unanue, E. R.,** Regulation of macrophage populations. I. Preferential induction of Ia-rich peritoneal exudates by immunological stimuli, *J. Immunol.*, 124, 1426, 1980.
503. **Walker, W. S., Hester, R. B., Grandour, D. M., and Stewart, C. C.,** Evidence of a distinct progenitor for the Ia-bearing (Ia^+) murine bone-marrow-derived mononuclear phagocyte, in *Heterogeneity of Mononuclear Phagocytes*, Landy, M. and Forester, O., Academic Press, New York, 1981.
504. **Scher, M. G., Beller, D. I., and Unanue, E. R.,** Demonstration of a soluble mediator that induces exudates rich in Ia-positive macrophages, *J. Exp. Med.*, 152, 1684, 1980.
505. **Beller, D. I. and Unanue, E. R.,** Regulation of macrophage populations. II. Synthesis and expression Ia antigens by peritoneal exudate macrophages is a transient event, *J. Immunol.*, 126, 263, 1980.
506. **Steeg, P. S., Moore, R. N., and Oppenheim, J. J.,** Regulation of murine macrophage Ia-antigen expression by products of activated spleen cell, *J. Exp. Med.*, 152, 1734, 1980.
507. **Steinmann, G., Mertelsmann, R., deHarven, E., and Moore, M. A. S.,** Ultrastructural demonstration of terminal deoxynucleotidyl transferase (TdT), *Blood*, 57, 368, 1981.
508. **Steinmann, G., Broxmeyer, H. E., deHarven, E., and Moore, M. A. S.,** Immunoelectronmicroscopic localization of lactoferrin in human monocytes, *Exp. Hematol.*, 8 (Suppl. 7), 104, 1980.
509. **Zucali, J. R., Broxmeyer, H. E., and Ulatowski, J. A.,** Specificity of lactoferrin as an inhibitor of granulocyte-macrophage colony-stimulating activity production from fetal mouse liver cells, *Blood*, 54, 951, 1979.
510. **Morris, T. C. M., McNeill, T. A., and Bridges, J. M.,** Inhibition of normal human *in vitro* colony forming cells by cells from leukaemic patients, *Br. J. Cancer*, 31, 641, 1975.
511. **Chiyoda, S., Mizoguchi, H., Kosaka, K., and Takaku, Y.,** Influence of leukaemic cells on the colony formation of human bone marrow cells *in vitro*, *Br. J. Cancer*, 31, 355, 1975.
512. **Chiyoda, S., Mizoguchi, H., Asano, S., Takaku, F., and Miura, Y.,** Influence of leukaemic cells on the colony formation of human bone marrow cells *in vitro*. II. Suppressive effects of leukaemic cell extracts, *Br. J. Cancer*, 33, 379, 1976.

513. **Goldman, J. M., Th'ng, K. H., Catowsky, D., and Galton, D. A. G.,** Production of colony stimulating factor by leukemic leukocytes, *Blood,* 47, 381, 1976.
514. **Knudtzon, S. and Mortensen, B. T.,** Interaction between normal and leukaemic human cells in agar culture, *Scand. J. Haematol.,* 17, 369, 1976.
515. **Hinterberger, W., Mittermayer, K., Kinast, H., and Paukovits, W. R.,** Action of humoral factors derived from acute and chronic myeloid leukemia cells on *in vitro* myelopoiesis, *Oncology,* 34, 193, 1977.
516. **Hinterberger, W., Frischauf, H., Kletter, K., Paukovits, W., and Bais, P.,** Humoral function of acute leukaemic blasts, *Scand. J. Haematol.,* 19, 121, 1977.
517. **Quesenbery, P. J., Rappeport, J. M., Fountebuoni, A., Sullivan, R., Zuckerman, K., and Ryan, M.,** Inhibition of normal murine hematopoiesis by leukemic cells, *N. Engl. J. Med.,* 299, 71, 1978.
518. **Handler, E. S., Handler, E. E., and Bacon, E. R.,** *In vitro* colony formation in bone marrow and spleen suspensions from rats with an acute myelogenous leukemia, *J. Lab. Clin. Med.,* 84, 249, 1974.
519. **Steinberg, H. N. and Handler, E. S.,** Leukemic host influence on normal erythrocyte and granulocytic colony formation in *in vitro* plasma clot diffusion chamber cultures, *Cancer Res.,* 39, 1575, 1979.
520. **Miller, A. M., Page, P. L., Hartwell, B. L., and Robinson, S. H.,** Inhibiton of growth of normal murine granulocytes by cocultured acute leukemic cells, *Blood,* 50, 799, 1977.
521. **Gordon, M. Y., Douglas, I. D. C., and Blackett, N. M.,** Effect of medium conditioned by acute myeloid leukaemia cells on normal marrow colony-forming ability and sensitivity to cytosine arabinoside, *Eur. J. Cancer,* 14, 661, 1978.
522. **Vincent, P. C. and Morris, T. C. M.,** Haemopoietic inhibitors in acute leukaemia, *Aust. N.Z.J. Med.,* 9, 455, 1979.
523. **Broxmeyer, H. E., Jacobsen, H., Kurland, J., Mendelsohn, N., and Moore, M. A. S.,** *In vitro* suppression of normal granulocyte stem cells by inhibitory activity derived from leukemia cells, *J. Natl. Cancer Inst.,* 60, 497, 1978.
524. **Broxmeyer, H. E., Grossbard, E., Jacobsen, N., and Moore, M. A. S.,** Evidence for a proliferative advantage of human leukemia colony forming cells (CFU-c) *in vitro, J. Natl. Cancer Inst.,* 60, 513, 1978.
525. **Broxmeyer, H. E., Grossbard, E., Jacobsen, N., and Moore, M. A. S.,** Persistance of leukemia inhibitory activity during remission of acute leukemia, *N. Engl. J. Med.,* 301, 346, 1979.
526. **Broxmeyer, H. E., Ralph, P., Margolis, V. B., Nakoinz, I., Meyers, P., Kapoor, N., and Moore, M. A. S.,** Characteristics of bone marrow and blood cells in human leukemia that produce leukemia inhibitory activity (LIA), *Leuk. Res.,* 3, 193, 1979.
527. **Broxmeyer, H. E., Koltun, L., Jacobsen, N., and Moore, M. A. S.,** Normal and leukemic hematopoiesis in diffusion chambers: comparison with *in vitro* culture systems, in *Diffusion Chamber Culture,* Cronkite, E. P. and Carsten, A. L., Springer-Verlag, Berlin, 1980, 110.
528. **Broxmeyer, H. E., Ralph, P., Gilbertson, S., and Margolis, V. B.,** Induction of leukemia-associated inhibitory activity and bone marrow granulocyte-macrophage progenitor cell alterations during infection with Abelson virus, *Cancer Res.,* 40, 3928, 1980.
529. **Dietz, M., Fouchey, S. P., Longley, C., Rich, M. A., and Furmanski, P.,** Spontaneous regression of Friend virus-induced erythroleukemia, *J. Exp. Med.,* 145, 594, 1977.
530. **Marcelletti, J. and Furmanski, P.,** Infection of macrophages with Friend virus: relationship to the spontaneous regression of viral erythroleukemia, *Cell,* 16, 649, 1979.
531. **Marcelletti, J. and Furmanski, P.,** A murine model system for the study of the human leukemia-associated inhibitory activity, *Blood,* 56, 134, 1980.
532. **Bognacki, J., Broxmeyer, H. E., deSousa, M., and LoBue, J.,** Isolation and biochemical characterization of leukemia associated inhibitory activity that supresses colony and cluster formation of cells, *Biochim. Biophys. Acta,* 672, 176, 1981.
533. **Harrison, P. M.,** Ferritin: an iron-storage molecule, Semin. Hematol., 14, 55, 1977.
534. **Aisen, P. and Listowsky, I.,** Iron transport and storage proteins, *Ann. Rev. Biochem.,* 49, 357, 1980.
535. **Clegg, G. A., Fitton, J. E., Harrison, P. M., and Treffry,** Ferritin: molecular structure and iron-storage mechanisms, *Prog. Biophys. Molec. Biol.,* 36, 56, 1980.
536. **Drysdale, J. W., Adelman, T. G., Arosio, P., Casareale, D., Fitzpatrick, P., Hazard, J. I., and Yokota, M.,** Human isoferritins in normal and disease states, *Semin. Hematol.,* 14, 71, 1977.
537. **Arosio, P., Yokota, M., and Drysdale, J. W.,** Structural and immunological relationships of isoferritins in normal and malignant cells, *Cancer Res.,* 36, 1735, 1976.
538. **Cragg, S. J., Jacobs, A., Parry, D. H., Wagstaff, M., and Worwood, M.,** Isoferritins in acute leukemia, *Br. J. Cancer,* 35, 635, 1977.
539. **Drysdale, J. W. and Singer, R. M.,** Carcinofetal human isoferritins in placenta and Hela cells, *Cancer Res.,* 34, 3352, 1974.

540. **Halliday, J. W., McKerring, L. V., and Powell, L. W.,** Isoferritin composition of tissues and serum in human cancers, *Cancer Res.*, 36, 4486, 1976.
541. **Mori, W., Asakawa, H., and Taguichi, T.,** Antiserum against leukemia cell ferritin as a diagnostic tool for malignant neoplasm, *J. Natl. Cancer Inst.*, 55, 513, 1975.
542. **Hazard, J. I., Yokoto, M., and Drysdale, J. W.,** Immunologic differences in human isoferritins: implications for immunologic quantitation of serum ferritin, *Blood,* 49, 139, 1977.
543. **Jones, B. M. and Worwood, M.,** An immunoradiometric assay for the acidic ferritin of human heart: application to human tissues, cells and serum, *Clin. Chim. Acta,* 85, 81, 1978.
544. **Moroz, C., Giler, S., Kupfer, B., and Urca, I.,** Lymphocytes bearing surface ferritin in patients with Hodgkin's disease and breast cancer, *N. Engl. J. Med.*, 296, 1172, 1977.
545. **Matzner, Y., Hershko, C., Polliack, A., Konijn, A. M., and Izak, G.,** Suppressive effect of ferritin on *in vitro* lymphocyte function, *Br. J. Haematol.*, 42, 345, 1979.
546. **Hancock, B. W., Bruce, L., May, K., and Richmond, J.,** Ferritin, a sensitizing substance in the leucocyte migration inhibition test in patients with malignant lymphoma, *Br. J. Haematol.*, 43, 223, 1979.
547. **Broxmeyer, H. E., Bognacki, J., Dorner, M. M., and deSousa, M.,** The identification of leukemia-associated inhibitory activity (L1A) as acidic isoferritins: a regulatory role for acidic isoferritins in the production of granulocytes and macrophages, *J. Exp. Med.*, 153, 1426, 1981.
548. **Broxmeyer, H. E., Bognacki, J., Dorner, M. M., deSousa, M., and Li, Lu,** Acidic isoferritins as feedback regulators in normal and leukemic myelopoiesis, in *Modern Trends in Human Leukemia IV,* Neth, R., Ed., Springer-Verlag, Berlin, 1981.
549. **Wagstaff, M., Worwood, M., and Jacobs, A.,** Properties of human tissue isoferritins, *Biochem. J.*, 173, 969, 1978.
550. **Olfsson, T. and Olsson, I.,** Suppression of normal granulopoiesis *in vitro* by a leukemia-associated inhibitor (LA1) of acute and chronic leukemia, *Blood,* 55, 975, 1980.
551. **Olfsson, T. and Olsson, I.,** Biochemical characterization of a leukemia-associated inhibitor (LA1) suppressing normal granulopoiesis *in vitro, Blood,* 55, 983, 1980.
552. **Pelus, L. M. and Strausser, H. R.,** Prostaglandins and the immune response, *Life Sci.*, 20, 903, 1977.
553. **Samuelsson, B., Granstrom, E., Green, K., Hamberg, M., and Hammerstrom, S.,** Prostaglandins, *Ann. Rev. Biochem.*, 44, 669, 1975.
554. **Lewis, G. P.,** Prostaglandins in inflammation, a review, *J. Ret. Soc.*, 22, 389, 1977.
555. **Williams, N. and Jackson, H.,** Limitation of macrophage production in long-term marrow cultures containing prostaglandin E, *J. Cell. Physiol.*, 103, 239, 1980.
556. **Humes, J. L., Bonney, R. J., Pelus, L. M., Dahlgren, M. E., Sadowski, S. J., Kuehl, F. A., Jr., and Davies, P.,** Macrophages synthesize and release prostaglandins in response to inflammatory stimuli, *Nature,* 269, 149, 1977.
557. **Kurland, J. I. and Bockman, R.,** Prostaglandin E production by human blood monocytes and mouse peritoneal macrophages, *J. Exp. Med.*, 147, 952, 1978.
558. **Kurland, J. I. and Moore, M. A. S.,** Modulation of hemopoiesis by prostaglandins, *Exp. Hematol.*, 5, 357, 1977.
559. **Kurland, J., Bockman, R., Broxmeyer, H. E., and Moore, M. A. S.,** Limitation of excessive myelopoiesis by the intrinsic modulation of macrophage-derived prostaglandin E, *Science,* 199, 552, 1978.
560. **Taetle, R. and Koessler, A.,** Effects of cyclic nucleotides and prostaglandins on normal and abnormal human myeloid progenitor proliferation, *Cancer Res.*, 40, 1223, 1980.
561. **Aglietta, M., Piacibello, W., and Gavosto, F.,** Insensitivity of chronic myeloid leukemia cells to inhibition of growth by prostaglandin E, *Cancer Res.*, 40, 2507, 1980.
562. **Pelus, L. M., Broxmeyer, H. E., Clarkson, B. D., and Moore, M. A. S.,** Abnormal responsiveness of colony forming cells from patients which chronic myeloid leukemia to inhibition by prostaglandin E, *Cancer Res.*, 40, 2512, 1980.
563. **Taetle, R., Guittard, J.-P., and Mendelsohn, M. J.,** Abnormal modulation of granulocyte/macrophage progenitor proliferation by prostaglandin E in chronic myeloproliferative disorders, *Exp. Hematol.*, 8, 1190, 1980.
564. **Jaffe, B. M., Behrman, H. R., and Parker, C. W.,** Radioimmunoassay measurement of prostaglandins E, A and F in human plasma, *J. Clin. Invest.*, 52, 398, 1973.
565. **Berenbaum, M. C., Cope, W. A., and Bundic, R. V.,** Synergistic effect of cortisol and prostaglandin E_2, *Clin. Exp. Immunol.*, 26, 534, 1976.
566. **Fontagne, J., Adolphe, M., Semichon, M., Zizine, L., and Lechat, P.,** Effect of *in vivo* treatment with indomethacin on mouse granulocyte-macrophage colony-forming cells in culture (CFUc): possible role of prostaglandins, *Exp. Hematol.*, 8, 1157, 1980.

567. **Passwell, J. H., Dayer, J-M., and Merler, E.,** Increased prostaglandin production by human monocytes after membrane receptor activation, *J. Immunol.,* 123, 115, 1979.
568. **Yamamoto, M., Takai, N. A., Rapoport, B., and Hinds, W. E.,** Modulation by thymus-derived (T) cells of thyroid cell-stimulated prostaglandin E release by human peripheral blood mononuclear cells, *Proc. Natl. Acad. Sci. U.S.A.,* 76, 6627, 1979.
569. **Hsueh, W., Gonzalez-Crussi, F., and Hanneman, E.,** Prostaglandin synthesis in different phases of phagocytosis in lung macrophages, *Nature,* 283, 80, 1980.
570. **Rouzer, C. A., Scott, W. A., Kempe, J., and Cohn, Z. A.,** Prostaglandin synthesis by macrophages requires a specific receptor-ligand interaction, *Proc. Natl. Acad. Sci. U.S.A.,* 77, 4279, 1980.
571. **Hamilton, J. A.,** Stimulation of macrophage prostaglandin and neutral protease production by phorbol esters as a model for the induction of vascular changes associated with tumor promotion, *Cancer Res.,* 40, 2273, 1980.
572. **Moore, R. N., Urbaschek, R., Wahl, L. M., and Mergenhagen, S. E.,** Prostaglandin regulation of colony stimulating factor production by lipopolysaccharide-stimulated murine leukocytes, *Infect. Immun.,* 26, 408, 1979.
573. **Goldyne, M. E. and Stobo, J. D.,** Synthesis of prostaglandins by subpopulations of human peripheral blood monocytes, *Prostaglandins,* 18, 687, 1979.
574. **Pelus, L. M. and Bockman, R.,** Increased prostaglandin synthesis by macrophages from tumor-bearing mice, *J. Immunol.,* 123, 2118, 1979.
575. **Stewart, W. E., II,** *The Interferon System,* Springer-Verlag, New York, 1979.
576. **Krim, M.,** Towards tumor therapy with interferons. Part I. Interferons: production and properties, *Blood,* 55, 711, 1980.
577. **Krim, M.,** Towards tumor therapy with interferons. Part II. Interferons: *in vivo* effects, *Blood,* 55, 875, 1980.
578. **Stewart, W. E., II, Blalock, J. E., Burke, D. C., Chany, C., Dunick, J. K., Falcoff, E., Friedman, R. M., Galasso, G. J., Joklik, W. K., Vileck, J. T., Younger, J. S., and Zoon, K. C.,** Interferon nomenclature, *J. Immunol.,* 125, 2353, 1980.
579. **McNeill, T. A. and Killer, M.,** The effect of synthetic double-stranded polyribonucleotides on haemopoietic colony-forming cells *in vivo, Immunology,* 21, 751, 1971.
580. **McNeill, T. A. and Fleming, W. A.,** The relationship between serum interferon and an inhibitor of mouse haemopoietic colonies *in vitro, Immunology,* 21, 761, 1971.
581. **Fleming, W. A., McNeill, T. A., and Killen, M.,** The effects of an inhibiting factor (interferon) on the *in vitro* growth of granulocyte-macrophage colonies, *Immunology,* 23, 429, 1972.
582. **McNeill, T. A. and Gressler, I.,** Inhibition of haemaopoietic colony growth by interferon preparations from different sources, *Nature,* 244, 173, 1973.
583. **Greenberg, P. L. and Mosny, S. A.,** Cytotoxic effects of interferon *in vitro* on granulocytic progenitor cells, *Cancer Res.,* 37, 1794, 1977.
584. **van't Hull, E., Schellekens, H., Lowenberg, B., and de Vries, M. J.,** Influence of interferon preparations on the proliferative capacity of human and mouse bone marrow cells *in vitro, Cancer Res.,* 38, 911, 1978.
585. **Gallien-Lartique, O., Carrez, D., de Maeyer, E., and de Maeyer-Guignard, J.,** Strain dependence of the antiproliferative action of interferon on murine erythroid precursors, *Science,* 209, 292, 1980.
586. **Ortega, J. A., Ma, A., Shore, N. A., Dukes, P. P., and Merigan, T. C.,** Suppressive effect of interferon on erythroid cell proliferation, *Exp. Hematol.,* 7, 145, 1979.
587. **Verma, D. S., Spitzer, G., Gutterman, J. U., Zander, A. R., McCredie, K. B., and Dicke, K. A.,** Human leukocyte interferon preparation blocks granulopoietic differentiation, *Blood,* 54, 1423, 1979.
588. **Taetle, R., Buick, R. N., and McCulloch, E. A.,** Effect of interferon on colony formation in culture by blast cell progenitors in acute myeloblastic leukemia, *Blood,* 56, 549, 1980.
589. **Iversen, O. H.,** The chalones, in *Handbook of Experimental Pharmacology, Tissue Growth Factors,* Baserga, R., Ed., Springer-Verlag, Berlin, 1981.
590. **Rytomaa, T. and Toivonen, H.,** Chalones: concepts and results, *Mech. Age. Dev.,* 9, 471, 1979.
591. **Rytomaa, T.,** Biology of the granulocyte chalone, in *Chalones,* Houck, J. C., Ed., North-Holland, Amsterdam, 1976, 289.
592. **Paukovits, W. R.,** *In vitro* biological and chemical properties of the granulocytic chalone, in *Chalones,* Houck, J. C., Ed., North-Holland, Amsterdam, 1976, 311.
593. **Maurer, H. R. and Laerum, O. D.,** Granulocytic chalone testing: a critical review, in *Chalones,* Houck, J. C., Ed., North-Holland, Amsterdam, 1976, 331.
594. **Chan, S. H.,** Influence of serum inhibitors on clony development *in vitro* by bone marrow cells, *Aust. J. Exp. Biol. Med. Sci.,* 49, 553, 1971.

595. **Chan, S. H., Metcalf, D., and Stanley, E. R.,** Stimulation and inhibition by normal human serum of colony formation *in vitro* by bone marrow cells, *Br. J. Haematol.*, 20, 329, 1971.
596. **Granstrom, M.,** Studies on inhibitors of bone marrow colony formation in normal human sera and during a viral infection, *Exp. Cell Res.*, 82, 426, 1972.
597. **Metcalf, D. and Russel, S.,** Inhibition by mouse serum of hemopoietic colony formation *in vitro, Exp. Hematol.*, 4, 339, 1976.
598. **Luban, N. L. and Miller, D. R.,** Serum inhibitors to granulopoiesis in thalassemia major, *Exp. Hematol.*, 6, 185, 1978.
599. **Mortensen, B. T., Knudtzon, S., and Schultz, H.,** Serum lipoprotein inhibitors of granulopoiesis in human bone marrow cultures, *Exp. Hematol.*, 7, 1, 1979.
600. **Knudtzon, S. and Mortensen, B. T.,** The effect of sonicated serum on growth of normal and leukaemic human cells in agar culture, *Scand. J. Haematol.*, 22, 296, 1979.
601. **Liu, Y. K., Stallard, S., Koo, V., and Dannaher, C. L.,** Serum inhibitor activity of granulocyte-macrophage colony formation in patients with cancer, *Cancer Res.*, 39, 1640, 1979.
602. **Dodge, W. H., Love, S. H., Bryant, D. L., and Mitchell, R. H.,** Properties of colony-stimulating and inhibiting activities of chicken serum, *Exp. Hematol.*, 8, 395, 1980.
603. **Fitchen, J. H. and Cline, J. J.,** Serum inhibitors of myelopoiesis, *Br. J. Haematol.*, 44, 7, 1980.
604. **Fitchen, J. H., Gale, R. P., and Cline, M. J.,** Serum inhibitors of *in vitro* hematopoiesis and graft outcome in bone marrow transplantation for aplastic anemia, *Transplantation,* 29, 223, 1980.
605. **Baker, F. L. and Galbraith, P. R.,** Mechanism of action of serum factors that regulate granulopoiesis *in vitro:* possible physiologic role of serum-inhibiting activity, *Blood,* 53, 304, 1979.
606. **Bryant, D., Smith, D., Sharma, S., and Dodge, W.,** Some circulating factors which influence granulocyte-monocyte production in the chick with myeloblastic leukemia, *Cancer Res.*, 40, 4031, 1980.
607. **Chervenick, P. A., Ellis, L. D., Pan, S. F., and Lawson, A. L.,** Human leukemic cells: *in vitro* growth of colonies containing the Philadelphia (Ph^1) chromosome, *Science,* 174, 1134, 1971.
608. **Moore, M. A. S. and Metcalf, D.,** Cytogenetic analysis of human acute and chronic myeloid leukemic cells cloned in agar culture, *Int. J. Cancer,* 11, 143, 1973.
609. **Aye, M. T., Till, J. E., and McCulloch, E. A.,** Cytological studies of granulopoietic colonies from two patients with chronic myelogenous leukemia, *Exp. Hematol.*, 1, 115, 1973.
610. **Moore, M. A. S., Ekert, H., Fitzgerald, M. G., and Carmichael, A.,** Evidence for the clonal origin of chronic myeloid leukemia from a sex chromosome mosaic: clinical, cytogenetic, and marrow culture studies, *Blood,* 43, 15, 1974.
611. Senn, J. S. and Price, G. B., Chronic myeloid leukemia: physical and functional similarities to acute leukemia, *Blood,* 49, 913, 1977.
612. **Moore, M. A. S., Spitzer, G., Williams, N., Metcalf, D., and Buckley, J.,** Agar culture studies in 127 cases of untreated acute leukemia: the prognostic value of reclassification of leukemia according to *in vitro* growth characteristics, *Blood,* 44, 1, 1974.
613. **Moore, M. A. S.,** *In vitro* culture studies in chronic granulocytic leukaemia, *Clin. Hematol.*, 6, 97, 1977.
614. **Moore, M. A. S.,** Predication of relapse and remission in AML by marrow culture criteria, *Blood Cells,* 2, 109, 1976.
615. **Moore, M. A. S.,** Agar cultures studies in CML and blastic transformation, *Ser. Haematol.*, 8, 11, 1975.
616. **Mertelsmann, R., Moore, M. A. S., Broxmeyer, H. E., Cirrincione, C. and Clarkson, B.,** The diagnostic and prognostic significance of the CFU-c assay in acute non-lymphoblastic leukemia (ANLL), *Cancer Res.*, 41, 4844, 1981.
617. **Greenberg, P.,** Clinical relevance of in vitro study of granulocytopoiesis, *Scand. J. Haematol.*, 25, 369, 1980.
618. **Spitzer, G., Dicke, K. A., McCredie, K. B., and Barlogie, B.,** The early detection of remission in acute myelogenous leukaemia by *in vitro* cultures, *Br. J. Haematol.*, 35, 411, 1977.
619. **Knudtzon, S.,** *In vitro* culture of leukaemic cells from 81 patients with acute leukaemia, *Scand. J. Haematol.*, 18, 377, 1977.
620. **Greenberg, P. L., Nichols, W. C., and Schrier, S. L.,** Granulopoiesis in acute myeloid leukemia and preleukemia, *N. Engl. J. Med.*, 284, 1225, 1971.
621. **Beran, M., Reizenstein, P., and Uden, A-M.,** Response to treatment in acute non-lymphatic leukaemia: prognostic value of colony forming and colony stimulating capacities of bone marrow and blood cells compared to other parameters, *Br. J. Haematol.*, 44, 39, 1980.
622. **Galbraith, P. R.,** Remission of acute myeloid leukemia: studies of *in vitro* colony formation by bone marrow cells, *Can. Med. Assoc. J.*, 110, 1147, 1974.

623. **Gustavsson, A., Olofsson, T., and Olsson, I.,** Oscillations of marrow culture growth in acute myeloid leukemia during remission induction and remission, *Acta Haematol.*, 62, 241, 1979.
624. **Vincent, P. C., Sutherland, R., Bradley, M., Lind, D., and Gunz, F. W.,** Marrow culture studies in adult acute leukemia at presentation and during remission, *Blood,* 49, 903, 1977.
625. **Dresch, C., Faille, A., Poirier, O., Balitrand, N., and Najean, Y.,** Bone marrow cell kinetics and culture in chronic and subacute myelomonocytic leukemia. Physiopathological interpretation and prognostic importance, *Leuk. Res.*, 4, 129, 1979.
626. **Verma, D. S., Spitzer, G., Dicke, K. A., and McCredie, K. B.,** *In vitro* agar culture patterns in preleukemia and their clinical significance, *Leuk. Res.*, 3, 41, 1979.
627. **Straus, D. J., Mertelsmann, R., Koziner, B., McKenzie, S., deHarven, E., Arlin, Z. A., Kempin, S., Broxmeyer, H. E., Moore, M. A. S., Menendez-Botet, C. J., Gee, T. S., and Clarkson, B.,** The acute monocytic leukemias: multidisciplinary studies in 45 patients, *Medicine,* 59, 409, 1980.
628. **Curtis, J. E., Cowan, D. H., Bergsagel, D. E., Hasselback, R., and McCulloch, E. A.,** Acute leukemia in adults: assessment of remission induction with combination chemotherapy by clinical and cell culture criteria, *Can. Med. Assoc. J.*, 113, 289, 1975.
629. **Smith, S. D., Uyeki, E. M., and Lowman, J. T.,** Colony formation *in vitro* by leukemic cells in acute lymphoblastic leukemia (ALL), *Blood,* 52, 712, 1978.
630. **Goldman, J. M., Shiota, F., Th'ng, K. H., and Orchard, K. H.,** Circulating granulocytic and erythroid progenitor cells in chronic granulocytic leukaemia, *Br. J. Haematol.*, 46, 7, 1980.
631. **Greenberg, P., Mara, B., Bax, I., Brossel, R., and Schrier, S.,** The myeloproliferative disorders, correlation between clinical evolution and alterations of granulopoiesis, *Am. J. Med.*, 61, 878, 1976.
632. **Spitzer, G., Verma, D. S., Dicke, K. A., Smith, T., and McCredie, K. B.,** Subgroups of oligoleukemia as identified by *in vitro* agar culture, *Leuk. Res.*, 3, 29, 1979.
633. **Lidbeck, J.,** *In vitro* colony and cluster growth in haemopoietic dysplasia (the preleukaemic syndrome). I. Clinical correlations, *Scand. J. Haematol.*, 24, 412, 1980.
634. **Lidbeck, J.,** *In vitro* colony and cluster growth in haemopoietic dysplasia (the preleukemic syndrome). II. Identification of a maturation defect in agar culture, *Scand. J. Haematol.*, 25, 113, 1980.
635. **Faille, A., Dresch, C., Poirier, O., Balitrand, N., and Najean, Y.,** Prognostic value of *in vitro* bone marrow culture in refractory anaemia with excess of myeloblasts, *Scand. J. Haematol.*, 20, 280, 1978.
636. **Faille, A., Najean, Y., Dresch, C., and Poirier, O.,** Cell culture studies in 19 cases of refractory anaemia: comparison of clinical data with *in vivo* erythrokinetic studies, *Scand. J. Haematol.*, 19, 39, 1977.
637. **Senn, J. S., Pinkerton, P. H., Price, G. B., Mak, T. W., and McCulloch, E. A.,** Human preleukaemia cell culture studies in sideroblastic anaemia, *Br. J. Cancer,* 33, 299, 1976.
638. **Senn, J. S. and Pinkerton, P. H.,** Defective *in vitro* colony formation by human bone marrow preceding overt leukaemia, *Br. J. Haematol.*, 23, 277, 1972.
639. **Sultan, C.,** *In vitro* studies of bone marrow in refractory anaemia, *Br. J. Haematol.*, 23, 177, 1972.
640. **Chu, J-Y.,** Granulopoiesis in Fanconi's aplastic anemia, *Proc. Soc. Exp. Biol. Med.*, 161, 609, 1979.
641. **Daneshbod-Skibba, G., Martin, J., and Shahidi, N. T.,** Myeloid and erythroid colony growth in non-anaemic patients with Fanconi's anaemia, *Br. J. Haematol.*, 44, 33, 1980.
642. **Standen, G., Philip, M. A., and Fletcher, J.,** Reduced number of peripheral blood granulocytic progenitor cells in patients with Down's Syndrome, *Br. J. Haematol.*, 42, 417, 1979.
643. **Price, T. H. and Dale, D. C.,** The selective neutropenias, *Clin. Haematol.*, 7, 501, 1978.
644. **Parmley, R. T., Crist, W. M., Ragab, H., Boxer, L. A., Malluh, A., Lui, V. K., and Darby, C. P.,** Congenital dysgranulopoietic neutropenia: clinical, serologic ultrastructural, and *in vitro* proliferative characteristics, *Blood,* 56, 465, 1980.
645. **Greenberg, P. L., Mara, B., Steed, S., and Boxer, L.,** The chronic idiopathic neutropenia syndrome: correlation of clinical features with *in vitro* parameters of granulopoiesis, *Blood,* 55, 915, 1980.
646. **Joyce, R. A., Boggs, D. R., and Chervenick, P. A.,** Neutrophil kinetics in hereditary and congenital neutropenias, *N. Engl. J. Med.*, 295, 1386, 1976.
647. **Greenberg, P. L. and Schrier, S. L.,** Granulopoiesis in neutropenic disorders, *Blood,* 41, 753, 1973.
648. **Faille, A., Dresch, C., Poirier, O., and Najean, Y.,** Granulopoiesis: studies of bone marrow culture in chronic granulocytopenia and comparison with granulocyte kinetics, *Biomedicine,* 26, 187, 1977.
649. **Olofsson, T., Olsson, I., Kostmann, R., Malmstrom, S., and Thilen, A.,** Granulopoiesis in infantile genetic agranulocytosis. In vitro cloning of marrow cells in agar culture, *Scand. J. Haematol.*, 16, 18, 1976.
650. **L'esperance, P., Brunning, R., and Good, R. A.,** Congenital neutropenia: *In vitro* growth of colonies mimicking the disease, *Proc. Natl. Acad. Sci. U.S.A.*, 70, 669, 1973.

651. **Parmley, R. T., Ogawa, M., Darby, C. P., Jr., and Spicer, S. S.,** Congenital neutropenia: neutrophil proliferation with abnormal maturation, *Blood,* 46, 723, 1975.
652. **Wiseman, L. L., Senn, J. S., Miller, R. G., and Price, G. B.,** Stem cell characterization of neutropenia: velocity sedimentation and mass culture analysis, *Br. J. Cancer,* 34, 46, 1976.
653. **Greenberg, P. L., Bax, I., Levin, J., and Andrews, T. M.,** Alteration of colony-stimulating factor output, endotoxemia, and granulopoiesis in cyclic neutropenia, *Am. J. Hematol.,* 1, 375, 1976.
654. **Wright, D. G., Fauci, A. S., Dale, D. C., and Wolff, S. M.,** Correction of human cyclic neutropenia with prednisolone, *N. Engl. J. Med.,* 298, 295, 1978.
655. **Greenberg, P., Mara, B., and Schrier, S.,** Alterations of granulopoiesis following chemotherapy, *Blood,* 44, 375, 1974.
656. **Moore, M.A.S., Hansen, J. A., Everson, L. K., O'Reilly, R., and Good, R. A.,** Hematologic analysis of clinical bone marrow grafting evaluated by *in vitro* cultures, *Transplant. Proc.,* 8, 647, 1976.
657. **Spitzer, G., Verma, D., Fisher, R., Zander, A., Vellekoop, L., Litam, J., McCredie, K. B., and Dicke, K. A.,** The myeloid progenitor cell—its value in predicting hematopoietic recovery after autologous bone marrow after transplantation, *Blood,* 55, 317, 1980.
658. **Elias, L. and Greenberg, P.,** Divergent patterns of marrow cell suspension culture growth in the myeloid leukemias: correlation of *in vitro* findings with clinical features, *Blood,* 50, 263, 1977.
659. **Park, C. H., Savin, M. A., Hoogstraten, B., Amare, M., and Hathaway, P.,** Improved growth of *in vitro* colonies in human acute leukemia using the feeding culture method, *Cancer Res.,* 37, 4595, 1977.
660. **Park, C. H., Amare, M., Savin, M. A., Goodwin, J. W., Newcomb, M. M., and Hoogstraten, B.,** Prediction of chemotherapy response in human leukemia using an *in vitro* chemotherapy sensitivity test on the leukemic colony-forming cells, *Blood,* 55, 595, 1980.
661. **Preisler, H. D.,** Prediction of response to chemotherapy in acute myelocytic leukemia, *Blood,* 56, 361, 1980.
662. **Metcalf, D. Moore, M. A. S., Sheridan, J. W., and Spitzer, G.,** Responsiveness of human granulocytic leukemic cells to colony-stimulating factor, *Blood,* 43, 847, 1974.
663. **Francis, G. E., Berney, J. J., Chipping, P. M., and Hoffbrand, A. V.,** Stimulation of human haemopoietic cells by colony stimulating factors: sensitivity of leukaemic cells, *Br. J. Haematol.,* 41, 545, 1979.
664. **Greenberg, P. L., Mara, B. and Heller, P.** Marrow adherent cell colony-stimulating activity production in acute myeloid leukemia, *Blood,* 52, 362, 1978.
665. **Weatherly, T. L., Fleisher, T. A., and Strong, D. M.,** Reduced granulocyte-macrophage colony-stimulating activity by mitogen-stimulated lymphocytes from patients with aplastic anaemia, *Br. J. Haematol.,* 43, 335, 1979.
666. **Kincade, P. W., Lee, G., Fernandes, G., Moore, M. A. S., Williams, N., and Good, R. A.,** Abnormalities in clonable B lymphocytes and myeloid progenitors in autoimmune NZB mice, *Proc. Natl. Acad. Sci. U.S.A.,* 76, 3464, 1979.
667. **Phillip, M. A., Standen, G., and Fletcher, J.,** The effects of surgical trauma on human granulopoiesis, *Br. J. Haematol.,* 44, 263, 1980.
668. **Bagby, G. C., Jr., Goodnight, S. H., Mooney, W. M., and Richert-Boe, K.,** Prednisone-responsive aplastic anemia: a mechanism of glucocorticoid action, *Blood,* 54, 322, 1979.
669. **Buick, R. N., Till, J. E., and McCulloch, E. A.,** Colony assay for proliferative blast cells circulating in myeloblastic leukaemia, *Lancet,* 1, 862, 1977.
670. **Chang, L. J. A., Till, J. E., and McCulloch, E. A.,** The cellular basis of self-renewal in cultures by human acute myeloblastic leukemia blast cell progenitors, *J. Cell. Physiol.,* 102, 217, 1980.
671. **Minden, M. D., Till, J. E., and McCulloch, E. A.,** Proliferative state of blast cell progenitors in acute myeloblastic leukemia (AML), *Blood,* 52, 592, 1978.
672. **Buick, R. N., Minden, M. D., and McCulloch, E. A.,** Self renewal in culture of proliferative blast progenitor cells in acute myeloblastic leukemia, *Blood,* 54, 95, 1979.
673. **Minden, M. D., Buick, R. N., and McCulloch, E. A.,** Separation of blast cells and T-lymphocyte progenitors in the blood of patients with acute myeloblastic leukemia, *Blood,* 54, 186, 1979.
674. **Buick, R. N., Messner, H. A., Till, J. E., and McCulloch, E. A.,** Cytotoxicity of adriamycin and daunorubicin for normal and leukemic progenitor cells of man, *J. Natl. Cancer Inst.,* 62, 249, 1979.
675. **Moore, M. A. S., Mertelsmann, R., and Pelus, L. M.,** Phenotypic evaluation of chronic myeloid leukemia, *Blood Cells,* 7, 217, 1981.
676. **Johnson, R. T. and Rao, P.,** Mammalian cell fusion. II. Induction of premature chromosome condensation in interphase nuclei, *Nature,* 226, 712, 1970.
677. **Hittleman, W. N. and Rao, P. N.,** Mapping G1 phase by the structural morphology of the prematurely condensed chromosomes, *J. Cell. Physiol.,* 95, 333, 1978.

678. **Hittleman, W. N. and Rao, P. N.,** Predicting response or progression of human leukemia by premature chromosome condensation of bone marrow cells, *Cancer Res.*, 38, 416, 1978.
679. **Hittleman, W. N., Broussard, L. C., and McCredie, K.,** Premature chromosome condensation studies in human leukemia. I. Pretreatment characteristics, *Blood,* 54, 1001, 1979.
680. **Hittelman, W. N., Broussard, L. C., McCredie, K. and Murphy, S. G.,** Premature chromosome condensation studies in human leukemia. II. Proliferative potential changes after induction therapy for AML patients, *Blood,* 55, 457, 1980.
681. **Easton, T. G., Valinsky, J. E. and Reich, E.,** Merocyanine 540 as a fluorescent probe of membranes: staining of electrically excitable cells, *Cell,* 13, 475, 1978.
682. **Valinsky, J. E., Easton, T. G., and Reich, E.,** Merocyanine 540 as a fluorescent probe of membranes: selective staining of leukemic and immature hemopoietic cells, *Cells,* 13, 487, 1978.
683. **Adamson, J. W., Singer, J. W., Calalano, P., Murphy, S., Lin, N., Steinmann, L., Ernst, C., and Fialkow, P. J.,** Polycythemia vera. Further *in vitro* studies of hematopoietic regulation, *J. Clin. Invest.*, 66, 1363, 1980.
684. **Hiraoka, A., Yamagishi, M., Ohkubo, T., Yoshida, Y., and Uchino, H.,** Relationship between *in vitro* colony-forming ability and expression of Ia-like antigen of acute nonlymphocytic leukemia (ANLL) cells, *Blood,* 56, 859, 1980.
685. **Kagan, W. A., Ascensao, J. A., Pahwa, R. N., Hansen, J. A., Goldstein, G., Valera, E. B., Incefy, G. S., Moore, M. A. S., and Good, R. A.,** Aplastic anemia: presence in human bone marrow of cells that suppress myelopoiesis, *Proc. Natl. Acad. Sci. U.S.A.*, 73, 2890, 1976.
686. **Ascensao, J., Kagan, W., Moore, M., Pahwa, R., Hansen, J., and Good, R.,** Aplastic anemia: evidence for an immunological mechanism, *Lancet,* 1, 669, 1976.
687. **Cline, M. J., Opelz, G., Saxon, A., Fahey, J. L., and Golde, D. W.,** Autoimmune panleukopenia, *N. Engl. J. Med.*, 295, 1489, 1976.
688. **Cline, M. J. and Golde, D. W.,** Immune suppression of hematopoiesis, *Am. J. Med.*, 64, 301, 1978.
689. **Amare, M., Abdou, N. L., Robinson, M. G., and Abdou, N. I.,** Aplastic anemia associated with bone marrow suppressor T-cell hyperactivity: successful treatment with antithymocyte globulin, *Am. J. Hematol.*, 5, 25, 1978.
690. **Gordon, M. Y.,** Circulating inhibitors of granulopoiesis in patients with aplastic anemia, *Br. J. Haematol.*, 39, 491, 1978.
691. **Abdou, N. I., NaPombejara, C., Balentine, L., and Abdou, N.,** Suppressor cell-mediated neutropenia in Felty's Syndrome, *J. Clin. Invest.*, 61, 738, 1978.
692. **Gordon, M. Y.,** Relevance of colony forming assays to bone marrow transplantation with particular reference to grafting for aplastic anaemia, *Br. J. Haematol.*, 42, 61, 1979.
693. **Bagby, G. C., Jr. and Gabourel, J. D.,** Neutropenia in three patients with rheumatic disorders. Suppression of granulopoiesis by cortisolsensitive thymus-dependent lymphocytes, *J. Clin. Invest.*, 64, 72, 1979.
694. **Faille, A., Barrett, A. J., Balitrand, N., Ketels, F., Gluckman, E., and Najean, Y.,** Effect of antilymphocyte globulin on granulocyte precursors in aplastic anemia, *Br. J. Haematol.*, 42, 371, 1979.
695. **Daneshbrod-Skibba, G., Shahidi, N. T., Becker, G. A., and Martin, J.,** Immune pancytopenia, *Br. J. Haematol.*, 43, 7, 1979.
696. **Nissen, C., Cornu, P., Gratwohl, A., and Speck, B.,** Peripheral blood cells from patients with aplastic anaemia in partial remission suppress growth of their own bone marrow precursors in culture, *Br. J. Haematol.*, 45, 233, 1980.
697. **Bacigalupo, A., Podesta, M., Mingari, M. C., Moretta, L., Van Lint, M. T., and Marmont, A.,** Immune suppression of hematopoiesis in aplastic anemia: activity of T lymphocytes, *J. Immunol.*, 125, 1449, 1980.
698. **Takaku, F., Suda, T., Mizoguchi, H., Miura, Y., Uchino, H., Nagai, K., Kariyone, S., Shibata, A., Akabane, T., Nomura, T., and Maekawa, T.,** Effect of peripheral blood mononuclear cells from aplastic anemia patients on the granulocyte-macrophage and erythroid colony formation in samples from normal human bone marrow *in vitro*—a cooperative study, *Blood,* 55, 937, 1980.
699. **Singer, J. W., Brown, J. E., James, M. C., Doney, K., Warren, R. P., Storb, R., and Thomas, E. D.,** Effect of peripheral blood lymphocytes from patients with aplastic anemia on granulocyte colony growth from HLA-matched and mismatched marrows: effect of transfusion sensitization, *Blood,* 52, 37, 1978.
700. **Singer, J. W., Doney, K. C., and Thomas, E. D.,** Coculture studies of 16 untransfused patients with aplastic anemia, *Blood,* 52, 37, 1978.
701. **Saunders, E. F. and Freedman, M. H.,** Constitutional aplastic anemia: defective haematopoietic stem cell growth *in vitro, Br. J. Haematol.*, 40, 277, 1978.

702. **Sullivan, R., Quesenbery, P. J., Parkman, R., Zuckerman, K. S., Levey, R. H., Rappeport, J., and Ryan, M.,** Aplastic anemia: lack of inhibitory effect of bone marrow lymphocytes on *in vitro* granulopoiesis, *Blood,* 56, 625, 1980.
703. **Broxmeyer, H. E., Pahwa, R., Jacobsen, N., Pelus, L. M., Ralph, P., Meyers, P. A., and Kapoor, N.,** Specific inhibitory activity against granulocyte-progenitor cells produced by non T-lymphocytes from patients with neutropenia, *Exp. Hematol.,* 8, 278, 1980.
704. **Pegoraro, L., Abrahm, J., Cooper, R. A., Levis, A., Lange, B., Meo, P., and Rovera, G.,** Differentiation of human leukemias in response to 12-0-tetradecanoylphorbol-13-acetate *in vitro, Blood,* 55, 859, 1980.
705. **Hoelzer, D., Kurrle, E., Schmucker, H., and Harriss, E. B.,** Evidence for differentiation of human leukemic blood cells in diffusion chamber culture, *Blood,* 49, 729, 1977.
706. **Hoelzer, D., Harriss, E. B., Bultman, B., Fliedner, T. M., and Heimpel, H.,** Differentiation into granulopoiesis in human acute leukemia and blast crisis in chronic myelocytic leukemia, in *Diffusion Chamber Culture,* Cronkite, E. P. and Carsten, A. L., Eds., Springer-Verlag, Berlin, 1980, 242.
707. **Lau, B., Staber, F. G., Netzel, B., Jager, G., Huhn, D., Thierfelder, S., Hiller, K., and Dormer, P.,** Granulopoietic activity of mononuclear blood cells from patients with cALL in diffusion chambers, submitted for publication.
708. **Nilsson, B., Olofsson, E., Olofsson, T., and Olsson, I.,** Proliferation and differentiation in diffusion chambers of marrow, blood and spleen cells from patients with chronic myeloid leukaemia during chronic phase and blastic transformation, *Scand. J. Haematol.,* 24, 381, 1980.
709. **Collins, S. J., Gallo, R. C., Gallagher, R. E.,** Continuous growth and differentiation of human myeloid leukemic cells in suspension culture, *Nature,* 270, 347, 1977.
710. **Collins, S. J., Ruscetti, F. W., Gallagher, R. E., and Gallo, R. C.,** Terminal differentiation of human promyelocytic leukemia cells induced by dimethyl sulfoxide and other polar compounds, *Proc. Natl. Acad. Sci. U.S.A.,* 75, 2459, 1978.
711. **Collins, S. J., Ruscetti, F. W., Gallagher, R. E., and Gallo, R. C.,** Normal functional characteristics of cultured human promyelocytic leukemia cells (HL-60) after induction of differentiation by dimethyl-sulfoxide, *J. Exp. Med.,* 149, 969, 1979.
712. **Gallagher, R., Collins, S., Trujillo, J., McCredie, K., Ahearn, M., Tsai, S., Metzgar, R., Aulakh, G., Ting, R., Ruscetti, F., and Gallo, R.,** Characterization of the continuous, differentiating myeloid cell line (HL-60) from a patient with acute promyelocytic leukemia, *Blood,* 54, 713, 1979.
713. **Collins, S. J., Bodner, A., Ting, R., and Gallo, R. C.,** Induction of morphological and functional differentiation of human promyelocytic leukemia cells (HL-60) by compounds which induce differentiation of murine leukemia cells, *Int. J. Cancer,* 25, 213, 1980.
714. **Breitman, T. R., Selonick, S. E., and Collins, S. J.,** Induction of differentiation of the human promyelocytic leukemia cell line (HL-60) by retinoic acid, *Proc. Natl. Acad. Sci. U.S.A.,* 77, 2936, 1980.
715. **Honma, Y., Takenaga, K., Kasukabe, T., and Hozumi, M.,** Induction of differentiation of cultured human promyelocytic cells by retinoids, *Biochem. Biophys. Res. Commun.,* 95, 507, 1980.
716. **Rovera, G., O'Brien, T. G., and Diamond, L.,** Induction of differentiation in human promyelocytic leukemia cells by tumor promoters, *Science,* 204, 868, 1979.
717. **Rovera, G., Olashaw, N., and Meo, P.,** Terminal differentiation in human promyelocytic leukemia cells in the absence of DNA synthesis, *Nature,* 284, 69, 1980.
718. **Huberman, E. and Callaham, M. F.,** Induction of terminal differentiation in human promyelocytic leukemia cells by tumor-promoting agents, *Proc. Natl. Acad. Sci. U.S.A.,* 76, 1293, 1979.
719. **Mendelsohn, N., Gilbert, H. S., Christman, J. K., and Acs, G.,** Effects of maturation on the response of human promyelocytic leukemia cells (HL-60) to the tumor promotor 12-O-tetradecanoylphorbol-13-acetate, *Cancer Res.,* 40, 1469, 1980.
720. **Mendelsohn, N., Michl, J., Gilbert, H., Acs, G., and Christman, J.,** L-Ethionine as an inducer of differentiation in human promyelocytic leukemia cells (HL-60), *Cancer Res.,* 40, 3206, 1980.
721. **Honma, Y., Fujita, Y., Okabe-Kado, J., Kasukabe, T., and Hozumi, M.,** Induction of differentiation of human promyelocytic leukemia cells (HL-60) by arginase, *Cancer Lett.* 10, 287, 1980.
722. **Niedel, J., Kahane, I., Lachman, L., and Cuatrecasas, P.,** A subpopulation of cultural human promyelocytic leukemia cells (HL-60) displays the formyl peptide chemotactic receptor, *Proc. Natl. Acad. Sci. U.S.A.,* 77, 1000, 1980.
723. **Crabtree, G. R.,** Fc receptors of a human promyelocytic leukemic cell line: evidence for two types of receptors defined by binding to the staphylococcal protein A-IgG complex, *J. Immunol.,* 125, 448, 1980.
724. **Gahmberg, C. G., Nilsson, K., and Andersson, L. C.,** Specific changes in the surface glycoprotein pattern of human promyelocytic leukemic cell line HL-60 during morphologic and functional differentiation, *Proc. Natl. Acad. Sci. U.S.A.,* 76, 4087, 1979.

725. **Boss, M. A., Delia, D., Robinson, J. B., and Greaves, M. F.,** Differentiation-linked expression of cell surface markers on HL-60 leukemic cells, *Blood,* 56, 910, 1980.
726. **Ip, S. H. C. and Cooper, R. A.,** Decreased membrane fluidity during differentiation of human promyelocytic leukemia cells in culture, *Blood,* 56, 227, 1980.
727. **Cabot, M. C., Welsh, C. J., Callaham, M. F., and Huberman, E.,** Alterations in lipid metabolism induced by 12-O-tetradecanoylphorphol-13-acetate in differentiating human myeloid leukemia cells, *Cancer Res.,* 40, 3674, 1980.
728. **Bodner, A. J., Tsai, S., Ting, R. C., Collins, S. J., and Gallo, R. C.,** Isolation and characterization of thioguanine resistant human promyelocytic leukemia cells, *Leuk. Res.,* 4, 151, 1980.
729. **Barnes, D. and Sato, G.,** Serum-free cell culture; a unifying approach, *Cell,* 22, 649, 1980.
730. **Brietman, T. R., Collins, S. J., and Keene, B. R.,** Replacement of serum by insulin and transferrin supports growth and differentiation of the human promyelocytic cell line, HL-60, *Exp. Cell Res.,* 126, 494, 1980.
731. **Olofsson, T. and Olsson, I.,** Suppression of normal granulopoiesis *in vitro* by a leukemia associated inhibitor (LAI) from a human promyelocytic cell line (HL-60), *Leuk. Res.,* 4, 437, 1980.
732. **Koeffler, H. P., Billing, R., Sparkes, R. S., and Golde, D. W.,** Antigens present on human myeloid leukemia cell lines, *Leuk. Res.,* 4, 69, 1980.
733. **Koeffler, H. P. and Golde, D. W.,** Acute myelogenous leukemia: a human cell line responsive to colony-stimulating activity, *Science,* 200, 1153, 1978.
734. **Koeffler, H. P. and Golde, D. W.,** Humoral modulation of human acute myelogenous leukemia cell growth *in vitro, Cancer Res.,* 40, 1858, 1980.
735. **Niskanen, E., Koeffler, H. P., Golde, D. W., and Cline, M. J.,** Responsiveness of a human myelogenous leukemia cell line (KG-1) to humoral factors *in vivo, Leuk. Res.,* 4, 203, 1980.
736. **Koeffler, H. P., Golde, D. W., and Lippman, M. E.,** Glucocorticoid sensitivity and receptors in cells of human myelogenous leukemia lines, *Cancer Res.,* 40, 563, 1980.
737. **Koeffler, H. P., Billing, R., Lusis, A. J., Sparkes, R., and Golde, D. W.,** An undifferentiated variant derived from the human acute myelogenous leukemia cell line (KG-1), *Blood,* 56, 265, 1980.
738. **Lozzio, B. B. and Lozzio, C. B.,** Properties and usefulness of the original K-562 human myelogenous leukemia cell line, *Leuk. Res.,* 3, 363, 1979.
739. **Sundstrom, C. and Nilsson, K.,** Establishment and characterization of a human histiocytic lymphoma cell line, *Int. J. Cancer,* 17, 565, 1976.
740. **Ralph, P., Moore, M. A. S., and Nilsson, K.,** Lysozyme synthesis by established human and murine histiocytic lymphoma cell lines, *J. Exp. Med.,* 143, 1528, 1976.
741. **Fibach, E., Landau, T., and Sachs, L.,** Normal differentiation of myeloid leukemic cells induced by a differentiation-inducing protein, *Nature,* 237, 276, 1972.
742. **Fibach, E., Hayashi, M., and Sachs, L.,** Control of normal differentiation of myeloid leukemic cells to macrophage and granulocytes, *Proc. Natl. Acad. Sci. U.S.A.,* 70, 343, 1973.
743. **Inbar, M., Ben-Bassat, H., Fibach, E., and Sachs, L.,** Mobility of carbohydrate-containing structures on the surface membrane and the normal differentiation of myeloid leukemic cells to macrophages and granulocytes, *Proc. Natl. Acad. Sci. U.S.A.,* 70, 2577, 1973.
744. **Lotem, J. and Sachs, L.,** Different blocks in the differentiation of myeloid leukemic cells, *Proc. Natl. Acad. Sci. U.S.A.,* 71, 3507, 1974.
745. **Fibach, E. and Sachs, L.** Control of normal differentiation of myeloid leukemic cells. IV. Induction of differentiation by serum from endotoxin treated mice, *J. Cell Physiol.,* 83, 177, 1974.
746. **Fibach, E. and Sachs, L.,** Control of normal differentiation of myeloid leukemic cells. VII. Induction of differentiation to mature granulocytes in mass culture, *J. Cell. Physiol.,* 86, 221, 1975.
747. **Lotem, J. and Sachs, L.,** Control of normal differentiation of myeloid leukemic cells. VI. Inhibition of cell multiplication and the formation of macrophages, *J. Cell. Physiol.,* 85, 587, 1975.
748. **Fibach, E. and Sachs, L.,** Control of normal differentiation of myeloid leukemic cells. XI. Induction of a specific requirement for cell viability and growth during the differentiation of myeloid leukemic cells, *J. Cell. Physiol.,* 89, 259, 1976.
749. **Vlodavsky, I., Fibach, E., and Sachs, L.,** Control of normal differentiation of myeloid leukemic cells. X. Glucose utilization, cellular ATP and associated membrane changes in D+ and D− cells, *J. Cell. Physiol.,* 87, 167, 1976.
750. **Fibach, E. and Sachs, L.,** Control of normal differentiation of myeloid leukemia cells. XI. Induction of a specific requirement for cell viability and growth during differentiation of myeloid leukemic cells, *J. Cell. Physiol.,* 89, 259, 1976.
751. **Lotem, J. and Sachs, L.,** Control of normal differentiation of myeloid leukemic cells. XII. Isolation of normal myeloid colony-forming cells from bone marrow and the sequence of differentiation to mature granulocytes in normal and D+ myeloid leukemic cells, *J. Cell. Physiol.,* 92, 97, 1977.

752. **Krystosek, A. and Sachs, L.,** Steroid hormone receptors and the differentiation of myeloid leukemic cells, *J. Cell. Physiol.*, 92, 345, 1977.
753. **Weiss, B. and Sachs, L.,** Indirect induction of differentiation in myeloid leukemic cells by lipid A, *Proc. Natl. Acad. Sci. U.S.A.*, 75, 1374, 1978.
754. **Maeda, S. and Sachs, L.,** Control of normal differentiation of myeloid leukemic cells. III. Inducibility for some stages of differentiation by dimethylsulfoxide and its disassociation from inducibility by MG1, *J. Cell. Physiol.*, 94, 181, 1978.
755. **Lotem, J. and Sachs, L.,** In vivo induction of normal differentiation in myeloid leukemia cells, *Proc. Natl. Acad. Sci. U.S.A.*, 75, 3781, 1978.
756. **Hoffman-Liebermann, B. and Sachs, L.,** Regulation of actin and other proteins in the differentiation of myeloid leukemic cells, *Cell,* 14, 825, 1978.
757. **Liebermann, D. and Sachs, L.,** Co-Regulation of type C RNA virus production and cell differentiation in myeloid leukemic cells, *Cell,* 15, 823, 1978.
758. **Lotem, J. and Sachs, L.,** Genetic dissociation of different cellular effects of interferon on myeloid leukemic cells, *Int. J. Cancer,* 22, 214, 1978.
759. **Lotem, J. and Sachs, L.,** Regulation of normal differentiation in mouse and human myeloid leukemic cells by phorbol esters and the mechanism of tumor promotion, *Proc. Natl. Acad. Sci. U.S.A.*, 76, 5158, 1979.
760. **Ichikawa, Y.,** Differentiation of a cell line of myeloid leukemia, *J. Cell. Physiol.*, 74, 223, 1970.
761. **Ichikawa, Y., Maeda, M., and Horiuchi, M.,** In vitro differentiation of Rauscher-virus-induced myeloid leukemia cells, *Int. J. Cancer,* 17, 789, 1976.
762. **Okabe, J., Honma, Y., and Hozumi, M.,** Differentiation of a resistant clone of mouse myeloid leukemia cells with dimethyl sulfoxide and ascitic fluids, *Jpn. J. Cancer Res.*, 68, 151, 1977.
763. **Honma, Y., Kasukabe, T., Okabe, J., and Hozumi, M.,** Glucocorticoid-induced differentiation of cultured mouse myeloid leukemia cells, *Jpn. J. Cancer Res.*, 68, 241, 1977.
764. **Maeda, M., Ichikawa, Y., and Azuma, I.,** Differentiation and production of colony-stimulating factor induced by immunostimulants in a leukemia cell line, *J. Cell. Physiol.*, 105, 33, 1980.
765. **Honma, Y., Kasukabe, T., Okabe, J., and Hozumi, M.,** Glucocorticoid binding and mechanism of resistance in some clones of mouse myeloid leukemic cells resistant to induction of differentiation by dexamethasone, *J. Cell. Physiol.*, 93, 227, 1978.
766. **Okabe, J., Hayashi, M., Honma, Y., and Hozumi, M.,** Differentiation of mouse myeloid leukemia cells is inhibited by a factor from nondifferentiating leukemia cells, *Int. J. Cancer,* 22, 570, 1978.
767. **Okabe, J., Honma, Y., Hayashi, M., and Hozumi, M.,** Actinomycin D restores *in vivo* sensitivity to differentiation induction of non-differentiating mouse myeloid leukemia cells, *Int. J. Cancer,* 24, 87, 1979.
768. **Nagata, K. and Ichikawa, Y.,** Requirements for RNA and protein synthesis in the induction of several differentiation-markers in a myeloid leukemia cell line, *J. Cell. Physiol.*, 98, 167, 1979.
769. **Hirai, K. I., Nagata, K., Maeda, M., and Ichikawa, Y.,** Changes in ultrastructures and enzyme activities during differentiation of myeloid leukemia cells to normal macrophages, *Exp. Cell Res.*, 124, 269, 1979.
770. **Honma, Y., Kasukabe, T., Okabe, J., and Hozumi, M.,** Replacement of serum by insulin, transferrin, albumin, phosphatidye choline, cholesterol, and some trace elements in cultures of mouse myeloid leukemia cells sensitive to inducers of differentiation, *Exp. Cell Res.*, 124, 421, 1979.
771. **Honma, Y., Kasukabe, T., Hozumi, M., and Koshihara, Y.,** Regulation of prostaglandin synthesis during differentiation of cultured mouse myeloid leukemia cells, *J. Cell. Physiol.*, 104, 349, 1980.
772. **Tomida, M., Yamamoto, Y., and Hozumi, M.,** Stimulation by interferon of induction of differentiation of mouse myeloid leukemic cells, *Cancer Res.*, 40, 2919, 1980.
773. **Maeda, M. and Ichikawa, Y.,** Production of a colony-stimulating factor following differentiation of leukemic myeloblasts to macrophages, *J. Cell. Physiol.*, 102, 323, 1980.
744. **Honma, Y., Kasukabe, T., and Hozumi, M.,** Changes in phospholipid composition during differentiation of cultured mouse myeloid leukemia cells, *Biochem. Biophys. Res. Commun.*, 93, 927, 1980.
775. **Nakayasu, M., Shimamura, S., Takeuchi, T., Sato, S., and Sugimura, T.,** A factor in human saliva that induces differentiation of mouse myeloid leukemia cells, *Cancer Res.*, 38, 103, 1978.
776. **Yamamoto, Y., Tomida, M., and Hozumi, M.,** Stimulation of differentiation of mouse myeloid leukemic cells and induction of interferon in the cells by double-stranded polyribonucleotidies, *Cancer Res.*, 39, 4170, 1980.
777. **Honma, Y., Kasukabe, T., Okabe, J., and Hozumi, M.,** Prolongation of survival time of mice inoculated with myeloid leukemia cells by inducers of normal differentiation, *Cancer Res.*, 39, 3167, 1979.
778. **Honma, Y., Kasukabe, T., and Hozumi, M.,** Inhibition of differentiation of cultured mouse myeloid leukemia cells by nonsteroidal antiinflammatory agents in counteraction of the inhibition by prostaglandin E, *Cancer Res.*, 39, 2190, 1979.

779. **Nakayasu, M., Shoji, M., Aoki, N., Sato, S., Miwa, M., and Sugimura, T.,** Enchancing effect of phorbol esters on induction of differentiation of mouse myeloid leukemia cells by human urinary protein and lipopolysaccharide, *Cancer Res.*, 39, 4668, 1979.
780. **Hozumi, M., Umezawa, T., Takenaga, K., Ohno, T., Shikita, M., and Yamane, I.,** Characterization of factors stimulating differentiation of mouse myeloid leukemia cells from a Yoshida, sarcoma cell line cultured in serum-free medium, *Cancer Res.*, 39, 5127, 1979.
781. **Yamamoto, Y., Tomida, M., and Hozumi, M.,** Production by mouse spleen cells of factors stimulating differentiation of mouse myeloid leukemic cells that differ from the colony-stimulating factor, *Cancer Res.*, 40, 4804, 1980.
782. **Sugiyama, K., Hozumi, M., and Okabe, J.,** Induction of differentiation of Rauscher virus-induced mouse myeloid leukemia cells with a factor(s) in ascitic fluid and inhibitors of nucleic acid and protein synthesis, *Cancer Res.*, 39, 1056, 1979.
783. **Takenaga, Hozumi, M., and Sakagami, Y.,** Effects of retinoids on induction of differentiation of cultured mouse myeloid leukemia cells, *Cancer Res.*, 40, 914, 1980.
784. **Fioritoni, G., Bertolini, L., Torlontano, G., and Revoltella, R.,** Cytochemical characteristics of leukopoietic differentiation in murine erythroleukemic (Friend) cells, *Cancer Res.*, 40, 866, 1980.
785. **Honma, Y., Kasukabe, T., and Hozumi, M.,** Relationships between leukemogenicity and *in vivo* inducibility of normal differentiation in mouse myeloid leukemia cells, *J. Natl. Cancer Inst.*, 61, 837, 1978.
786. **Tomida, M., Yamamoto, Y., and Hozumi, M.,** Inhibition of the leukemogenicity of myeloid leukemic cells in mice and *in vivo* induction of normal differentiation of the cells by poly (1) poly (c), *Jpn. J. Cancer Res.*, 71, 457, 1980.
787. **Honma, Y., Okabe, J., Kasukabe, T., and Hozumi, M.,** Survival of mice inoculated with non-differentiating myeloid leukemia cells is prolonged by the injection of an inducer of cell differentiation with a sensitizer, *Jpn. J. Cancer Res.*, 71, 543, 1980.
788. **Lotem, J. and Sachs, L.,** Potential pre-screening for theraputic agents that induce differentiation in human myeloid leukemic cells, *Int. J. Cancer,* 25, 561, 1980.
789. **Sachs, L.,** The differentiation of myeloid leukemia cells: new possibilities for therapy, *Br. J. Haematol.*, 40, 509, 1978.
790. **Sachs, L.,** Constitutive uncoupling of the controls for growth and differentiation in myeloid leukemia and the development of cancer, *J. Nat. Cancer Inst.*, 65, 675, 1980.
791. **Lotem, J., Lipton, J. H., and Sachs, L.,** Separation of different molecular forms of macrophage- and granulocytic-inducing proteins for normal and leukemic myeloid cells, *Int. J. Cancer,* 25, 763, 1980.
792. **Dexter, T. M., Garland, J., Scott, D., Scolnick, E., and Metcalf, D.,** Growth of factor-dependent hemopoietic precursor cell lines, *J. Exp. Med.*, 152, 1036, 1980.
793. **Todaro, G. J., De Larco, J. E., Marquardt, H., Bryant, M. L., Sherwin, S. A., and Sliski, A. H.,** Polypeptide growth factors produced by tumor cells and virus-transformed cells: a possible growth advantage for the producer cells, in *Hormones and Cell Culture,* Book A, Sato, G. H. and Ross, R., Eds., Cold Spring Harbor Laboratory, New York, 1979, 113.
794. **Todaro, G. J., Fryling, C., and De Larco, J. E.,** Transforming growth factors produced by certain human tumor cells: polypeptides that interact with epidermal growth factor receptors, *Proc. Natl. Acad. Sci. U.S.A.*, 77, 5258, 1980.
795. **De Larco, J. E. and Todaro, G. J.,** Growth factors from murine sarcoma virus-transformed cells, *Proc. Natl. Acad. Sci. U.S.A.*, 75, 4001, 1978.
796. **Todaro, G. J., De Larco, J. E., and Sporn, M. B.,** Retinoids block phenotypic cell transformation produced by sarcoma growth factor, *Nature,* 276, 272, 1978.
797. **Warner, N. L., Moore, M. A. S., and Metcalf, D.,** A transplantable myelomonocytic leukemia in Balb/c mice: cytology, karyotype and muramidase content, *J. Natl. Cancer Inst.*, 43, 963, 1969.
798. **Cline, M. J. and Metcalf, D.,** Cellular differentiation in a murine myelomonocytic leukemia, *Blood,* 39, 771, 1972.
799. **Metcalf, D., Moore, M. A. S., and Warner, N. L.,** Colony formation *in vitro* by myelomonocytic leukemic cells, *J. Natl. Cancer Inst.*, 43, 983, 1969.
800. **Metcalf, D. and Moore, M. A. S.,** Factors modifying stem cell proliferation of myelomonocytic leukemic cells *in vitro* and *in vivo, J. Natl. Cancer Inst.*, 44, 801, 1970.
801. **Broxmeyer, H. E.,** unpublished observations.
802. **Broxmeyer, H. E., and Winchester, R. J.,** unpublished observations.
803. **Broxmeyer, H. E. and Morrison, D. C.,** unpublished observations.
804. **Gentile, P., Broxmeyer, H. E. and Margolis, V. B.,** unpublished observations.
805. **Lu, L. and Broxmeyer, H. E.,** unpublished observations.
806. **Broxmeyer, H. E. and Pelus, H. M.,** unpublished observations.

807. **Pelus, L. M.,** unpublished observations.
808. **Hoelzer, D., Broxmeyer, H. E., and Bognacki, J.,** unpublished observations.
809. **Lu, L., Broxmeyer, H. E., Pelus, L. M., Moore, M. A. S., and Andreff, M.,** Detection of luxol-fast blue positive cells in human promyelocytic leukemia cell line, HL-60, *Exp. Hematol.,* 9, 887, 1981.

Chapter 7

MEGAKARYOCYTOPOIESIS: PROGENITOR POOL*

Alexander Nakeff

TABLE OF CONTENTS

*This work supported by Grant Numbers R01 AM/HL 28587 awarded by the National Institute of Arthritis, Diabetes, Digestive, and Kidney Diseases, DHHS. Alexander Nakeff is the recipient of Research Career Development Award HL 00440, awarded by the National Heart, Lung and Blood Institute, DHHS.

I. INTRODUCTION

Mammalian megakaryocytopoiesis is a unique and fascinating cell system whose uniqueness derives from its extreme contrasts.

Derived ultimately from small, morphologically unrecognized pluripotent and "committed" progenitor cells, megakaryocytes are clearly among the largest cells that are identified morphologically in hematopoietic tissue with cell diameters greater than 20 μm; indeed, their prefix "mega-" was aptly coined. In contrast to the predominant erythroid and myeloid elements, they and their progenitors constitute only an extremely small fraction (approximately 5×10^{-4} in rodent marrow, for example) of the cellular contents of these tissues. Furthermore, megakaryocytes contain a polyploid complement of deoxyribonucleic acid (DNA) constituting an increase greater than 32-fold that of diploid cells, and that is far beyond that observed in any other mammalian cell system; yet, the DNA remains contained within a single nucleus. We have only begun, in the most rudimentary fashion, to unravel the cellular mechanisms and modes of règulation that are responsible for this astounding redundancy in genetic information and can only speculate about the possible evolutionary advantage for such a fascinating development.

Megakaryocytes are also destined to self-destruct upon completion of a complex scheme of differentiation. During cytoplasmic development, they are truly incredible protein synthetic "factories" which individually produce, within a period of a few days, thousands of identical complex cytoplasmic structures, which upon their release into the peripheral circulation, constitute the blood platelets. The "birth" of platelets thus constitutes the "death" of the megakaryocyte.

Platelets, in contrast to their mother cells, are the smallest of the cells in peripheral blood (cell diameters of 1 to 2 μm) and yet next to erythrocytes constitute the second most plentiful. They are also among the most unique in mammalian tissues since they, together with erythrocytes, are anucleated. As with the polyploid nature of megakaryocytes, the evolutionary advantage of platelet anucleation remains speculative. Nevertheless, as cellular initiators of hemostasis that are also responsible fot the maintenance of vascular integrity, the physiologic importance of platelets to homeostasis is self-evident.

Following the first morphologic description of megakaryocytes almost 100 years ago, a large body of information, most of it qualitative and descriptive has been gathered on these cells through the prodigious efforts of a rather small group of investigators ("megakaryocytopoets?"). Nevertheless, even upon a cursory examination of this data, it is remarkable how deep our ignorance remains on fundamental questions of proliferation and differentiation. The most recent advances into understanding the previous "black box" of the megakaryocytic progenitor cell have, rather than clarified our previous concepts, possibly "raised our confusion to a higher level of incomprehension." We thus feel it essential in this treatise to assemble and critically analyze the most important aspects of this body of data with the view of proposing a new and hopefully more unifying concept of megakaryocytopoiesis. (See Chapter 12 on Thrombopoiesis, Volume II.)

II. PROGENITOR CELL COMPARTMENT

A. Cytokinetic Model of Megakaryocyte Production

The importance of the stem cell-megakaryocyte-platelet cell system lies in its production of blood platelets which are essential to the initiation of hemostasis and maintenance of the integrity of the blood vasculature. Platelets circulating in the peripheral blood are derived from megakaryocytes whose sole function it is to form platelets as anucleate fragments of their cytoplasm at the end stage of their maturation. Maturing megakaryocytes, in turn, are derived ultimately through a poorly understood process of differentiation or "commitment" of morphologically unrecognized progenitor cells. The latter cell compartment is composed of pluripotent stem cells capable of proliferation and eventually differentiation into either the erythrocytic, granulocytic-macrophage, lymphocytic or megakaryocytic cell lines, and cells committed solely to a given cell line, such as the progenitor cells of the megakaryocytic cell line. It is the latter compartment of cells which has received intensive interest of late and to which the focus of this section is directed.

A number of important technical innovations have contributed to recent advances in our understanding of the cell kinetics of hematopoiesis in general. Included among these are (1) the purification, assay, and mode of action of humoral regulators of hematopoiesis (erythropoietin and colony-stimulating activity [CSA]), (2) the establishment of clonogenic cell systems for erythrocytic, granulocytic-macrophage, and lymphocytic progenitor cells in culture to complement that for pluripotent stem cells in vivo, and (3) the use of gradient and, most recently, flow cytometric techniques for physically separating and defining various subpopulations of progenitors by functional cell assays. The impact of these advances is just beginning to be felt in the megakaryocyte-platelet system.[1,2] Various reviews and monographs adequately describe past efforts prior to these advances which have been limited to a descriptive analysis of the maturing megakaryocyte compartment and the process of platelet formation.[2a–17] Few incursions have been made into the direct study of specific humoral regulators and their cellular modes of action. The lack of quantitative cellular assays and the use of generally poor bioassays for such regulators are contributing factors in this respect. More recently, however, specific advances have generated much renewed interest in this cell system and its control, among which may be listed:

1. The characterization and, in some cases, the physical isolation of megakaryocytes based on differences in their size,[18–26] density, [20,24,27] and DNA content[25,28,29]
2. The establishment of clonogenic assays in vitro for studying megakaryocyte proliferation in rodent[30–36] and human marrow and blood[37–41] as well as in vitro techniques for supporting megakaryocyte differentiation through to possible platelet formation[27,33,34,42–45]
3. The cytochemical and immunofluorescent detection of megakaryocytes, and particularly their progenitors, in rodent marrow[46–49] and human marrow[39–41,50] although use of methanol-inhibitable phosphatase[82] is somewhat in dispute[51,52]
4. The isolation of a possible humoral platelet regulator,[53–56] its possible physiologic site of production,[57] and its production by human embryonic kidney cells[58] as well as the identification of potential regulators of megakaryocyte proliferation and differentiation[31,32,34,41,59–61]
5. The demonstration that megakaryocytes are capable of active, net synthesis of platelet-associated proteins and activities, including factor VIII antigen,[62] actin,[63] platelet-derived growth factor,[64] and thromboxane B2[26]
6. The discovery that the process of megakaryocytopoiesis in certain genetically-anemic mice is abnormal and may result from a specific genetic defect[65–71] whose possible origin has been traced back to the progenitor cell compartment[72]

A useful approach to the underlying complexity and uniqueness of this cell system is to compartmentalize those cells that are either morphologically or functionally distinguishable as shown schematically in Figure 1.

The pluripotent stem cell compartment is characterized by the following: (1) it has

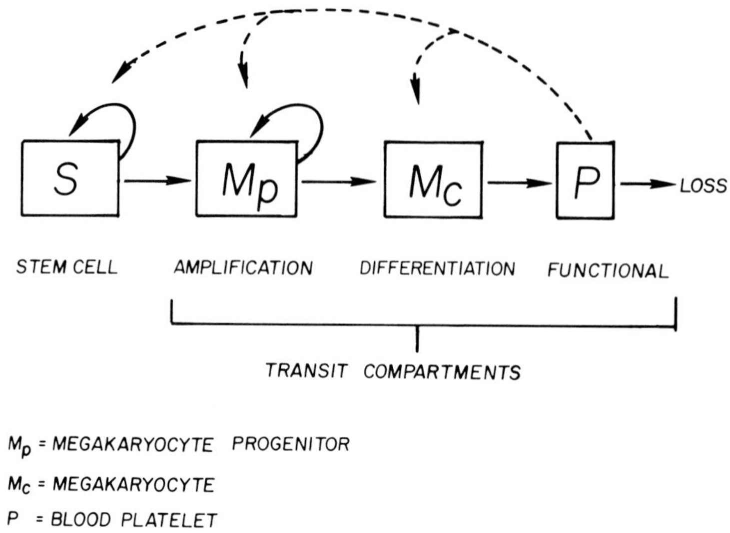

FIGURE 1. Schematical display of a simplified model of megakaryocytopoiesis indicating the major cell compartments and their functions. The loops within a compartment symbolize cell proliferation while the dotted lines denote feedback regulation.

cell input and is self-maintaining, i.e., cellular proliferation occurs within the compartment; (2) it supplies cells as output which either are, or give rise to, differentiated cells; and (3) it responds to regulation (either cell-to-cell or possibly long- or short-range humoral).

Although the three different transit cell compartments are rather straightforward as presented in Figure 1, they mask what must be a complex series of cellular events that take place normally under homeokinetic control. Certainly the most complex of the three is the amplification compartment (Mp) since it probably represents those cells that are capable of undergoing one or more mitotic cell divisions to increase the number of megakaryocyte progenitor cells as well as those that are capable of endoreduplicating their DNA content to produce populations of polyploid cells at several ploidy values. The initial step of ''commitment'' that draws a pluripotent stem cell into the amplification compartment is an obviously important and basic biological phenomenon. Its definition will probably have to await more direct approaches than those presently available since it is a common step taken by progenitors committed to other lines of differentiation which are generally better known, but have yet to yield much useful information in this regard. It is presently not clear whether progenitors that are not morphologically identified but that can be detected by either their acetylcholinesterase activity (in rodents) or their binding of specific antiplatelet antibodies, are capable of cell proliferation. There are no direct studies on this aspect although new approaches to this important question have been proposed.[73]

Upon leaving the amplification compartment, progenitors (Mp) become morphologically recognizable as megakaryocytes (Mc) and enter a period of cytoplasmic differentiation which procedes in the absence of any futher concomitant cell division. There is evidence, however, from flash-label-tritiated thymidine uptake studies and autoradiography that a small number of morphologically immature megakaryocytes are capable of endoreduplicative DNA synthesis. It would appear that megakaryocytes that can be identified by conventional cytology are in a stage of differentiation leading, at the end of about 2.5 days in rodents, to the eventual formation and release of about 5000 platelets from each megakaryocyte.[3,5] The peripheral blood platelets are thus the functional end-product of this complex series of steps and as such are either utilized in the maintenance of vascular integrity and microclot formation or die through senescence with a half-life in the rodent of about 1.5 days.

Several important factors, of course, have not been taken into consideration in this simplistic cell model. These include: (1) the relationship between cell mitosis and nuclear endoreduplication since megakaryocytes, being among the few uniquely polyploid mammalian cells, must be produced from progenitor cells capable of undergoing both proliferation in the conventional sense (i.e., mitosis) and a duplication of their DNA in the absence of cytokinesis (i.e., nuclear endoreduplication); (2) the demonstration that platelet protein synthesis (i.e., cytoplasmic differentiation) occurs in megakaryocytes at all ploidy classes, thus implying that nuclear proliferation and cytoplasmic differentiation are mutually exclusive processes[12,14,16] although this has been disputed;[74,75] (3) the observation that a small proportion of exclusively immature megakaryocytes incorporate tritiated thymidine and are thus capable of vestigial DNA synthesis[12,14,16] although the largest degree of DNA synthesis takes place in progenitors that have defied any morphologic characterization; (4) the specific cytochemical (acetylcholinesterase) and immunofluorescent marking of a class of progenitors that would otherwise have escaped detection by conventional cytological characterization since their relatively small size precluded their identification as a megakaryocytic cell;[46–48,75a,75b] and (5) a critical analysis of megakaryocyte kinetics that upon theoretical grounds leads to the inevitable conclusion that a class of progenitors must exist that contain a polyploid amount of DNA and yet are too small in size and nondescript in morphology to be classified as megakaryocytes.[9]

A more comprehensive cell model is presented schematically in Figure 2. Upon theoretical considerations, a committed progenitor cell compartment is proposed composed exclusively of diploid cells which are derived from the pluripotent stem cell and are capable of mitotic proliferation as depicted by the closed loop. The question of whether CFU-M comprise this compartment or that it may be composed of several subpopulations of cells rather than a single population remains moot at this time.

Progenitors would leave this compartment by undergoing endoreduplication (e$\underset{\rightarrow}{R}$) and thus enter the earliest polyploid progenitor compartment. Both sets of compartments would be composed of cells that are not morphologically identified by conventional cytology, but may possibly be detected by functional criteria. These include the degree of cell proliferation measured in a clonogenic assay in vitro or DNA content measured microspectrophotometrically on an individual cell basis or cytoplasmic markers, such as acetylcholinesterase (AChE) activity or platelet-associated protein (PAP) synthetic activity. The question of whether polyploid (4C and 8C) progenitors are capable of mitotic activity remains to be answered and is depicted by a closed loop enclosing a question mark for 4C and 8C progenitors. There is some question as to whether 16C and 32C progenitors can exist in a morphologically unrecognized state since it seems reasonable that their larger content of DNA would necessarily be reflected in a larger cell volume which is a major criterion for their morphologic identification. Odell and Jackson,[75c] Paulus,[75] and MacPherson[76] have combined microspectrophotometric analyses of the total DNA in individual megakaryocytes and autoradiography to show that the earliest megakaryocytes that can be recognized by conventional morphology have a ploidy value of at least 8C and that they can also incorporate tritiated thymidine. Recent work by Jackson[46] has identified progenitors in rat marrow that are morpholog-

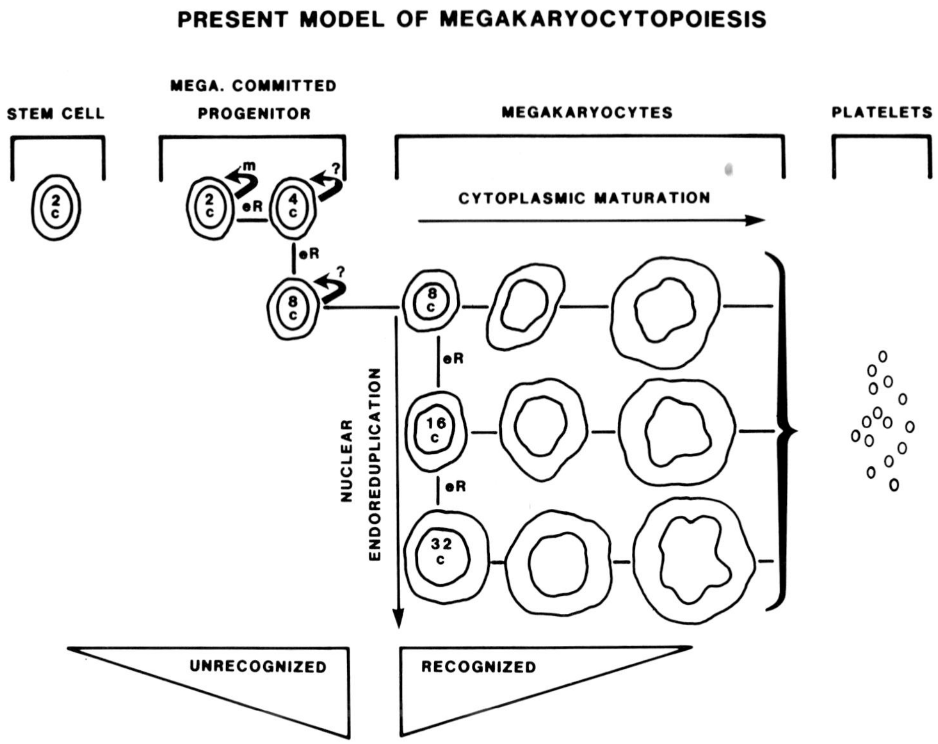

FIGURE 2. A working model of megakaryocytopoiesis. Proliferation indicated by closed loops although there is some question of this in polyploid progenitors.

ically unrecognized (i.e., very small), but that stain specifically for AChE activity and physiologically respond to platelet demand. Although no determination has been made of their ploidy, it may be that these cells have polyploid DNA values.

Since it is rather clear from numerous studies[75,75c,76] that platelet protein synthesis may begin in megakaryocytes at all ploidy levels from 4 to 32C, the "trigger" to initiate maturation may be responsible for increasing the overall cellular volume (basically cytoplasmic) in these cells such that polyploid progenitors with ploidy as low as 4C become morphologically recognizable. These cells could be depicted then as being the most immature, i.e., in Stage I of cytoplasmic maturation. This would account for the movement of morphologically unrecognized polyploid progenitor cells to the recognized and maturing cell compartment without any endoreduplicative step among these progenitors necessarily being a prerogative for recognition. On the other hand, it seems reasonable that some of the polyploid progenitors may go through one or more endoreduplicative steps before commencement of maturation as shown in Figure 2. The small number of immature megakaryocytes that label with tritiated thymidine within 30 min are probably in the process of endoreduplication.[76a] They are depicted in Figure 2 as a series of nuclear endoreduplicative steps leading from lower to higher ploidy within Stage I megakaryocytes. Megakaryocytes may also differentiate cytoplasmically, a process characterized by high rates of platelet protein synthesis directed towards the synthesis of platelet-associated proteins and the packaging and covering of intracellular platelet components with a plasma membrane; platelet release concludes the final stage of megakaryocyte differentiation.

The development and use of clonogenic assays for various classes of hemopoietic cell progenitors has provided a great deal of information and insight into the cellular kinetics and control of hematopoiesis.[77–79] Renewed interest and emphasis on the problem of the regulation of megakaryocytopoiesis has most recently been initiated with the advent of in vitro techniques for detecting population(s) of specific progenitor cells (colony-forming unit, megakaryocyte or CFU-M) that are responsible for colonial growth of megakaryocytes in plasma culture[32,33,36,80] and semisolid agar.[30,31,34,35] As megakaryocytes themselves are nonproliferative, the progenitor compartments, including CFU-M, are clearly the important areas in which homeostatic regulation is exerted. In this section, we will summarize the current state of our knowledge concerning the cellular composition and physiologic role of this progenitor cell compartment in terms of its proliferative activity and speculate upon its role in response to altered demands for peripheral blood platelets.

B. Cytokinetic Analysis

Advances over the past few years have made it possible to approach the question of the basic cellular biology defining the megakaryocytic progenitor cell compartment in an attempt to understand how complex control mechanisms regulate it at several levels including mitosis, nuclear endoreduplication, and cytoplasmic maturation. Some of these approaches are proven techniques such as autoradiography and microspectrophotometry of DNA content while others are relatively new, such as repopulation assays, clonogenic cell assays both in vivo and in vitro, cytochemical and immunological markers, and flow cytometric analysis. The viability of some of the newer approaches may be somewhat compromised by theoretical and technical limitations; yet, there is every reason to believe that we are on the threshold of what promises to be a rapid exploitation of this system using these new techniques.

1. Radioisotope Labeling

The application of tritiated thymidine labeling to megakaryocytes strengthened the concept that the morphologically recognized megakaryocytes were not mitotic, and at the same time opened up considerable controversy about the nature and cytokinetic behavior of the progenitor cell. In humans injected with tritiated thymidine, labeled megakaryocytes were observed to increase up to 5 days after a single exposure.[81] This observation was explained by the authors as reflecting an influx of labeled progenitor cells replacing the differentiated cells lost through platelet shedding.

When these studies were repeated in rats,[81a–81c] it was suggested that the immediate progenitor of the megakaryocyte was endomitotic,* and that differentiation preceded DNA synthesis in the absence of mitosis of the progenitor. This conclusion was based upon Ebbe and Stohlman's observation[81a] that the immature megakaryocyte labeling index increased with no concomitant change in the mean grain count of these cells. However, these authors also warned that the prolonged, high degree of megakaryocyte labeling was probably due to reutilization of labeled DNA from extruded red cell nuclei which also labeled with tritiated thymidine.[82]

To deal with this technical problem, Feinendegen et al.[81b] employed ^{125}I-D(5-iodo-2′-deoxyuridine) to label megakaryocyte DNA. This analog was not reutilized because of the iodine replacing the methyl group on the fifth carbon on the thymidine nucleus; although it can still be incorporated into DNA to a small extent, ^{125}I-deoxyuridine is rapidly catabolized upon hydrolysis of the DNA polymer. These experiments implicated

*The terms "endomitosis" and nuclear "endoreduplication" are used synonymously throughout this chapter to describe the duplication of DNA in the absence of cytokinesis. This is in keeping with their use in the literature on megakaryocytes, although reference to polyploidy in other cell systems may make a distinction between the processes described by those terms.

reutilization when it was observed that the labeling indices for the two compounds were identical during early periods following exposure, but that ^{125}I-deoxyuridine labeling decreased after several days while tritiated thymidine remained elevated. However, Feinendegen et al.[81b] reconfirmed the observation that proliferating cells, unidentified by morphological criteria, must reside kinetically between differentiating megakaryocytes and the pluripotent hemopoietic stem cell, since even 3 days after injection, 30% of the immature rat megakaryocytes were still labeled. This 3-day labeling period may represent the time spent by these progenitors in the proliferative compartment.

2. *Cell Markers*

The morphological identification of the megakaryocytic progenitor cell compartment remains to be defined. Recent advances, utilizing cytochemical and immunologic markers as well as electron microscopy, have begun to provide some measure of the heterogeneity and cellular complexity characterizing this early stage of differentiation.

a. Cytochemical

The early work of Zajicek[75a,75b] established the potential usefulness of the histochemical localization of acetylcholinesterase (AChE) activity in megakaryocytes of various species. In careful studies on the AChE content of individual megakaryocytes, Zajicek[75b] showed clearly that moving up the evolutionary scale from rodents through to humans resulted in a steady shift of positivity for this enzyme activity. Megakaryocytes were the only positive cells in rodents (erythrocytes being completely negative) with erythrocytes being the predominantly positive cells in humans and megakaryocytes exhibiting no activity. The function of this activity in megakaryocytes remains obscure. It is tempting to speculate that this activity may have some importance in mediating contractile megakaryocytic proteins since megakaryocytes have recently been shown to undergo dramatic shape changes in vitro in response to agents such as ADP.[83]

Jackson[46] utilized the simplified and more broadly applied technique of Karnovsky and Roots[84] for localizing the final enzyme product to identify a class of progenitor cells in rat bone marrow that was AChE-positive but otherwise too small ($<129\mu m^2$) to be classified as being megakaryocytic. These AChE-positive progenitors also responded physiologically to platelet demand. Their increase in number preceding the well-characterized increase in morphologically recognized megakaryocytes in rats recovering from an immune-induced thrombocytopenia suggested a mother-daughter relationship between the AChE-positive progenitors and their differentiated product, the megakaryocyte. This important finding and methodology was used subsequently by Nakeff and Daniels-McQueen[32] to more unequivocally identify megakaryocytic colonies in plasma culture, particularly those that were composed of immature megakaryocytic cells. Jackson[47] later showed that the same small cells that were AChE-positive also labeled specifically with a rabbit antirat platelet antibody conjugated with fluorescein isothiocyanate (FITC). This relationship was extended by Long and Henry.[48] They demonstrated that a thrombocythemia induced in rats by injections of fresh rat platelets resulted in a cessation of megakaryocytopoiesis preceded by a fall in the small, AChE-positive progenitors. These studies provided further evidence of a potential progenitor-product relationship alluded to earlier in Jackson's study.[47]

There still remained the question of whether the small, AChE-positive cells were capable of proliferative activity, i.e., could form megakaryocytic colonies in vitro, and to what degree these cells were polyploid. Studies by Nakeff and Floeh[27] using discontinuous bovine albumin density gradients to isolate rodent marrow megakaryocytes indicated that the small AChE-positive progenitors could be physically separated from the colony-formers (CFU-M) on the basis of density. The latter were characterized by a density profile with a peak at 1.076 g/mℓ whereas the small, AChE-positive cells displayed a density profile that overlapped that for the recognized megakaryocyte population with a peak at 1.1 g/mℓ. Unfortunately, no direct test of the proliferative activity of the small, AChE-positive cells is possible since the cells have to be fixed prior to the staining with acetylthiocholine in order to visualize the reaction product. Our attempts to demonstrate AChE activity in these progenitors in unfixed marrow cells suspended in the reaction mixture have been unsuccessful. We also do not know whether this treatment adversely affects the viability of these progenitors. In this regard, an interesting fluorescence technique has been published by Prince.[85] It utilizes a specific enzyme substrate that when acted upon by acetylcholinesterase becomes a fluorescent product. Although the sensitivity of this assay is in the nanogram range, the enzyme substrate used is not available commercially and must be synthesized. Whether the fluorescent reaction product will remain within the cell is also not known. Nevertheless, the availability sometime in the future of similar substrates specific for particular enzymes of interest that do not interfere with the target cell's viability raises the possibility of utilizing flow cytometry and cell sorting to isolate potential megakaryocytic progenitors for analysis of their ploidy and proliferative activity as outlined by Nakeff.[73] No information exists on the ploidy distribution of the small, AChE-positive progenitors since technical problems prevent simultaneous Feulgen staining and scanning microdensitometric analyses to be made of the DNA of cells that are AChE positive.[86]

In summary, it would appear that the small, AChE-positive progenitors may be a class of progenitors distinct from CFU-M, at least on the basis of buoyant density.[27] It is too premature to make an unequivocal statement about the nonproliferative role of the former since new techniques in the future may make it possible to test this relationship more directly. It could be that the small, AChE-positive progenitors are capable only of nuclear endoreduplication. If so, they might constitute a class of cells that has to be replenished by differentiation from the preceding CFU-M. These cells may themselves differentiate cytoplasmically into the most immature megakaryocyte compartment.

b. Immunological

In recent years, ever-increasing use is being made of fluoresceinated-immunologic probes specific for various hematopoietic progenitor cells. Monospecific antisera or monoclonal antibodies appropriately labeled with a fluorescent dye have been used which generally are specific for one or another membrane or cytoplasmic component of platelets.

Jackson[47] was the first to identify small cells in rat marrow that were labeled with a FITC-conjugated rabbit antirat platelet antiserum (RARPS) but that otherwise were not identified morphologically as megakaryocytes. He also showed that (1) the same population of cells stained for AchE activity, and (2) that this population exhibited a similar response as the small AchE-positive progenitors to an immune-induced thrombocytopenia. He concluded that the small AchE-positive cells and the small, RARPS-positive cells were probably the same population of megakaryocyte progenitors. Two other questions remain to be answered if the use of specific antiplatelet antibodies to probe progenitor populations is to be of value; namely, (1) what is the specific membrane structure or cytoplasmic protein determinant against which the antibody is being directed when it is raised in the rabbit to a cell concentrate of mouse platelets, and (2) what relation does the platelet determinant in the progenitor cell bear to the subsequent differentiation and possible proliferation of the target progenitor cell?

Clearly, the antibody raised to whole platelets is complex in that it is directed to numerous undefined antigenic determinants, even though it may be highly specific to platelets. Most recently, the work of McEver et al.[87] and Mazur et al.[40] has extended this approach to more specific antigenic determinants on human platelets. Specifically, McEver et al.[87] have produced a purified, monoclonal IgG (Tab) antibody directed to the glycoprotein IIb-IIIa complex on human platelets. The hybridoma technique involved the fusion of spleen cells from Balb/ C mice immunized with human platelets to a mouse myeloma cell line (Sp2/0-Ag 14). The monoclonal was used to demonstrate the presence on normal human platelets of the glycoprotein IIb-IIIa complex and its absence from the surface of human thrombasthenic platelets. The monoclonal binds to human megakaryocytes and may thus prove to be useful as a more specific marker of progenitor cells. Mazur et al.[41] applied an indirect immunofluorescent technique with a heterologous antihuman platelet glycoprotein antiserum to the identification in vitro of human bone marrow megakaryocyte colonies, especially those composed of small, morphologically unidentified megakaryocytic cells which previously had escaped detection.[37,38] Rabellino et al.[49] have presented preliminary results using a similar indirect immunofluorescence technique identifying small megakaryocytic progenitors that are positive for Factor VIII antigen and platelet-derived growth factor.

Inherent in these approaches which utilize platelet-associated protein markers is the underlying assumption that these phenotypic markers are expressed at a very early stage of megakaryocytic differentiation. It is at this stage that the positive cells remain undetected morphologically and are not just immature but still recognized megakaryocytes. It is probably safe to say that the use of fluoresceinated antibodies to specific platelet-associated proteins together with flow cytometry and cell sorting will be an area of active research over the next few years. The ability to isolate large numbers of megakaryocytes with high degrees of purity[24,26] and their subfractionation into various DNA classes[28] makes it possible for the first time to produce different classes of monoclonal antibodies specific to each ploidy class, if indeed different ploidy classes express different membrane antigenic determinants. A series of specific monoclonal antibodies together with flow cytometry might be used to isolate megakaryocyte subclasses for subsequent biochemical or enzymatic analysis.

3. *Platelet Repopulating Ability (PRA)*

This cellular approach to the study of stem cell differentiation into thrombocytopoiesis established by Goodman et al.[88] measures the capacity of progenitor cells to produce mature blood cells. This platelet repopulating ability (PRA) assay is similar to those devised earlier to measure the restoration of erythropoiesis[89,90] and granulopoiesis.[91] Here, the endogenous hematopoiesis of the recipient animals is first compromised. They are then engrafted with the hematopoietic tissue to be tested. In this PRA assay, Goodman et al.[88] counted blood platelets in irradiated (950R) C3H/HeJ mice 14 days after their engraftment with syngeneic bone marrow. The platelet counts obtained were proportional to the number of marrow cells injected and thus served as a measure of the ability of grafted megakaryocytic progenitor cells to support thrombocytopoiesis. An interesting observation was made comparing the similarity in response between the fraction of cells surviving 200 rad of whole-body radiation as measured by the PRA assay and that for the granulocytic repopulating ability, both assayed at various times after irradiation. Using direct clonogenic cell assays for the megakaryocytic (CFU-M) and granulocyte-macrophage (CFU-GM) progenitor cells, we have shown that they not only exhibit similar recovery kinetics following irradiation but also they have identical dose response relationships with a D_0 = 128 rad.[94]

Although repopulating assays have proven to be useful measures of committed progenitor cells, they are necessarily indirect. Thus, although relative sensitivities of various perturbations or agents for one or another repopulating cell line can be determined with these assays, the lack of a direct measure of the specific progenitor involved compromises the cell kinetic interpretation of the results.

4. Clonogenic Cell Assay

From previous theoretical considerations (Figure 2), it is reasonable to assume that there must exist a class of early megakaryocytic progenitors which are diploid and capable of cell division. These cells would, by definition, be the source from which the polyploid progenitors would derive and into which pluripotent stem cells would enter upon being committed to megakaryocytic differentiation. The ability of these cells to divide mitotically should be reflected in their ability to form colonies of megakaryocytes when injected into lethally irradiated syngeneic recipients and assayed microscopically in vivo as purely megakaryocytic spleen colonies or when placed in semisolid medium in tissue culture.

a. Spleen Colony Assay

The spleen colony assay of Till and McCulloch[93] was the first quantitative cellular assay for the pluripotent stem cell in rodent marrow. The assay measured the ability of stem cells in hematopoietic tissue to repopulate a syngeneic, lethally irradiated recipient as reflected in the number of splenic nodules that appeared some 9 to 10 days later. Each colony regardless of cell type cell bore a radiation-induced chromosomal marker, thus providing evidence of the clonal nature of each spleen colony. Each stemcell giving rise to a colony was referred to as a colony-forming unit, spleen or CFU-S.

The early work of Ebbe et al.[94,95] rested on the demonstration that the number of megakaryocytes, whether present singly or in a colony, and assayed in "representative" histological sections of spleens from lethally irradiated recipients injected with either normal or thrombocytopenic syngeneic marrow, was related linearly to the number of marrow cells injected. A large degree of variability was evident. The relationship of megakaryocytes (m) to spleen colonies (c) expressed as the m/c ratio was used in these studies as a measure of megakaryocyte production by the transplanted CFU-S. In an attempt to define more clearly the relationship between the number of circulating peripheral blood platelets and stem cell differentiation, Ebbe et al.[94,95] studied the stem cell response in bone marrow and spleen to thrombocytopenia. Bone marrow and spleen cells were obtained from CFI mice 1 day after they were rendered thrombocytopenic by several injections each of 0.1 mℓ of a 1:3 of 1:5 dilution of rabbit antimouse platelet serum (RAMPS) given intraperitoneally for either 2, 4, or 6 daily injections and then transplanted into lethally irradiated syngeneic recipients. The number of CFU-S in the spleen and femur of thrombocytopenic mice was increased over that for control mice injected with normal rabbit serum. Although the thrombocytopenia was able to modify the number of CFU-S directly, it had no effect on the ability of these CFU-S to differentiate, as indicated by an m/c ratio in the spleens of the irradiated recipients receiving either thrombocytopenic spleen or marrow cells that was observed to be unaffected by the depth and duration of the platelet demand in the donors. Also, this ratio was not significantly different from the control.

These results were interpreted to mean that the humoral mediator of platelet production (= thrombopoietin), which was produced in response to the thrombocytopenia, did not act directly on the pluripotent CFU-S. Rather, thrombopoietin acted on the committed megakaryocytic progenitor cell such that the resultant depopulation or proliferation in that compartment, in turn, affected the pluripotent stem cell compartment by local feedback mechanisms. In studies which were reported in abstract form,[96] we enumerated purely megakaryocytic spleen colonies. Stem cell-rich bone marrow fractions obtained by albumin density gradient centrifugation were obtained from mice made thrombocytopenic by three daily intravenous injections of RAMPS. Three days of induced thrombocytopenia was sufficient to increase the number of purely megakaryocytic colonies threefold, from 2% in the control (which received normal rabbit serum) to 6% in the marrow of thrombocytopenic mice. The number of CFU-S in the thrombocytopenic group was similar to that in the control. The colonies obtained were larger than in the control being composed of 10 to 30 megakaryocytes/colony. We interpret this data to indicate that a demand for platelets can modify the differentiation of marrow CFU-S and increase the degree of proliferation within these colonies.

More recently, McDonald et al.[97] tested the effect of a thrombopoietin preparation obtained from human embryonic kidney cells[58] on megakaryocytic spleen colony formation. Thrombopoietin treated recipients showed an increase in the number of megakaryocytic colonies in their spleens as compared to the appropriate controls, although the difference was not significant statistically. The number of CFU-S/spleen was unaffected as we had shown previously[96] although the number of megakaryocytes/spleen colony did increase, an observation also similar to what we had shown earlier.[96]

Goldberg et al.[98] studied whether hypertransfusion of platelets at different times after irradiation and transplantation of bone marrow cells would suppress megakaryocyte production in hematopoietic splenic colonies. CF1 mice were lethally irradiated (950R), injected with 10^5 normal, nucleated marrow cells, then injected with platelet concentrates sufficient to raise platelet levels about 2 to 2.5 × normal at early times (days 1 and 2), later times (days 6 and 7), and daily throughout the subsequent 10 day period prior to spleen colony harvest. Only the latter two treatments resulted in a reduction in the number of purely megakaryocytic colonies. In no case was there ever a significant change in the number of CFU-S. On the basis of these results, the authors concluded that the committed megakaryocyte progenitor cells (which were thought to be assayed only at times later than 3 to 4 days following marrow transplantation) were more sensitive to inhibition by increased platelet levels than CFU-S. It is generally agreed that the initial decrease in CFU-S during the first 2 days after transplantation into lethally irradiated, syngeneic recipients is partly due to differentiation of CFU-S and thus their loss from the assayable, pluripotent stem cell pool. However, it is not clear to what degree this early insensitive period of the stem cell to humoral influences is the result of differentiation or recruitment into a humorally insensitive part of the cell cycle. Although the spleen colony assay provides some measure of megakaryocyte production from the pluripotent stem cell, its interpretation of megakaryocyte progenitor cytokinetics is complex and may be misleading. This data should be interpreted with great caution.

b. Colony Formation In Vitro (CFU-M)

In an endeavor to assay functionally for these progenitors in vitro, we established the first successful set of conditions that permitted the culturing of megakaryocytic progenitors in thin layer agar cultures of stem-cell enriched mouse bone marrow following drug pretreatment of donors in vivo.[99] At about the same time, Porter and Gengozian[42] also reported the appearance of megakaryocyte-like cells in liquid cultures. These new experimental approaches seemed promising and subsequent efforts by our group[30,32] and independently by Metcalf et al.[31] resulted in the first reports of the successful growth of colonies in culture. Unequivocal identification of these colonies and their routine quantitation *in situ* proved equivocal in agar since more specific staining methods could not easily be applied. The successful culturing of megakaryocyte colonies in a plasma culture system[32] permitted the transfer of an entire microculture to a slide for *in situ* AChE staining as a specific cytochemical marker for rodent megakaryocytes and their progenitors. We entitled the progenitor giving rise to megakaryocyte colonies in this culture system, the colony-forming unit, megakaryocyte, or CFU-M. This work established the culture conditions and time course of appearance of these colonies and the cell dose range over which the assay could be used quantitatively. Subsequently, McLeod et al.,[33] used this system to report the growth of megakaryocyte colonies from mouse marrow in the presence of erythropoietin with subsequent platelet formation in vitro as revealed by electron microscopy.

We presented evidence of possible platelet formation in plasma culture at the light microscopic level,[44] and the effects of irradiation and drug treatment (cyclophosphamide) on CFU-M as well as other clonogenic marrow progenitors.[99] Williams et al.[34] established long-term (4 to 10 weeks) liquid cultures of CFU-M and megakaryocytes from mouse marrow. He demonstrated that medium from a mouse myelomonocytic leukemic cell line (WEHI-3) supported the growth of CFU-M from these cultures in agar which was "potentiated" by conditioned medium from the original liquid bone marrow cultures.

Williams et al.[100] have extended their studies to define the potentiator cells in more detail. They have identified them as being a population of adherent cells present in bone marrow, lung, bone shafts, and peritoneal exudates as well as certain macrophage cell lines (J774 and P388D1) which are capable of elaborating a potentiation activity that enhances the colony stimulating activity present in WEHI-3 cell conditioned medium.

The most recent work of Vainchenker et al.[37,38] and Mazur et al.[40,41] has established culture conditions that permit the growth of megakaryocyte colonies from fetal and adult human marrow as well as peripheral blood. Important work by Levin et al.[101,102] has amplified our ideas of the physiologic role played by CFU-M in response to platelet demand and provided insight into the ploidy distribution of megakaryocytes within colonies in vitro.[102] Chromosomal evidence has been provided by McLeod et al.,[103] growing CFU-M in the presence of eythropoietin that suggests the existence of a bipotential progenitor cell population prior to the CFU-M which can either differentiate into megakaryocytes or erythroid cells. Finally, the most recent report by Weinstein et al.[104] has provided a morphological and biochemical characterization of a long-term tissue culture line of cells derived originally from rat marrow that are identified tentatively as promegakaryoblasts.

These major developments are having a profound impact on our previous "blackbox" knowledge of the progenitor cells. Experimental tools are available that permit the quantitative analysis of proliferative events in culture and eventual differentiation steps that go to complete platelet formation. Thus regulatory mechanism can now be studied as well as the role of different stimulators and inhibitors of CFU-M.

Table 1 summarizes the cell properties of CFU-M that are known to date. It is evident that this culture system is being exploited rapidly.

The potential usefulness of the CFU-M lies in its use as an experimental method for quantitating the early megakaryocyte progenitors capable of proliferative activity within the theoretical framework presented in Figure 2. In addition, colony formation in vitro can be used to measure the potency and mechanism of action of both stimulatory and inhibitory "factors" on megakaryocytic proliferation. If we assume that colony formation in vitro is indicative of the series of cellular events that we have postulated previously as perspective cell models of events in vivo, then the technique itself may yield much important information on this question. The following discussion will attempt to summarize our present state of knowledge concerning CFU-M. It may be helpful at this point to consult a recent review[105] which examined a number of culture conditions that are essential for optimizing the growth of megakaryocyte colonies.

Table 1
CFU-M: CELL CHARACTERISTICS

Species	Property		Ref.
Mouse			
C57Bl	Sedimentation Velocity	4.2—4.3 mm/hr	31,35
B6D2F1	Density	1.076 g/mℓ	27
B6D2F1	Sensitivity to:		
	radiation	D_0 = 128 rad	92
	cyclophosphamide	D_{10} = 4 mg/mouse	92
Sl/Sl^D and W/W^v	Genetic control	Decreased number	72
C57BL	Modulation	Cholinergic	119
	Inhibition	Interferon	123
C57BL	Megakaryocytes in colonies	Polyploid	31,102
B6D2F1	Platelet response	Early	44,72
C57BL		No change marrow CFU-M to acute or chronic ↓ plat., but ↑ splenic CFU-M	101
B6D2F1		No effect of adding plat. (whole or frozen-thawed) to mice or directly to cultures	118
C57BL	Platelet formation in vitro	Electron microscopy	35
B6D2F1		Electron microscopy	34
B6D2F1		Light microscopy	44
Rat	Long-term BM culture line	Electron microscopy and anti-PAP antisera	104
Human	Stimulation EpO	Electron microscopy	37,38
	Ident. anti-PGP antisera	No effect Epo or HEK-CM	40
	Colony formation	Stimulation with aplastic anemia serum	41

Note: Abbreviations: Plat., platelets; i.v., intravenous; RAMP-gG, rabbit anti-mouse platelet gamma globulin; RAMPS, rabbit anti-mouse platelet serum; Epo, erythropoietin; PAP, platelet-associated protein; anti-PGP, anti-platelet glycoprotein antiserum; HEK-CM, conditioned media from long-term human embryonic kidney cell line.

i. Culture Methodology

A listing of the various culture conditions that have been used to establish CFU-M growth is presented in Table 2. In order to facilitate the morphologic identification of megakaryocytes, the thin-layer agar culture method[30,98] was adopted, and techniques were developed using agarase as an enzyme to dissolve the upper layer and permit cells to be harvested quantitatively and transferred to glass slides for staining and counting. This quantitative cell assay permitted megakaryocytes to be identified unequivocally, differentiated them from macrophages, and tested for their binding of specific FITC-labeled antiplatelet serum.[30] In addition, the stimulatory effect of thrombocytopenic

Table 2
CFU-M: CULTURE CONDITIONS

Mouse strain	Organ	Semi-solid medium	Culture medium	Serum	CM	Cells/culture ($\times 10^5$)	Day of assay	AChE stain	Minimum colony size	CFU-M/10^5	Colony size	Ref.
B6D2F1	BM	Plasma	L-15	HS (20%)	SPL PWM-CM	1	4—5	Yes	4	10	4—25	32
C57BL	BM	Bactoagar (0.3%)	Eagle's (Mod.)	FCS (15%)	SPL 2-MECM	0.75	7	±	2	6.4	2—40	31
	Spleen	Bactoagar (0.3%)	Eagle's (Mod.)	—	—	—	—	—	—	0.1—0.5	NR	
C57BL	BM	Plasma	NCTC 109	FCS (20%)	EpO—Sheep Human; Tp—	1	7	Yes	2	10	2—40	33
B6D2F1	BM	Bactoagar (0.2%)	McCoy's 5A	FCS (15%)	WEHI-3CM (10×)	0.75—1	7	±	3	7.5 ± 4.4	NR	34
					+BMCM					20.5 ± 5.7	10—15 20—30	
					WEHI-3CM +T_p-HEKC					15.1 ± 1.8	NR	
C57BL	BM	Bactoagar (0.25%)	Eagle's (Mod.)	FCS (20%)	SPL PWMCM	1	5	±	2	24 ± 1	2—25 (Loose)	35
	Spleen	Bactoagar (0.25%)	Eagle's (Mod.)	FCS (20%)	SPL PWMCM	1	5	±	2	5 ± 1	4—100 (Tight)	
	Blood	Bactoagar (0.25%)	Eagle's (Mod.)	FCS (20%)	SPL PWMCM	1	5	±	2	8 ± 1.5	4—100 (Tight)	
BALB/C	BM	Plasma	NCTC	HS (15%)	SPL PWMCM	0.4—2	7	Yes	4	50	NR	36

Note: Abbreviations: BM, bone marrow; L-15, Leibowitz's culture medium; HS, horse serum; SPL-PWM-CM, pokeweed mitogen-stimulated mouse spleen-cell conditioned medium; FCS, fetal calf serum; 2-ME, 2-mercaptoethanol; EPO, erythropoietin; Tp, thrombopoietin; WEHI-3, mouse myelomonocytic cell line; BMCM, bone marrow conditioned medium; HEKC, human embryonic kidney cells; NR, not reported; ± AChE, staining performed on few representative colonies plucked from medium but not routinely.

mouse serum on megakaryocyte differentiation in vitro was first reported,[99] and the ultrastructure of these cells in culture described.[43] Nevertheless, routine analysis of cultured megakaryocytes *in situ* was hampered by the presence of the agar itself since routine hematological stains (e.g., Romanovsky-type) could not be used effectively due to nonspecific binding.

The use of the plasma culture technique for erythroid (CFU-E) colony formation and the staining for hemoglobin on colonies *in situ* was an important advancement in colony analysis in vitro. This, together with the demonstration that rodent megakaryocytes could be stained specifically for AChE activity,[46] resulted in the establishment of the plasma culture technique and AChE staining of colonies *in situ* as the method of choice for growing megakaryocyte colonies and analyzing their subsequent patterns of colonial differentiation.[32,33] Nevertheless, Metcalf et al.[31] were able to pluck colonies of megakaryocytes out of agar cultures with finely drawn Pasteur pipettes for transfer to slides and subsequent staining with Feulgen to determine the distributions of DNA content among megakaryocytes within individual colonies using scanning microspectrophotometry. However, what is lost is the spatial distribution of cells within each colony as well as the relationship of megakaryocyte colonies to other colony types in the cultures. Levin et al.[102] carried this approach in agar culture one step further by removing all potential megakaryocytic colonies of greater than three megakaryocytes as first analyzed by inverted phase microscopy to slides for AChE staining. Mazur et al.[40] have used plasma clot cultures to grow human marrow megakaryocyte colonies. This culture method permitted the use of indirect immunofluorescence with a rabbit, antihuman platelet glycoprotein antiserum to identify the megakaryocytic origin of these colonies *in situ* for unequivocal quantitation. The plasma clot technique has an additional advantage: namely, that other committed marrow progenitors can also be cloned under similar conditions for those studies concerned with questions of cellular competition and inhibition at the level of these progenitors and their common, pluripotent stem cell.

Most recently, Nagasawa et al.[45] have established a liquid culture system for murine megakaryocyte colony formation. This advance permitted the first direct counting of platelets that were released into the culture supernatant. The analysis of platelet shedding from cloned CFU-M becomes a distinct possibility for the first time using this technique. An approach of this kind should provide data on the possible relationship between megakaryocyte differentiation in terms of the size and DNA content of cloned megakaryocytes and the properties and functions of the platelets eventually produced from each megakaryocytic subpopulation.

ii. Colony Identification

In agar culture, megakaryocyte colonies are distinguished mainly by their content of relatively small numbers of large (greater than 25 μm), refractile cells that upon their removal from the culture and AChE and DNA staining have been shown to be morphologically megakaryocytic.[30,31,101] In general, megakaryocytic cells in agar cultures must be identified either under phase microscopy with no prestaining or by removal from culture and staining with dyes such as orcein[31] or AChE.[101] This is not altogether satisfactory and may not only lead to possible misinterpretation with large "macrophages" in the same cultures, but also precludes the analysis of colony growth *in situ*. This limitation is circumvented in the plasma culture system where Romanovsky-type dyes such as Giemsa may be used as well as specific protein and enzyme markers. In addition, the possibility of analyzing every cell within a single megakaryocyte colony for various nuclear and cytoplasmic properties permits the construction of a complete colony "history" of proliferation and differentiation. It may be possible to study the interrelationship of mitotic and endomitotic processes by determining the DNA content of cells within a colony by microspectrophotometry of Feulgen-stained clots as a function of time and of various agents which may influence this relationship.

iii. Differentiation Patterns

When murine bone marrow is placed in plasma culture, the subsequent reappearance of morphologically recognized megakaryocytes over the remainder of the culture period must be the result of their differentiation from unrecognized committed progenitor cells. These megakaryocytes are present in colonies which may be either composed completely of megakaryocytic cells or be "mixed" in which megakaryocytes are present together with granulocytes and/or macrophages. Numerous megakaryocytes (usually ten times the number of CFU-M) are also present as single cells throughout the culture. These cells may be derived from polyploid progenitors solely by differentiation with no subsequent ability to undergo mitosis to form a colony;[44] the ability of these single megakaryocytes to endoreduplicate their DNA remains undetermined. The proportion of megakaryocytes found in "pure" and "mixed" colonies and singly depends to a great extent on the type of conditioned medium used to support proliferation.[30,44] To what extent single megakaryocytes may also represent those cells that have wandered away from a nearby colony is not clear since megakaryocytic cells in plasma cultures may be capable of extensive movement even in semisolid medium.[105a] Williams and Jackson[106] extended the original observation of Metcalf et al.[31] by demonstrating a bimodal distribution of cell sizes within individual megakaryocyte colonies in agar culture with large (greater than 25μm) and small (less than 25μm) cells presumably representing megakaryocytes and their progenitors respectively, since both cell types were AChE positive. This distribution of cell sizes in megakaryocyte colonies has also been confirmed by Levin et al.[102]

iv. Conditioned Media (CM)

Various CM have been shown to be capable of supporting murine and human CFU-M growth (Table 3). As has been discussed previously,[105] many different promoters have been used to obtain an active CM. Even when considering one promoter, namely pokeweed mitogen (PWM), there is much variation among different investigators including different amounts of PWM added, the length of time the promoter is present, the number and type of cells mixed with the PWM, and the optimal final concentration of the CM. Considering the quite different types of promoters that have been used, and even the different use of the same promoter by various laboratories, it is almost impossible to compare the potency and specificity of CM from the scientific literature. It is difficult to compare the specificity of the active moiety in these CM since some have been tested in the agar culture system while others have been used in plasma culture. In general, the "plating efficiency" for CFU-M is about the same at about 1 CFU-M/10^4 cells plated regardless of the type of CM used. It would be important to determine if any of these CM alone are able to preferentially alter the distribution of ploidy within colonies since possibly different factors may be necessary to stimulate CFU-M to undergo mitosis, endomitosis, and subsequent cytoplasmic maturation with platelet formation. Levin et al.[102] have determined the distribution of ploidy values in mouse megakaryocyte colonies stimulated by PWM-CM and measured the change in this distribution in those colonies produced by CFU-M elicited in response to an immune-induced thrombocytopenia.

The ability to raise CM in serum-free cell cultures as modified by Burstein et al.[35] is an important technical advance. The collection of large amounts of material with low protein content (basically, reflecting the active component elicited from the target cells)

Table 3
CFU-M: SOURCES OF CONDITIONED MEDIUM

Source	CM Cells: Concentration ($\times 10^6$ mℓ)	CM Cells: Promoters	Days of culture	Conc in CFU-M Culture	Ref.
Mouse					
B6D2F1 spleen	2	PWM-1/320 PHA-12.5μg/mℓ	2	10%	32
C57BL spleen	1.25	2-ME (50μM)	7—14	17%	31
		Epo (sheep = 2.1 U/mg) (human = 74.3 U/mg)	—	3U/mℓ	33
B6D2F1 BM + BALB/C	0.3—0.5		1—9 weeks	15.4%	66
WEHI-3 myelomono	1	2-ME (50μM) (10 ×= 700μg/mℓ)	7	7.7%	
C57BL spleen	2	PWM-1/320	7	20%	35
C57BL spleen	1	PWM-1/250	1	10%	36
Human kidney + BALB/C		Tp-HEKC + WEHI-3CM	>6 weeks	18—500 (U/mℓ) + 7.7%	118
C57BL/6J	2	PWM-1/320	7	17%	101
Rat		Long term culture line	6	—	104
Long Evans rat BM	4×10^5				
Human		Epo (sheep 2 U/mg) (human—70,000 U/mg)		3U/mℓ	38
		Urinary extract from aplastic anemic patients	—	2.8g/mℓ	41,61

makes it possible to attempt fractionation and purification using high pressure liquid chromatography as applied by Holley et al.[107] to the isolation of a kidney factor.

v. Serum Effects

Various sources of sera have been used successfully to support CFU-M growth including fetal calf serum (FCS),[30,31–33] horse serum,[44] and human AB serum.[37,38,40,41] In our experience, the use of FCS over the long run proved to be unsatisfactory in the plasma culture system which also contains bovine-derived protein in the form of citrated bovine plasma and bovine embryo extract;[44] the substitution of horse for 10% bovine serum rendered CFU-M growth more consistent for reasons that remain undetermined. In addition, we observed a more extensive display of platelet formation in vitro although platelet formation has been seen in cultures containing FCS.[33,34] As in most in vitro cell colony systems, different lots of sera can vary greatly in their ability to support CFU-M growth[105] so that pretesting of numerous sera lots is a prerequisite to maintain consistent colonial growth. The ability to work with a serum-free culture system or at least one with a defined serum requirement would be a substantial advancement and one that may permit the culturing of CFU-M to be adapted more successfully in other laboratories.

vi. Platelet Formation

Early work on demonstrating platelet formation electron microscopically in individual megakaryocytes in agar cultures indicated that these cells were not capable of completing their normal maturation and forming platelets because of the lack of some "maturation factor."[43] Subsequently, McLeod et al.[33] presented electron microscopic evidence that cells in megakaryocyte colonies grown in plasma culture with erythropoietin added could indeed form platelets. Whether the presence of different CMs which supported CFU-M growth was also responsible for stimulating megakaryocyte maturation is not completely understood. Whether megakaryocytes produced in culture are normal is still in question. Levin et al.[102] have presented evidence that megakaryocytes in agar colonies express only high ploidy profiles more indicative of the megakaryocyte response to increased platelet demand than of the "resting" state in marrow. Williams et al.[34] applied electron microscopy to megakaryocyte colonies stimulated by WEHI-3 CM which revealed normal megakaryocyte maturation with subsequent formation of platelets. In addition, Burstein et al.[35] and Nagasawa et al.[45] have provided additional evidence in liquid cultures. Vainchenker et al.[37,38] have presented ultrastructural evidence of platelet formation in human megakaryocytic colonies. The importance of the liquid culture system[45] for colony growth is that it permits released platelets to be collected easily for functional assays. Questions of whether states of abnormal megakaryocytopoiesis are the result of cellular maturation blocks or humoral deficiencies may soon be within our grasp experimentally in addition to more basic questions of how the entire sequence is regulated normally.

vii. Cell Cycle Status

The most widely used cytokinetic method for determining the proliferative state of clonogenic cell populations both of normal and tumor origin involves the so-called "suicide" technique. Cells are exposed to high doses of S-phase specific agents, such as tritiated thymidine or hydroxyurea, administered either in vivo or in vitro. These agents are incorporated into the DNA of cells that are in S phase and thus undergoing DNA synthesis. These cells are thus unable to complete subsequent mitoses to form a colony of progeny upon being retransplanted or replated. The fractional loss of survival of clonogenic cells following exposure to maximum or "plateau" doses of the S-phase specific agents is a measure of the fraction of the clonogenic cells that are in S phase during the time of exposure. Using this suicide technique, there is general agreement that most pluripotent stem cells or CFU-S in normal marrow are out of cell cycle or in a "resting" state. Generally, more granulocyte-macrophage clonogenic cells assayed in vitro are in cell cycle and thus fewer survive cytotoxic doses of S-phase agents than CFU-S. Data from four groups[35,36,72,106] is shown in Table 4.

Both in vivo and in vitro suicide technique with either tritiated thymidine, hydroxyurea, or cytosine arabinoside have been used to determine the fraction of CFU-M in DNA synthesis. Generally the data of Nakeff and Bryan[72] and Williams and Jackson[106] and Mizoguchi et al.[36] are in agreement that a substantial proportion of CFU-M are normally in cell cycle and are thus killed by S-phase agents. The data from these groups also indicates that more CFU-M are killed when exposed to these agents in vitro than in vivo which is in contrast to that of Burstein et al.[35] which indicates that only about 10% of CFU-M are normally in DNA synthesis. In their hands, the result is the same whether the assay was performed in vivo or in vitro. The reason for this discrepancy is not known but it may reflect a mouse strain difference. It has been shown[44] that there

Table 4
CFU-M: CELL CYCLE STATUS

Mouse strain	% in S-phase	Exposure of cells	Assay conditions	Ref.
B6D2F1	10—20	In vivo	HU = 50 mg/mouse; ARA-C = 10 mg/mouse—given i.v., assayed 3 hr later	72
	40—50	In vitro	HU = 2 mg/mℓ (26 m*M*); ARA-C = 1 mg/mℓ—assayed 1 hr later	
B6D2F1	9—23	In vivo	HU = 900 mg/kg (18 mg/mouse)—given i.p., assayed 3 hr later in 10-day regenerating marrow	106
	50—60	In vitro	^{3}H-Thymidine = 10 and 30 μCi/mℓ	
	55		HU = 2 m*M* —assayed 0.5—1 hr later	
C57BL	7 ± 1.5	In vivo	^{3}H-Thymidine = 1 mCi/mouse —assayed 0.5 hr later	35
	11 ± 2	In vitro	^{3}H-Thymidine = 20 and 200 μCi/mℓ	
BALB/C	30	In vitro	^{3}H-Thymidine = 200 μCi/mℓ —assayed 0.3 hr later	36

Note: Abbreviations: HU, hydroxyurea; ara-C, cytosine arabinoside; ^{3}H-Thymidine, tritiated thymidine, specific activity 15—24 Ci/mM; i.v., intravenous; i.p., intraperitoneal.

is a clear difference in the number of CFU-M assayed in femoral marrow of different mouse strains, including those used in Table 4. It is of interest to note that Williams and Jackson[106] obtained about the same degree of killing in vitro of CFU-M in "resting" marrow as CFU-M in 10-day regenerating marrow assayed in vivo where most of the proliferative cells would be expected to be in cell cycle. One would speculate that some type of cell surface contact of CFU-M during incubation in vitro may act as a trigger to stimulate these progenitors into cell cycle. The CFU-M are the only hematopoietic progenitor cells to our knowledge that show this in vivo-in vitro cell suicide difference which may be important to our understanding of the proliferative regulation of CFU-M. Williams and Jackson[106] suggest that changes in cell cycle and the fraction of cycling CFU-M may be an important regulatory response to an altered demand for functional platelets or megakaryocytes. It is apparent that more studies are needed to clarify the reason(s) for this difference and the discrepancy among the published proliferative data on CFU-M. Unfortunately, no data exists on the proliferative state of human CFU-M. No data is available on possible changes that might be induced in the fraction of cycling CFU-M in response to an accelerated platelet demand that might indicate the importance of this level of control to the subsequent absolute increase in the number of megakaryocytes that is observed following an immune-induced thrombocytopenia.

5. Regulation of Megakaryocyte Production: Role of CFU-M

An appreciation of the complexity of the control of megakaryocytic proliferation must acknowledge how little we know about the interplay of mitosis and endomitosis in early progenitors. The relationship between the degree of polyploidy and cytoplasmic maturation in megakaryocytes and how this relates to the ultimate release of hemostatically-functional blood platelets is important to elucidate. This scheme is obviously complex and not well understood. It may be somewhat premature to discuss the role of the CFU-M within the level of complexity in this scheme considering how recently the in vitro clonogenic assays were established. Nevertheless, the questions are clear.

1. What role do the stimulators and potentiators that have been defined in vitro as being essential for CFU-M growth, play in vivo, and how do they compare with those that have been shown to have an in vivo effect on platelet production?
2. Are the CFU-M a homogeneous cell population or are there subpopulations that are predominantly mitotic or endomitotic?
3. Do CFU-M comprise a physiological class of progenitor cells that responds to peripheral platelet demand?
4. If CFU-M respond to platelets, is the response direct or secondary to changes in megakaryocyte number?

There has been very recent activity in this area which is beginning to address itself to some of these questions. Although the information is incomplete, it might be useful to conceptualize progress in this area within the overall scheme of megakaryocyte differentiation as we known it presently.

a. Relationship to Platelet Production

A schematic model of potential control junctions is presented in Figure 3 which is based primarily on the present cell kinetic model of megakaryocytopoiesis. Control may be exercised at many different levels of differentiation involving distinctly unique mechanisms, such as cell cycle regulation and degree of recruitment, nuclear endoreduplication, cytoplasmic differentiation, and platelet production. Since mitotic activity is limited to the progenitor cell compartment, any increase in the flow of immature but morphologically recognized megakaryocytes conceivably may involve either an increase in the number of proliferating (mitotic) progenitors, a possible shortening of their cell cycle time, or a preferential shunting of endomitosis. Depending on the degree of the demand placed on this cell system, there may also be an increase in the rate of "commitment" of pluripotent stem cells into the megakaryocytic progenitor cell compartment. Other compensatory mechanisms that could be envisioned to meet the ultimate platelet demand probably involve the megakaryocyte cell compartment rather than its progenitor cells. Included in this latter category might be changes in the degree of polyploidy, megakaryocyte size, and rate of differentiation as well as the size and number of blood platelets produced from individual megakaryocytes. This would result in altered rates of platelet production and the production of platelets possibly altered in their functional expression, such as their degree of stickiness or their ability to initiate clot formation and retraction.

Summarized in Table 5 are the results of studies which have contributed to our present-day understanding of regulation. This information is keyed similarly to that presented in Figure 3 so that comparisons can be made.

It is not clear as to the degree to which each of these control junctions is governed separately and the degree to which they represent a cascade of response elicited originally at the earliest level of regulation, i.e., the pluripotent stem cell and passing through a sequence of proliferative and maturational events. Nevertheless, there is evidence that a number of the mechanisms at these junctions respond to both negative and positive feedback regulation. Ebbe[108] has discussed these various potential regulatory mechanisms in terms of humoral mediation through "thrombopoietin(s)." There is insufficient evidence to conclude that a single thrombopoietin is produced in response to a depletion of platelets that can act at many different levels or that there may exist numerous thrombopoietin subfractions each of which are targeted specifically to a single control junction. Efforts to purify potential thrombopoietins and the availability of new assay systems, such as clonogenic cell assays and cytochemical[46–48] as well as platelet-associated protein markers[24,49,62–64,109] will provide more direct information.

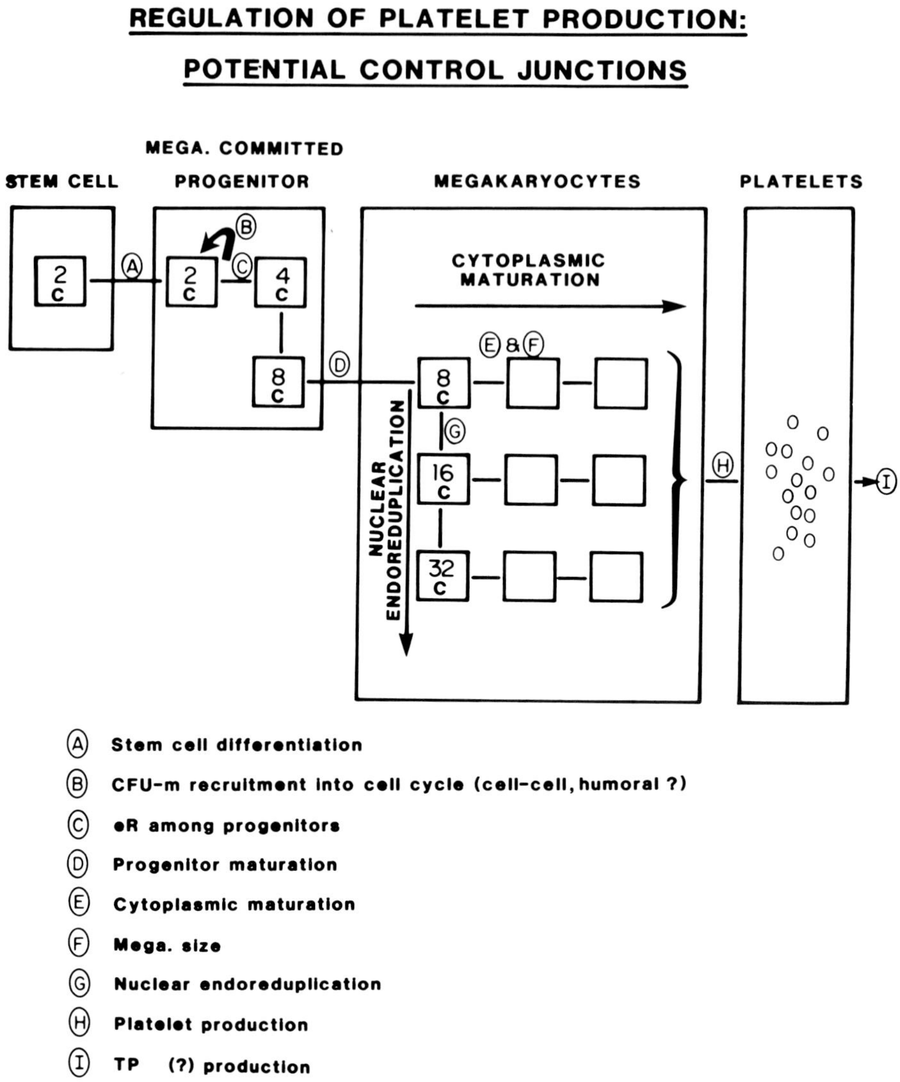

FIGURE 3. A model of potential regulatory junctions within the schematic model of megakaryocytopoiesis proposed in Figure 2. Abbreviations: eR, nuclear endoreduplication; Tp, thrombopoietin.

It should be noted that the degree and type of response that is elicited in response to platelet demand is dependent upon the degree and possibly the duration of the demand. For example, Jackson[46,47] has shown that an acute, immune-induced thrombocytopenia to platelet levels of less than 5% initially is essential to observe a significant change in the number of small AChE-positive progenitors. Harker[13] has also confirmed this for megakaryocyte nuclear changes (i.e., in the number of lobes) following either a 4- or 10-day continuous immune-induced thrombocytopenia. It has been reported that only increases in platelet levels of about three fold or greater can induce a significant suppression of megakaryocyte production.[12,14,97,110,111]

An important aspect of the heirarchy of cytokinetic responses elicited remains to be defined more precisely; namely, to what extent does the sequence of response at the various stages of progenitor and megakaryocyte differentiation represent a direct re-

Table 5
POTENTIAL CONTROL JUNCTIONS

		Ref.
A.	Megakaryocytic differentiation of pluripotent stem cell following:	
	Whole-body gamma irradiation	92, 124
	Immune-induced thrombocytopenia	72, 95, 96
	Suppression following thrombocytosis	97
	5-FU treatment	125
B.	Recruitment CFU-M into cell cycle:	
	↑ Kill after HU, Ara-C and ^{3}H-Thymidine in vitro	72, 106
	Kill during marrow regeneration	106
	Cylic neutropenia (man)	39
	Altered in Sl/Sl^D and W/W^v mice	72
C.	Degree nuclear endoreduplication (eR) among progenitors	46–48
D.	Progenitor differentiation:	
	↑ Early megs. after ↑ platelets	116, 117, 126–128
E.	Rate megakaryocytic cytoplasmic differentiation:	
	↓ Transit time after ↓ platelets	128, 129
	↑ Transit time after ↑ platelets	112
F.	Megakaryocyte size:	
	Increased after ↓ platelets	117, 126, 127, 129
	Decreased after ↑ platelets	127
	Increased in Sl/Sl^D mice and mediated by serum	66–69, 71
G.	Nuclear endoreduplication among immature megs:	
	↑ Mean ploidy after ↓ platelets	126, 127
	↓ Mean ploidy after ↑ platelets	126, 127
	↑ Mitotic index after ↓ platelets mediated by serum factor	59, 116, 130
H.	Platelet production:	
	Increased following ↓ platelets	7, 126
	Larger (younger?) platelets from megs. of higher ploidy	127
I.	Tp production:	
	Increased Tp after ↓ platelets	53–55
	Decreased Tp after ↑ platelets (rebound thrombocytosis)	54

Note: Abbreviations: Tp, thrombopoietin; megs, megakaryocytes; HU, hydroxyurea; ara-C, cytosine arabinoside; 5-FU, 5-fluorouracil.

sponse to the alteration in platelet level and to what degree is it a reflection of a secondary response to a change in the megakaryocyte compartment itself? In other words, is there evidence for auto-regulation of megakaryocytes and their progenitors separate from that aspect of the response that is platelet-mediated and thus possibly thrombopoietin-induced? Ebbe and Phalen[112] present a cogent discussion of this point. Clearly, a comprehensive analysis of the megakaryocytic response is essential at this time. Assay systems discussed previously should be applied in a time-course study following a clearly-defined perturbation. Mathematical models of megakaryocytopoiesis have been described by Wickmann.[113]

b. Nature of Growth Stimulators

Figure 4 presents a schematic summary of the growth stimulators that have been described to date within the context of the overall cytokinetic model of megakaryocytopoiesis described earlier. Megakaryocyte colony-stimulating activity (mega-CSA) has been reported in the supernatant from mouse spleen cell (MSpl) cultures stimulated with either pokeweed mitogen (mito.)[32,35,36,101] or 2-mercaptoethanol (2ME).[31,34] In ad-

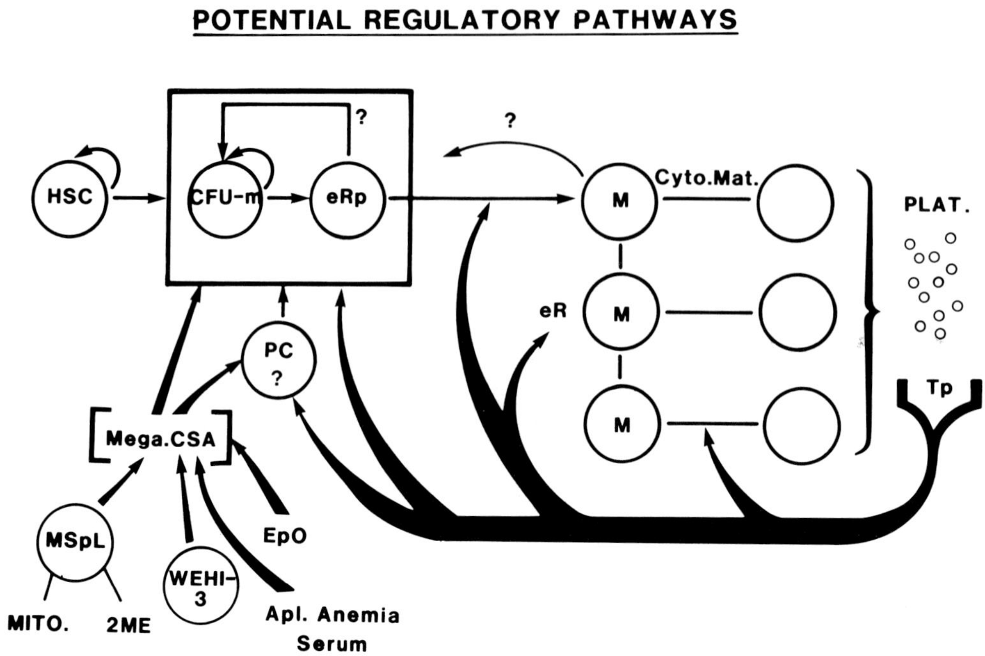

FIGURE 4. A diagrammatic representation of potential regulatory pathways in the megakaryocyte model proposed in Figure 3 showing the interactions between stimulators of megakaryocyte production both in vivo and in vitro. For abbreviations see the text.

dition, this activity has been identified in a mouse myelomonocytic cell line (WEHI-3).[34,100] It is not clear whether this potentiation reflects the fact that WEHI-3 CM is derived from a long-term tumor cell line (and not a normal cell as in the other studies) and thus needs the activity from the potentiating cells (PC) to be fully expressed.

The mega-CSA is thought to stimulate the progenitor compartment which is comprised of both mitotic cells (CFU-M) and nuclear endoreduplicating progenitors (eRp). Whether this mega-CSA stimulates both cell populations directly is not clear, although both an increase in megakaryocyte colonies (CFU-M) as well as single megakaryocytes is observed in the same cultures. The latter may be the product of the eRp progenitors which may only be capable of nuclear endoreduplication, although this has not been shown directly.[73]

The possibility that CFU-M may respond not only to a humoral control such as mega-CSA but also to cell-cell contact, possibly with the eRp cells, is indicated by the closed loop from the eRp to the CFU-M with a question mark placed above it. There also may be a possibility that the progenitor cell population responds to changes in the cellularity of the recognized megakaryocyte compartment as indicated by a second question mark. This mediation may involve cell-cell contact within the marrow structure or short-term humoral regulation.

There is a large body of experimental evidence that levels of platelets in peripheral blood are regulated through a humoral activity encompassed by the term "thrombopoietin."[13,114,115] As indicated in Figure 4, this material as thrombocytopenic mouse serum has been shown to alter the rate of cytoplasmic maturation of megakaryocyte[116,117] as well as the degree of megakaryocyte endomitosis.[59] What is less clear is the effect of this thrombopoietic activity on the progenitor cell compartment. McDonald et al.[58] have isolated a material from human embryonic kidney cells (HEKC-CM) in culture that has an activity in vivo that is identical to the active component in thrombocytopenic serum. Freedman et al.[80] have reported that this material stimulates CFU-M in plasma culture under these culture conditions, whereas Williams et al.[118] were not able to show potentiation in cultures to which this material was added over a broad dose range. Mazur et al.[41] were unable to demonstrate any activity of HEKC-CM in cultures of human megakaryocyte colonies. McDonald et al.[96] have demonstrated that this same material is capable of stimulating megakaryocytic colonies in vivo in the spleen colony assay.

It is only prudent to reserve judgement as to the capability of thrombopoietin either elicited in response to thrombocytopenia or as a CM from HEKC cultures, to stimulate megakaryocytopoiesis at all stages of differentiation including the pluripotent stem cell.

c. Cytokinetic Response to Platelet Demand

An important aspect of the CFU-M as a population of progenitor cells in marrow lies in their potential role as physiologic progenitors responsible for megakaryocyte production in vivo.

As summarized in Table 6, contradictory data has been obtained independently in two different laboratories[72,101] using similar cytokinetic analyses of CFU-M in mouse marrow and spleen as a function of time after an immune-induced thrombocytopenia. The data indicate that CFU-M in marrow increase rapidly within a few hours after platelet depletion.[72] This finding supports a direct response that precedes and accounts for the subsequent increase in small, AChE-positive progenitors and eventually megakaryocytes. Other investigators[101] find no significant increases in CFU-M throughout a 14-day period in marrow although there are significant increases in splenic CFU-M that follow rather than precede increases in the number of megakaryocytes. In the latter case, Levin et al.[101] propose that marrow CFU-M may not comprise a physiologically important progenitor population with respect to megakaryocyte production. Their response was not predictive of subsequent changes in the megakaryocyte and platelet populations.

The increase in splenic CFU-M may simply be reflecting either a response to initial depletions within the megakaryocytes themselves or an increased rate of influx of CFU-M from the pluripotent stem cell pool. More data will be needed to resolve this controversy although there are sufficient technical differences in culture techniques, mouse strains used, and the mode of inducing thrombocytopenia that these alone could explain the discrepancies.

Williams et al.[118] showed that the suppression of platelet production produced in vivo by the injection of either whole or frozen-thawed platelet suspensions or in vitro by the direct addition of the same materials to CFU-M cultures had no effect on the number of CFU-M assayed at different times after suppression.

In summary, these data are too equivocal to resolve the question of the in vivo physiologic importance of CFU-M in megakaryocyte cytokinetics.

d. Response to Other Perturbations

Nakeff et al.[99] have measured the radiation dose response of CFU-M to whole-body, ^{137}Ce-gamma irradiation and the administration of cyclophosphamide as a chemotherapeutic agent. CFU-M displayed a D_0 of 128 rad which was identical to that obtained for CFU-GM in the same mouse marrow but greater than the D_0 of 86 rad for CFU-S and 66 rad for the late erythroid progenitor (CFU-E). The recovery curve for CFU-M following 500 rad was more indicative of that for the CFU-S and CFU-GM than for the CFU-E. Thus these data could be interpreted to indicate that the CFU-M is a rather immature progenitor bearing a close relationship to the CFU-S and CFU-GM and being

Table 6
CFU-M: RESPONSE TO PLATELET DEMAND

Mouse strain	Platelet demand	Time period assayed	Number of CFU-M: Response	Number of CFU-M: Time of peak response	Ref.
B6D2Fl	↓ Platelets:				44, 72
	1 × RAMP-IgG (i.v.)	4 days	marrow: 2—3 fold ↑	2—4 hr	
C57BL	↓ Platelets:				101
	1 × RAMPS (i.v.)	14 days	marrow: no effect	—	
			spleen: 6-fold ↑	day 4	
	3 × RAMPS (i.v.) (days 0, 2, 4)	9 days	marrow: no effect	—	64
			spleen: 1.8 fold ↑	days 5, 9	
B6D2Fl	↑ Platelets:				
	In vivo:				
	1–5 × 10^9 q 48 hr × 5	11 days	marrow: no effect	—	
	1–5 × 10^8 q 24 hr × 3	4 days	marrow: no effect	—	
	In vitro:				
	Whole platelets: (10^8/1 mℓ culture)	7 days	marrow: no effect	—	
	Fr-Th platelets: (0.5—5 × 10^8/1 mℓ culture)	7 days	marrow: no effect	—	

Note: Abbreviations: RAMPS, rabbit anti-mouse platelet serum; Fr-Th, frozen-thawed.

dependent for its ultimate recovery on the integrity and survival of the pluripotent stem cell pool.

Burstein et al.[119] have shown that the growth of CFU-M in culture can be modulated by cholinergic antagonists. This growth, however, was not affected by adrenergic antagonists.

Nakeff and Bryan[72] have investigated the possible genetic control of CFU-M in two strains of genetically anemic mice, W/W^v and $S1/S1^D$. These strains had been shown to have a megakaryocyte defect that resulted in an altered production of new megakaryocytes.[65,66–70] We confirmed this result for the platelets and megakaryocytes in these mice and extended our analysis to indicate that the defect in these well may go back developmentally as far as the small, AChE-positive progenitors and the proliferative state of the CFU-M in these mice as compared to their normal littermates. Obviously, these models provide a powerful tool with which to investigate cellular control mechanisms that are under genetic regulation, since much is known of their megakaryocyte, erythroid, and pluripotent stem cell defects.

e. Role of Regulatory Cells

CFU-M have an incidence or "plating efficiency" that is at least a decade lower than CFU-GM and CFU-E but similiar to that for very immature erythroid progenitors (BFU-E). Since generally high cell concentrations of total marrow have to be plated to obtain reproducible colony growth, there has been concern regarding the regulatory role of cells other than those that are megakaryocytic on CFU-M proliferation.

Williams et al.[120] have used unit gravity sedimentation and density gradient techniques to isolate CFU-M from potential regulatory cells and then applied mixing experiments to examine their interaction. They have also extended their previous characterization of the potentiator cells[34,106] to define the radiation sensitivity and adherent properties of these cells.

Most recently, Castro-Malaspina et al.[121] have shown that human megakaryocytes themselves release a factor that stimulates the proliferation of bone marrow fibroblasts. They believe that this material may be distinct from the platelet-derived growth factor which Chernoff et al.[64] have recently demonstrated can be synthesized in guinea pig megakaryocytes.

If these data can be confirmed, then they will have profound implications for the possible regulation of proliferative activity in the megakaryocytic progenitor as outlined in Figure 5A.

C. Cytokinetic Models of the Progenitor Cell Pool

With the model in Figure 2 as a theoretical framework, the following discussion will attempt to speculate upon possible models of cellular proliferation operating in the progenitor compartments which may explain the pattern of differentiation observed in the megakaryocyte compartment.

1. Proliferation Limited to Diploid Cells

As a first approximation, it may be useful to consider the case of cell mitosis being limited solely to diploid progenitors as shown in Figure 5A. Diploid progenitors (CFU-M) capable of extensive mitotic activity would give rise to daughter cells, some of which may "switch" from a mitotic to an endomitotic cycle; in this model, the "switch" would be irreversible. The resulting tetraploid daughter cell could then either (1) cease further DNA synthesis which may constitute a signal for the cell to enter cytoplasmic maturation and thus be identified as a megakaryocyte, or (2) continue through successive rounds of DNA synthesis, each of which may have some predeter-

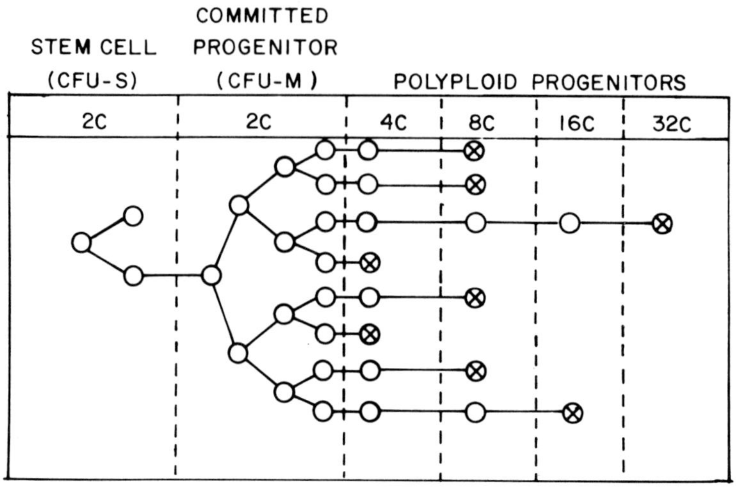

A

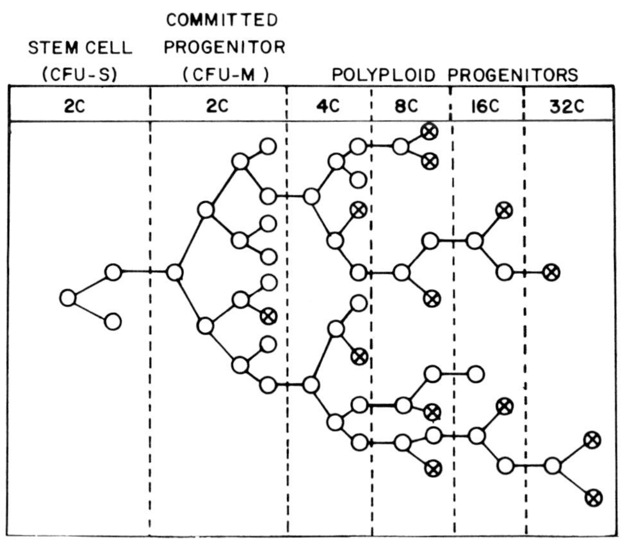

B

FIGURE 5. (A) Model megakaryocyte proliferation with mitotic activity limited solely to 2C committed progenitors. (B) Model of megakaryocyte proliferation with mitotic activity in both diploid and polyploid progenitors where the degree of mitotic activity decreases as they move from a lower to a higher ploidy class. Circles marked with crosses indicate commencement of cytoplasmic maturation and thus removal from the progenitor compartment into Stage I megakaryocytes.

mined probability of being terminated in favor of maturation as in (1). With rodent megakaryocytes being predominantly 16C in ploidy, most of the 4C cells would be capable of going through two additional rounds of DNA synthesis to become 16C cells; on the other hand, most of the 16C cells would cease DNA synthesis and mature cytoplasmically with only about 10% of these able to go through the last DNA synthetic cycle to form the rare 32C cells.

If indeed this were the correct in vivo model and in vitro colony formation mimicked this process, then an analysis of individual cells within single megakaryocyte colonies might reveal a profile of cellular DNA contents similar to that observed in the morphologically identified megakaryocyte compartment present in the original marrow of the donor mouse. Metcalf et al.[31] have shown that megakaryocytes in individual colonies exist at several ploidy values but it is clear from the data presented that this profile is not similar to that in the original marrow cell suspension. This has been confirmed by Levin et al.[102]

Another inherent assumption of the model implies that the polyploid progenitors are not morphologically recognizable. Thus, cells with ploidies possibly as high as 16C would still have cellular volumes not appreciably greater than the majority of diploid cells in marrow, an assumption which may on the surface be difficult to envision although flow cytometry may be a valuable tool here. In his model, Odell[12] has stated that cells with ploidies greater than 8C become morphologically identifiable as megakaryocytes at this ploidy level. However, it is conceivable that the manner in which polyploid levels of DNA are physically packed in the nucleus of a progenitor that has not commenced cytoplasmic maturation may obscure this distinction. Although the nucleus of the cell may be larger, its overall cell diameter which is used to identify these cells in marrow smears or sections may not be significantly increased.

It is not unreasonable to believe that there may very well be a degree of heterogeneity among progenitors with regard to their DNA content and extent of cytoplasmic maturation. This may obscure subtle though important differences measured at the level of overall cell diameters between progenitors with ploidy levels from 4 to 16C which happen to be at precisely the same stage of cytoplasmic differentiation. A more definitive answer to this important question may lie in the direct cell measurement of the DNA content of large numbers of ''small'' AChE-positive progenitors which otherwise would not have been recognized as being megakaryocytic by conventional morphology such as that used by Odell.[12] This approach may prove difficult since there are technical problems in staining cells for AChE activity, then destaining and restaining the same cells for their DNA content by the Feulgen reaction; other approaches such as analysis by flow cytometry[73] may prove to be more feasible and direct in that large enough numbers of cells may be processed (within a reasonable length of time) to lend a measure of satistical validity to the analysis of the very small fraction of these progenitors (less than $1{:}10^6$) that are present in normal bone marrow.

If progenitors with ploidy values of 8C or greater must be, by definition, megakaryocytes, it would be important to know the percentage of morphologically immature megakaryocytes of various ploidy some 30 min after a flash-label with tritiated-thymidine, at a time when about 24% of early megakaryocytes are labeled in mouse marrow.[122] Although no direct data are available, one might reasonably assume from the ploidy distribution of Stage I megakaryocytes, at least in rat marrow, that the largest proportion of these cells that are labeled should be 8C (greater than 80%). If the majority of these cells should have higher ploidy values, then this would provide additional evidence that progenitors may remain morphologically unrecognizable that have ploidies of greater than 4C since they were not observed in the early megakaryocyte compartment.

2. *Proliferation in Diploid and Polyploid Cells*

An alternative proposal would be to consider the more complex possibility of both polyploid and diploid cells being capable of mitosis and endomitosis as shown in Figure 5B. Let us first consider the case where movement of a cell to a higher ploidy has the effect of limiting its extent of mitotic proliferation. Here a small proportion of the diploid cells would be capable of differentiating out of the diploid compartment while the majority would divide mitotically, and some would leave by undergoing DNA synthesis in the absence of cytokinesis to thus enter the 4C pool of progenitors. Once there, the 4C cells would be capable of a somewhat more limited degree of mitotic activity than present in the preceding diploid compartment with more cells exiting this compartment as 4C, cytoplasmically immature megakaryocytes. A number would also be capable of becoming 8C cells, a ploidy level at which further mitosis is limited, with most cells commencing cytoplasmic differentiation and a minority going on to 16C (and 32C) progenitors. In these latter compartments, most of the cellular activity would be limited to either nuclear endoreduplication or subsequent cytoplasmic differentiation. This type of scheme would account for the spectrum of ploidy classes that has been determined in rat and mouse bone marrow.[28,75c]

On the other hand, it may be possible that increasing ploidy does not imply decreasing mitotic activity, but rather that various ploidy classes may have unique proliferative capabilities to account for the ploidy distributions observed in early megakaryocytes. In this case, 8C cells would not proliferate as extensively as 2C and 4C progenitors, but would be mainly responsible for providing 8C early megakaryocytes by maturation and 16C progenitors by nuclear endoreduplication. These 8C cells, however, would be able to proliferate extensively to provide a larger number of cells for differentiation as well as endoreduplication to 16 and 32C cells. This mechanism of differential proliferative capacity between 8C progenitors and the other ploidy classes would provide for the majority of 16C megakaryocytes observed in the cytoplasmically "early" compartment.

This model demands a far more complex control mechanism that would ensure this differential is maintained. Also, it is difficult to envision its response to either an increased or decreased demand for blood platelets. By analyzing for the movement of cells of various ploidy classes from the progenitor compartments and testing for their proliferative potentials, we may gain some insight into which of the above proposed mechanisms, or possibly even other mechanisms, may be involved.

REFERENCES

1. **Bessis, M.,** Megakaryocyte differentiation, *Blood Cells,* 5, 1, 1979.
2. **Evatt, B. E., Levine, R. F., and Williams, N. T.,** Eds., in *Megakaryocyte Biology and Precursors*: In Vitro, Cloning and Cellular Properties, Elsevier North Holland, Amsterdam, 1981.

2a. **Bessis, M.,** *Cytology of the Blood and Blood-Forming Organs,* Grune and Stratton, New York, 1956.

2b. **Bessis, M.,** The thrombocytic series, in *Living Blood Cells and Their Ultrastructure,* Bessis, M., Ed., Springer-Verlag, Berlin, 1973, 367.

3. **Cronkite, E. P.,** Regulation of platelet production, in Homeostatic Mechanisms, Brookhaven Symposia in Biology, No. 10, Brookhaven Laboratories, New York, 1958, 96.
4. **Odell, T. T., Jr. and Anderson, B.,** Production and life span of platelets, in *The Kinetics of Cellular Proliferation,* Stohlman, F., Jr., Ed., Grune & Stratton, New York, 1958, 278.
5. **Cronkite, E. P., Bond, V. P., Fleidner, T. M., Paglia, D. A., and Adamik, E. R.,** Studies on the origin, production and destruction of platelets, in, *Blood Platelets,* Johnson, S. A., Monto, R. W., Rebuck, J. W., and Horn, R. C., Jr., Eds., Little, Brown, Boston, 1961, 595.
6. **Odell, T. T., Jr. and Kniseley, R. M.,** The origin, life span, regulation and fate of blood platelets, in *Progress in Hematology,* Vol. 3, Tocantius, L. M., Ed., Grune & Stratton, New York, 1962, 203.
7. **Ebbe, S.,** Megakaryocytopoiesis and platelet turnover, *Ser. Haematol.,* 1, 65, 1968.

8. **Odartchenko, N. and Heiniger, H. J.,** Review on kinetics of megakaryocyte maturation, *Haematol. Lat.,* 12, 517, 1969.
9. **Ebbe, S.,** Megakaryocytopoiesis, in *Regulation of Hematopoiesis,* Gordon, A. S., Ed., Appleton-Century-Crofts, New York, 1970, chap. 56.
10. **Ebbe, S. and Phalen, E.,** Thrombocytopoietic regulatory mechanisms, in *Formation and Destruction of Blood Cells,* Greenwalt, T. J. and Jamieson, G. A., Eds., J. B. Lippincott, Philadelphia, 1970, 128.
11. **Ebbe, S.,** The megakaryocyte: maturation and self-renewal, in *The Platelet,* Brinkhous, K. M., Shermer, R. W., and Wostofi, F. K., Eds., Williams & Wilkins, Baltimore, 1971, 1.
12. **Odell, T. T., Jr.,** Megakaryocytopoiesis and its response to stimulation and suppression, in *Platelets: Production, Function, Transfusion and Storage,* Baldini, M. G. and Ebbe, S., Eds., Grune & Stratton, New York, 1974, 11.
13. **Harker, L. A.,** Control of platelet production, *Ann. Rev. Med.,* 25, 383, 1974.
14. **Odell, T. T., Jr. and Jackson, C. W.,** Megakaryocytopoiesis, in *Hematopoietic Cellular Differentiation,* Stohlman, F., Jr., Ed., Grune & Stratton, New York, 1970, 278.
15. **Ebbe, S.,** Biology of megakaryocytes, *Prog. Hemostasis Thromb.,* 3, 211, 1976.
16. **Odell, T. T., Jr.,** Megakaryocytopoiesis, in *Growth Kinetics and Biochemical Regulation of Normal and Malignant Cells,* Drewinko, B. and Humphrey, R. M., Eds., Williams & Wilkins, Baltimore, 1977, 563.
17. **Ebbe, S.,** Experimental and clinical megakaryocytopoiesis, *Clin. Haematol.,* 8, 371, 1979.
18. **Nakeff, A. and Maat, B.,** Separation of megakaryocytes from mouse bone marrow by velocity sedimentation, *Blood,* 43, 591, 1974.
19. **Pretlow, T. G. and Stinson, A. J.,** Separation of megakaryocytes from rat bone marrow cells using velocity sedimentation, in an isokinetic gradient of ficoll in tissue culture medium., *J. Cell. Physiol.,* 88, 317, 1976.
20. **Levine, R. F. and Fedorko, M. E.,** Isolation of intact megakaryocytes from guinea pig femoral marrow. Successful harvest made possible with inhibition of platelet aggregation; enrichment achieved with a two-step separation technique, *J. Cell Biol.,* 69, 159, 1976.
21. **Brown, W. M. and Axelrad, A. A.,** Effect of Friend leukemia virus on megakaryocytes and platelets in mice, *Int. J. Cancer,* 18, 764, 1976.
22. **Levine, R. F.,** Culture in vitro of isolated guinea pig megakaryocytes: recovery, survival, morphologic changes, and maturation, *Blood,* 50, 713, 1977.
23. **Sitar, G., Marini, G., Pellicciari, C., Casirola, G., and Ascari, E.,** Separation and enrichment of human megakaryocytes by velocity sedimentation on continuous albumin gradient, *Haematologica (Pavia),* 62, 119, 1977.
24. **Rabellino, E. M., Nachman, R. L., Williams, N., Winchester, R. J., and Ross, G. D.,** Human megakaryocytes. I. Characterization of the membrane and cytoplasmic components of isolated marrow megakaryocytes, *J. Exp. Med.,* 149, 1273, 1979.
25. **Seitz, R. and Wesemann, W.,** Studies in megakaryocytes: isolation from rat and guinea pig and incorporation of 5-hydroxytryptamine, *Eur. J. Cell Biol.,* 21, 183, 1980.
26. **Worthington, R. E. and Nakeff, A.,** Thromboxane synthesis in megakaryocytes isolated by centrifugal elutriation, *Blood,* 58, 175, 1981.
27. **Nakeff, A. and Floeh, D. P.,** Separation of megakaryocytes from mouse bone marrow by density gradient centrifugation, *Blood,* 48, 133, 1976.
28. **Nakeff, A., Valeriote, F., Gray, J. W., and Grabske, R. J.,** Application of flow cytometry and cell sorting to megakaryocytopoiesis, *Blood,* 53, 732, 1979.
29. **Levine, R. F., Bunn, P. A., Jr., Hazzard, K. C., Schlam, M. L.,** Flow cytometric analysis of megakaryocyte ploidy. Comparison with Feulgen microdensitometry and discovery that 8N is the predominant ploidy class in guinea pig and monkey marrow, *Blood,* 56, 210, 1980.
30. **Nakeff, A., Dicke, K. A., and Van Noord, M. J.,** Megakaryocytes in agar cultures of mouse bone marrow, *Ser. Haematol.,* 8, 4, 1975.
31. **Metcalf, D., MacDonald, H. R., Odartchenko, N., and Sordat, B.,** Growth of mouse megakaryocyte colonies *in vitro, Proc. Natl. Acad. Sci. U.S.A.,* 72, 1744, 1975.
32. **Nakeff, A. and Daniels-McQueen, S.,** *In vitro* colony assay for a new class of megakaryocyte precursor: colony-forming unit megakaryocyte (CFU-M), *Proc. Soc. Exp. Biol. Med.,* 151, 587, 1976.
33. **McLeod, D. L., Shreeve, M. M., and Axelrad, A. A.,** Induction of megakaryocyte colonies with platelet formation *in vitro, Nature,* 261, 492, 1976.
34. **Williams, N., Jackson, H., Sheridan, A. P., Murphy, M. J., Jr., Elste, A., and Moore, M. A.,** Regulation of megakaryopoiesis in long-term murine bone marrow cultures, *Blood,* 51, 245, 1978.

35. **Burstein, S. A., Adamson, J. W., Thorning, D., and Harker, L. A.,** Characteristics of murine megakaryocytic colonies in vitro, *Blood,* 54, 169, 1979.
36. **Mizoguchi, H., Kubota, K., Miura, Y., and Takaku, F.,** An improved plasma culture system for the production of megakaryocyte colonies *in vitro, Exp. Hematol.,* 7, 345, 1979.
37. **Vainchenker, W., Guichard, J., and Breton-Gorius, J.,** Growth of human megakaryocyte colonies in culture from fetal, neonatal and adult peripheral blood cells: ultrastructural analysis, *Blood Cells,* 5, 25, 1979a.
38. **Vainchenker, W., Bouquet, J., Guichard, J., and Breton-Gorius, J.,** Megakaryocyte colony formation from human bone marrow precursors, *Blood,* 54, 940, 1979b.
39. **Jacobsen, N. and Broxmeyer, H. E.,** Oscillations of granulocytic and megakaryocytic progenitor cell populations in cyclic neutropenia in man, *Scand J. Haematol.,* 23, 33, 1979.
40. **Mazur, E. M., Hoffman, R., Chasis, J., Marchesi, S., and Bruno, E.,** Immunofluorescent identification of human megakaryocyte colonies using an antiplatelet glycoprotein antiserum, *Blood,* 57, 277, 1981.
41. **Mazur, E. M., Hoffman, R., and Bruno, E.,** Regulation of human megakaryocytopoiesis: an *in vitro* analysis, *J. Clin. Invest.,* 68, 733, 1981.
42. **Porter, R. P. and Gengozian, N.,** *In Vitro* proliferation and differentiation of hemic precursor cells from marrow and blood of naturally chimeric marmosets, *J. Cell. Physiol.,* 79, 27, 1972.
43. **Nakeff, A., Van Noord, M. J., and Blansjaar, N.,** Electron microscopy of megakaryocytes in thin-layer agar cultures of mouse bone marrow, *J. Ultrastruct. Res.,* 49, 1, 1974.
44. **Nakeff, A.,** Colony-forming unit, megakaryocyte (CFU-M): its use in elucidating the kinetics and humoral control of the megakaryocytic committed progenitor cell compartment, in *Experimental Hematology Today,* Baum, S. J. and Ledney, D. G., Eds., Springer-Verlag, New York, 1977, 111.
45. **Nagasawa, T., Nakazawa, M., and Abe, T.,** A liquid culture system for murine megakaryocyte progenitor cells, *Blood,* 59, 250, 1982.
46. **Jackson, C. W.,** Cholinesterase as a possible marker for early cells of the megakaryocytic series, *Blood,* 42, 413, 1973.
47. **Jackson, C. W.,** Some characteristics of the rat megakaryocyte precursors identified using cholinesterase as a marker, in *Platelets: Production, Function, Transfusion and Storage,* Baldini, M. G. and Ebbe, S., Eds., Grune & Stratton, New York, 1974, 33.
48. **Long, M. W. and Henry, R. L.,** Thrombocytosis-induced suppression of small, acetylcholinesterase-positive cells in bone marrow of rats, *Blood,* 54, 1338, 1979.
49. **Rabellino, E. M., Levene, R. B., Leung, L. L. K., and Nachman, R. L.,** Human megakaryocytes. II. Expression of platelet proteins in early marrow megakaryocytes, *J. Exp. Med.,* 154, 88, 1981.
50. **Markovic, O. S. and Shulman, N. R.,** Megakaryocyte maturation indicated by methanol inhibition of an acid phosphatase shared by megakaryocytes and platelets, *Blood,* 50, 905, 1977.
51. **Messner, H. A. and Fauser, A. A.,** Identification of megakaryocytes in human bone marrow culture: nonspecificity of acid phosphatase, *Blood,* 55, 872, 1980.
52. **Firkin, F., Russell, S., and Orams, J.,** Identification of megakaryocytes in human bone marrow culture: nonspecificity of acid phosphatase, *Blood,* 55, 872, 1980.
53. **McDonald, T. P., Cottrell, M., Clift, R., and Love, K.,** Purification and assay of thrombopoietin, *Exp. Hematol.,* 2, 355, 1974.
54. **McDonald, T. P.,** Assay of thrombopoietin utilizing human sera and urine fractions, *Biochem. Med.,* 13, 101, 1975.
55. **Evatt, B. L., Shreiner, D. P., and Levin, J.,** Thrombopoietic activity of fractions of rabbit plasma: studies in rabbits and mice, *J. Lab. Clin. Med.,* 83, 364, 1974.
56. **Evatt, B. L., Levin, J., and Algazy, K. M.,** Partial purification of thrombopoietin from the plasma of thrombocytopenic rabbits, *Blood,* 54, 377, 1979.
57. **McDonald, T. P.,** Role of the kidneys in thrombopoietin production, *Exp. Hematol.,* 4, 27, 1976.
58. **McDonald, T. P., Clift, R., Lange, R. D., Nolan, C., Tribby, I. I. E., and Barlow, G. H.,** Thrombopoietin production by human embryonic kidney cells in culture, *J. Lab. Clin. Med.,* 85, 59, 1975.
59. **Odell, T. T., Jr., McDonald, T. P., Shelton, C., and Clift, R.,** Stimulation of mouse megakaryocyte endomitosis by plasma from thrombocytopenic rats, *Proc. Soc. Exp. Biol. Med.,* 160, 263, 1979.
60. **Burgess, A. S., Metcalf, D., Russell, S. H., and Nicola, N. A.,** Granulocyte/macrophage-, megakaryocyte-, eosinophil- and erythroid-colony-stimulating factors produced by mouse spleen cells, *Biochem. J.,* 185, 301, 1980.

61. **Enomoto, K., Kawakita, S., Kishimoto, N., Katayama, N., and Myake, T.,** Thrombopoiesis and megakaryocyte colony-stimulating factor in the urine of patients with aplastic anemia, *Br. J. Haematol.*, 45, 551, 1980.
62. **Nachman, R., Levine, R., and Jaffee, E. A.,** Synthesis of factor VIII antigen by cultured guinea pig megakaryocytes, *J. Clin. Invest.*, 60, 914, 1977.
63. **Nachman, R., Levine, R., and Jaffee, E.,** Synthesis of actin by cultured guinea pig megakaryocytes. Complex formation with fibrin, *Biochim. Biophys. Acta.* 543, 91, 1978.
64. **Chernoff, A., Levine, R. F., and Goodman, D. S.,** Origin of platelet-derived growth factor in megakaryocytes in guinea pigs, *J. Clin. Invest.*, 65, 926, 1980.
65. **Chervenick, P. A. and Boggs, D. R.,** Decreased neutrophils and megakaryocytes in anemic mice of genotype W/W^v, *J. Cell Physiol.*, 73, 25, 1969.
66. **Ebbe, S., Phalen, E., and Stohlman, F., Jr.,** Abnormalities of megakaryocytes in Sl/Sl^D mice, *Blood,* 42, 865, 1973.
67. **Ebbe, S., Phalen, E., and Stohlman, F., Jr.,** Abnormalities of megakaryocytes in $W\text{-}W^V$ mice, *Blood,* 42, 857, 1973.
68. **Ebbe, S., Phalen, E., and Howard, D.,** Parabiotic demonstration of a humoral factor affecting megakaryocyte size in Sl/Sl^D mice, *Proc. Soc. Exp. Biol. Med.*, 158, 637, 1978.
69. **Ebbe, S., Phalen, E., D'Amore, P., and Howard, D.,** Megakaryocytic responses to thrombocytopenia and thrombocytosis in Sl/Sl^D mice, *Exp. Hematol.*, 6, 201, 1978.
70. **Ebbe, S. and Phalen, E.,** Regulation of megakaryocytes in W/W^V mice, *J. Cell. Physiol.*, 96, 73, 1978.
71. **Ebbe, S., Phalen, E., and Ryan, M. K.,** The production of megakaryocytic macrocytosis by systemic factors in Sl/Sl^D mice, Proc. Soc. Exp. Biol. Med., 155, 243, 1977.
72. **Nakeff, A. and Bryan, J. E.,** Megakaryocyte proliferation and its regulation as revealed by CFU-M analysis, in *Hematopoietic Cell Differentiation,* Golde, D. W., Cline, J. M., Metcalf, D., and Fox, C. F., Eds., Academic, Press, New York, 1978, 241.
73. **Nakeff, A.,** Flow cytometric analysis of megakaryocytopoiesis: strategy for defining mitotic and endoreduplicative events in the committed progenitor compartment, *Blood Cells,* 6, 665, 1980.
74. **Paulus, J. M.,** Cytophotometric measurements of DNA in thrombopoietic megakaryocytes, *Exp. Cell Res.*, 53, 310, 1968.
75. **Paulus, J. M.,** DNA metabolism and development of organelles in guinea-pig megakaryocytes: a combined ultrastructural, autoradiographic and cytophotometric study, *Blood,* 35, 298, 1970.
75a. **Zajicek, J.,** Studies of the histogenesis of blood platelets, *Acta Haematol.*, 12, 38, 1954.
75b. **Zajicek, J.,** Studies on the histogenesis of blood platelets and megakaryocytes, *Acta Physiol. Scand.*, 40, Suppl. 138, 1957.
75c. **Odell, T. T., Jr., and Jackson, C. W.,** Polyploidy and maturation of rat megakaryocytes, *Blood,* 32, 102, 1968.
76. **MacPherson, G. G.,** Development of megakaryocytes in bone marrow of the rat: an analysis by electron microscopy and high resolution autoradiography, *Proc. R. Soc. London Ser. B,* 177, 265, 1971.
76a. **Odell, T. T., Jr., Jackson, C. W., and Friday, T. J.,** Megakaryocytopoiesis in rats with special reference to ploidy, *Blood,* 35, 775, 1970.
77. **Metcalf, D. and Moore, M. A. S.,** *Haemopoietic Cells,* North-Holland, Amsterdam, 1971.
78. **Metcalf, D.,** *Hemapoietic Colonies,* Springer-Verlag, Berlin, 1977.
79. **Till, J. E. and McCulloch, E. A.,** Hemopoietic stem cell differentiation, *Biochim. Biophys. Acta,* 605, 431, 1980.
80. **Freedman, M. H., McDonald, T. P., and Saunders, E. F.,** Differentiation of murine marrow megakaryocyte progenitors (CFU-M): humoral control *in vitro, Cell Tissue Kinet.*, 14, 53, 1981.
81. **Rubini, J. R., Cronkite, E. P., Bond, V. P., and Fleidner, T. M.,** The metabolism and fate of tritiated thymidine in man, *J. Clin. Invest.*, 39, 909, 1960.
81a. **Ebbe, S. and Stohlman, F., Jr.,** Megakaryocytopoiesis in the rat, *Blood,* 26, 20, 1965.
81b. **Feinendegen, L. E., Odartchenko, N., Cottier, H., and Bond, V. P.,** Kinetics of megakaryocyte proliferation, *Proc. Soc. Exp. Biol. Med.*, 111, 177, 1962.
81c. **Feinendegen, L. E., Bond, V. P., and Hughes, W. L.,** ^{125}I-DU (5-iodo-2'-deoxyuridine) in autoradiographic studies of cell proliferation, *Exp. Cell Res.*, 43, 107, 1966.
82. **Ebbe, S. and Stohlman, F., Jr.,** Effects of hypertransfusion and erythropoietin on labelling of rat megakaryocytes by tritiated thymidine, *Proc. Soc. Exp. Biol. Med.*, 116, 971, 1964.
83. **Leven, R. M. and Nachmias, V. T.,** The response of cultured megakaryocytes to adenosine diphosphate, in *Megakaryocyte Biology and Precursors: In Vitro Cloning and Cellular Properties,* Evatt, B. E., Levine, R. F., and Williams, N. T., Eds., Elsevier North Holland, Amsterdam, 1981, 261.

84. **Karnovsky, M. J. and Roots, L.,** A "direct-coloring" thiocholine method for cholinesterases, *J. Histochem. Cytochem.,* 12, 219, 1964.
85. **Prince, A. K.,** A sensitive fluorometric procedure for the determination of small quantities of acetylcholinesterase, *Biochem. Pharmacol.,* 15, 411, 1966.
86. **Odell, T. T., Jr.,** personal communication.
87. **McEver, R. P., Baenziger, N. C., and Majerus, P. W.,** Isolation and quantitation of the platelet membrane glycoprotein dificient in thrombasthenia using a monoclonal hybridoma antibody, *J. Clin. Invest.,* 66, 1311, 1980.
88. **Goodman, R., Grate, H. E., Hannon, E., and Hellman, S.,** Hematopoietic stem cells: effect of preirradiation, bleeding and erythropoietin on thrombopoietic differentiation, *Blood,* 49, 253, 1977.
89. **Hodgson, G.,** Erythrocyte ^{59}Fe uptake as a function of bone marrow dose injected in lethally irradiated mice, *Blood,* 19, 460, 1962.
90. **Gurney, C. W., Lajtha, L. G., and Oliver, R.,** A method for investigation of stem-cell kinetics, *Br. J. Haematol.,* 8, 461, 1962.
91. **Hellman, S. and Grate, H. E.,** Production of granulocyte progeny by transplanted bone marrow in irradiated mice, *Blood,* 30, 103, 1967.
92. **Nakeff, A., McLellan, W. N., Bryan, J., and Valeriote, F. A.,** Response of megakaryocyte, erythroid and granulocyte-macrophage progenitor cells in mouse bone marrow to gamma-irradiation and cyclophosphamide, in *Experimental Hematology Today, 1979,* Baum, S. J. and Ledney, G. D., Eds., Springer-Verlag, New York, 1979, 99.
93. **Till, J. E. and McCulloch, E. A.,** A direct measurement of the radiation sensitivity of normal mouse bone marrow cells, *Radiat. Res.,* 14, 213, 1961.
94. **Ebbe, S., Phalen, P., Overcash, J., Howard, D., and Stohlman, F., Jr.,** A difference between stem cells from marrow and spleen in initiating splenic megakaryocytopoiesis, *Proc. Soc. Exp. Biol. Med.,* 137, 233, 1971.
95. **Ebbe, S., Phalen, E., Overcash, J., Howard, D., and Stohlman, F., Jr.,** Stem cell response to thrombocytopenia, *J. Lab. Clin. Med.,* 76, 872, 1971.
96. **Nakeff, A.,** Control of hematopoietic stem cell differentiation into megakaryocytes both *in vivo* and *in vitro, Blood,* 49 (Abstr.), 589, 1972.
97. **McDonald, T. P., Cottrell, M., Congdon, C. C., Walaser, O., and Barlow, G. H.,** Stimulation of megakaryocytic spleen colonies in mice by thrombopoietin, *Life Sci.,* 22, 1853, 1978.
98. **Goldberg, J., Phalen, E., Howard, D., Ebbe, S., and Stohlman, F., Jr.,** Thrombocytotic suppression of megakaryocyte production from stem cells, *Blood,* 49, 59, 1977.
99. **Nakeff, A. and Dicke, K. A.,** Stem cell differentiation into megakaryocytes from mouse bone marrow cultured with the thin layer technique, *Exp. Hematol.,* 22, 58, 1972.
100. **Williams, N., Jackson, H., Ralph, P., and Nakoinz, I.,** Cell interactions influencing murine marrow megakaryocytes: nature of the potentiator cell in bone marrow, *Blood,* 57, 157, 1981.
101. **Levin, J., Levin, F. C., and Metcalf, D.,** The effects of acute thrombocytopenia on megakaryocyte-CFC and granulocyte-macrophage-CFC in mice: studies of bone marrow and spleen, *Blood,* 56, 274, 1980.
102. **Levin, J., Levin, F. C., Penington, D. G., and Metcalf, D.,** Measurement of ploidy distribution in megakaryocyte colonies obtained from culture with studies of the effects of thrombocytopenia, *Blood,* 57, 287, 1981.
103. **McLeod, D. L., Shreeve, M. M., and Axelrad, A. A.,** Chromosome marker evidence for the bipotentiality of BFU-E, *Blood,* 56, 318, 1980.
104. **Weinstein, R., Stemerman, M. B., MacIntyre, D. E., Steinberg, H. N., and Maciag, T.,** The morphological and biochemical characterization of a line of rat promegakaryoblasts, *Blood,* 58, 110, 1981.
105. **Nakeff, A.,** Examination of culture conditions for optimizing the growth of megakaryocyte colonies, in *Megakaryocyte Biology and Precursors: In Vitro Cloning and Cellular Properties,* Evatt, B. E., Levine, R. F., and Williams, N. T., Eds., Elsevier North Holland, Amsterdam, 1981, 111.

105a. **Axelrad, A. A.,** personal communication.

106. **Williams, N. and Jackson, H.,** Regulation of proliferation of murine megakaryocyte progenitor cells by cell cycle, *Blood,* 52, 1, 163, 1978.
107. **Holley, R. W., Bohlen, P., Fava, R., Baldwin, J. H., Kleeman, G., and Armour, R.,** Purification of kidney epithelial cell growth inhibitors, *Proc. Natl. Acad. Sci. U.S.A.,* 77, 5989, 1980.
108. **Ebbe, E.,** Thrombopoietin, *Blood,* 44, 605, 1974.
109. **Ryo, R., Proffitt, R. T., Roger, M. E., O'Bear, R., and Deuel, T. F.,** Platelet factor 4 antigen in megakaryocytes, *Thromb. Res.,* 17, 645, 1980.
110. **Ebbe, S., Stohlman, F., Jr., Donovan, J., and Howard, D.,** Megakaryocytopoiesis in the rat with transfusion-induced thrombocytosis, *Proc. Soc. Exp. Biol. Med.,* 122, 1053, 1966.

111. **Odell, T. T., Jr., Jackson, C. W., and Reiter, R. S.,** Depression of the megakaryocyte-platelet system in rats by transfusion of platelets, *Acta Haematol. (Basel),* 38, 34, 1967.
112. **Ebbe, E. and Phalen, E.,** Does autoregulation of megakaryocytopoiesis occur, *Blood Cells,* 5, 123, 1979.
113. **Wickmann, H. E., Gerhardts, M. D., Spechtmeyer, H., and Gross, R.,** A mathematical model of thrombopoiesis in rats, *Cell Tissue Kinet.,* 12, 551, 1979.
114. **Abildgaard, C. F. and Simone, J. F.,** Thrombopoiesis, *Semin. Hematol.,* 4, 424, 1967.
115. **Shreiner, D. and Levin, J.,** Regulation of thrombopoiesis, in *Haemopoietic Stem Cells,* Vol. 13, Ciba Foundation Symposium, Associated Scientific, Amsterdam, 1973, 224.
116. **Odell, T. T., Jr. and Shelton, C.,** Increasing stimulation of megakaryocytopoiesis with decreasing platelet count, *Proc. Soc. Exp. Biol. Med.,* 161, 531, 1979.
117. **Odell, T. T., Jr., Murphy, J. R., and Jackson, C. W.,** Stimulation of megakaryocytopoiesis by acute thrombocytopenia in rats, *Blood,* 48, 765, 1976.
118. **Williams, N., McDonald, T. P., and Rabellino, E. M.,** Maturation and regulation of megakaryocytopoiesis, *Blood Cells,* 5, 43, 1979.
119. **Burstein, S. A., Adamson, J. W., and Harker, L. A.,** Megakaryocytopoiesis in culture: modulation of cholinergic mechanisms, *J. Cell Physiol.,* 103, 201, 1980.
120. **Williams, N., Jackson, H. and Meyers, P.,** Isolation of pluripotent hemopoietic stem cells and clonable precursor cells of erythrocytes, granulocytes, macrophages and megakaryocytes from mouse bone marrow, *Exp. Hematol.,* 7(10), 524, 1979.
121. **Castro-Malaspina, H., Rabelline, E. M., Yen, A., Nachman, R. L., and Moore, M. A.,** Human megekaryocyte stimulation of proliferation of bone marrow fibroblasts, *Blood,* 57, 781, 1981.
122. **Odell, T. T., Jr., Burch, E. A., Jr., Jackson, C. W., and Friday, T. J.,** Megakaryocytopoiesis in mice, *Cell Tissue Kinet.,* 2, 363, 1969.
123. **Dukes, P. P., Izadi, P., Ortega, J. A., Shore, N. A., and Gomperts, E.,** Inhibitory effects of interferon on mouse megakaryocyte progenitor cells in culture, *Exp. Hematol.,* 8, 1048, 1980.
124. **Smith, P. J., Jackson, C. W., Whidden, M. A., and Edwards, C. C.,** Effect of hypertransfusion on bone marrow regeneration in sublethally irradiated mice. II. Enhanced recovery of megakaryocytes and platelets, *Blood,* 56, 58, 1980.
125. **Jones, B. C., Radley, J. M., Bradley, T. R., and Hodgson, G. S.,** Enhanced megakaryocyte repopulating ability of stem cells surviving 5-fluorouracil treatment, *Exp. Hematol.,* 8, 61, 1980.
126. **Harker, L. A.,** Kinetics of thrombopoiesis, *J. Clin. Invest.,* 47, 458, 1968.
127. **Penington, D. G. and Olsen, T. E.,** Megakaryocytes in states of altered platelet production: Cell numbers, size and DNA content, *Brit. J. Haematol.,* 18, 447, 1970.
128. **Odell, T. T., Jr., Jackson, C. W., Friday, T. J., and Charsha, D. E.,** Effects of thrombocytopenia on megakaryocytopoiesis, *Brit. J. Haematol.,* 17, 91, 1969.
129. **Ebbe, S., Stohlman, F., Jr., Donovan, J., and Overcash, J.,** Megakaryocyte maturation rate in thrombocytopenic rats, *Blood,* 32, 787, 1968.
130. **Odell, T. T., Jr. and Boran, D. A.,** The mitotic index of megakaryocytes of mice after acute thrombocytopenia, *Proc. Soc. Exp. Biol. Med.,* 155, 149, 1977.

INDEX

A

B

C

D

E

F

G

H

I

K

L

M

N

R

S

The Human Bone Marrow: Anatomy, Physiology, and Pathophysiology

Volume II

Editors

Sidney Trubowitz, M.D.
Veterans Administration Medical Center
East Orange, New Jersey
and
Professor of Medicine
CMDNJ-New Jersey Medical School
Newark, New Jersey

Stephen Davis, M.D.
Veterans Administration Medical Center
East Orange, New Jersey
and
Associate Professor of Medicine
CMDNJ-New Jersey Medical School
Newark, New Jersey

CRC Press, Inc.
Boca Raton, Florida

Library of Congress Cataloging in Publication Data
Main entry under title:

The Human bone marrow.

Bibliography: p.
Includes indexes.
1. Marrow—Diseases—Diagnosis. 2. Marrow—Biopsy, Needle. 3. Marrow—Examination.
4. Diagnosis, Cytologic. I. Trubowitz, Sidney, 1911– . II. Davis, Stephen, 1943– . [DNLM: 1. Bone marrow. WH 380 H918]
RC645.7.H85 616.4'1 81-18195
ISBN 0-8493-6105-2 (v. 1) AACR2
ISBN 0-8493-6106-0 (v. 2)

Direct all inquiries to CRC Press, Inc., 2000 Corporate Blvd., N.W., Boca Raton, Florida, 33431.

International Standard Book Number 0-8493-6105-2 (Volume I)
International Standard Book Number 0-8493-6106-0 (Volume II)

Library of Congress Card Number 81-18195
Printed in the United States

THE EDITORS

Sidney Trubowitz, M.D., is a graduate of Columbia College, Columbia University in New York City and received his medical degree from Rush Medical College (University of Chicago). On completion of his clinical training he was called to active duty and served in the Pacific Theatre during World War II for some 3 years. On his return to civilian life he spent a year at the National Transfusion Center in Paris and then joined the Veterans Administration Medical Center, East Orange, New Jersey where he served as Chief of the Hematology Section. He is Professor of Medicine, New Jersey College of Medicine, Newark New Jersey. His major research interests have centered on the alkaline phosphatase of granulocytes and on the structure and function of the bone marrow matrix. He is a member of the American College of Physicians, the American Society of Hematology, and the Royal Society of Tropical Medicine.

Stephen Davis, M.D., graduated magna cum laude from Brooklyn College of Pharmacy, Long Island University in Brooklyn, New York and obtained his doctorate in medicine at New York's Mount Sinai School of Medicine. His training in neoplastic and blood diseases was obtained at the National Cancer Institute (NIH), Bethesda, Maryland and the Tufts-New England Medical Center, Boston, Massachusetts. He served as Chief of the Oncology-Hematology Section at the Veterans Administration Medical Center, East Orange, New Jersey and Associate Professor of Medicine, New Jersey Medical School, Newark, New Jersey. His research interests are varied but have concentrated on normal and malignant lymphocyte biology, thymic hormones, and human and experimental lung carcinomas. He is also active in many scientific societies particularly the American Society of Clinical Oncologists, the American Society of Hematology, and the American Association for Cancer Research.

CONTRIBUTORS

Hal E. Broxmeyer, Ph.D.
Assistant Member
Sloan Kettering Institute for Cancer Research and
Assistant Professor
Cornell University
New York, New York

Professor Wenceslao Calvo, M.D.
Department of Clinical Physiology
University of Ulm
Federal Republic of Germany

Stephen Davis, M.D.
VA Medical Center
East Orange, New Jersey and
Health Research Institute
Fairleigh-Dickinson University
Madison, New Jersey and
Associate Professor of Medicine
CMDNJ-New Jersey Medical School
Newark, New Jersey

E. Kelemen, M.D., D.Sc.
Professor of Medicine
Semmelweis University Medical School
Budapest, Hungary

Alexander Nakeff, Ph.D.
Assistant Professor
Cancer Biology in Radiology
Mallinckrodt Institute of Radiology
Washington University School of Medicine
St. Louis, Missouri

Young K. Park, M.D.
Assistant Professor
CMDNJ-New Jersey Medical School
Attending Physician
VA Medical Center
East Orange, New Jersey

Pietro Rambotti, M.D.
Assistant Professor of Medicine
Instituto di Clinica Medica Generale e Terapia Medica del Universita di Perugia
Perugia, Italy

Nydia G. Testa, M.D., Ph.D.
Senior Research Scientist
Paterson Laboratories
Christie Hospital and
Holt Radium Institute
Manchester
Great Britain

Sidney Trubowitz, M.D.
VA Medical Center
East Orange, New Jersey and
Professor of Medicine
CMDNJ-New Jersey Medical School
Newark, New Jersey

TABLE OF CONTENTS
THE HUMAN BONE MARROW:
ANATOMY, PHYSIOLOGY, AND PATHOPHYSIOLOGY

Volume I

Volume II

TABLE OF CONTENTS

Volume II

Chapter 8

THE BONE MARROW ASPIRATE AND BIOPSY

Sidney Trubowitz and Stephen Davis

TABLE OF CONTENTS

I. INTRODUCTION

Hidden from view and widely dispersed in the internal cavities of the skeleton, the human marrow, despite its large size and impressive capacity, escaped the attention of both investigators and clinicians for many years. Hampered, too, by the poor quality of the sections prepared from the highly autolyzed material obtained at the post-mortem examination, pathologists and clinicians alike were willing to accept the dictum that blood is a perfect reflection of the marrow.

At the turn of the century, some physicians, notably the Italians, struck by the disparity of findings between the blood and marrow of individuals who had succumbed to pernicious anemia, initiated the early attempts at sampling marrow from live patients. The techniques employed were aggressive and were accomplished by trephining a core of bone from the epiphyseal end of the femur or tibia, permitting the operator to scoop out the soft, paste-like marrow for the preparation of both smears and sections.[1–3] The site selected by the early investigators was not wisely chosen, for the tibia in the healthy human adult contains variable quantities of red marrow and does not generally furnish samples representative of the red marrow under either normal or pathological conditions. Further, the technique was not without discomfort, requiring immobilization of the extremity for a week, and of course ran the serious risk of infection.[4] Obviously, the procedure received only limited application.

Unhappy with the tibial site, Seyfarth[5] developed a simple hand trephine for sampling the sternum: a site simpler to approach and one more likely to yield reliable material for examination. Ironically, Seyfarth was not interested in the hemopoietic function of the marrow, and developed his technique in his capacity as a physician in a hospital for tropical disease to aid him in the diagnosis of kala-azar and malaria.[6] The procedure, however, found some limited application in a number of hematologic institutions. Its major limitations were discomfort, and more seriously, from the point of view of the investigators, it was a one time procedure that could not be repeated on the same patient.

Though application of these techniques was limited, it became quite clear that the examination of the marrow sample from the sternum of the living patient could contribute significantly to the understanding of the normal hemopoietic process and its aberrations in disease. Thus, it was a happy event when Arinkin[7] introduced his method for the aspiration of marrow by a thin needle from the human sternum. Arinkin was impressed by Seyfarth's description of his biopsy material of the human sternal marrow and saw the potential of such a technique for the clinical investigator of hematologic disease and for the experimental investigator interested in marrow structure and function. He also saw the need for a simple procedure, requiring no special instrumentation and which would not cause much damage to skin or bone.

Arinkin[7] adapted a lumbar puncture needle for the task. Preliminary observations on the cadaver convinced him that the material obtained by aspiration was comparable to that secured by trephine. Careful anatomic studies of the sternum distinguished two basic types: a sternum with a broad manubrium but a spongiosa narrower in its midline than in its lateral portions, and a sternum with a marrow manubrium but more uniform spongiosa. He, therefore, recommended that the needle be inserted about 0.5 to 1.0 cm lateral to the midline in the first type and in the midline in the second. He also recognized that manubrium may occasionally be devoid of marrow, in which case the corpus sterni was recommended as a substitute site.

The technique is indeed simple. A needle is introduced into the manubrium, or into the corpus, immediately below the angle of Louis. On feeling the give of the compact lamellae, the stylus is removed and the marrow aspirated into a dry syringe. Rarely, the procedure may be foiled by an impenetrably hard bone. Arinkin[7] also called attention to the findings that the first few drops of the aspirate are rich in marrow tissue only to be diluted by contaminating blood on further aspiration. He also recognized the difficulty of obtaining samples from highly proliferating marrow, such as is encountered in acute leukemia.

The simplicity, utility, and safety of the needle aspiration of human sternal marrow led to its immediate acceptance and wide application. It did much to rekindle interest in morphologic hematology which had become rather dormant in that period. The 1930s saw the development of histochemistry, cell physiology, and electron microscopy—in brief, a shift of interest to the cell, its internal organization and structure, its chemistry and function. These rapidly developing advances were quickly applied to the study of the marrow cells provided by the needle aspiration technique,[8] and helped to narrow the gulf between morphology and function.

Needle puncture of the human sternum does carry some risk, and serious accidents, such as perforation into the mediastinum and laceration of the internal mammary artery, have been reported. Evidence has accumulated that marrow obtained by aspiration from different areas in the same person is of comparable composition if the sites are those that normally contain red marrow, such as ribs, sternum, vertebrae, and the iliac crest.[9,10] The iliac crest was recommended as a preferable site for the needle puncture of the marrow.[11,12] The safety of the procedure outweighed some of its disadvantages and it has become the preferred aspiration site in most institutions today.

Limitations of the aspiration technique in the recognition of certain disease states, such as Hodgkin's disease, non-Hodgkin's lymphoma, granulomatous disease, metastatic carcinoma, and myelofibrosis, and in the evaluation of bone marrow cellularity, particularly in the hypoplastic states, have led to increased utilization of needle core biopsies of the bone marrow. A variety of biopsy needles have been introduced;[13–16] a popular prototype is the Jamshidi biopsy needle.[17] The preferred biopsy site is the posterior superior iliac crest.

Methods for preparation of the marrow aspirate vary greatly. No standardized procedure has been achieved despite the fact that the technique has been widely used for the past 50 years. Smear, squashes, sections of clotted marrow, particle concentration for histologic preparation,[18,19] and buffy coat preparations are all used in varying measure. The biopsies can be processed for the customary usual histologic preparations or for thin epoxy-imbedded sections for both light or electron microscopy. Some of the basic information sought relates to marrow cellularity, the relative sizes of the hemopoietic compartments, and an evaluation of the maturation process.

Both the aspiration and the needle core biopsy of the marrow have their virtues and their limitations. The aspiration technique tends to destroy the histological relationships of the marrow sample and is plagued by considerable and variable contamination with peripheral blood, but it does provide simplicity, speed, and ease of preparation, and above all, excellent material for the cytological examination of intracellular detail. The cellular material provided by needle aspiration of the marrow lends itself readily for chromosome analysis, evaluation of stem cell compartments by tissue culture, and the study of living cells by phase microscopy and cinephotography. The needle core biopsy, on the other hand, preserves the histological relationships of the marrow sample and provides information in many circumstances where the aspiration technique fails, as in the recognition of granulomata, marrow infarction, necrosis, metastatic tumor, lymphoma and leukemia, and the identification of collagen, reticulin, amyloid, iron, etc. The biopsy specimen, after appropriate fixation, can be prepared for the familiar hematoxylin-eosin stained section, undecalcified plastic-embedded thin section for light microscopy. The biopsy specimen can also be prepared for electron microscopy, both transmission and scanning, and for cytochemical and marker studies.

The clinical application of the bone marrow examination requires planning and the development of a strategy for each individual patient which, based on the variety of techniques now available, is designed to achieve a projected goal. In some circumstances, neither the aspiration nor the needle core biopsy techniques may suffice. For example, in an attempt to define more precisely the functional capabilities of the mononuclear lymphoid cells of the marrow, Alley and MacDermott[20] had to use ribs, surgically removed at thoracotomy, to obtain sufficient marrow free of contamination with mononuclear cells of the peripheral blood to solve their specific problem.

II. BONE MARROW CELLULARITY

Early attempts at the quantitative assessment of the cellularity of the marrow have centered on the enumeration of the nucleated cells in the marrow aspirate or on the estimation of the fat content of the marrow, either from sections prepared from marrow particles or from biopsy, or from volumetric data obtained by centrifugation of the marrow aspirate.

The enumeration of the nucleated cell content of the marrow aspirate by a chamber count is the simplest and easiest approach to the problem.[21-32] Unfortunately, the marrow aspirate is not a homogeneously distributed material and is subject to considerable contamination with peripheral blood.[33] Despite rigid control of the variables that affect the enumeration such as standardization of pipettes, chambers, and quantity of marrow aspirated, the results of such counts, have been subject to wide fluctuation.

The volumetric method for the determination of bone marrow cellularity was introduced by Schleicher[34,35] following preliminary investigations by Stasney and Higgins[36,37] and by Schleicher and Sharp.[38] The procedure is based on the concept that under normal physiological conditions, hemopoietic tissue, fat, and the sinusuidal system bear a constant relationship to each other and that in pathologic states a reciprocal relationship exists between the hemopoietic cells and the fat. The procedure is simple: exactly 1.0 mℓ of marrow is aspirated, mixed with heparin and introduced into a Wintrobe hematocrit, centrifuged for 5 min at 1500 rpm. The marrow specimen separates into four gross zones, from top of tube down: fat, plasma, the myeloid-erythroid (M-E) layer, and the erythrocytes. The volume of each zone is read off the hematocrit scale and expressed as volumes per cent. The normal value for fat found to be 0.5 to 3.0 volumes/percent, mean: 1.0 volumes percent; plasma 39.0 to 48.5 volumes/percent, mean: 44 volumes/percent; the myeloid-erythroid layer 4.0 to 6.0 volumes/percent, mean: 5.0 volumes percent and the erythrocytes 45 to 54 volumes/percent, mean: 50 volumes/percent.

Limarzi[39] subsequently distinguished between a red and yellow fat zone. The procedure was evaluated by a number of investigators,[40-43] and the results of these studies suggested that, at best, the volumetric data give a very crude estimate of the marrow cellularity; that sections prepared from particles are superior to the volumetric data; but that the use of both together may be advantageous.

The anatomical approach to the estimation of marrow cellularity is based on the estimation of the relative areas of fat and hemopoietic cells in sections or squashes prepared either from particles retrieved from marrow aspirates or from the sections prepared from needle core biopsies. Purely qualitative estimates suffer from poor reproducibility due in large measure to the heterogeneous distribution of fat and cells in the marrow. Early investigators made use of the Whipple eyepiece and micrometer to aid in their attempts at some quantification.[35,42]

The proportions of bone, hematopoietic marrow, and fat in histologic sections of bone biopsies can be determined by a point counting method, using a Zeiss I integrating eyepiece containing a graticle of 25 randomly placed points. The principle on which the determination depends is based upon the fact that the number of points lying over any component in a section is proportional to the area of the component in the section and this in turn is proportional to its volume.[44]

The number of points projected on the object divided by 25 and multiplied by 100 is equal to the percentage of the surface occupied by the object measured. If 1600 points are examined for each sample (that is, a total of 64 microscopic fields) an absolute error of less than 1% is achieved. Hartsock, Smith, and Petty[45] utilized this image analyzing technique to determine the replacement of marrow hematopoietic tissue by adipose tissue in the iliac crest biopsies from 177 subjects of all ages who died suddenly but were hematologically normal. They found that the marrow fat increased steadily from a level of 20% at age 5 to 50% at age 35, remained stable between the ages 35 to 65, and then rose steadily to 67% at age 75. Dunnill, Anderson, and Whitehead[46] in a quantitative analysis of histologic sections of the second lumbar vertebra of 95 normal subjects found a striking change in the marrow cellularity with age. The volume of fat, expressed as a percentage of the total bone sample, increased from 15% in the first decade of life to 55% in the eighth. Meunier et al.,[47] in a study concerned with the effects of osteoporosis on marrow cellularity, measured the volume of bone and fat in 5-μm sections prepared from needle core biopsies of the ilium. They found a definite decrease in trabecular bone with age, falling from volumes of 26% at age 20 to 16% at age 65. With the fall in bone volume, an increase in marrow fat volume was noted, rising from 15% at age 20 to 60% at age 65. In osteopenic subjects much larger increments of adipose volume were found. Good correlation was found between marrow cellularity and bone volume; the more rarefied the bone, the less abundant was the marrow cell population. The authors speculated on the possible relationship of bone marrow to bone remodeling.

Automatic image analytic instruments are capable of extracting geometric and densitometric information from images.[48] Such instrumentation has been applied to the study of marrow cellularity of iliac bone biopsies, processed as 5-μm paraffin and thin epoxy-imbedded section.[49–53] Best results are obtained with the thin-sectioned expoxy-imbedded material. Marrow cellularity was found to decrease with age and the degree of physiologic osteopenia, for which appropriate correction could be made. The volume of adipose tissue in the sections prepared from normal human marrow was found to lie between 35% to 65%.

III. MEASUREMENT OF TOTAL MARROW VOLUME

Various estimates of total bone marrow cellularity have been made both in man and some laboratory animals. The methods used in these assays have been conveniently classified into three groups.[54]

Mechanik[55] made the first measurement of the marrow volume by macerating the bones of the skeleton. In the process of maceration the marrow was lost and the marrow volume therefore was assumed to be the difference in the weight of the skeleton pre- and post-maceration. Nye[56] modified the technique by impregnating the empty marrow cavities with agar. Now, from the increase in weight of the agar-filled bones over the weight of the macerated bone, the marrow volume for a number of animals—dogs,[57] guinea pigs,[58] and rats—determined by the agar impregnation technique was found to range between 1.56 to 1.7% of the body weight of the animal.

The total marrow cellularity can be obtained if the unit cellularity of the bone marrow is multiplied by the estimated total marrow volume. Pegg[54] collected the marrow from 12 ribs excised during thoracotomies and obtained an average of 1.2×10^9 cells presumed to be the marrow content of one rib. From the breakdown of Mechanik's data,[59] a rib marrow cellularity of 1.29×10^6 cells/mm^3 was calculated. The rib marrow cellularity of adults has been shown to be only one third as cellular as the marrow contained in other active hemopoietic sites.[60] Following correction for the difference in rib cellularity, and assuming a volume of 2%[54] for the hemopoietic marrow, the total marrow cellularity for man was calculated to be 8.1×10^9 cells/kg.

Osgood[61] based his calculation of the total marrow cellularity of man on five major assumptions: red cell production rate is derived from blood volume and red cell life span; total time for differentiation from last mitosis in normoblast stage until release from marrow is 48 hr; 25% of nucleated red cells are capable of mitosis; myeloid-erythroid ratio is 3:1; and finally, reticulocytes are delivered into the blood stream soon after their formation. His result, 46×10^9 cell/kg, is considerably overestimated, chiefly because the marrow reticulocyte stage was ignored. Marrow reticulocytes are approximately equal in number to the normoblasts.[62] On recalculation, including the marrow reticulocytes and assuming a myeloid-erythroid ratio of 2:1, the figure for the total marrow cellularity becomes 12.3×10^9 cells/kg, a result in closer agreement with other reports.

Patt[63] took a similar approach. He argued that in the steady state, production in the marrow and destruction in the periphery must be equivalent. If, then, one knew the number of cells in mitosis in a given series and the mitotic time, then the total number of cells in that series could be calculated. He assumed that mitotic time to be 45 min and accepted the published figure[64] for the percentage of cells in mitosis at any one time. His calculations revealed a total marrow cell population of 13.6×10^9 cells/kg.

Killman et al.[65] began his inquiry into the marrow cell population by determining the mitotic indices of specific cell types in normal human bone marrow. Of the mitotic figures counted, 69% were present in the erythroid precursors and 29% in the myeloid, namely the myeloblasts, promyelocyte, and myelocyte. The remaining mitotic figures were present in other marrow cells. The relative frequency of mitosis among the different hemopoietic cells was: normoblast, erythroblast, proerythroblast—9.5:4.1:1; and for myelocyte, promyelocyte, myeloblasts—7.8:2:1. Cells which resembled orthochromatic normoblasts on the basis of the hemoglobinization of the cytoplasm were considered to be polychromatophilic normoblasts if mitotic figures were present since it had been shown that typical small orthochromatic normoblasts do not synthesize DNA.[59] Thus, it was the mature cells of the marrow, normoblasts and myelocytes, which contributed most significantly, about 2/3 of the total number of mitoses in the marrow. If no difference in mitotic time exists at different levels of maturation, then the relative frequencies of the mitosis suggested five consecutive divisions for the erythroid cells and four to five for the granulocytic precursor cells.

The specific mitotic index, i.e., the fraction of a particular cell type in mitosis at any time is highest for the immature cells in the myeloid series and for the mature cells in the erythroid series. The specific mitotic index is five times greater for the erythroid cells than for the myeloid cells. Earlier reports on the number of mitotic figures in human marrow[66,67] were much lower than that reported by Killman et al.,[65] and were probably due to the use of smears rather than squash preparations.

Based on data obtained from tritiated thymidine incorporation of marrow cells[68–71] and assumptions relative to turnover time, multiplicative compartments, etc.,[59] and an estimated weighted mitotic time of 0.75 hr for the erythrocyte precursors and 0.51 hr for the granulocyte precursors, Killmann et al.[72] calculated a total mass of nucleated red cell precursors at 3.5×10^9 cells/kg and a total mass of neutrophils and their precursors at 8.5×10^9 cells/kg.

On the assumption that virtually all of the ^{59}Fe was recovered in the peripheral red blood cells following the intravenous administration of the transferin-bound isotope, Suit[73] proposed the use of ^{59}Fe as means of estimating the total marrow cellularity. Previous studies had shown that almost all of the administered ^{59}Fe is taken up by the marrow.[73,74] Suit[75] assumed that the ^{59}Fe content of the marrow 24 hr after its administration is the same as the amount of ^{59}Fe recovered from the red blood cells 5 days later, and is equal to 80% of the administered dose. In six subjects so studied, the erythrocyte precursor cells totaled 6 to 24×10^{10} cells per subject with a mean of 16 $\times 19^{10}$ cells. Assuming a myeloid-erythroid ratio of 2.5:1 and a mean body weight of 70 kg, a total bone marrow cellularity of 5.7×10^9 cells/kg (range 2.2 to 8.6×10^9 cells/kg) was obtained.

Donohue et al.[76,77] in similar fashion measured the total cellularity of the human bone marrow, but assumed a fixed value of 66% for the proportion of radioiron taken up by the bone marrow. They found a total marrow cellularity for man of 18×10^9 cell/kg, probably an overestimate resulting from their failure to account for the radioactivity present in the supernatant of their centrifuged marrow samples. Pegg[54] found a total marrow cellularity for the human marrow of 11.5×10^9 cells/kg, and Harrison[78] found 10.9×10^9 cells/kg; the calculations were based on an assumed 66% uptake of the injected radioiron.

Skarberg[79] blocked the recirculation of the radioiron in his assays of the total marrow cellularity by an intramuscular injection of an iron complex immediately after the administration of the ^{59}Fe, followed by oral iron sulfate daily for the next 12 days. Total marrow radioiron content was assumed to be equal to the total ^{59}Fe incorporation into the red blood cells 12 days later. Myeloid-erythroid ratios were determined from marrow smears and estimated at 3.7:1. The erythroid-megakaryocyte ratio was estimated from 4-μm sections of marrow and found to be 210:1. His results gave: total nucleated cell content of the marrow, 21×10^9 cells/kg; granulocyte precursors 13 $\times 10^9$ cells/kg; and megakaryocytes 0.016×10^9 cells/kg. The generation time of the erythroid precursors in polycythemia vera was unchanged from the normal.[80,81] In summary, despite limitations imposed by the inhomogeneity of the marrow tissue and the difficulties of quantitation and reproducibility, the techniques of needle aspiration and needle core biopsy of the human marrow have become the basic tools for the morphological study of the marrow. They have been of great value in the nosological classification and recognition of the primary hematologic disorders or of marrow involvement by tumor or lymphoma. Despite wide application in clinical practice during the past 50 years, little standardization has developed in the handling and processing of the marrow aspirates or in the establishment of normal values for the various parameters of interest and importance.

IV. CLINICAL EVALUATION OF MARROW ASPIRATES

An appeal for standardization of the marrow aspiration technique was made by Osgood[61] in his comprehensive review on the composition of the marrow cellularity. About a decade later Berman[82] proposed three standard puncture sites: the corpus sterni at the level of the second interspace; the anterior portion of the iliac bone; and the spinous process of the lumbar vertebrae.[83] He recommended the following format:

1. A "first drop smear." He well appreciated the effect of aspirate volume on the cellular content of the marrow sample and therefore proposed that more comparable and reproducible information could be garnered from smears prepared from the minimal volume of marrow aspirate, the first drop. The first drop smear was judged helpful in the evaluation of marrow cellularity and for the appreciation of fine cytological detail.
2. Centrifugation of the marrow aspirate for volumetrics data[40] to aid in the estimation of marrow cellularity; the preparation of smears from the myeloid-erythroid (buffy coat) layer for the generation of the myeloid-erythroid ratio, the maturation curve, and the mitotic index
3. Squash particle smears and imprints for the distribution of the marrow elements and overall cytological evaluation
4. Sections of the concentrated button of marrow particles to provide histologic appreciation of focal lesions, megakaryocyte number, and the fat cell/hemopoietic cell ratio; an estimate of marrow cellularity

Berman[82] reserved the needle core biopsy for those situations where the problem eluded solution by the simpler aspiration technique or in the event of failure to aspirate a suitable sample, the "dry" tap.

Many investigators[84–89] have argued that the needle core biopsy done concurrently with the marrow aspirate adds significantly to the morphological evaluation of the marrow. Brynes, McKenna, and Sundberg[90] in 1978 called for some standardization in the methods of preparation of the aspirated marrow samples for study. They recommended marrow aspiration and concurrent needle biopsy in all cases as the best approach to the thorough study of the marrow. They reemphasized the need for volumetric data, marrow buffy coat smears, squash particle smears, and particle sections. The handling of biopsy specimens was felt to be fairly uniform.

Perhaps more important than standardization is an appreciation of the limits as well as the usefulness of the cytologic data obtained from smears, particle squash smears, and buffy coat smears, and of the histologic evaluation obtained from the needle core biopsies, or particle sections, so that one can wisely select those techniques that can best furnish the basic data or the ancillary information required for the solution of the clinical problem. The basic information should include:

A. Marrow Cellularity

The marrow smears, buffy coat smears, volumetric data, and chamber counts do not give reliable and dependable evaluation of marrow cellular content. Section prepared from marrow particles give a good first approximation, limited primarily by the small sample size. Sections of a long needle core biopsy afford the best opportunity for a more reliable index of marrow cellularity, particularly if studied by a quantitative image analyzing method. The effects of age and osteopenia on marrow cellularity as well as the lack of homogeneity of the sample must be considered in the evaluation. A quantitative assessment of marrow cellularity is obviously time consuming without computer-aided equipment; a semiquantitative[91] approach may be selected in the more routine situation. The cellularity can be graded from 0, where the marrow section contains nothing but fat and there are no hematopoietic cells. In a 1 + marrow the section shows 1 to 3 cells between the fat cells; in a 2+ marrow, nests of 12 to 20 cells are seen between the fat cells; in a 3+ marrow, the hematopoietic cells are quite numerous, and less than ten but more than five fat cells are seen per microscopic field (magnification 200); and in 4+ marrow less than five fat cells/microscopic field are found. In the newborn, the normal marrow cellularity is in the 4+ range; in the adult, between 2 to 4+; and after the age of 60, 1 to 3+.

Marrow cellularity is a useful first approximation of marrow function or activity: the hypercellular marrow is seen as the morphologic expression of increased activity; the hypocellular marrow, of decreased function.

B. The Myeloid-Erythroid (M/E) Ratio

The M/E ratio helps define the relative sizes of the two major components of the hemopoietic compartment of the marrow. The M/E ratio is influenced by the degree of dilution of the sample with peripheral blood and is best obtained from first drop smears, squash particle smears, or sections. In general, the M/E ratio lies normally between 2:1 and 4:1, reflecting the predominantly granulocytic character of the marrow.

The M/E ratio, though a rough approximation, is nevertheless a useful measure of the activity of the erythroid and myeloid components of the marrow. Thus, in the presence of a normally cellular marrow and normal granulocyte production, a normal M/E ratio of 3:1 reflects normal erythropoietic activity. The reticulocyte index, obtained by correction of the reticulocyte count for hematocrit and maturation time,[92] is a measure of the effectiveness of the total marrow erythropoietic activity; hence, under normal conditions effective erythropoiesis would be characterized by a reticulocyte index of 1 and a M/E ratio of 3:1. Normal marrow cellularity, a very high M/E ratio, and corresponding decrease in the reticulocyte index should signal the presence of erythroblastopenia as seen, for example, in pure red cell anemia. Conversely, a hypercellular marrow, a reversed M/E ratio of 1:3, and a reticulocyte index of 5 reflects a marked expansion of the erythropoietic mass and red cell output as seen in severe hemolytic states. In general the M/E ratio is an expression of total marrow erythropoietic activity, and if erythropoiesis is effective a given production index can be anticipated as follows:

M/E ratio	Reticulocyte index
3:1	1
2:1 - 1:1	2-3
1:2 - 1:3	3-5

Lack of correspondence between the M/E ratio and the reticulocyte index suggests ineffective erythropoiesis. Thus, a hypercellular marrow, spinning in high gear with a M/E ratio of 1:3 and a reticulocyte index of 1 is obviously a highly ineffective marrow as typically seen in megaloblastic states.

The plasma iron turnover (PIT), derived from the half time clearance of intravenously injected radio labeled iron from the plasma, the serum iron, and the hematocrit and expressed as mg iron/100 ml whole blood/day is a measure of the iron uptake by the immature precursor red cells in the marrow. Red cell utilization is determined from the amount of radioiron in the circulating red cells 10 to 14 days later and is a measure of the productivity of the total erythropoietic activity. The PIT measures the number of erythroid precursors or the total marrow erythropoietic activity, and hence is comparable to the M/E ratio. The red cell utilization is a measure of red cell production and is thus equivalent to the reticulocyte index. The erythrocyte iron turnover (EIT) is derived from the PIT × red cell utilization and estimates the effectiveness of marrow erythropoietic activity.[93,94] Here we see two approaches, one physiologic and kinetic, the other morphologic and static, both clinically applicable in the evaluation of the functional state of the marrow. The fundamental aim of an analysis of the morphological data obtained from the examination of marrow specimens is the evaluation of marrow activity and function.

Similar reasoning can help in assessing the granulopoietic activity of the marrow. Assuming normal erythropoiesis, a hypercellular marrow and an increased M/E ratio, e.g., 6:1, reflect an increased leukoblastic activity which in turn suggests a leukocytic response to infection, a leukemoid reaction, or possibly chronic myelocytic leukemia. Production indices comparable to the reticulocyte index or clinically applicable kinetic measurements, such as ferrokinetic studies of erythropoiesis, are not currently available for the assessment of granulopoiesis. The morphological evaluation of granulopoiesis, in the clinical setting, is at best a crude, though useful, guide.

C. Megakaryocyte Number

The evaluation of the megakaryocyte mass and its efficiency is indeed difficult to accomplish with the available morphological techniques. Again marrow sections, or particle or needle biopsy can provide some approximation of the megakaryocyte density, reported to be 7.6 ± 2.7 megakaryocytes per square millimeter.[95] Marrow smears and the chamber counts are unreliable. Berman[42] recommended the use of a Whipple micrometer disk for scanning 50 consecutive fields of a marrow biopsy section. At a magnification of 600 dia he found 20 to 50 megakaryocytes per 50 fields.

Inefficient hematopoiesis is the result of either a quantitative or qualitative disturbance of maturation and/or replication of the hemopoietic elements. Aplasia or hypoplasia of the marrow is a quantitative defect in which the total marrow cellularity is reduced. Individual components of the hemopoietic compartment may be reduced to give rise to isolated cytopenias, such as erythrocytopenia in pure red cell anemia, or the thrombocytopenia of an amegakaryocytic marrow. Ineffective hematopoiesis due primarily to qualitative disturbances of maturation or replication has been designated dysplasia or dyshematopoiesis. The total cell content of the marrow may be normal or increased and the process recognized by the presence of the morphological changes of asynchrony of nuclear cytoplasmic maturation and mitotic aberrations. Dyshematopoiesis may be encountered in a wide variety of disorders but is the morphological hallmark of the megaloblastic states and the acute leukemias.[96]

D. Maturation Sequence

Under normal conditions the hemopoietic cells flow in an orderly sequence through the maturation process from the early to the late precursor cell. A rough guide of the maturation sequence of the recognizable precursor cells of the marrow can be gleaned from the comparison of relative sizes of the early and late compartments. In the erythroid series, the ratio E/N is about 1:3 to 1:4, where E includes the sum of proerythroblasts and erythroblasts and N, the sum of normoblast population, both polychromatiophilic and orthochromatic. Similarly, the ratio P/M is 1:2 to 1:2.5, where P is the proliferative pool of myeloblasts, promyelocytes, and myelocytes and N is the nonproliferative pool of metamyelocytes and segmented polymorphonuclear cells. Considerable variability in these ratios is introduced by contamination and dilution of the marrow sample by peripheral blood, perhaps more for the myeloid than for the erythroid series. The differential counts should be made from first drop smears or the squash particle smears.[97]

The determination of marrow cellularity and the maturation indices offer a reasonable initial morphologic approach to the evaluation of marrow function.

V. HISTOLOGICAL PREPARATIONS

Following the systematic evaluation of the hematopoietic compartment of the bone marrow, attention should be turned to the other functional subdivisions of the marrow, namely, the lymphocyte-plasma cell population, the monocyte-macrophage population, and the reticular, sinusodal, and mast cell populations. Estimation of iron collagen and reticulin content and a search for focal or diffuse infiltrative lesions such as granuloma, tumor, or lymphoma completes the examination.

The bone marrow examination has become an important tool for the diagnosis and evaluation of the patient with a hematologic disorder, for the staging of oncologic disease, and for the recognition of some infectious diseases such as histoplasmosis or kala azar. Optimal study requires careful planning both for the selection of the sampling techniques and the range of studies required. Thought must be given to the need for special cytogenetic procedures as well as the need for electron microscopy, tissue culture, or bacterial or fungal culture, etc. to aid in the resolution of the clinical problem.

For the technical details on specimen handling and preparation, staining, cytochemistry, and functional markers of the needle aspirate and needle core biopsy the reader is referred to References 90, and 98 to 103, for phase and interference microscopy Reference 104, for plastic-imbedded thin sections Reference 105, and for electron microscopy Reference 104.

REFERENCES

1. **Pianese, G.,** Sull anemia splenica infantile (anemia infantum a leishmannia), *Gazz. Int. Med. E. Chir.,* 3, 265, 1905.
2. **Ghedini, G.,** Neue Beitrage zur Diagnostik der Krankheiten der hamopoetischen Orgnae mittels Probepunktion des Knochenmarkes, *Wien. Klin. Wochenschr,* 2, 1840, 1920.
3. **Ghedini, G.,** Die Technik der Knochenmarkpunktion, *Wien. Klin. Wochenschr.,* 3, 284, 1911.
4. **Zadek, I.,** Knochenmarks Befunde im Lebenden bei kryptogenetische pernizioser Anämie, *Schweiz. Med. Wochenschr.,* 2, 1087, 1921.
5. **Seyfarth, C.,** Die Sternumtrepanation: eine einfache Methode zur diagnostisehen Entnahme von Knockenmark bei Lebenden, *Deutsch Med. Wochenschr.,* 1, 180, 1923.
6. **Segerdahl, E.,** Ueber Knochenmarkspunktionen, *Acta Med. Scand. (Suppl.),* 59, 173, 1934.
7. **Arinkin, M. I.,** Die intravitale Untersuchungsmethodik des Knochenmarks, *Fol. Haematol.,* 38, 233, 1929.
8. **Leitner, S. J.,** *Die Intravitale Knochenmarks,* Benno Schwake., Basel, 1945. (Contains an exhaustive list of references covering the 15 years following the introduction of the bone marrow aspiration technique.)
9. **Nordenson, N. G.,** Studies on the bone marrow from sternal puncture, Bortzells Esselte, Stockholm, 1935.
10. **Stasney, I. and Higgin, G.,** A cytologic study of the marrow in flat bone of man, *Fol. Haematol.,* 61, 344, 1939.
11. **Rubinstein, M. A.,** Aspiration of bone marrow from the iliac crest, *JAMA,* 137, 1281, 1941.
12. **Bierman, H. R.,** Multiple marrow aspirations in man from posterior ilium, *Blood,* 11, 370, 1956.
13. **Burkhardt, R.** Bone Marrow and Bone Tissue, Springer-Verlag, Berlin, 1971, 7.
14. **Notter, B. and Labhart, A.,** Die Knochenbiopsie, Beschreibung einer einfachen technik, *Achweiz. Med. Wochenschr.,* 82, 1263, 1953.
15. **Ellis, L. D., Jensen, W. H., and Westerman, W. P.,** Needle biopsy of bone and marrow, *Arch. Int. Med.,* 114, 213, 1964.
16. **Hellerberg-Rasmussen, I. and Sondergaard Petersen, H.,** Bone marrow biopsy with the bordier technique, *Scand. J. Haematol.,* 14, 123, 1975.
17. **Jamshidi, K. and Swaim, W. R.,** Bone marrow biopsy with unaltered architecture, *J. Lab. Clin. Med.* 77, 331, 1971.
18. **Rywlin, A. M., Marvan, P., and Robinson, N. J.,** A simple technique for the preparation of bone marrow smears and sections, *Am. J. Clin. Pathol.,* 53, 389, 1970.
19. **Miller, W. and Trubowitz, A.,** A simple method for the retrieval of human marrow tissue particles from aspirates, *Am. J. Clin. Pathol.* 38, 661, 1968.

20. **Alley, C. D. and MacDermott, R. P.,** Investigation of the blastogenic and cytotoxic capabilities of human bone marrow, differences between aspirate and rib marrow, *Blood,* 55, 669, 1980.
21. **Isaacs, R.,** Physiolgoic histology of the bone marrow; mechanisms of development of blood cells and their liberation into peripheral circulation, *Fol. Haematol.* 40, 395, 1930.
22. **Osgood, W. and Seaman, A. S.,** The cellular composition of the normal bone marrow as obtained by sternal puncture, *Physiol. Rev.,* 24, 46, 1944.
23. **Tuschinsky, M. D. and Kotlarenko, B. W.,** Ueber Knockenmark Veranderungen bei Flechtyphus mit Bemerkungen zur Methodkik der Diagnostischer Punktion des sternal markes, *Fol. Haematol.,* 46, 235, 1932.
24. **Gormsen, H.,** Der diagnostischer Wert der sternal punktion, *Ugesk. Laeger.* 102, 991, 1940.
25. **Gershenovich, R. S. and Titov, K. G.,** Sur le diagnostic precoce du kala-azar infantile au moyen de la ponction medullaire de sternum, *Arch. Med. d' Enf.,* 37, 147, 1934.
26. **Pitts, H. and Packham, E. A.,** Hematology of the sternal marrow and venous blood of pregnant and non pregnant women, *Arch. Int. Med.,* 64, 471, 1939.
27. **Greif, S.,** Methodisch Unterlagen zu einer quantitativem Auswertung des Sternal punkates, *Fol. Haematol.,* 59, 326, 1938.
28. **Schnetz, H. and Greif, S.,** Die Leukopenie bei Grippe in Sternalmark, *Aeitgchr. F. Klin. Med.,* 132, 178, 1937.
29. **Vogel, P., Erf., A., and Rosenthal, N.,** Hematologic observation on bone marrow obtained by sternal puncture, *Am. J. Clin. Pathol.,* 7, 498, 1937.
30. **Leitner, S. J.,** Die klinische Bedeutiung der intravitalen Knochenmarks untersuchung, *Fol. Haematol.,* 65, 1, 1941.
31. **Fieschi, A.,** Semeiolgoia del midolla osseo, Tipongrafia gia Coop Pavia, 1938.
32. **Fruhling, L. and Roger, S.,** Contribution a l'etude du monocyte, *Le Sang.,* 19, 111, 1948.
33. **Reich, E., Kolbrem, K.,** A quantative study of the variations of multiple sternal marrow samples taken simultaneously, *Am. J. Med. Sci.,* 24, 496, 1942.
34. **Schleicher, E. M. and Sharp, E. H.,** Rapid methods for preparing and staining bone marrow, *J. Lab. Clin. Med.,* 22, 949, 1937.
35. **Schleicher, E. M.,** The volumetric pattern of aspirated normal human sternal marrow of males, 18 to 40 years, *Am. J. Clin. Pathol.,* 14, 370, 1944.
36. **Stasney, J. and Higgins, J. M.,** Quantitative cytologic study of bone marrow of adult dog, *Am. J. Med. Sci.,* 193, 462, 1937.
37. **Stasney, J. and Higgins, J. M.,** Quantitative cytologic study of bone marrow of adult albino rat, *Anat. Rec.,* 63, 77, 1935.
38. **Schleicher, E. M. and Sharp, E. H.,** Rapid methods for preparing and storing bone marrow, *J. Lab. Clin. Med.,* 22, 949, 1937.
39. **Limarzi, L. R.,** Evaluation of bone marrow concentration techniques, modified method for simultaneous preparation and staining of blood and bone marrow films, *J. Lab. Clin. Med.,* 32, 732, 1947.
40. **Pizzolato, P. and Stasney, J.,** Quantitative cytologic study of multiple sternal marrow samples taken stimultaneously, *J. Lab. Clin. Med.,* 32, 741, 1947.
41. **Berman, J.,** A review of methods for aspiration and biopsy of sternal marrow, *Am. J. Clin. Pathol.,* 25, 385, 1953.
42. **Berman, L. and Axelrod, A. R.,** Evaluation of volumetric data obtained by centrifugation of aspirated sternol marrow of adult. I. Estimation of fat content, II. Estimation of cellularity of sternal marrow, *Am. J. Clin. Pathol.,* 7, 557, 1947.
43. **Marmont, H. and Fusco, F.,** Quantitative studies on aspirated human bone marrow with reference to the hematocrit patterns in major blood disorders, *Acta Med. Scand.,* 139, 387, 1951.
44. **DeLesse, M.,** Procède mécanique pour détérminer la composition des roches, *C. R. Acad. Sci. (D) Paris,* 25, 544, 1847.
45. **Hartsock, R. J., Smith, E. B., and Petty, C. S.,** Normal variations with aging of the amount of hematopoietic tissue in bone marrow from the anteroiliac crest, a study made from 177 cases of sudden death examined by necropsy, *Am. J. Clin. Pathol.,* 43, 326, 1965.
46. **Dunnill, M. S., Anderson, J. A., and Whitehead, R.,** Quantitative histological studies on age changes in bone, *J. Pathol. Bact.,* 94, 275, 1967.
47. **Meunier, P., Aaron, J., Edouard, C., and Vignon, G.,** Osteoporosis and the replacement of cell populations of the marrow by adipose tissue, *Clin. Orthopaed.,* 80, 147, 1971.
48. **Klein, J. E. and Serra, J.,** The texture analysis, *J. Micr.,* 95 (pt2), 349, 1972.
49. **Digabel, H. and Trebucket, C.,** Etude de la repartition spatiale des adipocytes a l'aide de l'analyseur de textures, *Pathol. Biol.,* 27, 218, 1979.
50. **Binet, J. C., Chomette, G., Debre, P., and D'Athis, P.,** L'utilisation de appareils a l'analyse automatique d' image dans la lecture de la biopsie de moelle, *Nouv. Rev. Francs. Hematol.,* 13, 436, 1973.

51. **Bryon, P. A., Gentilhomme, O., and Fiere, D.,** Eitude histologique quantitative du volume et de l'heterogeneite des adipocytes daus les insuffisiances myeloides globales, Pathol. Biol., 27, 209, 1979.
52. **Courpron, P., Meunier, P., Edouard, C., et al.,** Donnees histologicques quantitative sur le wiellissement osseux humain, *Rev. Du. Rhum.*, 40, 469, 1973.
53. **Heidrecheid, H., Charron, D., d'Athis, P., et al.,** Etude quantitative des adipocyte de la moelle dans l'; insuffisiance medullaire, *Pathol. Biol.*, 27, 215, 1979.
54. **Pegg, D. E.,** A quantitative study of bone marrow grafting; implications for human bone marrow infusion, *Br. J. Cancer,* 16, 400, 1962.
55. **Mechanik, N.,** Untersuchungen über das Gewichte des Knochenmarkes des Menschen, *Anat, Entwickl-Gesch.*, 79, 58, 1926.
56. **Nye, R. N.,** Bone marrow volume in rabbit, *Proc. Soc. Exp. Biol. Med.,* 29, 34, 1931.
57. **Fairman, E. and Whipple, G. H.,** Bone marrow volume in adult dogs, *Am. J. Physiol.* 104, 1352, 1933.
58. **Hudson, F.,** Bone marrow volume in guinea pigs, *J. Anat.,* 92, 150, 1958.
59. **Woodard, H. Q. and Holodney, E.,** A summary of the data of mechanik on the distribution of human bone marrow, *Phys. Med. Biol.,* 5, 57, 1960.
60. **Custer, R. P.,** Studies on structure and function of bone marrow, variability of hemopoietic pattern and consideration of method for examination, *J. Lab. Clin. Med.,* 17, 951, 1932.
61. **Osgood, E.,** Number and distribution of human hemic cells, *Blood,* 9, 1141, 1955.
62. **Donohue, D. M., Eabrio, B. W., and Finch, C. A.,** Quantitative measurement of hemopoietic cells of the marrow, *J. Clin. Invest.,* 37, 1564, 1958.
63. **Patt, H. M.,** A consideration of the myeloid-erythroid balance in man, *Blood,* 12, 277, 1957.
64. **Japa, J.,** A study of mitotic activity of normal human bone marrow, *Ant. J. Exp. Pathol.,* 23, 272, 1942.
65. **Killman, S. A., Cronkite, E. P., Fliedner, T. M., and Bond, V. P.,** Mitotic indices of human bone marrow cells, number and cytologic distribution of mitosis, *Blood,* 19, 743, 1962.
66. **Weicker, H.,** Die hemi-homoplastische Teilung des proerythroblasten: die Lösung des Staumzell problem der Erythropoese, *Fol. Haematol.,* 74, 49, 1956.
67. **Rohr, K.,** *Dos Menschliche Knochenmart,* Stuttgart, 3 Ause, Thieme, 1960.
68. **Bond, V. P., Fliedner, T. M., Cronkite, E. P., Rubini, J. R., and Robertson, J. S.,** Cell turnover in blood and blood forming tissues studies with tritiated thymidine, in *The Kinetics of Cellular Proliferation,* Stohlman, F. R., Ed., Grune and Stratton, New York, 1959.
69. **Cronkite, E. P., Bond, V. P., Fliedner, T. M., and Killman, S. A.,** The use of tritated thymidine in the study of hemopoietic cell proliferation, in *CIBA Foundation Symposium on Hemopoiesis,* Wolstenhome G. E. W. and O'Connor, M., Ed., Churchill, London, 1960.
70. **Cronkite, E. P., Bond, V. P., Fliedner, T. M., Rubini, J. R., and Killman, S. A.,** Studied on the life cycle of normal and neoplastic leucocytes by labeling DNA with tritiated thymidine, in *Transactions of the Ninth International Congress of Radiology,* Rajewsky, R., Ed., Stuttgart Thieme, Munich, 1960.
71. **Killman, S. A., Cronkite, E. P., Fliedner, T. M., Bond, U. P., and Brecher, G.,** Mitotic indices of human bone marrow cells, II. The use of mitotic indices for estimation of time parameters of proliferation in serially connected myeloproliferating cellular compartments, *Blood,* 21, 141, 1963.
72. **Killman, S. A., Cronkite, E. P., Fliedner, T. M., and Bond, U. P.,** Mitotic indices of bone marrow cells. III. Duration of some phases of erthrocytic and granulocytic proliferation computed from mitotic indices, *Blood,* 24, 267, 1964.
73. **Suit, H. D.,** A technique for studying the bone marrow cellularity in vivo using 59 Fe, *J. Clin. Pathol.* 10, 207, 1957.
74. **Huff, R. L., Hennessy, T. G., Harter, R. E., et al.,** Plasma and red cell iron turnover in normal subjects and in patients having various hematopoietic disorders, *J. Clin. Invest.,* 29, 1041, 1950.
75. **Suit, H. D., Laijtha, L. G., Oliver, R., and Ellis, F.,** Studies of the 59 Fe uptake by normoblasts and the failure of X-irradiation to affect uptake, *Br. J. Haematol.,* 2, 165, 1957.
76. **Donahue, D. M., Cabrio, B. W., and Finah, C. A.,** Quantitative measurements of hemopoietic cells of the marrow, *J. Clin. Invest.,* 37, 1564, 1958.
77. **Donohue, D. M., Raff, R. H., Hanson, M. L., Bitson, V., and Finch, C. A.,** Quantitative measurement of the erythrocytic and granulocytic cell of the marrow and blood, *J. Clin. Invest.,* 37, 254, 1962.
78. **Harrison, W. J.,** Total cellularity of the bone marrow in man, *Br. J. Clin. Pathol.,* 15, 254, 1962.
79. **Skarberg, K. O.,** Cellularity and cell proliferation in human bone marrow, I. An in vivo method to estimate the total marrow cellularity in man, *Acta Med. Scand.,* 195, 292, 1974.
80. **Skarberg, K. O., Cea, R., and Reizenstein, P., II.** Study on generation time and radiothymidine uptake of human red cell precursors, *Acta Med. Scand.,* 195, 301, 1974.

81. **Skarberg, K. O., Cea, R., and Reizenstein, P., III.** Studies on bone marrow cellularity and erythrocytes in primary and secondary polycythemia, *Acta Med. Scand.*, 195, 307, 1974.
82. **Berman, L.**, A review of methods for aspiration and biopsy of bone marrow, *Am. J. Clin. Pathol.*, 25, 385, 1953.
83. **Loge, J. P.**, Spinous process puncture, *Blood*, 3, 198, 1948.
84. **Block, M.**, Bone marrow examination, Aspiration or core biopsy, smear or section, hematoxylin-eosin or Romanowsky stain—which combination? *Arch. Pathol. Lab. Med.*, 100, 454, 197.
85. **Brunning, R. D., Bloomfield, C. D., McKenna, R. W., and Peterson, I.**, Bilateral tryphine bone marrow biopsies in lymphoma and neoplastic disease, *Ann. Int. Med.*, 82, 365, 1975.
86. **Dick, F., Bloomfield, C. D., and Brunning, R. D.**, Incidence, cytology and histopathology, of non-Hodgkin's lymphoma in the bone marrow, *Cancer*, 33, 1382, 1974.
87. **Ellman, L.**, Bone marrow biopsy in the evaluation of lymphoma, carcinoma and granulomatous disorders, *Am. J. Med.*, 60, 167, 1976.
88. **Frankel, K.**, Bone marrow aspiration and biopsy, *Am. J. Clin. Pathol.*, 66, 616, 1976.
89. **Neiman, R. S.**, The relative merits of bone marrow biopsy and particle section techniques, *Am. J. Clin. Pathol.*, 67, 308, 1977.
90. **Brynes, R. K., McKenna, R. W., and Sundberg, R. P.**, Bone marrow aspiration and trephine biopsy, *Am. J. Clin. Pathol.*, 70, 753, 1978.
91. **Diebold, J.**, Appreciation semi-quantitative de la richesse cellulaire des biopsies medullaires osseuses, *La Nouv. Press. Med.*, 4, 3193, 1975.
92. **Hillman, R. S. and Finch, C. A.**, *Red Cell Annual.*, F. A. Davis, Philadelphia, 1974, 60.
93. **Finch, C. A.**, Ferrokinetics in man, *Medicine*, 49, 17, 1970.
94. **Cook, J. D., Marsaglia, G., Eschbach, J. W., Funk, D. D., and Finch, C. A.**, Ferrokinetics, a biological model for plasma iron exchange in man, *J. Clin. Invest.*, 49, 197, 1970.
95. **Kronseder, A.**, *Das Verhalten der Megakaryocyten in Menschlichen Knochenmark unter mormalen und pathologischen Bedingungen*, Inauguraldiss, Munich, 1973.
96. **Lewis, S. M., and Verwilghen, R. L.**, *Dyserythropoiesis*, Academic Press, New York, 1977.
97. **Dresch, C., Faille, A., Poirier, O., and Kadouche, J.**, Cellular composition of granulocytic series in normal human bone marrow according to the volume of the sample, *J. Clin. Pathol.* 27, 106, 1974.
98. **Burkhardt, R.**, Bone marrow and bone tissue, *Color Atlas of Clinical Histopathology*, Springer-Verlag, Berlin, 1971.
99. **Block, M.**, *Text-Atlas of Hematology*, Lea and Febiger, Philadelphia, 1976.
100. **Vykoupil, K. F., Thiele, J., and Geoggii, A.**, Histochemical and immunohistochemical techniques on acrylate embedded bone biopsies, *Blut*, 32, 215, 1976.
101. **Senco, A.**, A new preparation method for several histopathological examinations on a single block, *Stain Tech.*, 53, 123, 1978.
102. **Jaffee, E. S., Braylan, R. C., Nanba, K., et al.**, Functional markers, A new perspective on malignant lymphoma, *Cancer Treat. Rep.*, 61, 953, 1977.
103. **Williams, W. J.**, Examination of the bone marrow, in *Hematology, 2nd ed.*, Williams, W. J., Beutler, E., Ersleu, A. J., and Rundles, R. W., Eds., McGraw-Hill, New York, 1977, 25.
104. **Bessis, M.**, *Living Blood Cells and Their Ultrastructure*, Springer-Verlag, New York, 1973.
105. **Beckstead, J. H. and Bainton, D. F.**, Enzyme histochemistry on bone marrow biopsies. Reactions useful in differential diagnosis of leukemia and lymphoma applied to 2-micro plastic section, *Blood*, 55, 386, 1980.

Chapter 9

PATHOPHYSIOLOGY OF ERYTHROPOIESIS

Sidney Trubowitz and Stephen Davis

TABLE OF CONTENTS

I. INTRODUCTION

Hematologists have long held to the view that hematopoiesis is maintained by a population of cells which are capable of self-renewal and differentiation into a population of mature blood cells which are doomed to ultimate extinction.[1] In this context, erythropoiesis is currently seen as an orderly, sequential, and continuous process of differentiation and amplification, beginning with the commitment of the multipotential stem cell toward erythroid differentiation and ending with the terminal maturation of the cells into functional erythrocytes. Although the process of differentiation is continuous and the cells involved in hemopoiesis heterogeneous, the erythron can be conveniently divided into a population of early cells, morphology not identifiable—but subject to analysis by functional assays—sensitivity to erythropoietin, and possessing burst-promoting activity as well as proliferative capacity; and a population of cells, morphologically recognizable, beginning with the proerythroblast and ending as erythrocytes, a population in which the terminal phases of maturation are completed.[2-4] For a discussion of the stem cells and the early erythroid progenitor cells see the chapter on erythropoiesis. The present discussion will deal with the morphologic and biochemical events in the recognizable compartment.

II. THE NORMAL TERMINAL MATURATION SEQUENCE

The proerythroblast (E_1) is the earliest recognizable red cell precursor in the Romanowsky stained smears of human marrow. It is a large round cell, some 20 to 25 μm in diameter with a high nuclear-cytoplasmic ratio, the nuclear diameter occupying about 80% of the cell diameter. The cytoplasm is deep blue, a measure of its RNA content. The nuclear margin is sharp and well defined; the chromatin is rather fine and homogeneously distributed, and rarely more than two nucleoli are present. The electron microscopic image confirms the presence of high concentrations of polyribosomes in the cytoplasm. Under very high magnification and resolution, ferritin molecules can be identified dispersed throughout the cytoplasm. Adjacent to the nuclear membrane, on the cytoplasmic side, within a site of nuclear indentation lie the centrosomes and a diminutive Golgi apparatus. At this stage hemoglobin synthesis has begun.

Some semantic confusion has arisen from the multitude of names that have been given to the various stages of the maturation sequence. It is important to remember that the descriptive designations were selected to serve as useful guides for the determination of a cell's progress in the maturation process. The boundaries between compartments are not sharp and a noncomittal number system such as E_1,E_2... such as has been suggested by Cronkite may be useful.

The next stage in the maturation sequence is the erythroblast (E_2). The erythroblasts are smaller than the proerythroblasts and measure on the average some 16 to 18 μm in diameter. The nuclear cytoplasm is apparent. The nucleoli are no longer visible and the chromatin is more compact and somewhat clumped. The cell contains many mitochondria, polyribosomes, and finely dispersed ferritin molecules.

With further maturation, increasing concentration of hemoglobin and concomitantly decreasing concentrations of RNA, the cytoplasm takes on a violet color, the result of the admixture of the red, eosinophilic stain of hemoglobin and the blue stain of the RNA. These cells are designated polychromatophilic normoblasts (E_3). These cells are about 9 to 12 μm in diameter. There is a further decrease in the nuclear cytoplasmic ratio; the nuclear chromatin is now compact and condensed. Freely dispersed as well as membrane-bound aggregates of ferritin are seen on electron microscopy.

Further hemoglobin synthesis and RNA degradation give rise to a cell which is small in size, has a markedly decreased nuclear cytoplasmic ratio and a highly pycnotic nucleus, and a predominantly pink cytoplasm with no visable basophilia. Large aggregates of hemosiderin are now present and can be visualized with the Prussion blue reaction. The margins of the cell show lumpy protrusions. This cell is the orthochromatic normoblast (E_4) which, following expulsion of the nucleus, becomes the reticulocyte.

The reticulocyte (E_5) remains in the marrow for 1 or 2 days and continues to synthesize hemoglobin. The reticulocyte contains polyribosomes which are responsible for the substantia filamentosa seen in the supravital stain.

The differentiation of the proerythroblast to a mature red cell is a continuous, uninterrupted process of protein synthesis, chiefly of hemoglobin and of small quantities of enzymes and other proteins required for the metabolic, transport, and specific membrane requirements of the cell. During the maturation sequence RNA is steadily degraded. Morphologically, then, the staining characteristics, namely, the degree of basophilia of the RNA and the eosinophilia of the hemoglobin, afford an insight into the progress of a given cell in the maturation sequence.

Concomitant with the tinctorial changes in the cytoplasm are changes in nuclear size, nuclear-cytoplasm ratio, and chromatin condensation. Thus, a morphologic synchronism is observed: a large nucleus, presence of nucleoli, and a fine chromatin pattern accompanies a deeply basophilic cytoplasm, while a pycnotic, highly condensed nucleus is seen with a fully hemoglobinized cytoplasm.

Since the cells in the recognizable compartment constitute a highly heterogeneous population in a constant state of differentiation, some problems in classification have arisen. Bessis[5] has suggested that the term orthochromatic normoblast be eliminated, and that all cells which contain ribosomes be considered polychromatophilic. In a similar vein, he recommended that the term reticulocyte be dropped and the cell renamed proerythrocyte. Wickramsinghe[6,7] argued that there is no simple method of distinguishing the polychromatophilic from the orthochromatic normoblasts and suggested that a nuclear diameter of 6 μm be used as a dividing line between the early polychromatophilic cells which incorporate tritiated thymidine and are capable of division from the late polychromatophilic cells whose nuclear diameter is less than 6 μm and in general do not incorporate thymidine and are not proliferative.

The selection of points on a maturation line is to some degree arbitrary and for the clinician who depends almost wholly on the examination of the Romanowsky stained smears of the marrow the old and widely used designations are quite satisfactory. It is important to keep in mind that the population of cells under any given designation are indeed heterogeneous and represent a field of cells. For the purposes of this discussion, using criteria established from the Romanowsky stained smears of marrow, the proerythroblasts include all cells with a high nuclear-cytoplasmic ratio, deep blue-staining cytoplasm, and the presence of nucleoli, two or less or even a recognizable remnant of one. The term erythroblast includes all cells with a blue cytoplasm, a somewhat condensed nucleus, and a complete absence of any nucleolar structure. The transition to the polychromatophic stage begins with the first detection of the eosinophilic stain of hemoglobin which renders the cytoplasm a shade of purple. The nuclei show greater condensation. With the disappearance of the blue stain of the ribosomes, the cell is labeled an orthochormatic normoblast. The cytoplasm is totally eosinophilic; the nucleus, small and pycnotic. The cytoplasm still contains ribosomes but these are no longer discernible in the light microscope. Admittedly, there is overlap between these cell populations; the divisions are not sharp, and the terms may be semantically incorrect. However, the classification has served the clinician well and is quite adequate for the clinical situation. The relative frequency of the different populations of cells as defined generates the E/N ratio which normally is about 1:3, where E includes all pro- and erythroblasts and N, all normoblasts, polychromatophilic and orthochromatic.

III. ERYTHROPOIETIN AND TERMINAL MATURATION

Erythropoietin, a glycoprotein of approximately 46,000 daltons, acts principally on the committed erythroid cell precursors in the unrecognizable compartment, the BFU-E and the CFU-E, which as they progressively differentiate augment their responsiveness to the hormone.[8–12] The proliferative capacity of the erythroid progenitor cells seems to decrease as they become progressively more sensitive to erythropoietin. The earlier cells show greater proliferative capacity and amplification of pool size. The more highly differentiated cells of the unrecognizable pool move into the recognizable pool as proerythroblasts.[13,14] Erythropoietin triggers the transcription of the specific RNA molecules and the ribosomes required for the erythroid maturation program in the highly hormone sensitive cells and at the same time stimulates proliferative and pool amplification of the early less sensitive cells.

The influence of erythropoietin on the erythroid cells of the recognizable compartment is less clear. The maturation process, once initiated, is believed to proceed on its own with little further influence from erythropoietin.[15,16] However, Stohlman[17] as well as Papayannopoulou and Finch[16] reported a shortening of the intermitotic time and an increase in the rate of hemoglobin synthesis in the maturing red cell precursor when stimulated by erythropoietin. Erythropoietin has been shown to shorten the maturation time and trigger the earlier release of the reticulocytes.[19–22] These studies suggested that under enhanced erythropoietin activity, maturation was accelerated and macrocytosis ensued as a result of a skipped terminal division in the presence of a relatively fixed generation time. Other studies on the action of erythropoietin on the recognizable red cell precursors have shown that the hormone can stimulate heme and globin synthesis throughout the maturation sequence; increase the synthesis of messenger, transfer and ribosomal RNA;[23,24] stimulate ALA synthetase activity,[25] and accelerate iron accumulation by the marrow cells.[26] Other biochemical effects such as glucose utilization, not directly concerned with hemoglobin synthesis, have been attributed to erythropoietin.[27,28] Whether all of the described activities ascribed to erythropoietin are due to the hormone itself or to contaminating substances will not be known until greater purification of erythropoietin is achieved. Whether all of the biochemical responses attributed to erythropoietin play a physiologically significant and direct role in the maturation of the erythrocyte awaits further clarification.

IV. RNA AND HEMOGLOBIN SYNTHESIS

Hemoglobin makes up some 95% of the red cell's proteins. Erythroid differentiation is essentially hemoglobin synthesis. Thorell[29] had shown quite early that the immature cells of the recognizable red cell precursors are rich in RNA and poor in hemoglobin, that the concentration of hemoglobin rises steadily, and that the concentrations of RNA falls as the cells become more and more mature. The proerythroblasts and erythroblasts synthesize RNA actively and in much larger amounts than the normoblasts.[30,31] Ribosomal and transfer RNA are apparently synthesized preferentially by the early cells and messenger RNA in the more mature cells.[32,33] The RNA turnover in the immature cells is high with a high rate of synthesis and breakdown; the RNA in the more mature cells is synthesized at a slow rate, but is more stable and the turnover rate is low.[30]

All of the recognizable red cell precursors including the early reticulocytes are engaged in protein synthesis. The rate of hemoglobin synthesis decreases progressively as the cells mature[28,30] hence the bulk of the hemoglobin is synthesized in the early red cell precursors most prominently in the early polychromatophilic normoblasts. The marrow reticulocytes synthesize but a small percentage of the hemoglobin of the cell.

V. THE ERYTHROID ISLAND

The maturing red cell precursors are frequently found in both human and other mammalian marrow samples arranged in compact clusters about a central reticular macrophage. These clusters, consisting of one or more rings of the maturing red cell precursors, have been considered to be structural entities of physiological significance and termed erythroblastic islands.[34,35] Erythroblastic islands are not commonly seen in smears prepared from normal human bone marrow and some doubt has therefore been cast on their importance in normal erythropoiesis. However, they are abundantly present in smears prepared from subjects with hemolytic anemia. The islands are easily identified, but are fragile and easily disrupted by the smearing process. Le Charpentier and Prenang[36] developed a relatively simple technique for the quantitative assessment of the erythroblastic islands and found a decrease in their number following transfusion-induced polycythemia in the rat and, conversely, a striking increase in the number of islands in response to experimentally induced hemolysis. It was noted, on examination of the isolated islands by scanning electron microscopy, that the central macrophage of the island tended to adhere and spread over glass surfaces, but maintained, nevertheless, its intimate connections with the surrounding erythroid precursors. The innermost ring of the erythroid precursors are generally the more immature forms. The more mature forms occupy the outer rings, with the reticulocytes in the outermost layer.

The significance of this relationship between the central macrophage and the maturing erythroid cells is not clear. Bessis and Breton-Gorius[35] have suggested a support function for the macrophage, that of a nursing cell capable of transferring iron,[37,38] removing the extruded nuclei, or possibly secreting regulatory substances. Ben-Ishay[39] commented on the morphologic similarity of erythroid colonies in culture with the erythroblastic island in the marrow. In a series of investigations he demonstrated that the central macrophage is resistant to chemical or radiation damage of the marrow. On regeneration of the marrow, erythropoiesis was found to begin in relationship to the macrophage. The nature of the exchange and communication between the macrophage and the surrounding red cell precursors is at the present unknown.

VI. EXPULSION OF THE NORMOBLAST NUCLEUS

The expulsion of the nucleus from the orthochromatic normoblast has been described dramatically by Bessis and Bricka[40] who studied the phenomenon with the aid of time-lapse microcinematography and phase optics. In their preparations nuclear expulsion was accomplished by the cell in 10 min at room temperature. The nucleus was seen to move to one side of the cell in apposition to the cell membrane; a furrow formed between the nucleus and the future reticulocyte; the cell then underwent active, convulsive movements; and in a process somewhat reminiscent of a mitotic division the nucleus was separated from the body of the cell, carrying with it a rim of cytoplasm and membrane.[40,41] The process has been studied by electron microscopy and a completely naked nucleus has not been seen. In all observations reported, a distinct membrane was distinguished about the cytoplasmic rim which occasionally contained mitochondria, vesicles, or Howell-Jolly bodies.[42–47]

Normoblasts in various stages of nuclear extrusion are frequently encountered in the Romanowsky stained smears of human bone marrow, particularly in the marrow response to severe hemolysis. It is believed that under normal conditions the nucleus is expelled intact without prior fragmentations or lysis. In contrast, karyorrhexis may be encountered frequently in those pathological states that are characterized by intramarrow death of the developing cells, e.g., megaloblastosis.

Simpson and Kling[44,48] suggested that the formation of pinocytotic vesicles was important in the denucleation process. In their electron microscope observations, the nucleus migrated toward the cell membrane from which it was separated by a thin layer of cytoplasm. Mitochondria aggregated about the opposite pole of the nucleus. Pinocytotic vesicles appeared in the same area, fused, elongated, and surrounded the nucleus and the mitochondria. The fused pinocytotic vesicles formed the limiting membrane that surrounds the extruded nucleus. Nuclear material could be identified in the cytoplasm of the late normoblasts adjacent to the nuclear membrane presumably extruded through the nuclear pores. Similarly, some hemoglobin might enter the nuclear domain. These findings were not considered to be manifestations of karyolysis; the extruded nuclei were always intact, surrounded by a hemoglobinized rim of cytoplasm and a limiting membrane. In the further maturation of the reticulocyte, the mitochondria were extruded from their peripheral position, assumed at the time of nuclear expulsion, again by the formation of pinocytotic vesicles which surrounded the mitochondria and subsequently fused with the cell membrane.

VII. MEMBRANE PROTEINS

The red cell membrane has served as a model for the study of the structural and chemical organization of the plasma membrane of the mammalian cell.[49–53] In recent years considerable information has been provided to help characterize the proteins of the erythrocytic membrane.[54–56] Most mammalian red cell membranes present seven to nine major fractions on gel electrophoresis, although some species differences do exist. These proteins include two polypeptides of molecular weight greater than 200,000, one of 43,000 (the three-spectrin polypeptides), a protein of molecular weight 90,000, and a sialoglycoprotein which in the human contains the MN, A, and B blood groups.[56] Most of the membrane proteins are confined to the cytoplasmic surface of the membrane; only two, the sialoglycoprotein and the 90,000-mol wt protein, are present on the cell surface, but probably penetrate to the inner surface as well.[49]

Major changes have been detected in the membrane proteins during the maturation processes.[57–66] Differences in the agglutinability of rabbit reticulocytes and erythrocytes with the plant lectin concanavalin A were attributed partially to differences in number of con A binding sites and to undefined changes in the membrane.[50] Dramatic changes were observed in the mobility of the lectin receptors and their topographical distribution in the various stages of chicken erythroid precursors. The lectins formed a distinct cap on the surface of the proerythroblasts, assumed a patchy appearance on the erythroblast, and then formed a homogeneous ring about the cells of the more mature erythroid stages.[59–60] During the course of erythroid maturation in the mouse, membrane protein synthesis becomes more and more restricted to lower molecular weight proteins. The more mature cells contain less membrane protein than the earlier cells. Thus, quantitative and qualitative changes in the surface membrane proteins have been detected during erythropoiesis. Distinctive changes in the membrane proteins from the normal have been found in the Freund virus infected erythroleukemic cells at comparable stages of maturation.[62,63]

Rabbit reticulocytes synthesize two predominant species of membrane proteins; the synthesis of the other major membrane polypeptides practically cease at this stage of differentiation.[64] Rabbit reticulocytes and erythrocytes contain one major protein fraction, polypeptide 3, accessible at the external surface of the membrane.[65]

Light and Tanner[65] compared the surface components of the bone marrow erythroid cells of the rabbit with the freely circulating erythrocytes. The set of proteins in the marrow erythroid cells was distinctly different from that found in the circulating red cells. The marrow cells contained little if any polypeptide 3 and displayed a set of distinctive glycoproteins which was present in the membrane of all the erythroid cell precursors until late in the development of the orthochromatic normoblast, close to the time of nuclear extrusion. Since the circulating reticulocytes and erythrocytes bear a different set of membrane polypeptides from those found in the marrow erythroid precursors, these investigators postulated that the marrow reticulocytes may serve as a transitional population in which there is a loss of the set of glycoprotein characteristics of the marrow cells and, concomitantly, synthesis of a new set of polypeptides which characterize the circulating cells. They proposed that surface membrane components may be important in keeping the erythroid precursor cells bound to their marrow environment and that the subsequent changes in the surface components which take place in the late orthochromatic normoblasts permits the egress of the reticulocyte into the sinusoids and its free circulation as an erythrocyte.[66]

Evidence has also been presented relating alterations of the surface membrane and the expulsion of the nucleus from the normoblast. Many investigators have been impressed by the remarkable similarity between the process of nuclear expulsion and cytokinesis.[40,43–45] This impression has been supported by the demonstrated inhibition of the nuclear extrusion by Colcemid®,[67] and the constant appearance of a furrow at the presumptive level of separation of the nucleus from the reticulocyte.[44,48] Both the free nuclei and the partially extruded nuclei are actively engulfed by the reticular macrophage.[68–72] Investigations on the membrane characteristics of the reticulocyte and the free nucleus revealed an inverse alteration of their properties. The reticulocyte displayed an increase in the negatively charged groups in its membrane and a decrease in the number of con A receptors, while the membrane of the extruded nucleus showed a decrease in this surface negativity and an increase in its con A receptors.[72] The decrease in negative charge on the surface of the extruded nucleus was considered to be the recognition signal for macrophage engulfment.[73,73a] Geyer et al.[74] found no change in surface charge during the enucleation process in the rabbit. They were, however, able to demonstrate a marked increase in the lectin binding sites about the surface of partially extruded nucleus and concommitant decrease about the surface of the future reticulocyte surface. However, they too suggested that it is the inverse structural alterations that provide the appropriate surface properties for the specific requirements of the enucleation phenomenon, namely macrophage recognition and engulfment of the extruded nucleus and the egress of the liberated reticulocyte.

VIII. ERYTHROKINETICS

The recognizable erythroid population can be logically divided into a transit population of early, more immature cells in which both proliferation and differentiation are actively at work and a late, more mature population, the orthochromatic normoblasts and the reticulocytes, which no longer divide but are still actively involved in the differentiation process, primarily hemoglobin synthesis. None of these subpopulations of cells is capable of selfmaintenance or renewal.[75] Just as sharp boundaries between the morphologic subtypes in a continuously differentiating cell population cannot be precisely defined, so too difficulty is encountered in setting a sharp division between those cells capable of replication and those that are not.

The early studies of the kinetics of cell proliferation relied heavily on the only identifiable morphologic structure associated with proliferative activity, namely, the mitotic apparatus. Japa[76] determined the mitotic index, the frequency of mitosis, in the marrow smears of three normal individuals and found 15 mitoses per 1000 cells in squashed marrow stained with acetocarmine and 5 per 1000 cells in the Romanowsky stained marrow smears. Rohr[77] cited the eariler reports on the mitotic index of the human marrow which covered a range for the erythroid cells of 0.01% to 2.0%. The mitotic index for the myeloid cells appeared in all instances to be lower and were found to range between 0.01% to 0.06%. In his own studies, Rohr found a mitotic index of 0.42% for the erythroid cells of which 48% were found in the proerythroblasts, 40% in the polychromatophilic normoblasts, and 6% in the orthochromatic normoblasts. He too found a lower index for the granulocytic precursors. A marked increase in the mitotic index of the red cell precursors was found in the hemolytic anemias and following bleeding. Fliedner et al.[78] estimated the mitotic index of the bone marrow of normal healthy individuals, of individuals with different hematologic disorders, and of a group of normal people who had been exposed to mixed neutron and gamma rays in a nuclear accident. They employed a hypotonic squash technique which gave higher indices but did not allow for the recognition of the different cell types. They reported a mitotic index of 0.09% in the normal human marrow and a significant elevation in polycythemia vera. The mitotic index of the accidently irradiated group declined sharply on the fourth postirradiation day and returned to normal levels at the end of four weeks. Killmann et al.[79] extended these studies with the projected aim of obtaining data on the mitotic index of the specific cell types in the normal human bone marrow to apply to the computations of time parameters of proliferation of the hemopoietic cells. They[79,80] confirmed their previously reported mitotic index, a mean mitotic index of 8.86 ± 0.73/1000 nucleated bone marrow cells: 6.15 mitoses/1000 cells were attributed to the erythroid cells and 2.5 mitoses/1000 cells to the myeloid precursors. The mitoses of the polychromatophilic normoblasts contributed more than two thirds of all of the erythroid mitoses. The relative frequency of mitoses in the erythroid cells compartments for proerythroblasts: erythroblasts: polychromatophilic normoblasts was estimated to be 1:4.1:9.5. No mitoses were found among the orthochromatic normoblasts.

In a follow up communication Killmann et al.[80,82] defined the information needed to use the measured mitotic indices for the estimation of the time parameters of the proliferation of the catenated cytologic compartments of the bone marrow and the restrictions imposed on the computations. From the information on the transit time of the orthochromatic normoblasts, given at an upper limit of 19 hr[82], an erythroid mitotic time of 0.75 hr was estimated. From this information Killmann et al.[80] computed the following ''best estimates'' of the compartment transit times of the precursor erythroid cell compartments: proerythroblasts—30 hr; erythroblasts—minimum transit time 12.4 hr, maximum transit time 63.5 hr; polychromatophilic normoblasts—minimum transit time 8.8 hr, maximum 25.0; the orthochromatic normoblasts at 19 hr as previously cited.

Boll and Mersch[83] attempted to arrive at an appreciation of the erythroid proliferation kinetics of the human marrow through the use of the mitotic index and marrow cultures which they hoped could find potential application to the clinical situation and routine diagnosis. They found a mitotic index of 1.47% for the normal erythroid precursor cells which doubled in response to iron deficiency and increased some 15-fold in hemolytic anemia. The index was also markedly elevated in the sideroblastic and megaloblastic anemias. A mild decrease in the index was found in polycythemia vera, in contrast to a marked increase observed in patients with erythrocytosis.

X-ray treatment was used by Knowlton and Widner[84] to prevent cells from entering prophase, but allowed cells in mitosis to continue through telophase. The time taken for the mitoses to disappear was taken as the equivalent to the mitotic duration. A mitotic time of 25 min was given by these authors for various tissues of the mouse and rat. This technique is obviously not easily applicable to man.

Colchicine is known to destroy the mitotic spindle and thus prevent the movement of the chromosomes from their metaphase position. Following the injection of an appropriate dose of colchicine new mitoses continue to appear but are arrested at metaphase. From the increase in mitotic index over a given time period, the mitotic duration can be calculated. Applying this technique to the erythroid and myeloid cells of the bone marrow of the rat, Dustin[85] calculated a mitotic duration of 43 min for these cells.

The morphologic mitotic index, stathmokinetic (colchicine) index, provides some insight into the sites and rate of mitosis. Information on erythrokinetics, however, has been considerably extended with the introduction of labeling techniques, notably, employing tritiated thymidine, which is incorporated during the S phase of the cell cycle. It provides good radioautographic localization and is hence an ideal method to show areas of cellular proliferation and to trace the postmitotic cells[81,86–88]. Radioiron is a specific marker of heme synthesis, which in turn is a specific marker of red cell maturation. Iron is incorporated by all of the recognizable erythroid cells and the label can be followed through the bone marrow into the peripheral blood.[89] Two windows are thus opened into the kinetics of erythropoiesis, one into the nucleus and the cell cycle, the other into the cytoplasm and the maturation process.

In man the S phase of the normoblasts has been estimated to be as little as 6 and as much as 17 hr and is believed to become progressively longer in the more mature forms.[90–93,18]

Radioiron uptake is greatest in the more immature erythroid cells and progressively decreases with increasing maturation of the cells, being least in the reticulocytes.[94–96] In man, 67% of the administered radioiron is assimilated by the nucleated erythroid precursors, 33% by the marrow reticulocytes and less than 1% by the circulating reticulocytes.[97] The time taken for all of the initially labeled cells to enter the peripheral circulation and reach a plateau level of maximum iron incorporation is equal to the total marrow transit time. The overall transit time from the proerythroblast to reticulocyte has been estimated at about 72 hr, during which interval some three to four divisions take place.[98] It was further postulated that cell division and cell maturation are independent processes.[98]

Lajtha and Suit[99] found, following in vitro exposure to radioiron, a very high concentration of ^{59}Fe in a proportion of the reticulocytes which they attributed to a skipped division. Lajtha and Oliver[100–102] proposed a kinetic model of the erythron which envisoned a balance between cytoplasmic differentiation and cell division. In this scheme, hemoglobin concentration assumed to be the critical factor in determining further cell proliferation. At a certain critical level of hemoglobin concentration (>27 pg/μg cytoplasm) nuclear pyknosis begins and the cells are unable to divide. Cytoplasmic differentiation continues until a final level of hemoglobin concentration is reached and the nucleus is extruded. The scheme also provided for a proportion of cells which presumably synthesize their hemoglobin more rapidly to arrive at a critical hemoglobin concentration, which eventuates in an earlier inhibition of cell division, the skipped division, and ultimately to the formation of larger erythrocytes.

Stohlman et al.[103] too, in their proposed model of the kinetics of erythropoiesis, speculated on the interrelationship of cytoplasmic differentiation and nucleic acid synthesis and cell division. They assumed a fixed interphase time and hence a fixed number of divisions for any given time interval. Again, in this scheme a critical cytoplasmic hemoglobin concentration shuts off nucleic acid synthesis and further cell division. Thus, when hemoglobin synthesis is accelerated, as following administration of high doses of erythropoietin to the experimental animal, or in the clinical situation of hemolysis, bleeding, or hypoxia, short-lived macrocytosis is observed. Conversely, when hemoglobin synthesis is slowed because of decreased availability of iron for heme synthesis or decreased globin chain synthesis as in thalassemia, additional divisions are possible with a resultant microcytosis. Although these conjectures remain hypothetical without supportive evidence, they are pleasing to the clinician in that they offer some intellectual insight into an area that has been purely empirical—the classification of the anemias based on red cell size.

A considerable volume of information has been accumulated in the past couple of decades on erythroid cell kinetics by Lord.[104] Data on the parameters of the kinetics of human erythropoiesis are limited; even less is known of the kinetics of the erythroid precursor cells in disease.

IX. THE RETICULOCYTE

The reticulocyte is the final product of the maturation sequence following extrusion of the nucleus from the orthochromatic normoblast. Endowed with polyribosomes and mitochondria, the reticulocyte continues to synthesize hemoglobin. The cell is recognized by the precipitation of the ribosomes into a filamentous network of granules by the so-called supravital dyes, brilliant cresyl blue or new methylene blue. The reticulocytes are easily identified in the living unstained state, particularly when viewed with the interference microscopy, by the presence of a pinched, purse-string-like area at one point on the surface of the cell and by its slow but constantly changing surface outpouchings. The number of reticulocytes in the bone marrow of rats, rabbits, and men is approximately equal to the total number of nucleated red cells.[105,106]

In man, the marrow reticulocytes take up about one third of the dose of administered radioiron, the circulating reticulocytes less than 1%. The time for marrow reticulocyte maturation has been put at 65 hr. Active hemoglobin synthesis occurs during the first day and a half when the marrow reticulocyte synthesizes about one quarter of the hemoglobin of the cell and then drops to a rate of hemoglobin synthesis of less than 5% in the final day before the release of the reticulocyte into the general circulation.[98,107] As the marrow reticulocyte undergoes further maturation, hemoglobin synthesis is accompanied by a decrease in RNA content, membrane lipids, and in the cell volume. Seip[106] stated that all marrow reticulocytes enter the blood at the same stage of development and remain in the blood during their further maturation, undergoing a further loss of membrane lipid, further shrinkage in cell volume and a total disintegration of ribosomal RNA and loss of mitochondria. The reticulocytes appear to spend a uniform maturation time in the blood, about 25 hr.[108] A maturation scheme for the reticulocytes was proposed by Heilmeyer and Westhauer,[109] in which the circulating reticulocytes were separated into four groups, according to the content of precipitated ribosomes seen on stained smears. Group I cells contain large dense clumps of granules; in group II, the granules assume a wreath-like appearance; in group III the clumps are scattered, and in group IV scattered granules remain.

The size of the circulating reticulocyte was determined by a photographic projection technique, a volume some 20% larger than that of the adjacent mature erythrocytes.[110] With active erythropoiesis following erythropoietin stimulation, hemoglobin synthesis is accelerated, an earlier cell release is triggered, and a more prolonged maturation time in the blood required. With sustained erythropoietin stimulation, striking increases in reticulocyte size occur, reaching levels twice that of the mature erythrocyte.[19,111–114]

Stohlman[114] attributed this macroreticulocytosis to skipped division in the maturation sequence. The macroreticulocytes were found to have a shortened life span and were followed by normal sized reticulocytes with continued erythropoietic stimulation. The early release of the marrow reticulocytes is recognized in the peripheral smear by the increased polychromasia of the red cells.[115] Normally, less than 5% of circulating reticulocytes are polychromatophilic, but with erythropoietin-induced stimulation of erythropoiesis the polychromatophilic erythrocyte population may rise to more than 20% of the circulating red cells. The increase in polychromatophilic erythrocyte may be presumed to be a manifestation of increased erythropoietin stimulation.[115] Clarkson and Moore[116] reported alterations in reticulocyte size in response to erythropoietin (phlebotomy) and to iron, folate, and B_{12} deficiency or treatment before change in the mean corpuscular volume of the erythrocyte could be detected. They also pointed out that the effects of iron and B_{12} deficiency or treatment could override the effect of erythropoietin. Stryckmans et al.[117] studied the maturation of the erythrocyte in the rat following stimulation of erythropoiesis. Following mild stimulation with erythropoietin, all of the reticulocytes appear to mature into normal red cells with normal life span. After marked marrow stimulation with erythropoietin the reticulocytes mature into red cells with a normal potential life span, but display a decreased mean circulating life span. There is no unanimity of opinion on the origin of the macroreticulocyte which is seen as the initial consequence of heightened erythropoiesis due to erythropoietin stimulation. Some consider the macroreticulocyte as a cell originating from a macronormoblast, probably the result of a skipped division, and distinct from normal reticulocytes, and not due to a shift of the marrow reticulocytes to the blood. Others[118] argue that the macroreticulocyte is due primarily to shift of the early reticulocytes into the periphery and is the result of the action of erythropoietin on hemoglobin synthesis modulated by other factors such as availability of iron[113,114] and the effect of the erythropoietin on the release of the reticulocytes into the sinusodal lumen.[111] In a clinical setting it is perhaps best to consider the macroreticulocyte as a ''shift'' cell until the more basic problems are resolved.

A morphological live-cell classification scheme of reticulocyte maturation has been proposed by Mel et al.[119] The cell which can be identified as the reticulocyte immediately after the expulsion of the nucleus and designated R_1 is characterized by its asymmetrical shape, motility and multilobularity. In the rat, and probably also in man, the R_1 reticulocytes constitute 25% of the normal bone marrow reticulocytes, but are not present in normal blood. With further maturation and remodulation the R_2 reticulocyte is recognized by a ''deep dished'' asymmetry, a few refractile granules (in phase contrast microscopy), and a loss of motility. A nonmotile reticulocyte, R_3, can be found which retains the reticulocyte asymmetry, but lacks granules or vesicles and is a transition form to the disc-shaped mature red cell. The percentage of R_1 forms is increased in the marrow in response to stimulation of erythropoiesis and is found to correlate in a linear fashion with the hematocrit in the range of 25 to 70%. The sum of the R_1 and R_2 cells, determined as live unstained cells, is equal to the number of reticulocytes identified by new methylene blue staining.

In summary, erythropoiesis begins in the bone marrow by the commitment of pluripotential cells to erythropoiesis. The cells of the committed cell population represent a continuum of cells in differentiation acquiring greater sensitivity to erythropoietin and decreasing proliferative capability. They finally emerge as proerythroblasts, the earliest cell of the recognizable population of marrow cells concerned chiefly with hemoglobin synthesis and differentiation into mature red cells. The recognizable erythroid precursors provide the clinician with the only window into the erythropoietic process. Morphological stages in the maturation sequence can be identified as the cells progress from the proerythroblasts (E_1) to erythroblasts (E_2), polychromatophilic normoblasts (E_3), and finally to orthochromatic normoblasts (E_4). The normal maturation sequence is characterized by a continuously decreasing nuclear-cytoplasmic ratio, decreasing cytoplasmic basophilia due to RNA degradation, and increasing eosinophilia reflecting hemoglobin synthesis. The ratio of early precursors (pro- and basophilic erythroblasts) to late erythroid precursors (the poly- and orthochromatic normoblasts) is about 1:3. Maturation of the recognizable erythroid precursors takes about 3 to 4 days during which time some four to five doublings take place. All of the recognizable erythroid precursors except the orthochromatic normoblasts are capable of division. On reaching a critical hemoglobin concentration the orthochromatic normoblast expells its nucleus to be a reticulocyte which remains in the marrow for an additional 2 to 2-1/2 days synthesizing an additional increment of hemoglobin and degrading all of the remaining RNA and mitochondria to enter finally the peripheral blood, where it undergoes further modulation to become a mature red cell. Considerable appreciation of this process can be gained from the morphologic assessment of smears prepared from the marrow aspirates. The final product of the maturation sequence, the red cell, its size, hemoglobinization, and shape is the result of an interplay between the various factors that enter into and control the synthesis of hemoglobin and the agents and material that enter into and control the replication process.

X. INEFFECTIVE ERYTHROPOIESIS

Ineffective erythropoiesis refers to the premature death of the recognizable red cell precursors in the marrow. Detection of ineffective erythropoiesis is made most reliably from the kinetic data obtained following in vivo tritium thymidine labeling. The indications are that the degree of ineffective erythropoiesis is minimal during normal erythropoiesis.[120,121] On a clinical level the term has been used to signal those anemias in which there is a discrepancy between the size of the erythroid precursor population and the number of reticulocytes delivered to the periphery. Clinical detection of ineffective erythropoiesis is approached through the comparison of the reticulocyte production index with the marrow M/E ratio or through the determination of the plasma iron turnover and the radioiron incorporation of the red cells.[122,123] The term dyserythropoiesis incorporates the concept of ineffective erythropoiesis by including, in addition to the quantitative abnormalities, the qualitative and morphological abnormalities of the circulating red cells which are the products of a faulty and abnormal maturation process.[124,125]

A. Dyserythropoiesis

The morphological features of dyserythropoiesis include nuclear budding and fragmentation, karyorrhexis, mitotic abnormalities, failure of cell separation, bi- and multinuclearity, and asynchrony of nuclear and cytoplasmic maturation. Basophilic stippling, ringed sideroblasts, and other aberrations of erythroid structure may be found. These features are easily recognized in the usual marrow preparation by light microscopy. The degree of abnormality varies considerably from minor disturbances such as can be found in the hemolytic anemias, infections, and severe iron lack anemias to a major and dominant expression seen in the congenital dyserythropoietic anemias.[126] Electron microscopic evidence suggests that disruption of the nuclear membrane is a fundamental defect which in turn may trigger some of the associated aberrations. The ultrastructural characteristics of dyserythropoiesis have been fully summarized and illustrated by Frisch and Broeckaert-Van Orshouen.[127]

The dyserythropoietic anemias have been separated into a primary group consisting of a variety of congenital disorders and secondary group in which dyserythropoiesis is found in association with other hematologic disorders.

B. Congenital Dyserythropoietic Anemia

1. Type I

Congenital dyserythropoietic anemia, type I[131] is an uncommon disorder, probably autosomal recessive, characterized by a moderate macrocytic anemia, splenomegaly, and secondary hemochromatosis and in which coexistent malformations, such as pigmentations of skin, abnormalities of the hand, or syndactyly may be found.

In the peripheral blood, anisocytosis, poikilocytosis, and basophilic stippling are almost always found. In the bone marrow marked erythroid hyperplasia is noted; the M/E ratio is reversed, 1:3 to 1:6; and large islands of normoblasts are encountered. The cells may be doubly nucleated, and small internuclear chromatin bridges which represent the single most typical abnormality, may be identified. Ultrastructural findings in addition, include dense nuclear chromatin separated by large masses of intervening cytoplasm.[129,130] The morphologic findings suggest a mitotic disturbance.

2. Type II(HEMPAS)

Congenital dyserythropoietic anemia, type II (HEMPAS)[131] is characterized by moderate anemia, mild jaundice, hepatosplenomegaly, and iron overload. The blood smear shows marked anisocytosis, poikilocytosis, and basophilic stippling. The marrow is markedly hypercellular with a reversed M/E ratio. Islands of normoblasts are seen and a very high percentage (10 to 35%) are doubly nucleated. The macrophages are loaded with iron and Gaucher cells may be observed.[132] Ultrastructurally, a linear structure (second membrane) parallel to and at distance of 40 to 60 nm at the inside of the cell may be present.[132] The red cells of HEMPAS are strongly agglutinated by anti i, less so by anti I. Characteristically, a positive acidified serum lysis test is observed.

3. Type III

Congenital dyserythropoietic anemia, type III,[133] is the rarest form of dyserythropoietic anemia, is characterized by a modest anemia (9 to 11 g/100 mℓ) and a variable clinical picture. The blood smear shows anisocytosis, macrocytosis, polychromasia, and basophilic stippling. The bone marrow is very abnormal, again with a reversed M/E ratio. Many multinucleated giant erythroblasts with as many as a dozen nuclear buddings and frequent karyorrhexis are present.

A group of rare variants of congenital dyserythropoietic anemia have been described.[134] Morphologic changes in the bone marrow similar to those already described, but usually less extreme may be seen in the megaloblastic states, sideroblastic anemias, thalassemia, aplastic anemia, paroxysmal nocturnal hemoglobinuria, etc.

C. Megaloblastosis

According to Ewing,[135] the first important observations on the changes in the bone marrow in pernicious anemia were made by Cohnheim in 1876. In a report of an autopsy examination of an individual who had succumbed to pernicious anemia, Cohnheim singled out the marked hyperplasia of the marrow, the almost complete absence of fat, and the presence of large numbers of cells which he considered to be megaloblasts and therefore proposed that the process represented a reversion to the embryonal type of blood formation. Ewing[135] carried Cohnheim's supposition a step further and argued that progressive pernicious anemia must be regarded as identical with or very closely related to a neoplasm involving the red cells. ''This is of course the fundamental nature of a tumor process in which the highly specialized properly functioning tissues are replaced by excessively cellular, poorly differentiated structures, subject to a great variety of degenerative changes.'' In brief, Ewing[135] visualized the essential lesion of pernicious anemia to be ''megaloblastic metaplasia of the marrow which is invariably present; is pathognomonic of the disease and in many respects resembles a tumor formation affecting the progenitors of the red cells.'' This concept dominated much of the early speculation on the nature of the megaloblast in pernicious anemia.[136] The weight of evidence that has accumulated during the past 50 years makes it abundantly clear that the megaloblast of pernicious anemia cannot be identified with the megaloblast of embryonic blood island formation,[140] and that the pathologic megaloblast is the morphologic expression of disordered DNA replication.

1. Morphology

The hallmark of megaloblastosis, regardless of whether it be folate or B_{12} deficiency or other disturbances of DNA synthesis, is asynchronism in the morphologic expression of nuclear and cytoplasmic differentiation at all levels of the maturation sequence. In this sense it does bear resemblance to a neoplastic process which struck the imagination of the early observers of this phenomenon.

The bone marrow is generally hypercellular with considerable reduction of its adipose component. Although all cells are involved in the pathologic process, the marrow is predominantly erythroid with an M/E ratio much in favor of the red cell precursors. In general, the degree of cellularity, the size of the population of the recognizable red cell precursors, and the frankness of the megaloblastic expression is related to the severity of the vitamin deficiency and to the degree of disordered DNA synthesis. The severity of the megaloblastic changes also correlates crudely with the red cell count: the lower the count the more extreme the morphologic changes. With increasing red cell counts the marrow changes become more subtle, and at counts above 3.5 to 4 million/mm^3 the changes may be difficult to discern with confidence. In the deficiency states, folate and B_{12}, the maturation sequence is shifted toward the more immature appearing cells as the vitamin deprivation increases: hemoglobinization becomes less apparent and erythropoiesis becomes increasingly inefficient.

The earliest recognizable megaloblast, a cell comparable to the proerythroblast of the normal erythropoietic maturation sequence, is a large cell, some 25 to 35 μm in diameter. The nucleus is large with a high nuclear-cytoplasmic ratio; the chromatin is diffusely and finely granular, the nucleoli faint and indistinct. The cytoplasm is deep blue in sharp contrast to the granular and finely clumped chromatin.

As the cell undergoes differentiation to a level comparable to the erythroblast, the nuclear-cytoplasmic ratio decreases sharply. The nucleus is at this point down to half or less of the cell diameter which itself decreased but slightly from its predecessor. The cytoplasm is now a lighter blue, the nuclear chromatin is now homogeneously granular with a diffusely stippled appearance.

With further maturation at a level now comparable with the polychromatophilic normoblast the cytoplasm assumes a purplish tone and the nuclear chromatin masses increase in size but remain rather diffusely distributed. When the megaloblast reaches the stage comparable to the orthochromatic normoblast the cell is now about 10 to 15 μm in diameter; the cytoplasm has an orange-yellow hue; and the nucleus though reduced in size is not fully pyknotic and still retains its clumped granular appearance. Thus, throughout the maturation sequence one sees evidence of a maturation asynchrony.

Secondary, but not pathognomonic, changes occur as the cells proceed in their maturation. Nuclear projections may appear to give the cell a multilobed appearance. Fragments of nuclear projections form the cytoplasmic Howell-Jolly bodies. Nuclear division without cell division may take place to produce large multinucleated cells, the gigantoblasts. The chromosomes of dividing megaloblasts appear to be slender and long in contrast to the short and more clumped appearance of the chromosome of the dividing normal erythroid precursors. Cell death is frequent and karyorrhexis and karyolysis commonly encountered. Megaloblasts which complete the maturation process emerge, following nuclear extrusion as macroovalocytes, the large oval shaped red cells so characteristic of the red cells of the peripheral blood in pernicious anemia or folate deficiency.

Phase contrast microscopic examination of the live megaloblast offers no particular advantages to the Giemsa stained preparations for purposes of diagnosis or for insights into the nature of the abnormality. The megaloblast can be readily distinguished in the living state; the beaded, diffusely clumped structure of the chromatin is striking, the small nucleoli being clearly visible even into late stages of maturation.

Electron microscopic studies of the megaloblast have uncovered a variety of intracellular anatomical aberrations which are not pathognomonic of the megaloblastic process. The significance, origin, and nature of these changes have not yet been elucidated.[138–140] The ultrastructural studies support the nuclear origin of the Howell-Jolly body whether formed from chromosome fragments separated during mitosis or by fragmentation of both hetero- and euchromatin of the resting nucleus.[141–143]

Megaloblastosis has been described classically in pernicious anemia and subsequently recognized as a manifestation of B_{12} and folate deficiency, regardless of cause.[144] Megaloblastosis may be encountered following administration of drugs that interfere with B_{12} and folate metabolism or B_{12} and folate absorption; drugs that interfere with DNA synthesis by inhibition of either purine or pyrimidine metabolism; in a variety of inherited metabolic abnormalities involving nucleotide synthesis such as the Lesch-Nyhan syndrome; and in neoplastic states such as erythroleukemia, or the preleukemic syndromes. The morphological lesion is identical in all of these clinical situations suggesting similar, fundamental biochemical defects.

The physiological and chemical processes that are responsible for the morphological configuration of the megaloblast are still incompletely understood. Beck[144] suggested that the nuclear/cytoplasmic asynchrony represented a state of unbalanced growth in which RNA and protein, that is hemoglobin synthesis, continue unabated while DNA synthesis and replication are sharply retarded. Beck directed attention to the remarkable changes in size of a *E. coli* mutant, cells of which, when grown on B_{12} deficient media, grew to be giants and in media heavily loaded with B_{12} were transformed into dwarfs.

2. *Kinetics*

The clinical impressions of bone marrow failure, significant ineffective erythropoiesis, and intramarrow death of red cell precursors are gleaned from the marrow examination; the reversed M/E ratio and markedly decreased reticulocyte production index was supported by the elegant studies of London and West[145] and of Finch et al.[146]

Messner et al.[147] demonstrated a decrease in the proliferation capacity of the megaloblasts in pernicious anemia. In normal erythropoiesis, the cells tend to double as they proceed from one maturation compartment to the next, from E_1 to E_5. In normal erythropoiesis the compartment sizes E_1 to E_5 bear a ratio of 1:2.3:5.1:9.9:20.[120] In megaloblastic erythropoiesis the relative compartment ratios are 1:2.2:3.3:2.1:3.8.[149] Two possibilities were raised to explain the delay in labeling indices of the more mature compartment E_4,E_5: either a prolonged turnover time or an inhomogeneity of the cell population, if turnover time is normal. Since an upper limit of 21 hr was found in the average generation time of one of the patients studied, Messner et al.[147] concluded that two populations of early polychromatophilic megaloblasts exist which are morphologically identical, but differ in their capacity to replicate. Death rate was presumed to be high in the cells incapable of division, whereas maturation continued apparently normally in the proliferating population of cells. Wickramsinghe et al.[7] detected two major disturbances in the megaloblasts of pernicious anemia: a slowing or arrest of DNA synthesis in some cells, and an accumulation of cells in G_2 suggesting a failure of the cells to enter mitosis. Since some of the arrested cells showed no protein synthesis, Wickramsinghe et al.[148] postulated that these cells probably suffer intramedullary death. These findings were explained by postulating an unequal distribution of B_{12} among the red cell precursors, by virtue of their geography and proximity to the sources of the vitamin and presumably other vital factors.[149]

Similar observations were made by Yoshida et al.[150] who also found a population of megaloblasts whose DNA value ranged about the 4C value, suggesting impaired or arrested synthesis DNA. They found a prolongation of the S period with or without prolongation of G_2. RNA and protein synthesis were, however, normal. The data on the cell cycle time and duration of phase in megaloblastosis are confusing and suggest considerable inhomogeneity of the cells in this regard.[91,151,152]

a. RNA and Protein Synthesis

Similar to the normal red cell precursors, megaloblasts show a progressive decrease in their mean RNA content and increasing concentrations of hemoglobin as the cells move through the maturation sequence.[154] However, varying proportions of both early and late polychromatophilic megaloblasts display depressed protein synthesis or complete cessation of protein synthesis.[148]

The concept that the megaloblast is the morphologic expression of a derangement in DNA synthesis and DNA replication, whatever the cause, is widely accepted and unchallenged. However, the mechanisms, biochemical and biophysical, that are responsible for the characteristic morphologic changes of the megaloblast are still largely unknown. The megaloblastic changes found in the proliferating cells of the hemopoietic tissues of the bone marrow in B_{12} and folate deficient states are not limited to the blood cells but also exist in other proliferating systems such as the gastrointestinal tract and lymphocytes stimulated by phytohemaglutinin.[154,155]

Das and Herbert[155a] in a recent review marshalled the information on the metabolic roles of B_{12} and folate and on the interrelationship of the two vitamins in support of the concept that both vitamins play a crucial role in the conversion of deoxyuridylate to thymidylate and that the failure of this reaction leads to a derangement in DNA synthesis.

The methylation of uridylate in its conversion to thymidylate is a rate-limiting reaction dependent on the presence of 5,10-methylene tetrahydrofolate. Following the transfer of its one carbon ligands, 5,10-methylene tetrahydrofolate is converted to the dihydrofolate compound which must be reduced again by dihydrofolate reductase to the tetrahydrofolate state before it can again resume its function as a one carbon donor. Tetrahydrofolate is regenerated by the conversion of serine to glycine under the influence of serine transhydroxymethylase. Decreased levels of 5,10-methylene tetrahydrofolate as a consequence of folate deficiency or inhibition of dihydrofolate reductase, e.g., methotrexate administration, or genetically deficient serine transhydroxymethylase causes the pathway from deoxyuridylate to thymidylate to run down. The fall in thymidylate concentration activates thymidylate kinase which can convert any available thymidine to thymidylate (salvage pathway).

The major form of circulating folate is the 5-methyl congener of tetrahydrofolate, which can be converted to tetrahydrofolate through only one reaction, the methylation of homocysteine to cysteine by the B_{12} dependent enzyme, homocysteine-5-methyltretrahydrofolate transferase. This B_{12} dependent reaction helps maintain the concentration of tetrahydrofolate in the cells and has been proposed as the key mechanism for the deranged DNA synthesis in B_{12} deficiency (the ''methyltetrahydrofolate trap'' hypothesis).[155] According to this hypothesis, B_{12} deficiency leads to a decrease in the conversion fate of 5-methyltetrahydrofolate to tetrohydrofolate thus producing a ''pile up'' of 5-methyltetrahydrofolate in the blood, a drop in the tetrahydrofolate in the cells and subsequent failure of the *de novo* synthesis of thymidylate from deoxyuridine. This interplay of B_{12} and folate is presumed to be the mechanism of megaloblastosis in pernicious anema.

b. Deoxyuridine Suppression Test

In an elegant study, Killmann[156] showed that the addition of deoxyuridine to cultures of normal bone marrow suppressed the incorporation of tritiated thymidine into DNA, but failed to do so in the cultures of bone marrow from subjects with pernicious anemia. This study became the basis of the deoxyuridine (dU) suppression test. Metz et al.[157] were able to correct the failure of thymidine incorporation into the DNA of megaloblasts due to B_{12} deficiency by the addition of B_{12} to the culture medium: megaloblasts due to folate deficiency did not respond to B_{12}. Large doses of folate corrected the thymidine incorporation of megaloblasts of either deficiency. Das et al.[158] utilized the dU suppression test to detect folate deficiency in patients with iron deficiency whose only hematologic manifestation of folate deficiency was hypersegmentation of the polymorphonuclear leucocytes.

Replication of mammalian DNA of normal cells occurs during the S phase with the unwinding of the double helix and the polymerization of the four deoxyribonucleoside triphosphates on the parental strands. Replication is not a continuous process beginning at one end and ending at the other. Rather, it is a discontinuous process initiated in smaller replicating units (replicons) and proceeds in opposite directions along the strand. The small fragments (the Okazaki pieces) are synthesized by extension of short RNA primers which are subsequently excised to leave gaps between the Okazaki pieces which are subsequently filled, thus joining the fragments to form the longer DNA molecules.[159–161]

Hoffbrand et al.[162] summarized the evidence in support of the argument that the lack of one or other of the four deoxyribonucleoside triphosphates, whether due to B_{12} folate deficiency or the action of drugs on nucleoside synthesis, or congenital abnormality of key enzymes in the synthesis of the nucleosides, impairs the ability of the cell to fill the gaps between the Okazaki pieces, leaving persistent single-stranded regions in the DNA molecules.[162] Drugs like hydroxyurea and fluorodeoxyuridine which are known to cause megaloblastosis and interfere with deoxyribonucleoside synthesis inhibit gap filling and ligation of the Okazaki pieces.[163–167] Using the lymphocytes from patients with megaloblastic anemia, stimulated to replicate DNA by phytohemagglutinin, Wickramsinghe et al.[168] were able to show a delay in the formation of chromosome-sized strands from the individual replicons in such cells and a delay in the replication fork movement.[169]

Although the emphasis has been on the changes in the red cell precursors it is clear that all proliferating cells suffer from an impairment of DNA synthesis and DNA replication in megaloblastosis. Both the granulocytic precursors and the megakaryocytes are affected in pernicious anemia and other megaloblastic states as witnessed by the leucopenia, thrombocytopenia, and the hypersegmentation of the polymorphonuclear cells so often present in these clinical situations. But the morphological characteristics of the megaloblastic myeloid precursors and the megakaryocytes are much less striking and dramatic than the eye-catching changes of the megaloblastic erythroid precursors. Giant metamyelocytes are, however, frequently seen in B_{12} and folate deficiency and help serve as markers for these disorders. The giant metamyelocyte appears to be a polyploid cell[177] which blocked at this stage of development, is destined to die in the marrow and does not appear in the peripheral blood.

How these abnormalities of DNA replication cause the morphological abnormalities seen in the megaloblastic state is not yet clear, but the possibility of chromosomal or other abnormality due to weak areas of single-stranded DNA, subject to either mechanical or enzymatic damage has been raised for further exploration.

XI. ANEMIAS

From the perspective of the bone marrow the anemias can be conveniently classified as the anemias arising from defects in the cytoplasmic maturation of the erythroid precursors; derangements in nuclear maturation; and a shortened survival of the circulating red cell, namely, hemolysis or inadequate production due to a quantitative reduction of the erythroid progenitors.[123]

A. The Cytoplasmic Maturation Defects

The disorders arising from defects in cytoplasmic maturation are essentially disorders due to disturbances in hemaglobin synthesis, and are recognized clinically by the production of red cells of low mean corpuscular volume. The prime clinical examples of disorders of cytoplasmic maturation are the iron lack anemias, the anemia of lead intoxication, sideroblastic anemias, and thalassemia.

1. Iron Lack Anemia

Iron is a rate-limiting substrate for heme synthesis. In its absence the concentration of heme declines and the intracellular level of protoporphyrin rises. Bone marrow macrophages normally accumulate masses of hemosiderin which can be readily identified by the Prussian blue reaction and has served as a means of estimating the nonheme iron in the aspirates of human bone marrow.[171] Gale et al.[172] calculated a total iron store of 288 mg or 0.24 μg of iron per mg marrow net weight (range 0.08 to 0.69 μg/mg) in the marrow of men (a calculation based on the marrow obtained from ribs resected during thorocotomy). Similar estimates, 0.25 μg/mg (SD ± 0.23) net weight of marrow were obtained from particles separated from the aspirate of human bone marrow.[173,174] Ferritin is readily recognizable on electron microscopy by virtue of its iron content and has been found to exist in both the reticular macrophages and the recognizable red cell precursors including the reticulocytes.[175]

The macrophages derive their iron from the digestion of aged red cells which had been engulfed by phagocytosis. Because of the anatomical relationships between the central reticular macrophage and the surrounding erythroblasts and the findings of pinocytotic vesicles in association with ferritin, Bessis and Breton-Gorius [176] proposed that preformed ferritin is transferred from the macrophage to the erythroblast and that the ferritin serves as a site of iron storage within the cytoplasm of the erythroblast. This hypothesis was challenged by Jandl and Katz[177] who presented data to show that the major pathway for iron transfer to the erythroid precursor cells is via circulating transferrin which attaches to a specific receptor site on the cell surface. The red cell precursors are capable of removing iron from transferrin and incorporating the iron into its cytoplasm.[178–180]

It is now well established that the erythroid precursor cells can synthesize apoferritin *de novo*.[181–184] The suggestion has been made[184] that the apoferritin is synthesized at the erythroblast surface in response to the transfer of the iron from the attached transferrin molecule and that the newly formed ferritin aggregates by a reversed pinocytosis-exocytosis.

During normal erthropoiesis, iron is transferred by plasma transferrin at the cell membrane of the red cell precursors. An intact, active mitochondrial electron transport system is required. Apoferritin synthesis is most active in the early recognizable precursor cells and declines and ultimately ceases with the subsequent maturation of the cells to reticulocytes. Iron incorporation into the apoferritin continues throughout the maturation sequence even into the reticulocyte.[183] The amount of apoferritin synthesized is related directly to the amount of iron delivered from the transferrin. The role of the intracellular ferritin is not clear, and may represent an intermediate in heme biosynthesis or simply a storage site of excess iron.

In the early erythroid precursor cells individual molecules of ferritin are found dispersed throughout the cytoplasm. With further maturation of the cells the ferritin molecules aggregate and subsequently form granules which can be made visible by the Prussian blue reaction. The normoblast with one or more Prussian blue staining granules, the sideroblast, makes up about 30 to 50% of all the normoblasts in the normal human marrow. In iron lack anemia the sideroblast population vanishes; the number of sideroblasts correlates with the level of the serum iron and the percent saturation of the transferrin.[185]

The sideroblast is capable of ridding itself of the excess iron by exocytosis and proceeding as a normoblast to mature into a reticulocyte and to an erythrocyte. On the other hand, the sideroblast may extrude its nucleus to become a reticulocyte with intracellular ferritin aggregates which can be recognized by special staining.[186] The iron-containing reticulocyte can shed its iron in a manner similar to the sideroblast or mature into a siderocyte, essentially an erythrocyte with iron granules which depend on the spleen for their removal.[194]

The bone marrow in iron-lack anemia shows normal cellularity. The M/E ratio is shifted in favor of the erythroid cells. The sideroblast population falls to practically zero levels and no stainable iron is detectable in the macrophages. Ineffective erythropoiesis is a prominent manifestation of this disorder.

2. *Sideroblastic Anemia*

The designation, sideroblastic anemia, includes a number of diverse, hereditary, and acquired conditions which present a common morphological abnormality, the ringed sideroblast. Electron microscopy has identified the abnormality as an overload with nonferritin iron of the mitochondria which tend to assume a perinuclear position in the more mature erythroid precursor cells.[195] The cells are readily recognized in the smears of marrow aspirate stained for iron with the Prussian blue reaction. A ring of blue granules, representing the iron loaded mitochondria, form a ring-like structure about the nucleus. The common biochemical pathway for the morphological abnormality is probably defective heme synthesis, in the synthesis of protoporphyrin, in the conversion of protoporphyrin to heme (defective hemoglobin synthetase), or damage to the mitochondria by iron overload.[187,189–195] How defective heme synthesis leads to mitochondria iron overload is unknown, but the presence of stainable iron in the mitochondria is distinctly pathological and not seen in the handling of iron by normal red cell precursors.

In the primary and hereditary sideroblastic anemia 40 to 70% of the normoblasts may be ringed. The mitochondria of these cells are distorted, swollen, and probably functionally abnormal.[196] The ringed sideroblast has difficulty in shedding the excess iron and many die in the bone marrow. Ineffective erythropoiesis is prominent. The siderocyte progeny of the ringed sideroblast is usually a hypochromic cell in which iron granules are seen at the margins of the hemoglobin. On electron microscopy these granules are iron-loaded, degenerating mictochondria.

The bone marrow findings of sideroblastic anemia include essentially normal cellularity, an M/E ratio in favor of the erythroid population, a marked increase in marrow macrophage iron, and the presence of many ringed sideroblasts.

The sideroblastic anemias have been divided into primary forms, such as the sex-linked hypochromic anemias, and into the acquired forms, such as refractory idiopathic sideroblastic anemia and a preleukemic form in which blast cells may be seen in hyperplastic marrow aspirates. Pelger-Huet-like cells and normoblasts may be present in the peripheral blood.[197–199] The secondary forms of sideroblastic anemia may be seen in alcoholics,[200] in lead intoxication, or following treatment with drugs like isoniazid or cycloserine. Ringed sideroblasts, usually in lesser numbers, may be seen in a wide variety of illnesses such as leukemia, carcinoma, hemochromatosis, rheumatoid arthritis, megaloblastic anemia, etc.

In summary it can be seen that in a cytoplasmic maturation disturbance in the red cell precursors, abnormal heme synthesis may be present in both iron lack and iron overload states. Ineffective erythropoiesis is present in both situations, but the marrow findings (absent sideroblasts and macrophage iron in one and the presence of ringed sideroblast and abundant macrophage iron in the other) readily separate the two conditions.

3. The Thalassemias

The thalassemias comprise a group of hereditary disorders in each of which the principal difficulty is an inability to produce sufficient quantities of one of the other globin chains.[201] Two main types of thalassemia are recognized, α thalassemia in which the deficient α chain synthesis and excess production of β and γ chains results in the formation of the tetramers, β_4 (hemoglobin H) and γ_4 (hemoglobin Bart's), and β thalassemia where diminished β chain production, continued γ chain synthesis, and excess α chain production give rise to the intraerythrocytic inclusions of the precipitated α_2 dimers and the continued production of fetal hemoglobin beyond the neonatal period.[202,203]

The clinical syndromes of thalassemia vary considerably in the severity of their clinical presentation, ranging from the symptomless carrier states, through the mild anemias of the heterozygotes to the severe, crippling, and lethal anemias of the homozygous forms. Microcytosis and hypochromia are the characteristic morphologic changes common to all of the thalassemic syndromes. Anisocytosis, poikilocytosis, basophilic stippling, and target cells are frequently present. The MCH is usually less than 27 pg and the MCV less than 70 μ^3.

In β thalassemia, the excess of α chains is presumed to be the major pathogenetic factor in effecting the abnormalities of the red cells. The uncombined α chains are highly unstable and are apparently readily oxidized to hemichromes which show an increased tendency to precipitate.[204] The precipitated α chains can be observed in the red cell precursors in the bone marrow, the degree of precipitation increasing with the increasing concentrations of hemoglobin in the maturing red cells.[205] It appears initially as a fine, diffuse dust-like material about the perinuclear zone of the early polychromatophilic normoblast and grows coarser, more granular, and finally forms large inclusions with increasing maturation of the red cell precursors. In the very severe forms of β thalassemia the inclusions may become as large as the nucleus of the mature orthochromatic normoblast. Such inclusions have been found to contain up to 75% of the total hemoglobin complement of the cell.[206] There is good correlation between the size of the inclusions and the number of normoblasts affected with the clinical severity of the disease. These morphological manifestations of the precipitated α chains are for the most part absent in the heterozygous states.

The mechanisms of cell damage by the precipitation of the excess α-chains are still highly unexplained. Some evidence has been presented to suggest that the oxidative denaturation of the α chains may generate excessive quantities of superoxide radical with a potential for the oxidation of cell proteins, lipids, and possibly DNA.[207,208] Lysosomal injury, through the release of proteolytic enzymes from the autophagic precipitates has been invoked as an additional mechanism of red cell injury.[206,209] The increased rigidity of the red cell caused by the precipitated α chains probably plays a minor role.

A number of other abnormalities has been detected in the red cell precursors and erythrocytes of the thalassemic patient, and has been concerned chiefly with the manifestations of iron overload and the accumulation of iron in the mitochondria of the normoblasts; the accumulation of PAS positive mucopolysaccharide (glycogen) chiefly in the polychromatophilic normoblasts and a cell membrane abnormality characterized by an increased potassium flux.[210] Abnormalities in the maturation of the red cell precursors, notably an increase in the proportion of erythroblasts in the S phase and corresponding decrease of cells in G_1 have also been demonstrated.[209]

In severe cases of β-thalassemia the bone marrow exhibits a marked increase in cellularity with an enormous expansion of the marrow space. The M/E ratio is reversed and decreased to levels indicative of an increase in the red cell mass to 20 to 30 times greater than normal. There is a marked increase in the number of late erythroblasts and polychromatophilic normoblasts. In the heterozygote some increase in cellularity is present and the M/E is more modestly decreased down to levels of about 1:2. The cell diameter of all of the red cell precursors is smaller than normal. Macrophage iron is markedly increased and ringed sideroblasts may be present. In severe forms of the disease Gaucher-like cells may be observed.

Ineffective erythropoiesis appears to be the major disturbance responsible for the anemia. The severity of the anemia is aggravated by the coexistant shortened red cell survival in the homozygote; red cell survival in the heterozygote tends to be normal.[208,211,212]

The homozygous α-thalassemia, hemoglobin Bart's hydrops fetalis, is an invariably fatal disease. Most of the afflicted infants are stillborn or die soon after birth. The red cells are large but hypochromic, but some microcytes and target cells are present. Seventy to eighty percent of the total hemoglobin is Bart's; no A hemoglobin is present.

The bone marrow is markedly hyperplastic, the M/E ratio reversed. The erythroid compartment of the marrow is markedly increased and extramedullary hematopoiesis is found in the liver and spleen. The marrow iron is markedly increased.

Hemoglobin-H disease (α-thalassemia - 1, α thalassemia·2) is generally a mild clinical disorder characterized by the presence of large amounts of hemoglobin H, about 25% of the total hemoglobin, and the presence of inclusion bodies in the circulating red cells following their incubation with brilliant cresyl blue or new methylene blue. Microcytosis, marked hypochromia, basophilic stippling, and target cells are characteristically present.

Like the excess α-chains in β-thalassemia, hemoglobin H is unstable and forms hemichromes which tend to precipitate.[213] The red cell injury caused by the precipitated hemoglobin is probably responsible for the shortened red cell survival.

Bone marrow aspiration reveals increased cellularity and reversal of the M/E ratio, the bone marrow macrophage iron is usually increased. Modest ineffective erythropoiesis has been demonstrated.[214]

In summary, the unbalanced globin synthesis of the thalassemias unfolds a constellation of pivotal findings common to all of the thalassemic syndromes—defective hemoglobinization of the red cells, microcytosis, hyperplasia of the erythroid compartment of the bone marrow, ineffective erythropoiesis, and varying degrees of hemolysis.

4. Lead Poisoning

An anemia, usually mild, characterized by hypochromia of the red cells, an elevated reticulocyte count and basophilic stippling is a frequent accompaniment of chronic lead intoxication.[215] Lead has a particular affinity for red cells and for the red cell precursors. Of the lead in the peripheral blood, 95% is bound to the erythrocytes. The bone marrow lead concentration is some 50 times greater than the lead concentration of the blood.[216] The white cells and platelets do not appear to be altered.[216]

Lead affects the metabolism of the red cell and the synthesis of hemoglobin at many points. Lead can depress the activity of three important mitochondrial enzymes in the heme pathway—δ-aminolevulinic acid synthetase, δ-aminolevulinic acid dehydrase and heme synthetase to cause an accumulation of free protoporphyrin in the red cells and the excretion of delta aminolevulinic acid and copropophyrin in the urine. In severe lead poisoning porphobilinogen may be elevated.[217,218]

Lead causes swelling of the mitochondria and disorganization of the cristae,[216,219] accumulation of mitochondrial iron, and the formation of abnormal sideroblasts. Isolated mitochondria incubated with lead form extremely dense granules in the matrix around the cristae and other regions of the inner membrane, suggesting mitochondrial damage, decreased ATP formation, and interference in the gradient across the mitochondrial membrane.[220]

Lead also depresses globin synthesis and the degree of suppression is dependent on the concentration of lead. The depression of α-chain synthesis is greater than that for β-chain synthesis. This in vitro effect of lead can be corrected by the introduction of hemin, but the α-chain inhibition tends to persist.[221] The action of lead on globin synthesis may well be due to its action on heme synthesis[222] and RNA. These effects of globin synthesis observed in vitro were not duplicated in in vivo studies on lead-burdened workers.[221] It is of interest that Albahary[216] suggested a similarity between the globinopathy of lead poisoning and thalassemia minor.

Basophilic stippling, though not pathognomonic of the anemia of lead poisoning, is seen frequently in the more severe cases of this disorder and has been shown to be due to the aggregation of intracellular RNA.[223] Paglia et al.[224] demonstrated inhibition of pyrimidine 5′-nucleotidase of red cells by exposure to low levels of lead. Valentine et al.[225] had previously reported on the presence of marked basophilic stippling and a large accumulation of intraerythrocytic nucleotides in the hemolytic syndrome associated with the congenitally determined decrease in pyrimidine specific 5′-nucleotidase. They attributed the accumulation of the nondiffusible nucleotides to the inability of the cell to dephosphorylate and that the accumulated pyrimidine nucleotides by a feedback mechanism retarded the breakdown of RNA which on aggregation was responsible for the basophilic stippling. Valentine et al.[226] subsequently reported on a patient suffering from severe lead poisoning who mimicked in all detail the clinical and laboratory findings of the hemolytic anemia associated with the congenitally deficient pyrimidine 5′-nucleotidase deficiency.

Chronic lead poisoning can cause significant membrane changes of the red cells[220] and blunt the erythropoietic response to hypoxia.[227] The pathogenesis of the anemia associated with lead poisoning is obviously highly complex. The major manifestation is ineffective erythropoiesis and maturation failure. The bone marrow is hypercellular and essentially erythroblastic. There is an increase in the proportion of polychromatophilic normoblasts some of which may show basophilic stippling and PAS-positive inclusions. The morphologic abnormalities become more pronounced with hemoglobin synthesis. Macrophage iron is increased and ringed-sideroblast usually in small numbers, may be present. The anemia may be further aggravated by an accompanying hemolytic component.

B. The Nuclear Maturation Defects

1. The Megaloblast Anemias

The anemia resulting from nuclear maturation defects is characterized by macrocytosis of the red cells with elevations of the mean corpuscular volume well beyond 100, and megaloblastic hematopoiesis in the bone marrow, the features of which have been previously discussed. The diagnosis of megaloblastosis can be made most easily by examination of the bone marrow aspirate. The cause of the megaloblastosis, whether B_{12} or folate deficiency, the DiGuglielmo syndrome of an acute myeloblastic leukemia, treatment with oncologic agents like methotrexate etc., must be systematically investigated and determined by appropriate tests.

C. Hemolytic Disorders

Hemolysis, or decreased survival of the circulating red cell, may be due to an intrinsic defect in the red cell such as membrane abnormalities in hereditary spherocytic and elliptocytic anemia, paroxysmal nocturnal hemoglobinuria, etc.; an enzyme deficiency, such as glucose-6-phosphate dehydrogenase deficiency, pyruvate kinase deficiency, etc., an abnormal hemoglobin such as sickle cell hemoglobin, the presence of unstable hemoglobin, or to some external influence on a normal red cell such as the immunologically induced defects of the membrane leading to lysis or phagocytosis of the erythrocyte; or toxic agents such as phenylhydrazine, drugs, infections, etc. The mean corpuscular volume is generally normal or slightly elevated; the reticulocyte production index is elevated.

The bone marrow reflects the heightened red cell output, displaying marked increase in bone marrow cellularity and a reversal of the M/E ratio. Iron stores are normal or somewhat increased. In severe hemolytic states large clusters of normoblasts usually surrounding macrophages (blood islands) are frequently encountered, and some evidence of dyserythropoiesis may be present.

D. Marrow Failure

In absolute terms, the term ''marrow failure'' implies an inability of the marrow to meet the demand of a normal red cell output—in relative terms, an inability to respond as fully to the same stimulus for increased red cell production as a normal marrow. In marrow failure, the marrow may be functionally normal but the stimulus for erythroid production may be defective, inactivated, or deficient, or the stimulus may be adequate and normal but the marrow response may be inadequate as a result of normal but quantitatively diminished erythroid cell proliferation or qualitatively abnormal maturation of the erythroid precursor cells.

1. Anemia of Chronic Disease

Relative bone marrow failure is commonly present in a variety of unrelated disorders, such as chronic infections, chronic granulomatous disease, malignancy, renal failure, collagen vascular disease, etc. The anemia accompanying these disorders is usually of moderate severity, rarely falling below 7 to 8 g per 100 mℓ and in all cases associated with a low serum iron, reduced iron binding capacity, and an increase in storage iron. The anemia is rarely symptomatic and overshadowed by the underlying disease. Early on the red cells are normochronic and normocytic, but with prolongation of the syndrome, the red cells become more hypochromic and microcytic with an MCV falling generally in the upper seventies.

The pathogenesis of the anemia of chronic disorders is not completely understood and attention has been focussed chiefly on the role of erythropoietin and iron metabolism. The bone marrow is generally morphologically normal except as modified by the underlying disease: cellularity and M/E ratios tend to be normal. Bone marrow macrophage iron is increased, but the percentage of sideroblasts is decreased.[167] Bone marrow examination may therefore be helpful in distinguishing the anemia of chronic disorders from iron lack anemia.

2. Aplastic Anemia

The aplastic anemias are discussed elsewhere in detail. The bone marrow in classic aplastic anemia[228] is hypoplastic. The bone marrow consists almost wholly of fat cells; the cellular elements are markedly reduced. Bone marrow aspiration usually yields inadequate material for examination. The bone marrow biopsy is indispensable for the appropriate evaluation of the disorder. Islands of active cellular proliferation may be seen as well as an increase in lymphocytes and mast cells. Recent application of image analysis for the quantitative estimation of marrow cellularity may aid in the recognition of the less severely affected hypocellular anemias. Anemia and pancytopenia may be seen with a normo- or hypercellular marrow, the expression of ineffective hematopoiesis.

3. Pure Red Cell Anemia

Pure red cell anemia is characterized by anemia, reticulocytopenia, and a marrow which is normally cellular with almost complete disappearance of the recognizable erythroid precursor cells. The M/E ratio is thus heavily loaded in favor of the myeloid elements. Myeloid and megakaryocytic maturation are normal.

Pure red cell anemia is seen in children as in the Blackfan-Diamond syndrome whose lymphocytes have been shown to inhibit the CFU-E colony formation of normal marrow[229,230] in some cases but not in others.[231,232] The role of lymphocyte inhibition of the erythroid stem cell population in this disorder has yet to be elucidated.

Adult pure red cell anemia is seen in association with thymoma, myasthenia gravis, and other autoimmune states. An IgG fraction from the serum of such patients has been shown to inhibit heme synthesis in cultures of autologous and normal bone marrow. Not all patients with the adult pure red cell anemia have demonstrable antibodies for erythroblasts or erythropoietin in their sera. Pure red cell anemia has been subdivided into type I, in which an antibody against the red cell precursors is present; type II, a rare form in which an antibody against erythropoietin can be demonstrated; and type III, presumably a preleukemic condition in which no immunologic abnormality has been documented.[213,214]

XII. POLYCYTHEMIA

Polycythemia rubra vera is presumably a clonal disease of the pluripotential stem cell.[235] Proliferation of the erythroid precursors is independent of erythropoietin control.[236,237] The bone marrow of patients with polycythemia vera is characteristically hypercellular, although a normally cellular marrow may be encountered occasionally. The megakaryocyte number appears to be increased, but essentially parallels the overall hyperplasia of the marrow. Again, the reticulin content of the marrow correlates with the degree of hyperplasia. Macrophage storage iron is markedly reduced, generally absent. The maturation sequence of all hemopoietic cell lines appears morphologically normal. The bone marrow biopsy is a valuable adjunct in the diagnosis of polycythemia vera.[218]

In the secondary polycythemias the morphological characteristics are only moderately altered. Cellularity is modestly increased with a modest shift of the M/E ratio in favor of the red cells. The megakaryocytes and granulocytes are unaffected. The maturation sequence is normal.

REFERENCES

1. **Schwartz, E.,** Maturation and proliferation in normo and megaloblastic erythropoiesis, *Acta Med. Scand.* 139, 445,1951.
2. **Testa, N. G.,** Erythroid progenitor cells, their relevance for the study of haematologic disease, *Clin. Haematol.,* 8, 311, 1979.
3. **Wickramsinghe, S. N.,** Normal erythropoiesis, mechanisms of disturbance in disease in *Dyserythropoiesis,* Lewis, S. M., Verwilghen, R. L., Eds., Academic Press, New York, 1977, 21.
4. **Quesenberry, P. and Levitt, L.,** Hemopoietic stem cells, *N. Engl. J. Med.* 301, 755, 1973.
5. **Bessis, M.,** *Living Blood Cells and Their Ultrastructure,* translated by Weed, R. J., Springer-Verlag, New York, 1973.
6. **Wickramsinghe, S. N., Chalmer, D. G., and Cooper, E. H.,** Disturbed proliferation of erythropoietic cells in pernicious anemia, *Nature,* 215, 189, 1967.
7. **Wickramsinghe, S. N., Cooper, E. H., and Chalmers, D. G.,** A study of erythropoiesis by combined morphologic, quantitative cytochemical and autoradiographic methods, normal human bone marrow, vitamin B_{12} deficiency and iron deficiency anemia, *Blood,* 31, 304, 1968.
8. **Krantz, S. B. and Jacobson, L.,** *Erythropoietin and the Regulation of Erythropoiesis,* University of Chicago Press, 1970.
9. **Wagemaker, G.,** Induction of erythropoietin responsiveness in vitro, *Hemopoietic Cell Differentiation,* Golde, D. W., Clime, J. M., Metcalf, D., and Fox, C. F., Eds., Academic Press, New York, 1978, 109.
10. **Iscove, N. N.,** The role of erythropoietin in regulation of population size and cell cycling of early and late erythroid precursors in mouse bone marrow, *Cell Tissue Kinet,* 10, 323, 1977.
11. **Eaves, C. J., Humphries, R. K., and Eaves, A. C.,** *In vitro* characterization of erythroid precursor cells and the erythropoietic differentiation process, in *Cellular and Molecular Regulation of Hemoglobin Switching,* Stomatoyannopoulus, A., and Nienhuis, A. W., Eds., Grune and Stratton, New York, 1979, 251.
12. **Adamson, J. W., and Brown, J. E.,** Aspects of erythroid differentiation and proliferation, in, *Molecular Control of Proliferation and Differentiation,* Papaconstinou, J. and Rutter, W. D., Eds., Academic Press, New York, 1978, 161.
13. **Gregory, C. J.,** Erythropoietin sensitivity as a differentiation marker in the hemopoietic system, studies of three erythropoietic colony responses in culture, *J. Cell. Physiol.,* 89, 289, 1976.
14. **Peschle, C.,** Erythropoiesis, *Ann. Rev. Med.,* 31, 303, 1980.
15. **Chui, D. H., Djaldetti, M., Marks, P. A., and Rifkind, R. A.,** Erythropoietin effects on fetal mouse erythroid cells, I. cell population and hemoglobin synthesis, *J. Cell. Biol.* 51, 585, 1971.
16. **Terada, M., Marks, P. A., and Rifkind, R. A.,** Erythroid cell differentiation, *Mol. Cell. Biochem.,* 21, 33, 1978.
17. **Stohlman, F.,** Regulation of erythropoiesis in *Regulation of Hematopoiesis,* Vol. 1, Gordon, A. S., Ed., Appleton-Century-Crofts, New York, 1970, 317.
18. **Papayannopoulou, T. and Finch, C. A.,** On the *in vivo* action of erythropoietin, a quantitative analysis, *J. Clin. Invest.,* 51, 1179, 1972.

19. **Hillman, R. S.,** Characteristics of marrow production and reticulocyte maturation in normal man in response to anemia, *J. Clin. Invest.,* 48, 443, 1969.
20. **Tarbutt, R. G.,** Cell population kinetics of the erythroid system in the rat, the response to protracted anemia and to continuous X-irradiation, *Br. J. Haematol.,* 16, 9, 1969.
21. **Fisher, J. E., Lajtha, L. G., Buttoo, A. S., et al.,** Direct effects of erythropoietin on the bone marrow of the isolated perfused hind limbs of rabbits, *Br. J. Haematol.,* 11, 342, 1965.
22. **Glass, J., Lavidor, L. M., and Robinson, S. H.,** Studies of murine erythroid cell development, synthesis of heme and hemoglobin, *J. Cell. Biol.,* 65, 298, 1975.
23. **Gross, M. and Goldwasser, E.,** On the mechanism of erythropoietin induced differentiation, characterization of the ribonucleic acid formed as a result of erythropoietin action, *Biochemistry* 8, 1795, 1969.
24. **Pavlov, A. P.,** Molecular aspects of action of endogenous erythropoietin, the effects of erythropoietic stimuli on synthesis of ribonucleic acids in rabbit bone marrow, *Biochim. Biophys. Acta,* 195, 156, 1969.
25. **Bottomly, S. S. and Smithee, G. E.,** Effect of erythropoietin on bone marrow δ amino-levulinic acid synthetase and heme synthetase, *J. Lab. Clin. Med.,* 74, 445, 1969.
26. **Hrinda, M. E. and Goldwasser, E.,** On the mechanism of erythropoietin induced differentiation. VI. induced accumulation of iron by marrow cells, *Biochim. Biophys. Acta,* 195, 165, 1969.
27. **Peets, E. A. and Gordon, A. S.,** Effect of erythropoietin on glucose utilization by bone marrow cells, *Life Sci.* 7, 591, 1968.
28. **Dukes, P. P., Takaku, F., and Goldwasser, E.,** *In vitro* studies on the effect of erythropoietin on glucosamine—1—^{14}C incorporation into rat bone marrow cells, *Endocrinology,* 74, 960, 1968.
29. **Thorell, B.,** Studies on formation of cellular substances during blood cell formation, Acta Med. Scand. [Suppl.], 200, 1947.
30. **Torelli, U., Grossi, G., Artusi, T., et al.,** RNA and protein metabolism in normal human erythroblasty and granuloblasts, *Acta Haematol.,* 32, 271, 1964.
31. **Schmid, J. R., Kiely, J. M., Tauxe, N. J., and Owens, C. A.,** *In vitro* DNA and RNA synthesis in human bone marrow cells, a study of 12 normal subjects and 12 patients with lymph plasmocytic disorders, *Blood,* 27, 310, 1966.
32. **Evans, M. J. and Lingrel, J. B.,** Hemoglobin messenger ribonucleic acid ribonucleic synthesis of 95 and ribosomal ribonucleic acid during derythroid cell development, *Biochemistry,* 8, 3000, 1969.
33. **Gaskill, P. and Kabat, D.,** Unexpectedly large size of globin messenger ribonucleic acid, *Proc. Natl. Acad. Sci. (U.S.A.),* 68, 72, 1971.
34. **Bessis, M.,** L'ilôt érythroblastique, unité functionelle de la moelle osseuse, *Rev. Hématol.,* 13, 8, 1958.
35. **Bessis, M. and Breton-Gorius, J.,** Nouvelles observations sur l'ilôt érythroblastique et la rhophéocytose de la ferritine, *Rev. Hématol.,* 14, 165, 1959.
36. **Le Charpentier, V. and Prenant, M.,** Isolement de l'ilòt érythroblastique, *Nouv. Rev. Franç d' Hématol.,* 15, 119, 1975.
37. **Bessis, M. and Breton-Gorius, J.,** Iron metabolism in the bone marrow as seen by electron microscopy, a critical review, *Blood,* 10, 635, 1962.
38. **Tanaka, Y., Brecher, G., and Bull, B.,** Ferritin localization on the erythroblast cell membrane and rhopheocytosis in hypersiderotic human bone marrow, *Blood,* 28, 758, 1966.
39. **Ben-Ishay, Z.,** The erythroid island, structure and function, *Pathobiol. Annu.,* 7, 63, 1977.
40. **Bessis, M. and Bricka, M.,** Aspect dynamique des cellules du sang, son etude par la microcinematographie en contrase de phase, *Rev. Hematol.,* 7, 407, 1952.
41. **Rind, H.,** Kinetik der erythroblasten, *Fol. Haematol.,* 74, 202, 1956.
42. **Pease, D. C.,** An electron microscopic study of the bone marrow, *Blood,* 11, 501, 1956.
43. **Jones, O. P.,** Electron microscopic studies of the nuclear membrane in mitotic erythroblasts, Proc. 8th International Congress Hematology PHQ, Pacific Press, Tokyo, 1960.
44. **Simpson, C. F. and Kling, J. M.,** The mechanism of denucleation in circulating erythroblasts, *J. Cell. Biol.,* 36, 103, 1968.
45. **Skutelsky, E. and Danon, D.,** An electron microscopic study of nuclear elimination from the late erythroblast, *J. Cell. Biol.,* 33, 625, 1967.
46. **Awai, M., Okada, S., Takebayashi, S., et al.,** Studies on mechanism of denucleation of the erythroblast, *Acta Haematol.,* 39, 193, 1968.
47. **Arlic, D., Gordon, A. S., and Rhodin, J. A. G.,** An ultrastructural study of erythropoietin induced red cell formation in mouse spleen, *J. Ultrastruct. Res.,* 13, 516, 1965.
48. **Simpson, C. F. and Kling, I. M.,** The mechanisms of mitochondrial extrusion from phenyl hydrazine induced reticulocytes in the circulating blood, *J. Cell. Biol.,* 36, 103, 1968.
49. **Steck, T.,** The organization of protein in the human red blood cell membrane, *J. Cell Biol.,* 62, 1, 1974.

50. **Rosenberg, S. A. and Guidotti, G.,** The proteins of the erythrocyte membrane, structure and arrangements in the membrane, in *Red Cell Membrane Structure and Function,* Jamieson, G. A. and Greenwalt, T., Eds., J. B. Lippincott, Philadelphia, 1969, 93.
51. **Guidotti, G.,** Membrane proteins, *Annu. Rev. Biochem.,* 1, 731, 1972.
52. **Singer, S. J. and Micolson, G. L.,** The fluid model of the structure of cell membranes, *Science,* 175, 720, 1972.
53. **Wallach, D. F. H.,** The disposition of proteins in the plasma membranes of animal cells, *Biochim. Biophys. Acta,* 265, 61, 1972.
54. **Fairbanks, G., Steck, T., and Wallach, D. F. H.,** Electrophoretic analysis of the major polypeptides of the human erythrocyte membrane, *Biochemistry,* 10, 2606, 1971.
55. **Marchesi, V. T. and Steers, E.,** Selective solubilzation of a protein component of the red cell membrane, *Science,* 159, 203, 1969.
56. **Wenzler, R. J.,** A glycoprotein in human erythrocyte membrane in *Red Cell Membrane Structure and Function,* Jamieson, C. A. and Greenwalt, T., Eds., J. B. Lippincott, Philadelphia, 1969, 57.
57. **Ackerman, G. A. and Waksai, S. D.,** Ultrastructural localization of Concavalin, a binding sites on the surface of differentiatiating hemopoietic cells, *Cell Tissue Res.,* 159, 331, 1974.
58. **Inoue, M., Mori, M., Seno, S., et al.,** Structural difference in sites on surface membrane of mature and immature erythrocytes, *Nature,* 250, 247, 1974.
59. **Chan, L. N., Wacholz, M., and Sha Afi, R. I.,** Changes in membrane structure and function during chick embryonic erythropoiesis, *Membrane Biochem.,* 1, 159, 1978.
60. **Chan, L. N. and Oliver, J. M.,** Changes in number, mobility and topographic distribution of lectin receptors during maturation of chick erythroid cell, *J. Cell Biol.,* 69, 647, 1976.
61. **Fischer, S., Nunex, T., and Fifer, M.,** Studies of plasma membranes during maturation of mammalian erythrocytes, *Fed. Proc.,* 34, 1875, 1975.
62. **Glass, J., Fischer, S., Lavidor, L. M., and Nunez, T.,** External surface membrane proteins in normal and neoplastic murine erythroid cells, *Cancer Res.,* 37, 1497, 1977.
63. **Freeman, W. H. and Ackerman, G. A.,** Ultrastructural localization of Con A binding sites on guinea pig bone marrow cells with gold labeled horseradish peroxidase, *Anat. Rec.,* 187, 581, 1977.
64. **Lodish, H. F. and Small, B.,** Membrane proteins synthesized in rabbit reticulocytes, *J. Cell. Biol.,* 65, 51, 1975.
65. **Light, N. D. and Tanner, M. J. A.,** Changes in surface membrane components during the differentiation of rabbit erythroid cells, *Biochem. J.,* 164, 565, 1977.
66. **Sreschner, D., Mishan-Dahan, H., Kaab, M., and Hertzberg, M.,** Interaction between membrane properties and protein synthesis, *Exp. Cell. Res.,* 108, 321, 1977.
67. **Skutelsky, E. and Danon, D.,** Comparative study of nuclear expulsion from the late erythroblast and cytokinesis, *Exp. Cell. Res.,* 60, 427, 1970.
68. **Skutelsky, E. and Danon, D.,** On the expulsion of the erythroid nucleus and its phagocytosis, *Anat. Res.,* 173, 123, 1972.
69. **Seki, M., Yoneyama, T., and Shirosawa, H.,** Role of the reticular cells during maturation process of the erythroblasts, I, denucleation of erythroblasts by reticular cells; electron microscopy study, *Acta Path. Jpn.,* 15, 295, 1965.
70. **Seki, M., Yoneyama, T., and Shirosawa, H.,** Role of reticular cells during maturation process of the erythroblasts II, further observation on the denucleation process, *Acta Path. Jpn.,* 15, 387, 1965.
71. **Seki, M., Yoneyama, T., and Shirosawa, H.,** Role of the reticular cells during the maturation process III the fate of the phagocytosed nucleus, *Acta Pathy. Jpn.,* 15, 387, 1965.
72. **Campbell, F. R.,** Nuclear elimination from the normoblasts of fetal guinea pig liver as studied in electron microscopy and serial section techniques, *Anat. Rec.,* 160, 539, 1968.
73. **Skutelsky, E. and Danon, D.,** Variation in distribution of con A receptors sites and anionic groups during red cell differentiation, *J. Cell. Biol.,* 71, 218, 1976.

73a. **Skutelsky, E. and Danon, D.,** Reduction in surface charge as an explanation of the recognition by macrophages of nuclei expelled from normoblasts, *J. Cell. Biol.,* 43, 8, 1969.

74. **Geyer, G., Linss, W., Meyer, H. W., et al.,** Alterations of the enucleating glycocolyx, *Acta Histochem.,* 64, 26, 1979.
75. **Alpen, E. L. and Cranmore, D.,** Observations on the regulation of erythropoiesis and on cellular dynamics by ^{59}Fe autoradiography in *Kinetics of the Regulation of Red Cell Proliferation,* Stohlman, F., Jr., Ed., Grune and Stratton, New York, 1959, 200.
76. **Japa, J.,** A study of the mitotic activity of normal human bone marrow, *Br. J. Exp. Pathol.,* 23, 272, 1946.
77. **Rohr, K.,** *Das Menschliche Knochenmark,* 3rd Ed., Thieme, Stuttgart 1960, 101.
78. **Fliedner, T., Cronkite, E. P., Bond, V. P., et al.,** The mitotic index of human bone marrow in healthy individuals and irradiated human beings, *Acta Haematol.,* 22, 65, 1969.

79. **Killmann, S. A., Cronkite, E. P., Fliedner, T. M., and Bond, V. P.,** Mitotic indices of human bone marrow cells. I. number and cytologic distribution of mitoses, *Blood,* 19, 743, 1962.
80. **Killman, S. A., Cronkite, E. P., Fliedner, T. M., et al.,** Mitotic indices of human bone marrow cells. II. the use of mitotic indices for estimation of time parameters of proliferation in serially connected multiplicative cellular compartments, *Blood,* 21, 141, 1963.
81. **Bond, V. P., Fliedner, T. M., Cronkite, E. P., et al.,** Cell turnover in blood and blood forming tissues studied with tritiated thymidine, in *The Kinetics of Cellular Proliferation,* Stohlman, F. R., Ed., Grune and Stratton, New York, 1959, 188.
82. **Killmann, S. A., Cronkite, E. P., Fliedner, T. M., and Bond, V. P.,** Mitotic indices of human bone marrow cells. III. duration of some phases of erythrocytic and granulocyte proliferation computed from mitotic indices, *Blood,* 24, 207, 1964.
83. **Boll, I. and Mersch, G.,** Morphologische Untersuchungen zur Proliferationskinetik der normalen und pathologischen Erythropoiese in vitro, *Blut,* 17, 193, 1968.
84. **Knowlton, N. P., Jr. and Widner, W. R.,** The use of X-rays to determine the mitotic and intermitotic time of various mouse tissues, *Cancer Res.,* 10, 59, 1950.
85. **Dustin, P., Jr.,** The quantitative estimation of mitotic growth in the bone marrow of the rat by the stathmokinetic (colchicine) method, in *The Kinetics of Cellular Proliferation,* Stohlman, F., Jr., Ed., Grune and Stratton, New York, 1959, 50.
86. **Cronkite, E. P., Bond, V. P., Fliedner, T. M., and Rubini, J. R.,** The use of tritated thymidine in the study of DNA synthesis and cell turnover in hemopoietic tissues, *Lab. Invest.,* 8, 263, 1959.
87. **Leblond, C. P., Messier, B., and Kopriwa, B.,** Thymidine H^3 as a tool for the investigation of the renewel of cell populations, *Lab. Invest.,* 8, 296, 1959.
88. **Messier, B.,** Histological localization of tritium labeled thymidine, 3rd Cancer Conf., Academic Press, New York, 1958.
89. **Hennessy, T. G. and Huff, R. L.,** Depression of a tracer iron uptake curve in rat erythrocytes following total body irradiation, *Proc. Soc. Exp. Biol. Med.,* 73, 436, 1950.
90. **Lord, B. I.,** Measurement of the duration of DNA synthesis in erythroid cells of the bone marrow using a double labelling auto radiographic technique designed especially for use with haemaopoietic tissues, *Cell. Tiss. Kinet.,* 3, 13, 1970.
91. **Dormer, P.,** Erythropoietic proliferation in normal and anemic man, a new approach using ^{14}C autoradiography, *Prog. Histochem. Cytochem.,* 6, 1, 1974.
92. **Monette, F. C., Lo Bue, J., Gordon, A. S., et al.,** Erythropoiesis in the rat, differential rates of DNA synthesis and cell proliferation, *Science,* 162, 1132, 1968.
93. **Hanna, I. R. A., Tarbutt, R. G., and Lamerton, L. F.,** Shortening of the cell cycle time of erythroid precursor in response to anemia, *Br. J. Haematol.,* 16, 381, 1969.
94. **Harris, E. B.,** *In vivo* uptake of radioactive iron by the erythroid cells of rat bone marrow in *Advance in Radiobiology,* Proc. 5th Int. Conf., Hevesy et al., Eds., Charles C. Thomas, Springfield, 1, 26, 1957.
95. **Myare, E.,** Iron uptake and hemoglobin synthesis by human erythroid cells in vitro, *Scand., J. Clin. Invest.,* 16, 212, 1964.
96. **Ward, H. P., Tauxe, W. N., and Kiely, J. M., Jr.,** ^{59}Fe autoradiography of bone marrow culture from normal subjects and patients with uremia and pernicious anemia, *Br. J. Haematol.,* 12, 99, 1966.
97. **Lambardini, J., Papyannopoulou, T., Cook, J. D., et al.,** Marrow radio iron kinetics, *Haematologia,* 7, 301, 1973.
98. **Stohlman, F., Jr.** Observations on the kinetics of red cell proliferation, in *The Kinetics of Cellular Proliferation,* Stohlman, F., Ed., Grune and Stratton, New York, 1959, 328.
99. **Lajtha, L. G. and Suit, A. D.,** Uptake of radioactive iron by nucleated red cells in vitro, *Br. J. Haematol.,* 1, 55, 1955.
100. **Lajtha, L. G. and Oliver, R.,** Studies of the kinetics of erythropoietin, a model of the erythron in *Ciba Found. Symp. Haemopoiesis,* Wolstenholme, G. E. W., O'Connor, M., Eds., J. A. Churchill, London, 1969, 289.
101. **Lajtha, L. G.,** Recent studies in erythroid differentiation and proliferation, *Medicine,* 43, 625, 1964.
102. **Lajtha, L. G. and Oliver, R.,** Studies on the kinetics of erythropoiesis, a model of the erythron in *Haemopoiesis,* Wolstenholme, G. E. W., O'Connor, M., Eds., Little, Brown, Boston, 1960, 289.
103. **Stohlman, F. R., Jr., Lucarelli, G., Howard, D., et al.,** Regulation of erythropoiesis. XVI. Cytokinetic patterns in disorders of erythropoiesis, *Medicine,* 13, 651, 1964.
104. **Lord, B. J.,** Kinetics of the recognizable erythrocyte precursor cells, *Clin. Haemaol.,* 8, 335, 1979.
105. **Reiff, R. H., Nutter, J. Y., Donohue, M., and Finch, C. A.,** The relative number of marrow reticulocytes, *Am. J. Clin. Pathol.,* 30, 199, 1958.
106. **Seip, M.** Reticulocyte studies, *Acta Med. Scand. [Suppl.],* 282, 146, 1953.

107. **Shattil, S. J. and Cooper, R. A.,** Maturation of macroreticulocyte membranes *in vivo, J. Lab. Clin. Med.,* 79, 215, 1972.
108. **Lowenstein, L. M.,** The mammalian reticulocyte, *Int. Rev. Cytol.,* 8, 1135, 1959.
109. **Heilmeyer, L. and Westhauer, R.,** Reifungsstudien an uberlebenden Reticulocyten *in vitro* und ihre Bedeutung fur die taglichen haemproduktion *in vivo, Z. Klin. Med.,* 121, 361, 1932.
110. **Killmann, S. A.,** On the size of the normal human reticulocytes, *Acta. Med. Scand.,* 176, 529, 1964.
111. **Chamberlain, J. K., Weiss, L., and Weed, R. I.,** Bone marrow sinus cell packing, a determinant of cell release, *Blood,* 46, 91, 1975.
112. **Brecher, G. and Stohlman, F., Jr.,** Reticulocyte size and erythropoietic stimulation, *Proc. Soc. Exp. Biol. Med.,* 107, 887, 1962.
113. **Jacobs, P. and Finch, C. A.,** Iron for erythropoiesis, *Blood,* 37, 220, 1971.
114. **Stohlman, F., Jr.,** Erythropoiesis, *N. Engl. J. Med.,* 167, 342, 1962.
115. **Perrotta, A. L. and Finch, C. A.,** The polychromatophilic erythrocyte, *Am. J. Clin. Pathol.,* 57, 471, 1972.
116. **Clarkson, D. R. and Moore, E. M.,** Reticulocyte size in nutritional anemias, *Blood,* 48, 669, 1976.
117. **Stryckmans, P. A., Cronkite, E. P., Giacomelli, G., et al.,** The maturation and fate of reticulocytes after *in vitro* labeling with tritiated thymidine, *Blood,* 31, 33, 1968.
118. **Brecher, G., Haleym, J. E., Prenant, M., and Bessis, M.,** Macronormoblasts, macroreticulocytes and macrocytes, *Blood Cells,* 1, 547, 1975.
119. **Mel, H. E., Prenant, M., and Mohandas, N.,** Reticulocyte motility and form, studies on maturation and classification, *Blood,* 49, 1001, 1977.
120. **Cronkite, E. P., Gliedner, T. M, Stryckmans, P., et al.,** Flow patterns and rates of human erythropoiesis and granulocytopoiesis, *Ser. Haemat.,* 5, 51, 1965.
121. **Giblett, E. R., Coleman, D. H., Pirzio-Biroli, G., et al.,** Erythrokinetics, Quantitative measurements of red cell production and estruction in normal subjects and patients with anemia, *Blood,* 11, 291, 1956.
122. **Haurani, F. I. and Tocantins, L. M.,** Ineffective erythropoiesis, *Am. J. Med.,* 31, 519, 1961.
123. **Finch, C. A.,** *The Red Cell Manual,* University of Washington, Seattle, 1971, 13.
124. **Lewis, S. M.,** Dysplastic anemias, *Nouv. Rev. Fran. Hematol.,* 12, 375, 1972.
125. **Lewis, S. M. and Verwilghen, R. L.,** Dyserythropoiesis and dyserthropoietic anemia, *Br. J. Haematol.,* 23, 1, 1972.
126. **Lewis, S. M. and Frisch, B.,** Congenital dyserythropoietic anemia, Electron microscopy, in *Congenital Disorders of Erythropoiesis,* Ciba Found. Symp. 37 (new series), Porter, R. and Fitzsimons, P. W., Eds., Elsevier, Amsterdam, 1976, 171.
127. **Frisch, B. and Broeckaert-Van Orshoven, A.,** Ultrastructure of normal and abnormal erythropoiesis, in *Dyserythropoiesis,* Lewis, S. M. and Verwilghen, R. L., Eds., Academic Press, New York, 1977, 271.
128. **Heimpel, H. and Wendt, F.,** Eine neue Variante der kongenitalen dyserythropoietischen Anamie, *Schweiz. Med. Woschenshr.,* 97, 1470, 1967.
129. **Breton-Gorius, J., Daniel, M., Clauvel, J., and Dreyfus, B.,** Anomalies ultrastructurales des erythroblasts et des erythrocytes dan six cas de dyserythropoiese congenitale, *Nouv. Rev. Fran. Hematol.,* 13, 23, 1973.
130. **Lewis, S. M., Nelson, D. A., and Pitcher, C. S.,** Clinical and ultrastructural aspects of congenital dyserthropoietic anemia type. I. *Br. J. Hematol.,* 23, 113, 1972.
131. **Crookston, J. H., Crookston, M. C., Burnie, K. L., et al.,** Hereditary erythroblastic multinuclearity associated with a positive acidified serum test in a type of congenital dyserythropoietic anemia, *Br. J. Haematol.,* 17, 11, 1969.
132. **Verwilghen, R. L., Lewis, S. M., Dacie, J. V., et al.,** HEMPAS congenital dyserythropoietic anemia type II, *Q. J. Med.,* (new series), 42, 257, 1973.
133. **Wolf, J. A. and Hofe, F. H.,** Familial erythroid multinuclearity, *Blood,* 6, 1274, 1951.
134. **Van Dorpe, A.,** Dyserythropoietic anemia, 3rd meeting, European and African Division Int. Soc. Hemato., London, Abstract 20, 1975.
135. **Ewing, J.,** *Clinical Pathology of the Blood,* 2nd ed., Lea & Febiger, New York, 1903, Chap. 7, 202.
136. **Piney, A.,** The genesis of pernicious anemia, Zeitschr. f. Konstitutionslehre, 10, 659, 1924.
137. **Jones, O. P.,** Morphologic, physiologic, chemical and biologic distinction of megaloblasts, *Arch Pathol.,* 35, 752, 1943.
138. **Ito, K., Ito, N., Sato, S., and Katsonuma, H.,** Electron microscopic study of the megaloblast in pernicious anemia, *Acta Haematol., Jpn.,* 23, 20, 1964.
139. **Verwilghen, R. L., Broeckhart-Van Orshoven, A., and Heynen, M. J.,** Dyserythropoiesis and annulate lamellae, *Br. J. Haematol.,* 30, 307, 1975.

140. **Wickramsinghe, S. N. and Bush, V.**, Electron microscope and high resolution autoradiographic studies of megaloblastic erythropoiesis, *Acta Haematol.*, 57, 1, 1977.
141. **Discombe, G.**, L'origine des corps de Howell-Jolly et des anneaux de Cabot, *Sang*, 19, 262, 1948.
142. **Koyama, S.**, Studies on Howell-Jolly body, *Acta Haematol. Jpn.*, 23, 20, 1960.
143. **Rondanelli, E. G., Trenta, A., Maeliulo, E., et al.**, Morphogenese des micronoyaux supplementaire (pseudocorps de Jolly) dans les cellules erythropoietiques irradies, *Acta Haematol.*, 35, 232, 1966.
144. **Beck, W.**, The metabolic basis of megaloblastic erythropoiesis, *Medicine*, 43, 715, 1964.
145. **London, L. M. and West, R.**, The formation of bile pigment in pernicious anemia, *J. Biol. Chem.*, 184, 369, 1950.
146. **Finch, C. A.**, Coleman, D. H., Motulsky, A. G., et al., Erythrokinetics in pernicious anemia, *Blood*, 11, 807, 1965.
147. **Messner, H., Fliedner, T. M., and Cronkite, E. P.**, Kinetics of erythropoietic cell proliferation in pernicious anemia, *Ser. Haematol.*, Vol. 2, 4, 44, 1969.
148. **Wickramsinghe, S. N., Chalmers, D. G., and Cooper, E. H.**, Arrest of cell proliferation and protein synthesis in megaloblasts of pernicious anemia, *Acta Haematol.*, 41, 65, 1969.
149. **Wickramsinghe, S. N.**, Kinetics and morphology of hemopoiesis in pernicious anemia, *Br. J. Haematol.*, 22, 111, 1972.
150. **Yoshida, Y., Todo, A., Shigeru, S., et al.**, Proliferation of megaloblast in pernicious anemia as observed from nucleic acid metabolism, *Blood*, 31, 292, 1968.
151. **Wickramsinghe, S. N. and Longland, J. E.**, Rate of incorporation of tritiated thymidine into DNA of normoblasts and megaloblastic bone marrow cells in vitro, *Acta Haematol.*, 52, 14, 1974.
152. **Beck, W. S.**, Metabolic feature of cobalamin deficiency in man, in *Cobalamin Biochemistry and Pathophysiology*, Babior, B. M., Ed., John Wiley & Sons, New York, 1974, 403.
153. **Wickramsinghe, S. N.**, RNA content of megaloblasts in pernicious anemia, *Scand. J. Haematol.*, 7, 398, 1970.
154. **Das, K. C. and Hoffbrand, A. V.**, Studies of folate uptake by phytohaemagglutinin stimulated lymphocytes, *Br. J. Haematol.*, 19, 203, 1970.
155. **Das, K. C. and Hoffbrand, A. V.**, Lymphocyte transformation in megaloblastic anemia, Morphology and DNA synthesis, *Br. J. Haematol.*, 19, 459, 1970.
155a. **Das, K. C. and Herbert, V.**, Vitamin B_{12} folate interrelations, *Clin. Haematol.*, 5, 697, 1976.
156. **Killmann, S. A.**, Effect of deoxyuridine on incorporation of tritiated thymidine; difference between normoblasts and megaloblasts, *Acta Med. Scand.*, 175, 483, 1964.
157. **Metz, J., Kelly, A., Swett, V. C. et al.**, Deranged DNA synthesis by bone marrow cells from vitamin B_{12} deficient humans, *Br. J. Haematol.*, 14, 575, 1968.
158. **Das, K. C., Herber, V., Gelman, N., and Longo, D. L.** Unmasking covert folate deficiency in iron deficient subjects with neutrophil hypersegmentations, d U suppression tests on lymphocytes and bone marrow, *Br. J. Haematol.*, 39, 352, 1978.
159. **Huberman, J. A. and Riggs, A. D.**, On the mechanisms of DNA replication in mammalian chromosomes, *J. Mol. Biol.*, 32, 327, 1968.
160. **Edenburg, H. J. and Huberman, J. A.**, Eukaryocytic chromosome replication, *Annu. Rev. Genet.*, 9, 245, 1975.
161. **Alberts, B. and Bernglanz, R.**, Recent excitement in the DNA replication problem, *Nature*, 269, 655, 1977.
162. **Hoffbrand, A. V., Ganeshaguru, K., Hooton, J. W. L., and Tripp, E.**, Megaloblastic anemia, initiation of DNA synthesis in excess of DNA chain elongation as the underlying mechanisms, *Clin. Haematol.*, 5, 727, 1976.
163. **Magnusson, G.**, Hydroxyurea induced accumulation of short fragments during polyoma DNA replication I Characterization of fragments, *J. Virol.*, 12, 600, 1973.
164. **Laipis, P. J. and Levine, A. J.**, DNA replication in SV 40 infected cells, the inhibition of a gap filling step during the discontinuous synthesis of SV 40 DNA, *Virology*, 56, 580, 1973.
165. **Martin, R. F., Radford, I., and Pardee, M.**, Accumulation of short DNA fragments in hydroxyurea treated mouse L cells, *Biochim. Biophys. Res. Commun.*, 74, 9, 1977.
166. **Salzman, N. P. and Thoren, M. M.**, Inhibition in the joining of DNA intermediates to growing simian virus 40 chains, *J. Virol.*, 11, 721, 1975.
167. **Chan, A. C. and Walker, I. G.**, DNA synthesis in L cells in the presence of 5 fluorodeoxyuridine, *Biochim. Biophys. Acta*, 395, 422, 1975.
168. **Wickramsinghe, R. G. and Hoffbrand, A. V.**, Defective DNA synthesis in megaloblastic anemia, studies employing velocity sedimentation in alkaline sucrose density gradients, *Biochim. Biophys. Acta*, 563, 46, 1979.
169. **Wickramsinghe, R. G. and Hoffbrand, A. V.**, Reduced rate of DNA replication fork movement in megaloblastic anemia, *J. Clin. Invest.*, 65, 26, 1980.

170. **Wickramsinghe, S. N. and Pratt, J. R.**, Myelocyte proliferation in pernicious anemia, *Acta Haematol.*, 44, 37, 1970.
171. **Rath, L. E. and Finch, C. A.**, Sternal marrow hemosiderin, *J. Lab. Clin. Med.*, 33, 81, 1948.
172. **Gale, E., Torrance, J., and Bothwell, T. H.**, The quantitative estimation of total iron stores in human marrow, *J. Clin. Invest.*, 42, 1076, 1963.
173. **Miller, W. L. and Trubowitz, S.**, A simple method for the retrieval of human marrow tissue particles from aspirates, *Am. J. Clin. Pathol.*, 50, 661, 1968.
174. **Trubowitz, S., Miller, W. L., and Zamora, J. C.**, The quantitative estimation of nonheme iron in human marrow aspirates, *Am. J. Clin. Pathol.*, 54, 71, 1970.
175. **Bessis, M.**, Living Blood Cells, Springer-Verlag, New York, 1973, 118.
176. **Bessis, M. and Breton-Gorius, J.**, Iron metabolism in the bone marrow as seen by electron microscopy, *Blood,* 19, 635, 1962.
177. **Jandl, J. H. and Katz, J. H.**, The plasma-to-cell cycle transferrin, *J. Clin. Invest.*, 42, 314, 1963.
178. **Morgan, E. M. and Appleton, T. C.**, Autoradiographic localization of ^{125}l labeled transferrin in rabbit reticulocytes, *Nature,* 223, 1371, 1969.
179. **Hemmaplardh, D., Kailis, S. B., and Morgan, E. M.**, The effects of inhibitors of microtubule and cirofilament function on transferrin and iron uptake by rabbit reticulocytes and bone marrow, *Br. J. Haematol.*, 28, 53, 1974.
180. **Loh, T. T. and Morgan, E. H.**, The effect of concavalin A on transferrin and iron uptake by rabbit reticulocytes, *Exp. Cell. Res.*, 91, 87, 1975.
181. **Eylar, E. M. and Matioli, G.**, Apoferritin synthesis in human erythroid cells in thalassemia, *Nature,* 208, 661, 1965.
182. **Tanaka, Y. and Brecher, G.**, Bidirectional transport of ferritin in guinea pig erythroblasts *in vitro, Blood,* 35, 793, 1970.
183. **Yamada, H. and Gabuzda, T. G.** Erythroblast ferritin synthesis, structure and function in developing erythroid cells, *J. Lab. Clin. Med.*, 83, 478, 1974.
184. **Tanaka, Y. and Brecher, G.**, Effect of surface digestion and metabolic inhibitors on appearance of ferritin in guinea pig erythroblasts *in vitro;* evidence for production of a poferritin on the erythroblast cell membrane, *Blood,* 37, 211, 1971.
185. **Bainton, D. F. and Finch, C. A.**, The diagnosis of iron deficiency anemia, *Am. J. Med.*, 37, 62, 1964.
186. **Deiss, A. and Kurth, D.**, Circulating reticulocytes in normal adults determined by the new methylene blue methods, *Am. J. Clin. Pathol.*, 53, 481, 1970.
187. **Cartwright, G. E. and Deiss, A.**, Sideroblasts, siderocytes and sideroblastic anemia, *N. Engl. J. Med.*, 292, 185, 1975.
188. **Bessis, M. and Jensen, W. N.**, Sideroblastic anemia, mitochondrial and sideroblastic iron, *Br. J. Haematol.*, 11, 49, 1965.
189. **Kushner, J. P., Lee, G. R., Wintrobe, M. M., and Cartwright, G. E.**, Idiopathic refractory sideroblastic anemia, clinical and laboratory investigation of 17 patients and review of the literature, *Medicine,* 50, 139, 1971.
190. **Hines, J. D. and Grasso, J. H.**, The sideroblastic anemias, *Semin. Hematol.*, 7, 186, 1970.
191. **Hoffbrand, A. V., Konopka, L., and White, M. J.**, Sideroblastic anemia, *Br. J. Haematol.*, 28, 138, 1974.
192. **Hoffbrand, A. V.**, Sideroblastic anemia, in *Dyserythropoiesis,* Lewis, S. M. and Verwilghen, R. L., Eds., Academic Press, New York, 1977, 136.
193. **Aoki, Y., Urata, G., Wada, O., and Takaku, F.**, Measurement of delta-amino levulinic acid synthetase activity in human erythroblasts, *J. Clin. Invest.*, 53, 1326, 1974.
194. **Bottomley, S. S., Tanaka, M., and Self, Y.**, Delta-aminolevulinic acid synthetase activity in normal bone marrow and in patients with idiopathic sideroblastic anemia, *Enzyme,* 16, 138, 1973.
195. **Brown, E. G.**, Evidence for the involvement of ferrous iron in the biosynthesis of amino-levulinic acid by chicken erythrocyte preparations, *Nature,* 182, 313, 1958.
196. **Aoki, Y.**, Multiple enzymatic defects in mitochondria in hematological cells of patients with primary sideroblastic anemia, *J. Clin. Invest.* 66, 43, 1980.
197. **Linman, J. W. and Saarni, M. I.**, The preleukemic syndromes, *Sem. Hematol.*, 11, 93, 1974.
198. **Pierre, R. V.**, Preleukemic states, Sem. Hematol., 11, 73, 1974.
199. **Linman, J. W. and Bagby, G. C., Jr.**, The preleukemia syndrome, clinical and laboratory features, natural course and management, *Blood Cells,* 2, 11, 1976.
200. **Hines, J. D. and Cowan, D.**, Studies on the pathogenesis of alcohol induced sideroblastic bone marrow abnormalities, *N. Engl. J. Med.*, 283, 441, 1970.
201. **Weatherall, D. J. and Clegg, J. B.**, 2nd ed., *The Thalassemia Syndromes,* Blackwell, Oxford, 1972.

202. **Wickramsinghe, S. N., McElwain, T. J., Cooper, E. H., and Hardisty, R. M.,** Proliferation of erythroblasts in beta thalassemia, *Br. J. Haematol.*, 19, 719, 1970.
203. **Wickramsinghe, S. N., Leisky, E., and Moffatt, B.,** Effect of α chain precipitations on human marrow function in homozygous B-thalassemia, *Br. J. Haematol.*, 25, 123, 1973.
204. **Rachmilewitz, E. A.,** The formation of hemichromes from oxidized hemoglobin subunits, *Ann. N.Y. Acad. Sci.*, 165, 171, 1969.
205. **.Yataganas, X. and Fessas, P. H.,** The pattern of hemoglobin precipitations in thalassemia and its significance, *Ann. N.Y. Acad. Sci.*, 165, 407, 1969.
206. **Yataganas, X., Fessas, P. H., and Gahrton, G.,** Quantification of α chain excess in erythocytes in B-thalassemia by microinterferometry, *Br. J. Haematol.*, 22, 117, 1972.
207. **Winterbourn, C. C. and Carrell, R. W.,** Studies of hemoglobin denaturation with heinz body formation in the unstable hemoglobins, *J. Clin. Invest.*, 54, 678, 1974.
208. **White, J. M.** Dyserythropoiesis in thalassemia, in *Dyserythropoiesis*, Lewis, S. M. and Verwilghen, R. L., Eds., Academic Press, New York, 1977, 133.
209. **Wickramsinghe, S. N.,** Erythropoiesis in B thalassemia, in *Congenital Disorders of Erythropoiesis*, Porter, R. and Fitzsimmons, D. W., Eds., CIBA Found. Symp. 37, (new series) Elsevier, Amsterdam, 1976, 221.
210. **Fessas, P. H. and Loukopoulos, D.,** The B thalassemias, *Clin. Haematol.*, 3, 411, 1974.
211. **Sturgeon, P. and Finch, C. A.,** Erythrokinetics in Cooley's anemia, *Blood*, 12, 64, 1957.
212. **Cazzola, M., Alesandrino, P., Barosi, G., et al.,** Quantitative evaluation of the mechanisms of the anemia in heterozygous B thalassemia, *Scand. J. Haematol.*, 23, 107, 1979.
213. **Rachmilewitz, E. A. and Harari, E.,** Slow rate of haemichrome formation from oxidized haemoglobin Bart's (γ_4), a possible explanation for the unequal quantities of hemoglobin H (B_4) and bart's in alphathalassemia, *Br. J. Haematol.*, 22, 357, 1972.
214. **Wasi, P., Na-Nakorn, S., and Pootrakul, S. N.,** The thalassaemias, *Clin. Haematol.*, 3, 383, 1974.
215. **Waldron, H. A.,** The anemia of lead poisoning, a review, *Br. J. Ind. Med.*, 23, 83, 1966.
216. **Albahary, C.,** Lead and hemopoiesis, the mechanism and consequence of the erythropathy of accupational lead poisoning, *Am. J. Med.*, 52, 367, 1972.
217. **Goldberg, A.,** Lead poisoning as a disorder of heme synthesis, *Semin. Hematol.*, 9, 124, 1968.
218. **Goldberg, A.,** Annotation, lead poisoning and haem biosynthesis, *Br. J. Haematol.*, 23, 521, 1972.
219. **Heynen, M. J.,** Experimental dyserythropoiesis, in *Dyserythropoiesis*, Lewis, S. M. and Verwilghen, R. L., Eds., Academic Press, New York, 1977, 315.
220. **Walton, J. R.,** Granules containing lead in isolated mitochondria, *Nature*, 273, 100, 1973.
221. **Piddington, S. K. and White, J. M.** The effect of lead on total and B chain synthesis; *in vitro* and *in vivo*, *Br. J. Haematol.*, 27, 415, 1974.
222. **Hunt, T., Vanderhoff, G. H., and London, I, M.,** Control of globin synthesis, the role of heme, *J. Mol. Biol.*, 66, 471, 1972.
223. **Jensen, W. N., Moreno, G. D., and Bessis, M.,** An electron microscopic description of basophilic stippling in red cells, *Blood*, 25, 933, 1965.
224. **Paglia, D. E., Valentine, W. N., and Dahlgren, J. G.,** Effect of low level lead exposure on pyrimidine 5′nucleotidase in the pathogeneisis of lead-induced anemia, *J. Clin. Invest.*, 56, 1104, 1975.
225. **Valentine, W. N., Fink, K., Paglia, D. E., et al.,** Hereditary hemolytic anemia with human erythrocytic pyrimidine 5′nucleotidase deficiency, *J. Clin. Invest.*, 54, 866, 1974.
226. **Valentine, W. N., Paglia, D. F., Fink, F., and Modakoro, G.,** Lead poisoning association with hemolytic anemia, basophilic stippling, erythrocyte pyrimidine 5′nucleotidase deficiency and intra erythrocytic accumulation of pyrimidines, *J. Clin. Invest.*, 58, 926, 1976.
227. **Arbrecht, P., Mounw, D., Vander, A., and Kalitis, K.,** The effect of chronic low-level lead poisoning on erythropoietin response to hypoxia, *Proc. Soc. Biol. Med.*, 158, 109, 1978.
228. **Ehrlich, P.,** Ueber einen Fall von Anamie mit Bemerkungen uber regenerative Veranderungen des Knochenmarks, *Charite-Ann*, 13, 300, 1888.
229. **Hoffman, R., Zanjani, E. D., Lutton, J. D., Zalusky, B., and Wasserman, L. R.,** Suppression of erythroid-colony formation by lymphocytes from patients with aplastic anemia, *N. Engl. J. Med.*, 296, 10, 1976.
230. **Hoffman, R., Zanjani, E. D., Vila, J., Zalusky, R., Lutton, I. D., and Wasserman, L. R.,** Diamond-Blackfan syndrome, Lymphocyte mediated suppression of erythropoiesis *Science*, 193, 899, 1976.
231. **Nathan, D. G., Clark, J. B., Hillman, D. G., Alter, B. P., and Houseman, D. E.,** Erythroid precursors in congenital hypoplastic (Diamond-Blackfan) anemia, *J. Clin. Invest.*, 61, 589, 1978.

232. **Freedman, M. H. and Saunders, E. F.,** Diamond-Blackfan syndrome, evidence against cell mediated suppression, *Blood,* 51, 1125, 1978.
233. **Krantz, S. B. and Zaentz, S. D.,** Pure red cell aplasia, in *The Year in Hematology,* Gordon, A. S., Silber, R., and LoBue, J., Eds., Plenum Press, New York, 1977, 153.
234. **Peschle, C., Marmont, A., Perugini, S., et al.,** Physiopathology and therapy of adult pure red cell anemia, in *Aplastic Anemia,* Hibinok, T., Takata, F., and Shaldidi, N. T., Eds., University Tokyo Press, 1976, 285.
235. **Adamson, J. W., Fialkow, P. J., Murphy, S., et al.,** Polycythemia vera, stem cell and probable clonal origin of the disease, *N. Engl. J. Med.,* 295, 916, 1976.
236. **Adamson, J. W.,** The erythropoietin-hematocrit relationship in normal and polycythemic man: Implications of marrow regulation, *Blood,* 35, 597, 1968.
237. **Zanjani, E. D., Lutton, J. D., Hoffman, R., and Wasserman, L. R.,** Erythroid colony formation by polycythemia vera bone marrow in vitro, *J. Clin. Invest.,* 59, 84, 1977.
238. **Ellis, J. T., Silver, R. T., Coleman, M., and Geller, S. A.,** The bone marrow in polycythemia vera, *Semin. Hematol.,* 12, 433, 1975.

Chapter 10

PATHOPHYSIOLOGY OF GRANULOPOIESIS

Sidney Trubowitz and Stephen Davis

TABLE OF CONTENTS

I. INTRODUCTION AND GRANULOCYTOPOIESIS

The origin of the human granulocytic cells, the neutrophil, eosinophil, and the basophil, is presumed to be a pluripotential stem cell which on commitment to a granulocytic destiny, becomes sensitive to a variety of regulatory influences which control the amplification and the differentiation of these cells into the recognizable precursors of granulocytic development. Further differentiation of the precursor cells in the marrow into mature granulocytes invokes the familiar morphologic events of nucleolar involution, nuclear chromatin condensation, decreasing nuclear/cytoplasmic ratios, change in nuclear shape and size, and the concomitant cytoplasmic alterations of decreasing basophilia and increasing granule content.

The earliest precursor cell of human granulopoiesis was identified by Naegeli[1] at the begining of the century and designated by him as the myeloblast. In the usual Romanowsky stained smears, the myeloblast (M_1) is a relatively undifferentiated cell of moderate size, some 15 μm in diameter, with a high nuclear/cytoplasmic ratio. The nucleus is round with a fine chromatin network in which a number, usually two to five, of distinct nucleoli are embedded. The cell has a narrow rim of deep blue cytoplasm and contains no visible granules. The peroxidase reaction, as observed by light microscopy is negative. Myeloblasts, so defined, are uncommon in the normal human marrow and constitute at best about half to one percent of the total population of granulocytic cells of the marrow. It is clearly difficult to distinguish and securely separate the myeloblast from other undifferentiated marrow cells. Distinction can be made by electron microscopic examination of cytochemically reacted marrow sections for peroxidase in which the reaction product can be found on the rough surface endoplasmic reticulum and in the Golgi cisternae of the myeloblasts. An occasional peroxidase positive granule, the azurophilic granule, may be encountered.[2]

With the appearance of granules in the cytoplasm of the cells, as observed on light microscopy, the cell has arrived at the promyelocyte (M_2) stage of granulocytic maturation. The promyelocyte is considerably larger than the myeloblast. The nuclear/cytoplasmic ratio has decreased; the cytoplasm is light blue; and scattered, fine, azurophilic granules are clearly visible. The nucleus is round and tends to assume a somewhat eccentric position toward one pole of the cell. The nucleoli are indistinct, but some nucleolar structure may be recognized. The nuclear chromatin shows minimal clumping and condensation.

With further maturation, the cytoplasmic basophilia disappears; the granules increase considerably in number and the nucleus assumes a more eccentric position. The nucleus is now more often ovoid than round and displays a slight indentation on its margin facing the interior of the cell. The cytoplasm at the nuclear indentation and immediately above it appears clear and practically devoid of granules and is the site of the cell's Golgi complex and its central bodies. The central bodies or centrioles are paired cylindric structures 1500 Å in diameter, some 3000 to 5000 Å long and made up of nine groups of three microtubules arranged in a spiral. A satellite, some 600 to 900 Å in diameter, arises from each of the microtubule groups. Cytoplasmic microtubules originate from the satellite region.[3] The nuclear chromatin is now coarse and highly condensed and the nucleoli are no longer visible. The nuclear cytoplasmic ratio is smaller and at this level of granulocytic maturation the cell has arrived at the myelocyte (M_3) stage of its development.

Further granule formation finally crowds the central bodies of the cell into the nucleus, converting the slightly indented ovoid nucleus of the myelocyte into the horseshoe-shaped structure of the metamyelocyte (M_4). Again one is struck by the sparse population of granules in the cytoplasmic extension into the nucleus. On phase microscopic examination of the living metamyelocyte one can readily appreciate the molding of the plastic nuclear structure by the rigid juxta-nuclear centrosomes as they rock to and fro along the nuclear margin with the movement of the cell. The nuclear chromatin is now highly condensed; the metamyelocyte is a fully functional neutrophilic granulocyte, and its further maturation in the marrow into the ultimate product of granulocytopoiesis, the segmented neutrophil, involves primarily further condensation and lobulation of the nucleus.

Specific differentiation into polymorphonuclear neutrophils, eosinophils, and basophils begins quite early in the maturation sequence, probably at the late myeloblast or early promyelocyte level.[3] Under the light microscope the differentiation of cells into the different granulocytes, recognized by their characteristic staining properties of the granules, is discernible at the myelocyte stage at the very earliest, which led early investigators to believe that the programming for neutrophilic, eosinophilic, and basophilic differentiation came late in the maturation sequence.

In summary, the recognizable precursor cells of granulopoiesis in the normal human bone marrow, as seen in Romanowsky stained preparations of the marrow, can be related to a point in the maturation sequence beginning with the myeloblast and ending with the segmented polymorphonuclear leucocyte. The myeloblast is difficult to identify, but characteristically has a large nuclear/cytoplasmic ratio, and deep blue cytoplasm and nucleoli. With the appearance of granules, a population of promyelocytes is identified. The cytoplasm is now light blue and remnants of nucleoli remain. On total disappearane of the cytoplasmic basophilia, the myelocyte is identified which, on indentation of its nucleus by the juxta-nuclear centrosomes is converted into the metamyelocyte. Lobulation of the nucleus signals the end of the maturation process.

The myeloblast, promyelocyte, and myelocyte are all capable of cell division and together constitute the mitotic or proliferative pool of granulocytes. The metamyelocytes are no longer capable of cell division and together with the band and segmented cells form the postmitotic or nonproliferative pool. The number of cells found in these pools in human marrow aspirates, whether prepared as smears or squashes, is quite variable, due in some measure to varying admixtures of peripheral blood granulocytes. The ratio of cells in the proliferative pool (myeloblasts, promyelocytes, and myelocytes) to those in the nonproliferative pool (metamyelocytes, bands, and segmented cells) in the normal human marrow lies somewhere between 1:2 to 1:3. Although the measurement is admittedly crude, it does afford some insight into the state of the maturation process. The preponderant cell of the proliferative pool is the myelocyte.

A. Ultrastructure and Granule Formation

The application of cytochemistry and electron microscopy to the study of the structural changes that accompany granulocytic development has greatly expanded our comprehension of the process and of granule formation, the hallmark of granulocytic differentiation. Early studies recognized morphologic heterogeneity of the granules of the guinea pig,[3] rabbit,[4,5] and human neutrophil.[6,7] Further, these studies suggested that large dense granules are seen predominantly in the early precursor cells and that smaller less dense granules are more common in the late, more mature forms. This shift in the nature of the granule during maturation was substantiated in the rabbit by histochemical means.[8] The granules in the immature cells were shown to be rich in sulfated mucopolysaccharide and basic proteins, while the smaller granules in the more mature cells lacked these components.[9] Electron microscopic examination of rabbit bone marrow revealed a population of large dense granules in the immature neutophil precursors which appeared to be reduced in number in the later, more mature cells as a second population of smaller, less dense granules made their appearance. The less dense granules increased in number to become the predominant granule of the fully mature neutrophil.[10,11] Similar observations were made in the developing neutrophils of human marrow.[12]

Peroxidase cytochemistry and ultrastructural analysis permitted Bainton and Farquhar[13,14] to elucidate the mechanism of granule formation in the rabbit granulocyte and the mechanism of the shift in granule production. They emphasized the role of the Golgi complex in the process. The formation of the primary azurophilic granule was found to be confined to the promyelocyte. The process begins as a condensation of dense material on the inner concave surface of the Golgi cisternae. Small dense cored vacuoles, measuring some 240 nm are pinched off. The free vacuoles tend to coalesce and form a multicored vesicle. Aggregation of the cored material forms a lobulated mass which becomes more compact and thus forms the mature azurophilic granule. At the myelocyte stage of maturation the formation of primary granules ceases and the synthesis of the enzymes and proteins of the secondary or specific granules begins. Now, finely granular material condenses at the outer or convex face of the Golgi comples. Small granules, about 90 nm in diameter are released from the outer cisternae. The small immature granules fuse to form the more or less spherical specific granules which are 300 to 500 nm in diameter. The secondary granules were shown to possess alkaline phosphatase activity which has been employed as a marker for the specific granule.[10,11,13–15]

The myeloid precursor cells, like all protein and enzyme producing cells,[16–18] synthesize their specific proteins and enzymes for granule packaging on the ribosomes of the rough endocytoplasmic reticulum. The newly synthesized proteins are transferred to the cavities of the endocytoplasmic reticulum and transported to the Golgi complex where the material is concentrated and granulogenesis, as outlined, proceeds[19–21] The process of granule formation is similar in all of the myeloid cells, neutrophils, eosinophils, and basophils. The differences in the different granulocytes reside primarily in the differences of the proteins, enzymes, and other substances synthesized and packaged.

With some modification the model for granulogenesis outlined by Bainton and Farquhar[13,14] appears to be applicable to man as well.[22] In the human myeloblast the rough surface endocytoplasmic reticulum contains reaction product for peroxidase and the Golgi cisterne may contain a few peroxidase positive granules. In the myelocyte, peroxidase positive reaction product can be found in the endocytoplasmic reticulum, the Golgi cysternae and in all of the forming granules.[22,24] A large population of azurophilic, peroxidase positive primary granules are formed during the promyelocyte stage. The granules are for the most part spherical and measure about 500 nm in diameter.

At the end of the promyelocyte stage, an abrupt disappearance of peroxidase reaction product from the secretory apparatus (that is, from the rough endocytoplasmic reticulum, the Golgi complex, and the vesicles of the cell) marks the transition to the myelocyte stage of maturation. At this point the formation of the primary granules ceases and the creation of the specific or secondary granules begins. Primary granules do not become secondary granules. A new wave of protein synthesis begins and the formation of the smaller, less dense specific granules follows. The human specific granules do not form reaction product for peroxidase and can be identified by their lactoferrin content. The formation site on the Golgi complex is less clearly marked in the human myelocyte than it is in the rabbit's but the ultrastructural images of the human myelocyte suggest that, as in the rabbit, the granules arise from the convex surface of the Golgi complex.[25]

In the subsequent, nonproliferative stages of granulocytic development the smaller secondary granules become more numerous. In the mature polymorphonuclear neutrophil the specific granules outnumber the azurophilic granules about two to one, a result primarily of continued specific granule formation in the myelocyte as the content of azurophilic granules is diluted by cell division.

The broad aspects of granulogenesis in the neutrophil of man and the rabbit as described above are apparently valid for most animals examined to date. There are undoubtedly species differences involving differences in granule composition, nature of involvement of the Golgi complex and the variety of granules formed. Thus, the existence of a tertiary granule in the rabbit neutrophil has been proposed. The tertiary granules are pleomorphic, often grouped in clusters, and, though peroxidase positive, appear to be biochemically distinct from both the primary and secondary granules.[26] A third granule is thought to exist in the guinea pig granulocyte.[27] This granule is nucleated and felt to be a second type of azurophilic granule. Some doubt has also been cast on the participation of the Golgi complex in the guinea pig neutrophil in the formation of the primary or secondary granules.[27] Other investigators have described different forms of peroxidase positive azurophilic granules, but the relationship between these two structures is still undefined.[28–31]

B. Composition of Granule Formation

Isolation of the granules of the rabbit neutrophil by centrifugation on a density gradient has for the most part confirmed the heterogeneity of the granule population, and the presence of two predominant populations of granules, the azurophil and specific.[32–37] The biochemical data obtained from the assays of the granule fractions and the information obtained from the cytochemical studies of the cell[3,10,13,14] have made it abundantly clear that the azurophilic granules represent a special type of primary lysosome. They contain a variety of acid hydrolases, myeloperoxidase, about one third of the lysozyme activity of the neutrophils, acid mucosubstances, cationic antibacterial proteins, and neutral proteases. By contrast, the secondary granules contain alkaline phosphatase, lactoferrin, and lysozyme. The two granules operate at different pH optima, the primary at an acid and the secondary at an alkaline pH.

The alkaline phosphatase of the rabbit specific granule has been shown to be associated with the granule membrane. Lactoferrin is probably a more specific marker. The membrane obtained from the two populations of rabbit neutrophil granules, though morphologically similar in ultrastructural appearance, showed distinct differences in cholesterol phospholipid ratios and protein components.[38] These membrane differences have been attributed to the difference in origin of the two granules in the Golgi complex,[39] and may account for the differences in interaction of the two granules with the membrane of the endocytic vacuole.

Basically similar data have been obtained from cell fractionation and cytochemical studies of human neutrophil granules.[40–45] Again, a question has arisen about the localization of the alkaline phosphatase activity. Centrifugation techniques identify the enzyme in a lighter membrane fraction distinct from the granules. The composition of the human neutrophilic granules again reinforces the essentially lysosomal character of the primary granules which contain acid hydrolases, myeloperoxidase, neutral proteases, acid mucosubstances, and cationic proteins. The major constituents of the specific granules are lactoferrin and lysozyme; no hydrolases are present.

Although granule formation is the major activity of the cell during its course through the maturation process, other developmental attributes are required to achieve a functional neutrophil capable of locomotion, chemotaxis, phagocytosis, and bacterial killing. Specific membrane characteristics and both actin and myosin are necessary for normal neutrophil function. Lichtman and Weed[46] found a progressive increase in the ability of the neutrophilic surfaces to adhere to glass or plastic surfaces with increasing maturation. Myeloblasts and promyelocytes showed minimal adhesiveness on glass or plastic, a low propensity to aggregate, a slow rate of cell spreading, minimal pseudopod extension and motility, and a very slow rate of phagocytosis. At the myelocyte level of maturation, surface adhesiveness and phagocytosis, though not prominent, become evident. The mature neutrophil, on the other hand has a lower negative charge and displays a higher degree of deformability and adhesiveness. About 90% of the polymorphonuclear and band cells, and about 50% of the metamyelocytes stick to glass or plastic surfaces. The less mature cells show a decreasing capacity for adhesiveness. About 20 to 30% of myelocytes, 10% of promyelocytes, and about 2% of myeloblasts adhere to glass or plastic. Lichtman and Weed[46] suggested that the membrane changes are related to neutrophil function, particularly locomotion and phagocytosis, and are necessary for contact with particulate surfaces and for egress from the marrow.

Differences in the surface characteristics of the mature neutrophils and their precursors have been demonstrated by the binding of plant lectins and certain cationic binding agents.[47–52] Binding sites for the Fc portion of IgG and for the third component of complement have been identified on the cell surface of the mature neutrophil.[53–55] Specific receptors for chemotactic peptides have also been detected on the surface of human polymorphonuclear leucocytes.[56]

Motility and locomotion of the neutrophil are the functional expressions of highly developed specific proteins in the microtubules and microfilaments associated with the cell membrane. The depolymerization and repolymerization of the microtubules mediate functions concerned with cell orientation, while the microfilaments are involved in the directed, amoeboid movement of the cell. Myosin from guinea pig polymorphonuclear leukocytes has been isolated and purified and found to resemble myosin of skeletal muscle in many respects including the size of its heavy chains, morphological characteristics, pattern of ATP-activation, etc. The granulocyte myosin filaments are smaller than the myosin filaments of muscle and on binding with actin form polarized arrowhead structures.[57,58] The developmental sequence of the membrane proteins, surface charge, the microtubular and microfilamentous structures during the process of granulocyte maturation have yet to be elucidated. However, Altman and Stossel[59] have shown that myeloblasts and promyelocytes have no phagocytic capability; myelocytes and metamyelocytes are modestly phagocytic, whereas the mature neutrophils are most actively phagocytic of opsonized particles. In the presence of unopsonized particles the mature neutrophils of the marrow reserve pool have an ingestion defect when compared with the neutrophils on release from the marrow. Active, directed amoeboid movement is observed first at the end of the myelocyte phase of the maturation sequence.

C. Kinetics of Granulocytopoiesis

The kinetics of the neutrophilic granulocyte is concerned with the dynamic relationship between production, distribution, survival, and the ultimate fate of the cell. In vivo investigations of neutrophil kinetics have depended heavily on the use of isotopic labels, principally ^{3}H-thymidine[60–62] and labeled diisopropylfluorophosphate (DF^{32}P).[63,64] Radioactive chromium, ^{51}Cr[65–67] and technetium (^{99}Tc^{m}) have also been employed.[68,69] Although a considerable body of information has been developed through their use a satisfactory label for clinical application is not yet available.[70,71] The in vitro approach to the study of neutrophil kinetics and the regulation of granulopoiesis was made possible by the introduction of the semisolid culture methods[72–74] and the intraperitoneally implanted diffusion chambers.[75,76] For a complete review of the in vitro techniques and their application see Reference 77.

In the adult human, granulocytes are produced exclusively in the marrow where they originate from a stem cell pool consisting of a concatenated series of morphologically unrecognizable cells. The more advanced committed cells are fed into the recognizable pool of myelocytes where both cell amplification and maturation take place.

The pluripotential stem cell compartment of the marrow can be assayed in the mouse,[78] but not yet in man. The committed stem cell compartment of man and of the laboratory animal can be measured by the semisolid colony or diffusion chamber culture methods.[79]

Determination of the absolute number of precursor cells in the recognizable marrow compartments and the determinations of their transit time through these compartments have been challenging problems. The estimates of these parameters of neutrophil production reported by Cronkite and Vincent[80] were based on the following assumptions: the generation time for all dividing cells in the proliferating pool is the same; the generation time is about 24 hr; and all granulocytopoiesis is effective. From the reported distribution of the cells in the compartments of the proliferative pool[81] it was concluded, on the basis of the above stated assumptions, that one doubling division at the myeloblast and promyelocyte level and two at the myelocyte level would provide the ratio of cells found. The transit time from the stem cell through the proliferative pool requires an average of 5 days.

The absolute number of cells in each of the marrow granulocytic compartments has been estimated from the M/E ratio of the marrow, determined from either marrow cell suspensions[82] or marrow sections[82–86] and from the absolute number of the red cell precursors determined from their radioiron uptake. The M/E ratio derived from the analysis of marrow sections is believed to be more reliable than the M/E ratio obtained from cell suspensions of marrow, due principally to the cell injury and cell lysis encountered during preparation of the suspension. Utilizing the data obtained from autoradiographic analysis[80] and the cell distribution data reported by Dancey et al.,[85] Vincent[86] calculated the size of the myeloblastic compartment at 4×10^{7} cells per kg body weight and the compartment transit time at 14 hr; the promyelocytic compartment at 12×10^{7} cells per kg with a compartment transit time of 19 hr; and the myelocytic compartment at 199×10^{7} cells per kg with a compartment transit time of 102 hr. Similar values were reported by Finch et al.:[87] 2.1×10^{9} cells per kg body weight for the proliferative pool, a transit time through the pool of 5 days and a production rate of 0.85×10^{9} cells per kg per day.

Upon completion of its residence in the proliferative pool the neutrophil precursor enters the nonproliferative pool as a metamyelocyte and undergoes further maturation, without amplification, into a band cell and finally a segmented neutrophil. The cellularity of the metamyelocyte compartment has been estimated at 160×10^7 cells per kg with a compartment transit time of 30 hr; the compartment of band cells at 267×10^7 cells per kg with a compartment of segmented neutrophils at 378×10^7 cells per kg and a transit time of 72 hr.[86] Finch et al.'s[87] estimate of the postmitotic pool size is 5.6 $\times 10^9$ cells per kg with a transit time for the pool of 6.6 days. Thus, the total time for neutrophil maturation from stem cell to segmented neutrophil is some 10 to 11 days. The principal cell of the proliferative pool is the myelocyte, which makes up some 90% of the pool's cell population. The ratio of the proliferative pool to the nonproliferative pool is about 1:3.

The nonproliferative pool of metamyelocytes, bands, and segmented neutrophils forms a large storage reservoir of functional cells which can be released into the circulating pool on demand. This marrow reserve pool is about 15 times larger than the total number of neutrophils in the circulation. A shift of the reserve pool into this circulation is presumed to be responsible for an increase in the band cell population in the peripheral blood. Endotoxin, following a brief initial neutropenia due to the margination of the neutrophils, triggers a release of the marrow reserve pool.[88] Glucocorticoids initiate an early leucocytosis by impeding neutrophil egress from the circulating pool and stimulate a subsequent release of cells from the marrow reserve.[89] The glucocortoids also prolong the residence time in the blood of the circulating neutrophils. Etiocholanolone can also release the cells from the reserve pool.[90] These agents have been employed in a clinical setting to assess the adequacy of the marrow reserve pool for purposes of treatment[91,93] or for the investigation of the neutropenic state.[94] Dale et al.[95] evaluated the various agents capable of producing a neutrophilic leukocytosis in man. They found that the glucocorticoids, endotoxin and etiocholanolone, caused a peak leukocyte response in 4 to 6 hr, and that endotoxin, on average, produced a rise of 6000/mm^3 neutrophils above the base value and glucocorticoids about 4000/mm^3 neutrophils above the base value. Etiocholanolone produced the least vigorous neutrophil response of the agents employed. They recommended the use of glucocorticoids as the least noxious, yet sufficiently reliable agent for the evaluation of the state of the marrow reserve pool in man.

II. KINETICS OF THE BLOOD NEUTROPHILS

Under normal conditions bone marrow production and release of neutrophils maintain the blood neutrophil count within fairly narrow limits. The marrow also has great capacity for augmented neutrophil production to meet the tissue demand for these cells. The blood neutrophil count varies considerably among individuals and has been shown to range between values of 1830 to 7250 per mm^3 (medium value 3650).[96] The total circulating pool of neutrophils can be readily calculated from the blood neutrophil count and the total blood volume.

The development of labeling techniques for autologous neutrophils made possible the measurement of their disappearance rate from the blood and their compartmentalization into a marginated pool.[63,64,82,83,85] About 50% of autologously labeled neutrophils disappear from the circulation immediately after reinfusion.[97] The rate of disappearance of the labeled cells is rapid, its manner, random. The measured half time clearance of neutrophils from the blood is 6.7 hr (range 4 to 10 hr).[98] The disappearing cells are thought to stick to the endothelial surfaces of small vessels and in this fashion create a pool of marginated neutrophils.[99–101] The marginated pool is approximately equal in size to the circulating pool with which it is in equilibrium. The neutrophils can be mobilized from the marginated pool by adrenalin or exercise, a phenomenon recognized by Naegeli more than 50 years ago as the Verschiebungsleukozytose.[102] The marginated neutrophil has two options: it can reenter the circulating pool to marginate elsewhere or exit from the capillary bed to enter the tissues from which it cannot return. It is abundantly clear that neutrophils can enter an inflammatory area in large numbers as witnessed clinically in abscess formation, empyemas, or experimentally in the Rebuck window.[103] Whether neutrophils enter tissue in any significant number under inflammatory-free conditions has not been settled. Cronkite[104,105] calculated the exit rate of neutrophils per unit area of capillary bed and estimated the number of neutrophils that should be present per unit volume of tissue, assuming different tissue life span. Januar and Cronkite[106] could find no extravascular neutrophils either by light or electron microscopy in pathogen-free mice. The fate of the neutrophil may depend on the state of the animal: in the pathogen-free animal or infection-free man the aged neutrophils die in the blood stream and are removed by the macrophages; in the nonpathogen-free animals, activated chemotactic factors attract the neutrophils into the tissues where the cells complete their life span.

In summary, the blood neutrophils exist in a circulating and a marginated pool the sum of which is the total blood granulocyte pool. The neutrophils in the two pools are in dynamic equilibrium. In a steady state condition the size of the pools has been estimated at 2.2, 2.7, and 4.9 $\times$ 10^{10} cells for the circulating, marginated, and total blood granulocyte pools, respectively.[98] The half time residence of the neutrophil in the circulating pool is 6.7 hr. Thus, for a normal man with a total blood granulocyte pool of 4.9 $\times$ 10^{10} cells, the granulocyte turnover rate is 4.8 $\times$ 10^9 neutrophils per hr.

Much useful information has been obtained from kinetic measurements of the functional capacity of the marrow. Their application to the clinical problems of granulocytopoiesis has been limited, but improvements in techniques should make future clinical application profitable.

III. ABNORMALITIES OF GRANULOCYTOPOIESIS

A. Neutrophil Function

The prinicipal functions of granulocytopoiesis are to provide neutrophils in sufficient numbers to stem bacterial invasion and to endow the neutrophil with the necessary machinery for locomotion, oxidant generation, phagocytosis, and degranulation—in brief, the central processes to the successful execution of neutrophil function, namely bacterial killing. To trigger these events, the cell membrane of the neutrophil must be equipped with a cytoskeleton and receptors for chemotaxins and for opsonized bacteria.[107,108]

The cytoskeleton of the neutrophil consists of microtubules, approximately 240 Å in diameter, which emanate from the central bodies of the cell which, as has been previously described, lie in the concavity of the indented nucleus. The cytoplasmic microtubules originate from the vicinity of the centrioles and radiate from the central area of the cell in all directions toward the plasma membrane. The microfilaments lie immediately below and adjacent to the plasma membrane. The microfilaments are about 60 Å in diameter and are most conspicuous in the protrusions and ruffled regions of the membrane. These fibers concentrate in regions of increased surface activity as seen in locomotion or phagocytosis. A third variety of cytoskeletal fiber has been recognized and designated the intermediate or 100-Å filament. Its constitution and function are unknown.

Tubulin is the principal component of the microtubule. It is a protein dimer of two nonidentical subunits. The microfilaments contain actin, a globular protein of about 42,000 daltons, and myosin, which consists of both heavy and light chains. Colchicine binds with tubulin and causes rapid and complete disassembly of the cytoplasmic microtubules. Similar disruption of the microtubular assembly can be accomplished by vinblastine, vincristine, griseofulvin, or podophyllotoxin as well as by glutathione oxidizing agents. Disruption of the microfilaments system has thus far been accomplished with but one agent, cytochalasin B.[109–120]

Assuming then the presence of a normal mature neutrophil, an opsonized bacterium, and a chemotactic gradient derived from the complement system, the following sequence of events are set into motion. The chemotactic factor, e.g., fragments of C_3 and C_5, bind to membrane receptors and induce the rapid assembly of microtubules from the centrioles. The neutrophil moves by means of lamellipodia in directed fashion up the chemotactic gradient to bind the opsonized bacterium to appropriate surface receptors. Microfilaments are immediately brought into the region of binding, endocytosis and internalization of the bacterium follow, and a phagocytic vacuole is created.[120] At the same time a membrane-initiated generation of oxidants and a metabolic oxygen burst take place. The specific granules attach immediately to the phagosome and discharge their contents into the vacuole, and the azurophilic granules subsequently bind onto the phagocytic vacuole and in turn empty their charge of lysosomal enzymes and protein.[121–124]

Bacterial killing is effected by two independent systems, one oxygen dependent and the other oxygen independent. The oxygen-dependent oxidase is presumably activated by the liganding of the opsonized particle and superoxide anion and hydrogen peroxide are formed. A metabolic shift from the anaerobic Meyerhof-Embden pathway to the aerobic hexose-monophosphate shunt is simultaneously triggered. The hydrogen peroxide produced by these mechanisms serves as a substrate for the myeloperoxidase liberated from the azurophilic granules which, with a halogen cofactor can oxidize bacterial proteins and lipids, produce chloramine, or iodinate bacterial proteins. Singlet oxygen and hydroxy radicals derived from the interaction of superoxide anion and hydrogen peroxide also contribute to their antimicrobial property to the field.[125–127] The oxygen-independent system depends on the antimicrobial activity of lactoferrin, lysozyme, the cationic proteins from the specific granules, and the low intravacuolar pH.[130]

B. Qualitative Abnormalities

Abnormalities of neutrophil function may be due to qualitative alterations of the cell, a result of defective maturation,[131–133] or quantitative inadequacy of neutrophil numbers due either to production failure or excessive peripheral destruction of neutrophils.[134]

Abnormalities of maturation may produce structural and/or functional alterations under a variety of congenital and acquired conditions.[135–137]

1. Pelger-Huet Anomaly

The Pelger-Huet anomaly is a defect in the process that normally leads to lobulation of the nucleus. It is transmitted as an autosomal dominant and is seen clinically in the heterozygous state in about 1 of 5000 blood smears examined. The bone marrow shows an increase in the percentage of metamyelocytes in the postmitotic compartment. The metamyelocyte and band forms show similar chromatin clumping. Lobulation rarely proceeds beyond the two lobed, particularly striking and characteristic pince-nez spectacle form. In the blood, 50% of the neutrophils are band forms and the remainder bilobed. At most, 2% of the circulating neutrophils may have three segments. Many variations may be encountered, depending primarily on the degree of inhibition of lobule formation, but in all instances the characteristic nuclear clumping helps in the recognition of the disorder. Neutrophil function is apparently not affected and the carriers of the trait do not show increased susceptibility to infection.

The homozygous form of the hereditary Pelger-Huet anomaly is rare. In the cases reported, more than 90% of the circulating neutrophils have a small round nucleus. The deeply staining clumped chromatin, consisting usually of about eight to twelve fragments, is held together by lighter staining chromatin in the shape of a ball.

The Pelger-Huet anomaly may be acquired and has been seen in an assortment of clinical conditions, particularly chronic infections, preleukemia, and in the leukemias. The acquired or pseudo Pelger-Huet cell cannot be distinguished from the hereditary forms morphologically but one usually finds a greater percentage of the homozygous forms.[138]

2. *Hereditary Constitutional Hypersegmentation of the Neutrophil*

A rare familial disorder, probably autosomal dominant, in which the neutrophils show a marked shift to the right in the mean lobe count has been reported.[139] The majority of the cells in the blood have four or more lobes and in the marrow the promyelocytes and myelocytes have a somewhat flattened, indented nucleus. Apparently the hypersegmentation has no deleterious effects on neutrophil function in the hereditary anomaly but is strikingly similar to the acquired hypersegmentation seen in the megaloblastic states where neutrophil function is definitely compromised.

3. *Hereditary Giant Neutrophils*

Neutrophils with a diameter 17 μm or greater have been encountered in severe sepsis, marked leucocytosis, and following chemotherapy for carcinoma. A family has been described in which the affected members have 16 giant neutrophils per 1000 neutrophils. The anomaly appears to be harmless.[140]

4. *May-Heggelin Anomaly*

This disorder of maturation is expressed clinically by leukopenia, mild thrombocytopenia, large bizarre platelets, and the presence of intracytoplasmic inclusions in the cytoplasm of the neutrophils. The inclusions are located at the rim of the cell adjacent to the plasma membrane. The inclusions are rod or cone shaped, stain grey-blue with the Romanowsky stains and intensely red with pyronine, but contain no lipids or polysaccharides. The disorder is familial, probably autosomal dominant, and often clinically silent.[141–150]

The intracytoplasmic inclusions in the neutrophils of the May-Heggelin anomaly appear to be identical with the inclusions known as Döhle bodies. First described as an acquired phenomenon in scarlet fever,[151] Döhle bodies have been subsequently found in acute infections and toxic processes, in severe burns,[152] and following chemotherapy for malignant disease.[153] The inclusions are probably derived from ribonucleic acid and ribosomal structures and appear as dense fibrils, about 50 Å in diameter on ultrastructural examination.[146] Jenis et al.[147] found the inclusions in the May-Heggelin anomaly to be aggregates of rod-like structures. They postulated that at the myelocyte stage of development the lipoprotein membranes of the stacked cisternae of the rough endocytoplasmic ribosomes subsequently unfold into an ordered paracrystalline array of beaded rods and filaments. Bessis[148] described the acquired Döhle bodies as free ribosomes or parallel sacs of ergostoplasm and raised some question about the identity of the acquired Döhle body with the inclusions seen in the May-Heggelin anomaly. The evidence suggests that both are derived from the ribosomal nucleic acids. The structural defect has been thought by some investigators to be the result of a focal failure in cytoplasmic maturation.[145,148,149] In the bone marrow Döhle bodies are present in myelocytes and promyelocytes as well as in the more mature neutrophilic cells.

5. Chediak-Higashi Syndrome

This anomaly is characteristically seen in young, blond children with photophobia (oculocutaneous albinism) who are remarkably susceptable to pyogenic infection. The characteristic feature of the syndrome is the presence of large azurophilic granules, often 2 to 5 μm in diameter lying free in large cytoplasmic vacuoles. The nuclei are frequently deformed by the cytoplasmic vacuoles. In the marrow aspirates the megakaryocytes and red cell precursors appear normal. The promyelocytes and myelocytes contain vacuoles with round bodies which become larger and coarse as the cells mature;[154–158] comparable genetic abnormality has been reported for the aleutian mink,[159] partial albino hereford cows,[160] beige mice,[161] killer whales,[162] and the Persian cat.[163]

Species related differences in the neutrophil granules have been reported. In man, the abnormal granules are present in almost all of the mature neutrophils. The granules are azurophilic, react positively to periodic acid-Schiff and sudan black staining and demonstrate acid phosphatase and peroxidase activity. On electron microscope a reticulated array of membrane-like material, often with myelin figures, is usually seen.[164–166] Freeze fracture studies reveal the presence of two types of granules: a massively enlarged primary lysosome and an irregularly contoured granule thought to be the product of fused smaller granules.[167]

The abnormal properties of the Chediak-Higashi neutrophils include impaired chemotaxis,[128] decreased mobilization,[168] impaired degranulation, and impairment of in vitro bactericidal capacity.[169] Impressed by the similarity of these abnormal functions of the Chediak-Higashi neutrophil and the abnormalities of the neutrophils of colchicine-treated animals, Oliver et al.[170,171] studied the response of Chediak-Higashi neutrophils to concanavalin A capping. They found that Chediak-Higashi neutrophils form concanavalin caps spontaneously and that concanavalin A failed to trigger centriole-induced microtubule assembly. They, therefore, proposed that the central defect in the Chediak-Higashi syndrome might reside in an abnormality of the microtubules. This suggestion received considerable support by their demonstration that elevating the cyclic GMP levels of the cell with cholinergic agonists corrected the chemotactic and bactericidal defects, and restored as well the centriole-associated microtubules formation. These findings have been successfully applied to the clinical control of the human Chediak-Higashi syndrome by the administration of 200 mg of ascorbic acid daily.[172,173] Ascorbic acid has been shown to increase leucocyte cyclic GMP.[174]

6. The Lazy Leukocyte Syndrome

This rare disorder of the neutrophil, so named because of the severe impairment of in vitro chemotaxis and random motility, is characterized clinically by severe neutropenia and recurrent sinusitis, stomatitis, and otitis media.[175] The neutrophils are morphologically normal on customary Giemsa stain. Granulocyte maturation in the bone marrow is morphologically normal. Bone marrow cellularity is normal, with a normal quantitative relationship between the postmitotic and proliferative pools. However, endotoxin fails to release the marrow reserve pool and epinephrine fails to release the marginated pool. The lazy neutrophils do not migrate into a Rebuck window. The basic defect of the lazy leukocyte is thought to reside in an abnormality of the microfilamentous system.[176]

Isolated instances of neutrophil dysfunction related to cytoskeletal abnormalities have been reported. Boxer et al.[177] described a child with severe recurrent infections whose neutrophils showed severe impairment of chemotaxis and phagocytosis. Neutrophil actin dysfunction was considered to be the basic disturbance. Gallin et al.[178] reported on an unusual occurrence in a 7-year-old child of repeated severe infections associated with marked impairment of neutrophil function as evidenced by diminished adherence to nylon, decreased degranulation, decreased bacterial killing, and decreased random or directed motility. Ultrastructural study revealed a striking increase in microtubules which was associated with a 400% increase in intracellular cyclic GMP.

7. Abnormalities of the Neutrophil Granules

A hereditary form of myeloperoxidase deficiency has been recognized.[179–181] Presumably transmitted as an autosomal recessive, the abnormality appears to be clinically silent with little propensity for infection. The neutrophils of myeloperoxidase deficiency lack the early microbicidal activity which is apparently myeloperoxidase dependent, but the later myeloperoxidase independent systems are sufficient to achieve bacterial killing and protect the individual. In the hereditary form of the disease, myeloperoxidase is absent in the neutrophils in the blood and the precursors in the marrow.

Acquired forms of myeloperoxidase have also been reported[182–185] and are probably more commonly seen in the preleukemia syndromes. Both myeloperoxidase positive and negative cells are present in blood and marrow.

Lack of lactoferrin in the specific granules of the neutrophil is associated with recurrent infection. The majority of the patients described had morphologically abnormal neutrophils characterized by decreased lobulation with nuclear blebs, absent alkaline phosphatase reaction, and reduced chemotaxis.[186–190]

8. Disorders of Oxidant Generation

This hereditary disease of early childhood is characterized by recurrent and severe staphylococcal (aureus) and enteric bacterial infections that can present with involvement of any organ. Lymphadenopathy and hepatosplenomegaly, a result of the chronic infection, is often present. The disorder may be transmitted genetically as either sex-linked or as an autosomal recessive.[191,192]

The neutrophils of this disorder are morphologically normal and display normal random and directed motility, chemotaxis, phagocytosis, and degranulation, and are normal in number. The morphological aspects of neutrophil maturation in the marrow are normal. Holmes et al.[193,194] provided the first important insight into the nature of this disease when they demonstrated that the neutrophils of chronic granulomatous disease are indeed capable of bacterial ingestion, but incapable of killing catalase-positive bacteria. Subsequently, it was shown that the respiratory burst associated with phagocytosis of bacteria could not be elicited in the neutrophils of chronic granulomatous disease.[195,196]

a. Chronic Granulomatous Disease

The normal neutrophil response to perturbation of its plasma membrane is a burst of oxygen consumption, and the subsequent production of a field of products resulting from oxygen reduction (superoxide anion, hydrogen peroxide, etc.) and hexose monophosphate shunt activation. The neutrophils of chronic granulomatous disease fail to generate superoxide anion in response to ligand binding.[197] The findings suggest an absence of an important membrane-associated enzyme activity, involving either an absent of functionless mutant oxidase enzyme or a defect in the triggering mechanism.[198]

b. Glucose-6-Phosphate Dehydrogenase Deficiency

Variants of G-6-PD deficiency which involve the neutrophils as well as the red cells can mimic the neutrophil defect of chronic granulomatous disease[100,203] The neutrophils of both chronic granulomatous and glucose-6-phosphate dehydrogenase deficiency fail to reduce nitroblue tetrazolium following phagocytic stimulation. Distinction of the two diseases rests on the measurement of glucose-6-phosphate dehydrogenase activity of the red cells and neutrophils and the stimulation of the hexose monophosphate shunt by methylene blue.[202] The enzyme activity is obviously normal in chronic granulomatous disease and absent in G-6-PD deficiency and similarly, the shunt pathway can be stimulated by methylene blue in the neutrophil of chronic granulomatous disease in vitro, but not in G-6-PD deficient neutrophils.

C. Quantitative Abnormalities of the Neutrophil

1. The Neutropenias

Neutropenia may be seen as a regular feature of the pancytopenia of bone marrow failure or as an isolated phenomenon in a variety of congenital and acquired clinical situations. By definition, neutropenia is present when the neutrophil count of the blood falls below 1200 cells/mm^3. Increased risk of infection is rarely seen with neutrophil counts above 1000 cells/mm^3; moderate risk exists with counts ranging between 500 to 1000 cells/mm^3; and grave risk to infection is present when the neutrophil count falls to levels below 500 cells/mm^3.

Logically neutropenia may be attributed to a quantitative decrease in the precursor cells in the marrow or to abnormal maturation and ineffective granulocytopoiesis; impaired mobilization of the marrow reserve pool; excessive margination, or excessive peripheral utilization; or destruction. However, in a given clinical situtation the pathophysiological mechanisms may not be readily defined or more than one cause may be operative.[131]

Neutropenia is a regular feature of bone marrow aplasia whether idiopathic or the sequel of marrow injury from the direct toxic action of drugs, chemicals or ionizing radiation. In this circumstance the neutropenia most often accompanies an anemia and thrombocytopenia. The bone marrow biopsy is characteristically hypoplastic with marked reduction in the hemopoietic elements. Pancytopenia and marrow aplasia have been associated with hepatitis[204] and possibly other bacterial or viral infections. Kinetic measurements of the blood and marrow granulocytes show a decrease in both the circulating and the marginated pool, a normal or slightly reduced half-time circulation in the blood, a reduced marrow reserve pool, and decreased granulocyte turnover. For a more detailed discussion of bone marrow aplasia, see the chapter on Aplastic Anemia.

The isolated neutropenias can be congenital or acquired.[131] Congenital neutropenia comprises a group of disorders, some benign, others grave, some constant, others cyclic.

a. Hereditary Neutropenia (Kostmann's Syndrome)

Kostmann's syndrome is an uncommon autosomal recessive disorder in which the blood neutrophil population falls to vanishing low levels.[205,206] The bone marrow aspirate is hyperplastic with a marked increase in the proliferative pool of granulocytes. Myelocytes and promyelocytes make up more than 50% of all of the nucleated cells in the smears. The myeloid cells often show excessive lobulation, vacuolization of the cytoplasm, and coarse granulation (toxic granulation). Abnormal mitotic behavior, such as tetraploidy or doubly nucleated metamyelocytes, may be encountered. A mild increase in plasma cells and reticulum macrophages may be present. The anatomical findings suggest an inhibition of maturation. Kostmann[207] found that the serum of a patient with hereditary neutropenia inhibited myelopoiesis of normal cells in culture. Decreased numbers of CFU-C have been found in the marrow of these patients and the colonies that do develop are either monocytic or eosinophilic.[208–210] Inhibitors of myelopoiesis, or a decrease in colony-stimulating factor may be additional problems in some cases.[211]

A host of other chronic neutropenic states, usually appearing in children or young adults, has been reported under a bewildering array of designations and eponyms, such as benign familiar neutropenia (Gansslen),[212] familial severe neutropenia (Hitzig),[213] neutropenia and pancreatic insufficiency (Schwachman),[214] and Kostmann syndrome described above.[215,216] These disorders are uncommon and the findings are so variable in individual subjects of any group under study, as well as in a given individual at different time periods, that a rational classification has been indeed difficult to construct. The bone marrow aspirates in these disorders as reported by Dale et al.[217] are generally normally cellular and show a relative increase of myeloid elements, predominantly of myelocytes. The postmitotic pool is decreased in size and mature polymorphonuclear leucocytes are scanty. The marrow reserve pool responds to endotoxin. Leukokinetic studies and assays for CFU-C have given essentially normal values. These studies are made difficult by the severe neutropenia. Colony-stimulating activity is normal and no inhibitors or antineutrophil antibodies have been detected. The bone marrow findings suggest ineffective granulocytopoiesis, but the responsible factors are still largely unknown. Various hypothesis that have been proposed include autoimmune[218] and microenvironmental mechanisms.[219]

b. Drug-Induced Neutropenias

Drugs are the most common offenders in the production of neutropenia. The list of drugs that can cause this problem is prodigious and includes many commonly used and valuable medications.[220] Severe leukopenia, after variable periods of drug ingestion, sets the stage for infection. Bone marrow examination done early usually reveals a total disappearance of the myeloid elements, at times depletion only of the more mature elements, leaving the myelocytes and promyelocytes as the predominant myeloid population.

On removal of the offending agent hematologic recovery begins with proliferation of the early precursor cells and an expansion of the proliferative compartment of the marrow. Maturation proceeds in an orderly fashion with reconstitution of the postmitotic pool and release of mature neutrophils into the peripheral blood.

Two basic mechanisms are responsible for the neutropenia: one is immunologic, the other, direct suppression of the marrow. The aminopyrine-induced agranulocytic angina of Schultz[221] is the classic example of immune-induced neutropenia. Other drugs like sulfonamides, quinine, and the antithyroid drugs have a similar mechanism of action. Antineutrophil antibodies are present in the serum and presumably destroy the neutrophils of blood and marrow.[222] Bone marrow examination reveals usually a depleted postmitotic pool. Myelocytes remain as the predominant myeloid cell.

Phenothiazine-induced neutropenia is the best-studied example of a neutropenia due to direct suppression of marrow activity.[223] The disorder is dose dependent and generally requires a total dose of 10 to 20 grams of phenothiazine for its initiation. Marrow examination shows an absence of the myeloid cells. The phenothiazines interfere with DNA synthesis of the marrow cells.

c. Immune Neutropenia

Iso-Immune—The development of maternal antibodies to the fetal neutrophil antigens can be responsible for neutropenia and subsequent infection a few days after birth. Akin to erythroblastosis, the leukoagglutinins are formed by the mother against antigens present on the fetal neutrophil, but not on her own. A least two neutrophil-specific antigen systems have been identified.[224,225] The bone marrow shows a depletion of the marrow reserve pool.[226]

Auto-Immune—Isolated patients have been reported in whom a serum factor was present which was capable of agglutinating normal neutrophils. Neutropenia of less than 1000 cells/mm^3 is the sole hematologic abnormality. The bone marrow reveals a normal or hyperplastic proliferative pool with decrease in the mature neutrophils.[123]

Felty's syndrome—Neutropenia, associated with arthritis and splenomegaly occurs in about 1% of patients with long-standing rheumatoid arthritis. Bone marrow examination shows myeloid hyperplasia with depletion of the postmitotic pool. The mechanism for the neutropenia is not clear and multifactorial but the presence of antinuclear antibodies in a high percentage of the patients suggests an immune process.[227,228]

d. Cyclic Neutropenia

This disorder, frequently in a familial setting, is distinguished clinically by recurring periods of neutropenia during which upper respiratory or other infection appears.[229,230] Recurring severe neutropenia, usually in 3-week cycles, is the hallmark of the syndrome. Cyclic fluctuations have been found in these patients for all hemopoietic elements, i.e., white blood cells, platelets, and reticulocytes.[232] Hemopoiesis in these patients proceeds in a wave-like fashion with the bone marrow oscillating between hypo- and hyperproliferation.

The cause of cyclic neutropenia is not clear. Morley[232] found an oscillation of the neutrophil values of some normal men recurring over a 2- to 3-week cycle. He argued that the oscillation is the result of an inherent time delay in the negative feedback control of granulopoiesis. Cyclic neutropenia could therefore be the result of an exaggeration of the normal cycling. King-Smith and Morley[233] developed a computer model for granulopoiesis which contained two feedback loops and which could simulate normal and abnormal granulopoiesis. Morley and Stohlman[234] on the strength of this model were able to induce cyclic neutropenia in dogs by producing bone marow repression with cyclophosphamide. This concept was also invoked to explain the cyclic leukocytosis of chronic myelogenous leukemia.[235]

Cyclic neutropenia occurs in the gray collie syndrome,[236] a lethal disease of young collie dogs characterized by lack of hair pigmentation and intestinal malabsorption. The neutropenic cycle-length averages 10 to 12 days. The syndrome has many features in common with the human disease. This animal model for cyclic neutropenia was extensively investigated by Dale et al.[237–239] It was further shown that the transplantation of normal marrow into afflicted dogs dampens the cyclic fluctuations of the neutrophils[240] and conversely and disease can be transferred by the transplantation of marrow from afflicted animals to normal dogs.[241] Dale et al. postulated defect in regulation at the stem cell level.[242]

2. *Leukocytosis and Leukemoid Reactions*

Leukocytosis, or more specifically neutrophilia, has served the physician during the past half century and more as a herald of infection, inflammation, or leukemia. Leukocytosis has been defined as a total leukocyte count greater than 10×10^9 cells per liter or a neutrophilia (including band and segments neutrophils) greater than 7×10^9 cell per liter.[96] Leukemoid reaction refers to peripheral blood findings suggestive of leukemia. The characteristic elements of a leukemoid reaction are leukocytosis and the presence of mature cells of one or more types, but low or normal leucocyte counts may be encountered.[243] For some, any leucocyte count greater than 50×10^9 cells per liter is leukemoid, even in the absence of immature forms in the peripheral blood.[244] The term "leukoerythroblastic reaction" has been used to describe the presence of immature, nucleated red cells in the peripheral blood in association with immature granulocytic elements.

a. Neutrophilia

An increase in the number of circulating neutrophils may result from an increase in marrow production; a release of the marrow reserve pool; a shift of the marginated pool into the circulating pool; or a prolonged residence of the neutrophil in the blood. In the clinical setting, neutrophilia is most commonly associated with infection, inflammatory conditions, or the presence of tumor. The factors that control the production and maturation of the neutrophils in the marrow and the mechanisms concerned with the release of the neutrophils from the marrow under normal steady state conditions and in the neutrophilia of infection are still incompletely understood. The evidence strongly suggests that, in addition to the regulation by local microenvironmental factors and cell-to-cell interactions,[245] humoral substances provide further regulatory control in dampening or stimulating granulopoiesis and in the egress and release of the neutrophils from the bone marrow.[246,247]

Bacterial products, notably endotoxin, after their administration or release from a site of infection, decrease the number of circulating neutrophils within the first 2 to 3 hr followed by a return of the neutrophil count to base line values, and finally between the fourth and sixth hr to a doubling of the neutrophil count.[248] The initial fall in the neutrophil count has been attributed to margination and the subsequent increase in the neutrophil count to the release of the marrow reserve pool. Endotoxin mediates its effect on the marrow reserve pool through an intermediate, the neutrophil releasing factor, a protein of low molecular size.[249,250] Factors capable of stimulating the production and maturation of the neutrophils appear in the serum coincident with the neutrophil releasing factors.[250] Whether these properties, neutrophil release and stimulation of granulocytopoiesis, reside in one or more substances is not known, although some evidence for the separation of these factors has been presented.[251–253] The release of the marrow reserve pool fills the immediate demand for neutrophils at the inflammatory site, but the sustained and adequate supply of neutrophils must be met by an increase in granulocyte production by shortening of the generation time and increasing the number of divisions in the proliferative compartment, the delayed response loop. With continued demand for neutrophils the committed stem cell compartment expands.[80,86]

The bone marrow response to infection is characterized by an initial fall in the number of segmented neutrophils followed by an increase in the marrow cellularity with an increasing M/E ratio. The percentage of myelocytes and promyelocytes increases and the ratio of the proliferative: nonproliferative compartments shifts from the steady state 1:3 to a ratio of 1:1. In a highstress, acute infection like pneumococcal lobar pneumonia, the left shift of the myeloid elements may indeed be striking with promyelocytes making up some 20 to 25% of the white cell population. Myeloblasts are, however, uncommon and rarely exceed 2 to 3%. With subsidence of the infection the myelocytes fall from their high levels of about 25% to about 6 to 8 and the segmented cells increase from about 5 to 30%. The bone marrow picture varies considerably but, in general, an increase in the M/E ratio in a moderately hypercellular marrow with a left shift of the myeloid cells together with the blood neutrophilia suggest a response to infection or inflammation. The examination of the marrow aspirate or biopsy for the assessment of granulocyte production has serious limitations. The more sophisticated techniques which rely on white cell labeling do not find easy application in the clinical situation but the information on granulopoiesis that has been acquired by these techniques does aid the clinician in his evaluation of the morphologic information obtained from the marrow examination. Despite its limitations the marrow examination provides the physician with a useful and practical approach to the assessment of granulocyte production.

In chronic inflammatory conditions, such as the chronic granulomatous diseases, rheumatoid arthritis, tumor, etc. the bone marrow is moderately hyperplastic with a moderate left shift of the myeloid cells, accompanied by a definite increase in plasma cells and the reticular macrophages. On rare occasions the offending agent like *Histoplasma capsulatum* or *Leishmania donovani* may be found in the reticulum macrophages.

b. The Leukemoid Reactions

The leukemoid reactions[254] refer to the presence of immature cells of a given cell type in the peripheral blood and hence can be myeloid, lymphoid, or monocytoid in character. The myeloid leukemoid reactions are far and away the most common of all of the leukemoid reactions encountered and of primary concern in the present discussion. The diagnosis is established by the recognition of myelocytes in the routine peripheral blood smear. The severity of the leukemoid reaction varies considerably from the usual presentation of occasional myelocytes in the peripheral blood smear to the more striking picture of nucleated precursor red cells associated with immature myeloid cells. The leukoerythroblastic reaction may indeed resemble and indeed on rare occasions be difficult to distinguish from chronic myelogenous leukemia.

Leukemoid reactions, like leukocytosis, are seen in association with infections,[255,256] malignant disease,[257–259] inflammatory disease, and a variety of miscellaneous conditions.[260] The tuberculosis-associated leukemoid reactions have received considerble attention and appear to be related to activity of the tuberculous infection or its dissemination.[261,262]

c. Leucoerythroblastic Reactions

The leucoerythroblastic reaction was always considered to be an expression of infiltration and replacement of the marrow and compensatory myeloid hyperplasia in spleen, liver, and lymph nodes from which the immature hemopoietic cells were presumably released. Carcinomas of lung, prostate, and stomach, are the more common tumors that can either metastasize diffusely throughout the marrow or incite a myelofibrotic or osteoblastic reaction. The bone marrow examination may show tumor cells, hypercellularity with increase in the granulocytic precursors, plasmacytosis, an increase in the reticulum cells, and eosinophils. More recent reviews of the problem do confirm that 30 to 50% of patients who present with a leucoerythroblastic reaction do have marrow infiltrations but 50% of this group are leukemic. In the remainder of the patients, 50 to 70% of the total, infection, hemolytic anemia, bleeding, and other miscellanous conditions are responsible for the peripheral blood reaction. The true incidence of the leucoerythroblastic reaction is not known, and bias probably played some role in skewing the figures toward the infiltrative lesions of the marrow.[263,264]

Rare instances of congenital neutrophilia and leukemoid reactions have been reported. Hereditary neutrophilia is probably an autosomal dominant disease characterized by persistant neutrophilia of morphologically and functionally normal cells. The subjects appear to be clinically well, but have enlarged livers and spleens and expanded marrows to produce the widened diploë and the hair-on-end image on X-ray examination of the skull. The leucocyte alkaline phosphatase scores are high as are the serum B_{12} levels. The peripheral blood neutrophils are all mature cells; none are younger than band forms. The bone marrow is hypercellular; the M/E ratio is 15:1 with a marked shift to the left of the total granulocyte population in the marrow.[265]

Rare instances of congenital leukemoid reaction have been reported, some with thrombocytopenia and a megakaryocytosis,[266] and others with leucoerythroblastic reactions, bone marrow hyperplasia, and with an increase in all cell types of the myeloid series and an increase in the number of megakaryocytes.[267,268]

Persistant neutrophilia can follow splenectomy or be associated with functional asplenia. Spencer et al.[269] observed a patient with a neutrophilia of 11 to 26,000 cells for 11 years. There were Howell-Jolly bodies in the red cells and the spleen did not visualize on radiologic examination. The bone marrow was moderately hypercellular, the M/E ratio was normal, and the megakaryocytes were slightly increased.

Unexplained, apparently harmless leucocytosis in the absence of any known stimulus for an elevation of the white blood cell count has been described as chronic idiopathic leucocytosis. The leucocyte alkaline phosphatase is normal and no morphological marrow abnormality has been detected.[270] An elevated granulocyte turnover rate was found in seven patients with idiopathic leukocytosis.[271]

3. Myelofibrosis and Osteomyelosclerosis

a. Clinical Features

Classically, myelofibrosis is defined by a triad of findings, splenomegaly, marrow replacement by reticulin and collagen fibers, and a leukerythroblastic reaction. The clinical features of myelofibrosis have been covered in a number of reviews.[272–275] Splenomegaly is present early in the disease, is rarely absent,[276] and develops slowly and insidiously. Ward and Block[272] correlated the size of the spleen with the duration of the disease and noted that the enlargement of the spleen proceeded roughly at the rate of 1 cm/yr below the left costal margin. Myeloid metaplasia predominantly of the red pulp is the outstanding histologic feature of the spleen and involves all three lines of hematopoiesis. Numerous megakaryocytes, both in the cords and sinusoids, and erythroblastic foci are conspicuously evident. Myelocytes are less prominently displayed and are found usually between the sinusoids and the cords. The splenic aspirate is densely crowded with both red and white cell precursors and megakaryocytes. Different stages of maturation are present. Erythropoiesis in most cases is partially megaloblastic, a typical feature of all hepatic and splenic erythropoiesis, regardless of cause.[268] As in the marrow, large erythroblastic islands about a reticulum cell may be present. The liver is usually enlarged and on microscopic examination has prominent myeloid metaplasia; the spleen is similarly affected, but to a lesser extent.[277,278]

The disease may be preceded by polycythemia for several years, and a history of polycythemia vera is obtained in a large number of patients. The hemoglobin levels gradually decline to dip to the anemic levels, normochromic in character and detected in most patients at the initial examination. The initial white blood cell count may be normal, or increased, and in a small number of cases leucopenic. Basophilia and eosinophilia are common. The platelet count may be markedly elevated, but is more frequently normal, and thrombocytopenia is usually present in the late stages of the illness. The characteristic alterations of the blood picture are qualitative. Anisocytosis, polychromasia, and poikilocytosis are common and the presence of tear-drop red cells suggests the diagnosis of myelofibrosis. Nucleated red blood cells are almost invariably present, chiefly as orthochromatic normoblasts, but earlier forms may be encountered. With elevation of the white blood cell count, increasing numbers of myelocytes are seen. Promyelocytes and myeloblasts may also appear. Abnormally large platelets may be seen, particularly in the presence of thrombocythemia and intact large circulating megakaryocytes may be found in the peripheral blood. The neutrophil alkaline phosphatase score is elevated in the majority of cases of myelofibrosis and may be of aid in the differentiation of this disease from chronic myelocytic leukemia. However, about a fifth of the patients with myelofibrosis have diminished neutrophil alkaline phosphatase activity, usually at levels somewhat higher than the neutrophil scores of chronic myelocytic leukemia.[279] Mitus et al.[280] related the low enzyme activity to the greater immaturity of the circulating white cell precursors in a group of patients with the low neutrophil alkaline phosphatase score. In a subsequent study on the surgically removed spleens of four patients with myelofibrosis, two of whom had a high neutrophil alkaline phosphatase score and two a low score, Mitus et al.[281] found greater cytologic immaturity of the granulocytic precursors, greater distortion of the splenic architecture, and a striking increase in fibrous tissue in spleens of the low score patients. They concluded that a low neutrophil alkaline phosphatase score was indicative of a more advanced myelofibrotic disease which on morphological and cytochemical grounds resembled chronic granulocytic leukemia.

b. Bone Marrow Findings

The conversion of the bone marrow into a fibrotic mass is the most dramatic histologic feature of myelofibrosis if not, perhaps, the primary pathogenetic event of idiopathic myelofibrosis. Fibrosis, of the marrow may occur as sequel of marrow injury by ionizing radiation,[282,283] toxic chemicals,[284] bacterial infection (notably tuberculosis), and metastatic carcinoma.[285,286] These secondary forms of myelofibrosis usually offer no difficulty in diagnosis. Of greater concern, in terms of diagnosis, is the marrow fibrosis that accompanies chronic granulocytic leukemic[287] and the acute leukemias, both myeloblastic[288] and lymphoblastic.[289] The cause of the fibrosis in idiopathic myelofibrosis and in chronic granulocytic leukemia is not known, but is presumed to be due to disordered proliferation of the fibroblasts similar to the disordered proliferation of the hemopoietic cell lines. Recent cytogenetic evidence does not support this speculation.[290,291] Jacobson et al.[290] studied a young woman, heterozygous for glucose-6-phosphate dehydrogenase deficiency, who was found to have myelofibrosis. The enzyme in the patient's red cells, white cells, and platelets was all of type A, whereas the enzyme in the cells of skin cultures and in fibroblast of marrow cultures consisted of both types A and B. They concluded that the proliferation of the hemopoietic cells in myelofibrosis is clonal and that the fibroblast reaction was a secondary phenomenon. Similarly, the fibroblasts obtained from culture of the marrow of patients with Ph positive chronic myelocytic leukemia were Ph negative.[291] Hoshi and Weiss[292] proposed, on the basis of their ultrastructural observations on saponin-induced myelofibrosis in the rabbit, that an injury to the wall of the vascular sinus is the basic lesion which leads to a defect in the marrow blood barrier, and hence, to a leucoerythroblastic blood picture and a diminished blood supply which sets the stage for the marrow necrosis and fibrosis. They also found the reemergence of hemopoietic foci in the fibroblastic areas. Lewis and Pegrum[293] found immune complexes both within the cytoplasm of phagocytic cells and the serum of patients with myelofibrosis. The basic lesion of myelofibrosis is proliferation of the three hemopoietic cell lines. The process begins with marked trilinear proliferation. Bone marrow examination at this time reveals a highly cellular specimen with almost complete absence of fat cells. Large clusters of red cell precursors can be seen throughout the section. The megakaryocytes are numerous and large and are frequently grouped. The neutrophils and their precursors are also increased but diffusely distributed. At this stage, the reticulin content of the marrow may be normal or slightly increased. As the marrow cellularity continues to increase the fat cells disappear. The marrow cell population remains unchanged and a diffuse increase of reticulum fibers is now evident. The sinusoids appear to be normal, but decrease in number as the capillaries increase. As the process continues the number of red cell elements declines; granulocytopoiesis tends to become more immature. The megakaryocytes remain prominently grouped in the fibrous tissue and in the sinusoids. Dense bundles of collagen and new bone form in apposition to the original trabeculae which retain their lamellar birefringence and can be distinguished from the nonbirefringent new bone by polarizing microscopy. Ultimately, the normal hemopoietic cells disappear to be replaced by reticulum cells, mast cells, lymphocytes, and fibroblasts. Dense collagen and reticulin fill the marrow spaces. The sinusoids dilate, a few fat cells reappear, and some blood forming cells may be found in the lumen of the sinuses. Bone tissue can occupy a large volume of the total marrow space.[281–284] The tempo of evolution of the lesion of myelofibrosis varies considerably between individuals and among different anatomical sites in the marrow of the same individual. The lesions tend to start in the flat bones and gradually extend into the yellow marrow of the long bones.[294–297]

The clinical cause of idiopathic myelofibrosis is quite variable. In the majority of patients the disease progresses slowly leading finally to a transfusion-dependent anemia, thrombocytopenia, and elevated white blood cell counts with many immature forms. Death is usually due to an intercurrent infection, bleeding, or cardiac failure. In a minority of patients, perhaps 5 to 10%, transformation to an acute myeloblastic leukemia occurs.[298,299] Conversion of myelofibrosis to chronic myelocytic leukemia is probably not part of the natural history of the disease. Tumors of extramedullary hematopoiesis, often as extension of the bone marrow into adjacent tissues, may develop, and such tumors arising from the vertebral marrow may compress the spinal cord or nerve trunks.[300]

The possibility of an acute variant of myelofibrosis was offered by Lewis and Szur[301] to describe an illness characterized by pancytopenia, circulating blast cells, marked fibrosis of the bone marrow with increased numbers of megakaryocytes, and a rapid fatal course. Whether indeed, malignant myelosclerosis is a variant of idiopathic myelofibrosis[302–304] or an unusual presentation of acute myeloblastic leukemia with marked fibrosis of the marrow has not been resolved.[305,306] Bearman et al.[307] concluded from their experience and from a review of the literature that acute myelofibrosis can be distinguished on clinical and pathological grounds. They characterized the marrow of such patients as hyperplastic with prominent increase in reticulin and immaturity of the cells in all hemopoietic lines. Confusion is further compounded by reports of the conversion of both chronic myelocytic leukemia and myelofibrosis into an acute micromegakaryoblastic leukemia in which numerous small and large megakaryocytes are present in the bone marrow, associated with an increase in reticulin.[308–310]

4. *Chronic Myelocytic Leukemia*

The disease begins insidiously. It is sometimes discovered fortuitously in an asymptomatic patient whose neutrophil counts have been found to be unexpectedly high with slight shifts toward immaturity of the cells. There has been little opportunity to study such patients in detail. In our own experience, the initial neutrophil counts of such asymptomatic patients were in the range of 12 to 15,000 cells/mm^3 of which 5 to 15% were metamyelocytes. Splenomegaly was not detected, but the bone marrow was invariably hyperplastic with an increase in the M/E ratio to 8 to 10:1. The percentage of metamyelocytes and myelocytes was slightly increased and the cells appeared morphologically normal. The neutrophil alkaline phosphatase scores were frequently low. The marrow resembled the reactive marrow response of the neutrophilia seen in infection, but was generally more cellular.

After a variable period of time, from a few months to a year or more from the onset of the illness, the neutrophil counts approach 80 to 100,000 cells/mm^3. The metamyelocytes comprise 25 to 35% of the total count and a small number of myelocytes make their appearance. Anemia may or may not be present, but the patients are often symptomatic as a result of their highly hypermetabolic state. Thrombocytosis is frequently present. The spleen is usually enlarged. The bone marrow is highly cellular with almost complete disappearance of fat. The M/E ratio is very high, upward of 10 to 30 or more to one due in large measure to the marked expansion of the granulocytes, but also to a concommitant decrease in the red cell precursors. The myelocyte compartment is considerably enlarged; the number of promyelocytes and blast cells is modestly increased.

With advancing disease, untreated, the neutrophil count may rise to levels well above 200,000 cells/mm^3. Anemia is almost always present; the spleen is enlarged further; and the patients are highly symptomatic. The peripheral blood smears now resemble smears prepared from bone marrow aspirates; the myelocytes reach 20 to 30% of the myeloid population. A small number of promyelocytes and blast cells are also present. Treatment produces a considerable reduction in the granulocyte population, a return or erythropoiesis in the marrow, a reduction in spleen size, and marked improvement in the patient's well being. A conversion to normal marrow is usually not accomplished; moderate hypercellularity and increased M/E ratios remain, and the neutrophil alkaline phosphatase scores tend to remain low.

Despite treatment chronic myelocytic leukemia proceeds inexorably to greater immaturity of the granulocytic precursors. The blast cells increase strikingly, often existing in groups or sheets. The megakaryocytes are filled with PAS positive debris and may resemble the typical Gaucher cells.[311] The reticulin fibers in the marow may now be quite prominent, as the reticulin fibers increase steadily with the progression of the disease. This late stage of chronic myelocytic leukemia has been designated by Gralnick et al. as the accelerated phase.[312] The peripheral blood picture mirrors in many respects the bone marrow smears. Smears prepared from the simultaneous bone marrow and splenic aspirates are almost identical.

The terminal phase of chronic myelocytic leukemia is the blast crisis or metamorphosis. The marrow is hyperplastic, but completely replaced by blast cells. The normal hemopoietic elements have disappeared and the picture is now indistinguishable from acute leukemia. Blast cell crisis may occur at any time in the course of the illness but usually appears late about 2 to 5 years after the onset of the disease. It is now well established that the blast cell which appears in the blast cell transformation is most often of myeloid origin, in about 70% of cases, or of lymphoblastic origin. Indeed a mixed population of myeloblastic and lymphoblastic cells may exist in a single individual.[313–315] In general, chronic myelocytic leukemia runs its course in about 2 to 5 years, but its tempo does vary and atypical presentations are not unusual.[316]

The differential diagnosis of the leucoblastic response of the bone marrow, on purely morphological grounds between idiopathic myelofibrosis and chronic myelocytic leukemia, may indeed be difficult, and indeed has caused considerable confusion in the separation of these entities. Cell kinetic studies, though of considerable interest, have not been too useful in this regard. Current leukocyte labeling techniques are not easily applicable to the clinical situation and the results of such studies have been highly variable, depending on the stage of the illness.[317–319] In the Romanowsky stained smears the granulocytic cells in both chronic myelocytic leukemia and myelofibrosis do not differ much from normal. Bessis[320] however, states that morphological abnormalities do exist in chronic myelocytic leukemia best defined by electron microscopy but that "an experienced eye can detect many abnormalities, including clean cut evidence as asynchrony of nuclear cytoplasmic development" in a stained blood smear.

The neutrophil alkaline phosphatase activity is depressed in the great majority of cases of chronic granulocytic leukemia. A large percentage of patients with idiopathic myelofibrosis have high neutrophil phosphatase scores, and elevated scores are invariably present in the leukemoid reaction of infection, carcinoma, Hodgkin's disease, hemolysis, and polycythemia vera. The significance of these shifts in the neutrophil alkaline phosphatase has not been elucidated. The low neutrophil alkaline phosphatase activity of chronic granulocytic leukemia is probably not due to an absence of the enzyme or of the specific granules.[321] The granulocytic cells of the peripheral blood and bone marrow undergo maturation when cultured in diffusion chambers and previously negative cells do develop neutrophil alkaline phosphatase.[322] The question of whether the neutrophil alkaline phosphatase is related to the aging of the cell or to its physiologic maturation has still not been satisfactorily answered.[323–327]

The differentiation of chronic myelocytic leukemia from myelofibrosis should not be made solely on the morphological information gleaned from the bone marrow examination. Every effort should be made to obtain all of the necessary clinical and laboratory data that best define these disorders. The neutrophil alkaline phosphatase activity, though not pathognomonic of either condition, offers some aid in the evaluation of these disorders.

The Philadelphia chromosome is present in the granulocytic, erythrocytic, and thrombocytic precursors of the large majority of patients with chronic myelocytic leukemia and is absent in idiopathic myelofibrosis. The Philadelphia chromosome has been identified as chromosome number 22 whose long arms are missing and it is hence defined as 22,22q.[328] The missing material of chromosome 22 is translocated to the long arms of chromosome 9 (9q+). In about 8% of patients, the translocation may be to a chromosome other than 9.[329,330] The Philadelphia chromosome is not present in cultures of circulating lymphocytes or in the fibroblast cultures of marrow. It should be sought in metaphases of bone marrow cells or in the replicating precursor cells when present in blood. The Philadelphia chromosome is a highly characteristic marker for chronic myelocytic leukemia, though one must bear in mind that a small percentage of cases, perhaps 10 to 15% are negative for the Philadelphia chromosome. Thus, the presence of granulocyte hyperplasia of the marrow, a low neutrophil alkaline phosphatase score and the Philadelphia chromosome in the marrow cells are the most reliable criteria for the identification of chronic myelocytic leukemia.

5. *Acute Myeloblastic Leukemia*

Acute myeloblastic leukemia is characterized by the infiltration of blood and marrow by abnormal early granulocytic precursors. Though the predominant cells are granulocytic in origin, abnormalities of differentiation of erythrocytic, monocytic, and megakaryocytic precursors are frequently present in the bone marrows of patients with acute myeloblastic leukemia. The disease is presumed to originate in the pluripotential stem cell, thus accounting for its varied morphologic expression and its overlap between the different hemopoietic cell lines.[331]

The recognition of acute leukemia by examination of the traditional Romanowsky stained smears of blood and marrow is usually fairly straightforward. The marrow is generally hyperplastic, almost completely replaced by blast cells, atypical by virtue of nuclear cytoplasmic asynchronism at the expense of the erythrocytic and megakaryocytic precursors. However, the attempt to identify the ancestral lines of the leukemic blasts or their variants from the Giemsa stained smear alone may be frustrating and frequently requires the concerted application of cytochemical, cytogenetic, histological, ultrastructural, and immunologic technics for the successful solution of the task. Despite the greatly expanded armamentarium of sophisticated techniques, the blast cells of a small, possibly 2 to 5% group of patients with acute leukemia defy precise categorization and remain unclassifiable.

The myeloblasts of acute myeloblastic leukemia have all the characteristics of young cells, that is a large nucleus and nuclear/cytoplasmic ratio. Two to four nucleoli occupy a considerable volume of the nucleus. The cells may be small or large, and show considerable heterogeneity of nuclear shape. Cytoplasmic basophilia may be modest or abundant and a few azurophilic granules may be present.

Auer bodies are small rod- or needle-shaped structures in the cytoplasm of leukemic cells, generally under one μm in length. They are azurophilic and considered highly specific for acute myeloblastic or monocytic leukemia. They are found in about 1 to 5% of the cells examined.[48] The rods, like the azurophilic granules, stain for peroxidase and contain, as do the granules, both neutral and basic proteins and hence are thought to arise from fusion of the azurophilic granules. Ultrastructural studies of the Auer bodies have revealed a crystalline structure with apparently varying periodicity.[332–337] Tulliez and Breton-Gorius[338] concluded from their studies on the Auer bodies of ten cases of acute myeloblastic leukemia that three types of Auer bodies exist. In promyelocytic leukemia the Auer bodies consisted of a hexagonal arrangement of hollow tubes. In acute myeloblastic leukemia the Auer bodies consisted of a regular linear arrangement of protein with well-defined periodicity. A third type of Auer body, consisting of large granules containing many micro-Auer bodies was found in a subclass of acute myeloblastic leukemia with giant inclusions. The authors suggested that the Auer bodies may be heterogeneous structures of which type I may be uniquely related to the coagulopathy associated with acute promyelocytic leukemia.[339–341]

A unique ellipsodal particle, the so-called Phi body, with peroxidase activity has been found to be exclusively present in the cytoplasm of the blast cells of acute myeloblastic leukemia.[333,334] The Phi body was originally observed in the course of cytochemical investigations of the peroxisomes in mouse salivary glands. The spindle-shaped structures were found to be crystalloid in character. It was postulated that they arose from spherical microbodies which became ellipsoidal as a result of the internal pressures exerted by the developing crystalloid. It was also suggested that the azurophilic granules may transform into Phi bodies and that these bodies may be responsible for the Auer rods.[342] Hanker et al.[343] found Phi bodies in 33 of 36 patients with active acute myeloblastic leukemia. The Phi bodies were not observed in nine patients with acute lymphoblastic leukemia and in six patients with the blast crisis of chronic myelocytic leukemia. The Phi bodies disappeared in five patients who achieved a full clinical remission only to reappear when the patients relapsed. The Phi bodies were also demonstrated in the leucocytes obtained from the gingiva, vagina, and cerebrospinal fluid of leukemic subjects, and hence these bodies may serve as a useful marker for the detection of cells in the sancutary areas. In the patients studied by Hanker et al.[343] Auer rods were observed in the Romanowsky stained smears infrequently and with great difficulty.

In 1976 a classification of the acute leukemias was formulated by the French-American-British (FAB) cooperative group as a basis for the more precise categorization of these patients for study.[344,345] The classification was based on the traditional morphological characteristics of the Romanowsky stained films of blood and marrow, supplemented by the application of certain cytochemical reactions.

The myeloid leukemias were separated into six main groups (M_1 to M_6) categorized by the direction of differentiation along one or more cell lines and the degree of maturation of the cells. The patients in groups M_1, M_2, M_3 showed predominantly granulocytic differentiation and differed only in the degree of maturation of their cells. In group M_4 differentiation proceeded along both granulocytic and monocytic lines; group M_5 predominantly monocytic and M_6 predominantly erythroblastic. The further application of immunochemical markers and ultrastructural examination has assisted greatly in the more precise categorization of these disorders.[346,347]

a. Myeloblastic Leukemia Without Maturation (M_1)

The bone marrow is heavily infiltrated with nongranular blast cells which contain one or more nucleoli. A small number of the blast cells, about 3% may contain azurophilic granules or an Auer rod. On electron microscopic examination, the cells show dilated, rough endoplasmic reticulum, and rare primary granules. Maturation does not proceed beyond the blast phase.

b. Myeloblastic Leukemia with Maturation (M_2)

The cells are now typically granulocytic by conventional, cytochemical, or ultrastructural examination. About 50% of the cells are myeloblasts and promyelocytes. The promyelocytes contain many azurophilic granules. The cells usually contain nucleoli and varying amounts of cytoplasm. Single Auer rods may be present. Sudan black B stains are often helpful in identifying the granulocytic cells and the Auer rods. The esterase stains may aid in distinguishing the myeloblasts from monocytes. The polymorphonuclear cells may resemble Pelger-Huet cells; they may lack peroxidase activity; and they may appear to be free of granules.

c. Hypergranular Promyelocytic Leukemia (M_3)

The promyelocytes of acute promyelocytic leukemia draw immediate attention by their strikingly heavy granulation which fills the moderately abundant blue cytoplasm. The nuclei are round to oval, sometimes bilobed or reniform with several prominent nucleoli. The granules are large, coarse, and azurophilic. Fine dust-like granules are present in some cells. Auer rods are frequent, often stacked in bundles or in a mesh. Electron microscopy reveals numerous dilated cisternae containing electron dense material as well as the characteristic azurophilic granules and Auer rods. More than 35 to 40% of the bone marrow cells are abnormal promyelocytes. Bleeding and disseminated intravascular coagulation are common in these patients, particularly in those patients with promyelocyte concentrations in the marrow greater than 50%.[348]

Evidence has accumulated to suggest a close association between acute promyelocytic leukemia (M_3) with a specific chromosome translocation involving chromosomes 15 to 17 [t (15q+;17q−)].[349–354] This chromosome abnormality has not been observed in other leukemic states and is present in approximately 90% of patients with acute promyelocytic leukemia;[353] but other studies indicate an uneven geographical distribution of the anomaly.[354] Golomb et al.[355] reported on three patients with acute leukemia whose clinical course was complicated by disseminated intravascular coagulation and whose blast cells showed reniform and bilobed nuclei and dust-like granules. On electron microscopic examination the blast cells were found to contain many small granules, less than 250 nm in diameter and extremely dilated rough endoplasmic reticulum. Since the 15:17 translocation was demonstrated in all of the patients, Golomb et al.[355] suggested that these patients constituted a distinct subset of acute promyelocytic leukemia which they designated as microgranular.

Similar experiences have been reported by other observers.[345,356] The variant has been recognized and incorporated into the FAB classification of the leukemias.[357] Because of its reniform or bilobed nucleus and paucity of cytoplasmic granules on light microscopy the "microgranular" blast cell may be confused with the monoblast, and in some instances the micrograngular blast was reported to give a positive esterase reaction.[358] Electron microscopy and cytogenetic studies may prove to be indispensable techniques for the identification of the M_3-variant. In general, the M_3-variant has a higher leucocyte count, about 200×10^9 cells/per liter, than the classical acute promyelocytic leukemia.

d. Myelomonocytic Leukemia (M_4)

In the myelomonocytic leukemias differentiation along both granulocytic and monocytic lines is evident and the proportion of monocytes and promonocytes exceeds 20% of the nucleated cells of the marrow. Specific cytochemical reactions and ultrastructural examinations are often necessary to aid in the identification of the monocytes. The myelomonocytic leukemias have been further subdivided into:

Monocytic poorly differentiated leukemia (M_{5a})—Again, confirmation of the monocytic character of the cells by the cytochemical fluoride-inhibited esterase reaction and ultrastructural examination is required. The marrow in the condition is completely replaced by monoblasts which have an abundant basophilic cytoplasm with one or more pseudopodial buds and rare azurophilic granules. The nucleus has a lacy chromatin pattern and large prominent nucleoli.

Differentiated monocytic leukemia (M_{5b})—The predominant bone marrow cell in this subset of monocytic leukemia is the promonocyte accompanied by both monoblasts and monocytes. The promonocyte has a large nucleus with condensed chromatin and a slightly basophilic cytoplasm with abundant fine azurophilic granules.

An occasional Auer rod may be present in the monocytic leukemias. The granulocytic compartment is quite small, rarely more than 10% of the nucleated cells of the marrow. The close association of granulocytic and monocytic differentiation is highlighted by a report on the induction of differentiation of promyelocytes from acute promyelocytic leukemia into monocyte macrophages by phorbolester tumor promoters.[359]

e. Erythroleukemia (M_6)

The bone marrow in erythroleukemia is principally erythroid, the M/E ratio ranging from 1:1–1:3. The red cell precursors are frankly megaloblastic. Myeloblasts and promyelocytes make up 30% or more of the nucleated red cells. Early in the illness the percentage of myeloblasts and promyelocytes may be quite low and a diagnosis of leukemia may be difficult to validate. With progression of the disease the myeloblast population increases, the erythroid cells decrease and the marrow picture assumes the more typical aspects of myeloblastic leukemia (M_1,M_2) or myelomonocytic leukemia (M_4).

The following cytochemical studies should be routinely employed in addition to the Romanowsky stain in the evaluation of the marrow and blood of the patient suspected of having acute leukemia: Sudan black B or myeloperoxidase, esterase with fluoride inhibition, periodic acid-Schiff-hematoxylin (PAS). The myeloblasts and promyelocytes are typically positive for Sudan black B and myeloperoxidase, and of particular importance in distinguishing these cells from the blast cells of acute lymphoblastic leukemia. The myeloblasts give a diffuse reaction with PAS and a positive reaction with naphthol AS or ASD-acetate esterase reaction (NASDA) unaffected by exposure to sodium fluoride. The monoblasts and promonocytes also react positively with NASDA, but the reaction is inhibited by sodium fluoride. The erythroblasts normally do not stain with esterase or PAS stains. However, the erythroblasts of erythroleukemia may give a positive PAS reaction. The lymphoblasts of acute lymphoblastic leukemia are typically negative when stained for lipid (Sudan black), myeloperoxidase and esterase, but the cells do demonstrate, following PAS staining, a positive granular reaction without diffuse staining. The bone marrow biopsy permits more precise evaluation of the marrow cellularity than does the marrow aspirate, and its use in the diagnosis of leukemia and lymphoma has been considerably enhanced by improved techniques of fixation, plastic embedding, and application of cytochemical and traditional staining procedures.[360] The improved histological preparations provide another dimension in the total evaluation of the marrow disorders.

For a review of the earlier literature on the fine structure and cytochemistry of the acute leukemia see Reference 361.

IV. EOSINOPHIL

A. Morphology and Nature of the Granule

The eosinophil is readily distinguished from the neutrophilic and basophilic granulocytes by its large acidophilic granules, a property of their rich arginine content.[362] The evidence suggest that the eosinophil, in common with the other granulocytes, originates from an early premyeloblastic cell rather than from a common granulocytic precursor with undifferentiated granules.[3,7,11,363–366]

The mature eosinophil is larger than the neutrophil, about 12 to 17 μm in diameter.[367] Its nucleus is most often bilobed, showing less lobulation than the neutrophilc nucleus,[368] and its cytoplasm contains more ribosomes, vesicles, and more fully developed Golgi complex as well as more and larger mitochondria, but fewer and larger granules.[369] The eosinophil viewed with the aid of the scanning electron microscope is a spherical cell whose surface is covered by microvilli which possess no distinguishing characteristics.[370]

The specific granules of the eosinophil possess a highly characteristic ultrastructure both in man and in the common laboratory animal. In general, the eosinophil granule has been described as a membrane-bound structure in which one or more crystalloid inclusions are imbedded. The crystal, the internum or core of the eosinophilic granule, is reported to be a cubic lattice with a repeat of about 30 Å in rodents, and about 40 Å in man.[371–373] The core protein is an arginine-rich, basic protein with an approximate molcular weight of 11,000 daltons. This major basic protein accounts for more than 50% of the granule's protein content and is responsible for the highly characteristic acidophilic staining property of the cell. A second population of smaller, homogeneous appearing granules are about one fifth to one third the size of the specific granules and react positively for arylsulfatase and acid phosphatase.[373,375]

The early eosinophilic granules appear as large homogeneous electron-dense bodies in the promyelocytes of the human and rabbit bone marrow. At the myelocyte stage of development crystals appear and two morphologically distinct granules can be identified. With increasing maturation of the cell the number of granules lacking crystals decreases markedly. Bainton and Farquhar[376] believe that these differences in granule structure represent differences in granule type, whereas Hardin and Spicer[377] consider the crystalloid granule as a more mature form of the larger homogenous granule. On further maturation to the metamyelocyte state increasing numbers of micrograules appear and are thought to be morphologically and cytochemically distinct.[378]

In a study of the leucocytes of the rat bone marrow by electron microscopy and peroxidase cytochemistry, Bentfield et al.[379] demonstrated peroxidase reaction product in the rough endoplasmic reticulum, the Golgi complex, and in the cytoplasmic granules of the immature cells of the neutrophils, eosinophils, basophils, and the monocytes. In the fully mature neutrophils and monocytes two distinct populations of peroxidase positive and peroxidase negative granules were present. In the mature eosinophil all of the granules were peroxidase positive. Observations on the basophil were uncertain.

The contents of the isolated granules of the rat and the horse eosinophil have been examined by Archer and Hirsch.[380] They identified a number of lysosomal enzymes in the extracted protein of the eosinophilic granule. On disruption of the granules, cathepsin, ribonuclease, arylsulfatase, and beta-glucuronidase were released in soluble form, while acid and alkaline phosphatase were only partially solubilized. The peroxidase activity remained in the insoluble debris of the granules.

Archer et al.[381] subsequently extracted and partially purified a hemoprotein with the spectral properties of a peroxidase from rat eosinphils. The peroxidase was found to be distinct from the peroxidase of the neutrophil, but similar to the peroxidase of milk and horseradish. Thus, though the eosinophil and neutrophil arise from a common progenitor cell a separate genetic control of peroxidase synthesis is suggested.

Eosinophilic peroxidase and neutrophilic myeloperoxidase can be distinguished immunologically.[381] Strikingly, the eosinophils in patients with hereditary myeloperoxidase deficiency contain abundant peroxidase, though the enzyme is completely absent in the neutrophils and the monocytes.[179,382,383] The reverse situtation has been described in which the eosinophil peroxidase is absent in the face of continued peroxidase activity in the neutrophils and the monocytes.[181,384,385] The speculation has also been raised that the eosinophilic peroxidase may reside in the core of the granule, or that, indeed, the granule crystal may be crystallized peroxidase protein. This hypothesis has not been supported by combined ultrastructural and cytochemical studies.[46,60,386]

Further investigations on the contents of the eosinophilic granule have revealed that the eosinophil lacks lysozyme and that the small amount of alkaline phosphatase which had been found on biochemical analysis of the isolated eosinophil granule is due to contamination by neutrophils.[387] Williams et al.[387] have been able to demonstrate alkaline phosphatase reaction product on the outer surface of eosinophils obtained from the peritoneal exudate of rats. A similar localization of alkaline phosphatase reaction product has been reported for human polymorphonuclear leucocytes.[388]

The eosinophil is relatively rich in histaminase, kininase, arylsulfatase, and phospholipase D; enzymes which have the potential to inactivate important mediators of inflammation.[389–391] The eosinophil surface possesses unique sites to which specific antisera can be directed. Receptors for the Fc portion of IgG and for C_3 have been detected on 10 to 50% of eosinophils from normal subjects.[392–396] The presence of the receptors may reflect the level of maturation of these cells.

Thus, though the eosinophil and the neutrophil arise from a common precursor, the two cells differ significantly from each other in structure, cell surface characteristics, in some elements of their enzyme content, their metabolic activity, and life span.[397–399] Of further interest in this regard, is the report of L'Esperance et al.[208] describing eosinophilia in a patient with congenital neutropenia. Further, colonies arising in cultures from the ''lymphocyte'' fraction of human peripheral blood are either neutrophilic or eosinophilic; mixed cultures were not seen.[340]

B. Kinetics

Eosinophil kinetics mirrors much of what has been described for the neutrophil but has been more difficult to investigate because of the relatively small size of the eosinophil population. In the marrow one can identify a proliferative pool of promyelocytes and myelocytes and postmitotic nonproliferative pool of metamyelocytes and mature eosinophils. About 50 to 70% of the eosinophils in the marrow are in the mature postmitotic reserve pool.[401]

The cell cycle time of the rat eosinophilic precursor is about 22 to 23 hr; the marrow transit time is approximately 5 to 6 days.[402] Both the transit time and the cell cycle time are shortened in the presence of an experimental trichinella infection. The marrow transit time of the eosinophil in man has been estimated at about three days.[403,404] Like the neutrophil, the residence time of the eosinophil in the blood is quite brief with a half-time clearance of 3 to 8 hr,[405] but lengthened in the hypereosinophilic syndrome to 44 hr.[406] Eosinophils circulate, marginate, are capable of demargination, recirculation, further maturation in the spleen, and finally egress into tissues.[407–409]

The eosinophils may be found in tissues, notably lung, intestinal tract, skin, and uterus in abundant numbers.[410] The blood marrow ratio of eosinophils in the guinea pig has been estimated at 1:400, and for man at 1:100.[411] The eosinophil can apparently survive in tissues for several days[412] where they are either removed by macrophages[413] or shed into the respiratory or intestinal tracts.[414,415]

The normal human marrow contains more eosinophils than any other tissue or organ, though these cells represent but a minor population estimated at about 4% of the total granulocytes of the marrow.[416] The eosinophils also constitute about 4% of the circulating granulocytes. An increased peripheral demand for eosinophils is met by an expansion of the eosinophil population in the marrow. The eosinophils in the marrow can increase some eight- to ten-fold within the normal range of marrow granulocyte cellularity.[417]

C. Eosinophilia

Reactive blood eosinophilia is commonly seen in association with allergic hypersensitivity states, parasitic infections, tumors, pruritic skin eruptions, etc. It is accompanied usually by a more prominent marrow eosinophilia. In general, the mature and less mature eosinophils increase simultaneously in the marrow and few eosinophilic promyelocytes are found. The marrow eosinophil response usually precedes the blood eosinophilia and subsides before the blood eosinophil counts return to normal. The percentage of eosinophils in the marrow parallels the percentage of eosinophils in the blood throughout the period of eosinophilia, but prominent marrow eosinophilia may be encountered with normal or modestly elevated eosinophil counts. Eosinophils with mixed acidophilic and basophilic granules are frequently found in the marrow smears in the presence of reactive eosinophilia. Such blue-gray granules are seen occasionally in eosinophils of normal human marrow and probably do not represent a maturation disturbance.

Studies on the regulation of eosinophil production have perforce been carried out in animal models utilizing tetanus toxoid, trichinella, or schistosomal antigens for the eosinophilic stimulus. These studies have clearly demonstrated a central role for the thymus-derived lymphocytes in the eosinophil accumulations. Evidence has also been presented to suggest the existence of a specific humoral factor which can stimulate eosinophil production. The hypothesis has therefore been projected that the T lymphocytes, in response to an appropriate antigen, release a lymphokine which is an eosinophilopoietin and can stimulate the proliferation of the marrow eosinophils.[418–422]

Eosinophilia is also seen in association with infiltrative lesions in such organs as the stomach, intestines, prostate, or skin but more frequently in the lung in the form of the more benign Loeffler's syndrome or the more severe chronic eosinophilic pneumonia. These disorders are characterized by local tissue accumulations of eosinophils with or without concommittant blood eosinophilia. The marrow invariably responds dramatically to steroid adminstration.

1. The Hypereosinophilic Syndrome

An uncommon, progressive, and sometimes fatal eosinophilic syndrome associated with pulmonary and cardiac abnormalities, neurologic lesions, lymphadenopathy, and hepatosplenomegaly has been recognized and described as eosinophilic leukemia, or disseminated eosinophilic collagen disease.[423–425] The peripheral blood and the marrow eosinophil appear to be morphologically normal. The marrow is hyperplastic with an increase in the myeloid elements, but predominantly eosinophilic. The argument concerning the leukemic or nonleukemic nature of the illness has not been resolved. Chromosomal abnormalities have been detected and presented as evidence for the malignant nature of the syndrome.[426]

The major basic protein of guinea pig eosinophils are cytotoxic and can injure or kill schistosomules,[427] murine ascites tumor cells, and newborn larvae of trichinella.[428] The major basic protein can also injure cells from the intestine, skin, trachea, etc. and in concentrations that are found in tissues infiltrated with eosinophils in disease.[429] This mechanism may be responsible for the cardiac damage in the hypereosinophilic syndrome. Eosinophils have also been known to be neutrotoxic.[430]

V. BASOPHIL

A. Morphology

The basophil is the smallest of the granulocytic cells averging about 10 to 12 μm in diameter, but a smaller population of cells averaging 6 to 8 μm may also be seen in human blood and tissue. The basophil is readily distinguished in the Romanowsky stained smears of blood and marrow by their dense population of large blue-black granules. Basophils exhibit sluggish mobility and advance by moving the nucleus forward rather than the cytoplasm. The basophil nucleus is either band or bilobed.

The basophil is also the least common of the human granulocytes. They represent but 0.8% of the blood granulocytes and about 0.3% of the marrow granulocytic cells.[431] More accurate chamber counts give values of about 40 to 70 cells per mm^3 for normal human blood.[429] There appears to be a striking inverse relationship between the number of basophils and mast cells in the different species. Thus, rats and mice are extremely rich in tissue mast cells but are strikingly deficient in basophils.[433]

On an ultrastructural examination,[434,435] the human basophil contains abundant glycogen and the characteristically large round or oval granules, about 1.2 μm in their largest dimension, in its cytoplasm. Each granule is filled with particles of fairly uniform size which are fairly uniform in any given granule but vary in size in different granules of the same cell. The largest of the intragranular particles is about 200 Å in diameter and randomly distributed in the center of the granules. The granule is surrounded by a unit membrane beneath which a few rows of the particles are arranged in concentric fashion. A fairly large number of fibers, 100 to 150 Å in diamter, are present in the cytoplasm arranged in bundles or in criss-cross patterns. Hastie[434] described tubulovesicular structures on the basophil surface, myelin figures both in and adjacent to the granule; and the presence of Charcot-Leyden-like crystals in the granules, and proposed the existence of a second class of granules. The ultrastructural characteristic of the basophil granule varies with the species. The guinea pig granule may show a banded pattern, hexagonal array or a rectangular lattice.[436]

Basophils are produced in the bone marrow in a manner comparable to the other granulocytes. In all probability a committed basophil precursor is responsible for the basophilic line of cells, but supportive evidence for this proposal has been meager.[437,438] Both by light and by electron microscopic examination, the specific basophilic first appears in the myelocyte. The granules arise in the Golgi region of the early myelocyte, appear first as small vacuoles which pinch off from the cisternae. By a process of fusion the small vesicular granules coalesce to form large granules whose internal contents condense and form a filamentous array.[439]

The major biochemical components of the basophilic granule are histamine, lipoprotein, and an acid mucopolysaccharide thought to represent heparin. Basophils release on degranulation a low-molecular weight protein (about 1100 daltons) which can activate platelet aggregation. The proteins of the basophilic granules lack hydrolytic enzymes.[440–443]

The tissue mast cell has been considered closely related to the basophil in its acidic nature, metachromasia, and content of histamine and heparin. Structural differences in the granules and the presence of proteolytic enzymes in the mast cells have served to separate these two cell types. Recently, evidence has been presented for the bone marrow origin of the tissue mast cells.[444,445] Zucker-Franklin[446] described cells in the peripheral blood of two patients with chronic myelocytic leukemia and one with agnogenic myeloid metaplasia which possessed the characteristic ultrastructural features of both basophils and mast cells and proposed a common origin and close kinship for the two cells.

Basophil production may be regulated by a basophil-stimulating factor derived from T lymphocytes on stimulation by specific antigens.[447] Utilizing a guinea pig model for basophilia[448] Denburg, Davison, and Bienenstuck[447] derived data in support of the existence of a basophilopoietin.

B. Basophilia

In certain inflammatory states, the tissue basophils are believed to be increased. Thus, basophils are reported to accumulate on the cover slips of a Rebuck window in patients with ulcerative colitis, regional ilieitis, and interstitial cystitis.[449] Blood basophilia is not usually found in ulcerative colitis. Information on bone marrow response in these disorders is surprisingly scanty. Blood basophilia has been described in hypersensitivity states and in myxedema. The highest levels of circulating basophils are usually associated with chronic myelocytic leukemia and agnogenic myeloid metaplasia. The basophils appear mature and few immature basophils are present both in blood and marrow. Dvorak et al.[450] reported on a patient with chronic myelocytic leukemia who developed a picture of so-called basophilic leukemia with 85% basophils in his peripheral blood. The basophils were mature but showed on electron microscopy striking evidence of degranulation in the form of fused granules (anaphylactic type of degranulation) and the formation of pinocytotic vesicles and vacuoles.[443] This type of degranulation was not reported by Zucker-Franklin in her study of the basophils in chronic myelocytic leukemia.[446] Knowledge of the physiological marrow response to the demand for basophils in tissues or of the proliferative abnormalities of the basophils in pathological states is still quite fragmentary.

REFERENCES

1. **Naegeli, O.,** Ueber rotes Knochenmark und Myeloblasten, *Dtsch. Med. Wochenschr.*, 3, 287, 1900.
2. **Bainton, D. F.,** Differentiation of human neutrophilic granulocytes: normal and abnormal, in *Prog. Clin. Biol. Res.*, 13, 1, 1977.
3. **Bessis, M.,** *Living Blood Cells and Their Ultrastructure*, Springer-Verlag, New York, 1973, 310.
4. **Wetzel, B. K., Horn, R. G., and Spicer, S. S.,** Fine structural studies on the development of heterophil, eosinophil and basophil granulocytes in the rabbit, *Lab. Invest.*, 16, 349, 1967.
5. **Wetzel, B. K.,** The comparative fine structural studies and cytochemistry of developing granulocytes with special reference to the rabbit, in *Regulation of Hematopoiesis*, Gordon, A.S., Ed., Appleton, New York, 1970, 819.
6. **Pease, D. C.,** An electron microscopic study of red bone marrow, *Blood*, 11, 501, 1956.
7. **Florey, H. W.,** Inflammation, in *General Pathology*, 3rd ed., Florey, H. W., Ed., W. B. Saunders, and Philadephia, 1962, 68.
8. **Bessis, M. and Thiery, J. P.,** Electron microscopy of human white blood cells and their stem cells, in *International Review of Cytology*, Vol. 12, Bourne, G. H., 2nd Danielli, J. F., Eds., Academic Press, New York, 1961, 199.
9. **Horn, R. G. and Spicer, S. S.,** Sulfated mucopolysachardie and base proteins in certain granules of rabbit, *Lab Invest.*, 13, 1, 1964.

10. **Horn, R. G., Wetzel, B. K., and Spicer, S. S.,** Fine structural localization of nonspecific acid and alkaline phosphatases in rabbit meyloid elements, *J. Appl. Physics,* 34, 2517, 1963.
11. **Wetzel, B. K., Spicer, S. S., and Horn, R. G.,** Fine structural localization of acid and alkaline phosphatase in cells of rabbit blood and bone marrow, *J. Histochem. Cytochem.,* 15, 311, 1967.
12. **Capone, R. J., Weinreb, E. L., and Chapman, C. B.,** Electron microscopic studies of normal human myeloid elements, *Blood,* 23, 300, 1964.
13. **Bainton, D. F. and Farquhar, M. G.,** Origin of granules in polymorphonuclear leucocytes. Two types derived from opposite faces of the Golgi complex in developing granulocytes, *J. Cell. Biol.,* 28, 277, 1966.
14. **Bainton, D. F. and Farquhar, M. J.,** Differences in enzyme content of azurophilic and specific granules of polymorphonuclear leucocytes. II. Cytochemistry and electron microscopy of bone marrow cells, *J. Cell. Biol.,* 39, 299, 1968.
15. **Wetzel, B. K., Horn, R. G., and Spicer, S. S.,** Cytochemical localization of nonspecific phosphatase activity in rabbit myeloid elements, *J. Histochem. Cytochem.,* 11, 812, 1963.
16. **Jamieson, J. D. and Palade, G. E.,** Intracellular transport of secretory proteins in the pancratic exocrine cell. I. Role of the peripheral elements of the Golgi complex, *J. Cell. Biol.,* 34, 597, 1967.
17. **Carol, G. and Palade, G. E.,** Protein synthesis; storage and discharge in the pancreatic exocrine cell: an autoradiographic study, *J. Cell. Biol.,* 20, 473, 1964.
18. **Palade, G.,** Intracellular aspects of the process of protein synthesis, *Science,* 189, 347, 1975.
19. **Beams, H. W. and Kessel, R. G.,** The Golgi apparatus: structure and function, *Int. Rev. Cytol.,* 23, 259, 1968.
20. **Fedorko, M. E. and Hirsch, J. G.,** Cytoplasmic granule formation in myelocytes. An electron microscopic radioautographic study on the mechanism of formation of cytoplasmic granules in rabbit heterophilic myelocytes, *J. Cell, Biol.,* 29, 307, 1966.
21. **Young, R. W.,** The role of the Golgi complex in sulfate methabolism, *J. Cell. Biol.,* 57, 175, 1973.
22. **Bainton, D. F., Ullyot, J. L., and Farquhar, M. G.,** The development of neutrophilic polymorphonuclear leucocytes in human bone marrow, *J. Exp. Med.,* 136, 907, 1971.
23. **Breton-Gorius, J. and Guichard, J.,** Etude au microscope electronique de la localisation des peroxydases dans les cellules de la moelle osseuse humaine, *Nouv. Rev. Fr. Hematol.,* 9, 678, 1969.
24. **Ackerman, G. A. and Clark, M. A.,** Ultrastructural localization of peroxidase activity in normal human bone marrow cells, *Zellforsch, Mikroskop. Anat.,* 117, 463, 1971.
25. **Bainton, D. F.,** Differentation of human neutrophilic granulocytes: normal and abnormal, in *The Granulocytes: Function and Clinical Utilization,* Greenwalt, T.J. and Jamieson, G. A., Eds., Alan R. Liss, New York, 1977, 1.
26. **Murata, F. and Spicer, S. S.,** Morphological studies of rabbit heterophilic leucocytes and evidence for tertiary granules, *Lab. Invest.,* 29, 65, 1973.
27. **Brederoo, P. and Daems, W. T.,** The ultrastructure of guinea pig heterophil granulocytes and the heterogenity of the granules of the development in the bone marrow, *Cell Tissue Res.,* 194, 183, 1978.
28. **Breton-Gorius, J. and Reyes, F.,** Ultrastructure of human bone marrow cell maturation, *Int. Rev. Cytol.,* 46, 251, 1976.
29. **Scott, R. E. and Horn, R. G.,** Ultrastructural aspects of granulocyte development in humans, *Lab. Invest.,* 23, 202, 1970.
30. **Watanabe, Y. and Enomote, Y.,** Fine structure of human neutrophilic granulocytes and leukemic cells, in *Eighth International Congress of Electron Microscopy,* Vol. II, Sanders, J.V., Goodchild, V.J., Eds., Canberra, 1974, 416.
31. **Payne, D. N. and Ackerman, G. A.,** Tertiary granule formation in human developmental neutrophils revealed by S^{35} ultrastructural autoradiography, *J. Cell. Biol.,* 63, (Abstr.), 261, 1974.
32. **Cohn, Z. A. and Hirsch, J. G.,** The isolation and properties of the specific cytoplasmic granules of rabbit polymorphonuclear leucocytes, *J. Exp. Med.* 112, 983, 1960.
33. **Fedorko, M. E. and Morse, S. I.,** Isolation, characterization and distribution of acid mucopolysaccharides in rabbit leucocytes, *J. Exp. Med.,* 121, 39, 1965.
34. **Zeya, H. I. and Spitznagel, J. A.,** Antibacterial and enzymatic basic proteins from leucocytic lysosomes: separation and identification, *Science,* 112, 1085, 1963.
35. **Bagglioni, J., Hirsch, J. G., and DeDuve, C.,** Resolution of granules from rabbit heterophil leucocytes into distinct populations by zonal sedimentation, *J. Cell. Biol.,* 40, 529, 1969.
36. **Zeya, H. I. and Spitznagel, J. C.,** Characterization of cationic protein-bearing granules of polymorphonuclear leucocytes, *Lab, Invest.,* 24, 229, 1971.
37. **Bretz, U. and Baggiolini, M.,** Association of the alkaline phosphatase of rabbit polynorphonuclear leucocytes with the membrane on the specific granules, *J. Cell. Biol.,* 59, 696, 1973.

38. **Nachman, R., Hirsch, J. G., and Baggiolini, M.,** Studies on isolated membranes of neutrophil and specific granules from rabbit polymorphonuclear leucocytes, *J. Cell. Biol.,* 54, 133, 1972.
39. **Bainton, D. F., Nichols, B. A., and Farquhar, M. G.,** Primary lysosomes of blood leucocytes, *Frontiers Biol.,* 45, 3, 1976.
40. **Olsson, I.,** Isolation of human leucocyte granules using colloidal silicapolysaccharide density gradients, *Exp. Cell. Res.,* 54, 325, 1969.
41. **West, B. C., Rosenthal, A. S., Beib, A. N., and Kimball, H. R.,** Separation and characterization of human neutrophil granules, *Am. J. Pathol.,* 77, 41, 1974.
42. **Bretz, U. and Baggiolini, M.,** Biochemical and morphological characterization of azurophilic and specific granules of human neutrophilic polymorphonuclear leucocytes, *J. Cell. Biol.,* 63, 251, 1974.
43. **Avila, J. L. and Convit, J.,** Studies on human polymorphonuclear leucocytes. II. Comparative study of the physical properties of primary and specific granules, *Biochim. Biophys. Acta,* 293, 409, 1973.
44. **Spitznagel, J. K., Dalldorf, F. G., Leffel, M. S., et al.,** Character of azurophils and specific granules purified from human polymorphonuclear leukocytes, *Lab. Invest.,* 30, 774, 1974.
45. **Dewald, B., Rinkler-Ludwig, R., Bretz, U., and Baggiolini, M.,** Subcellular localization and heterogeneity of neutral proteases in neutrophilic polymorphonuclear leucocytes, *J. Exp. Med.,* 141, 709, 1975.
46. **Lichtman, M. A. and Weed, R. I.,** Alterations of cell periphery during granulocyte maturation and relationship to cell function, *Blood,* 39, 301, 1972.
47. **Ackerman, G. A. and Clark, M. A.,** A cytochemical evaluation of pyroantimonate binding to the plasmalemma of blood and bone marrow cells and its relationship to cellular maturation, *J. Histochem. Cytochem.,* 20, 880, 1972.
48. **Ackerman, G. A.,** Microscopic and histochemical studies on Auer bodies in leukemic cells, *Blood,* 5, 847, 1950.
49. **Ackerman, G. A.,** Ultrastructure and cytochemistry of the developing neutrophil. *Lab. Invest.,* 19, 299, 1968.
50. **Ackerman, G. A.,** Surface differeniation of hemopoietic cells demonstrated ultrastructurally with cationized ferritin, *Cell Tissue Res.,* 159, 23, 1975.
51. **Ackerman, G. A. and Waksal, S. D.,** Ultrastructural localization of concanavalin A binding sites on the surface of differentiating hemopoietic ells, *Cell Tissue Res.,* 150, 311, 1974.
52. **Parmley, R. T., Martin, B. J., and Spicer, S. S.,** Staining of blood cell surfaces with a lectin-horse radish peroxidase method, *J. Histochem. Cytochem.,* 21, 912, 1973.
53. **Henson, P. M.,** The adherence of leucocytes and platelets induced by fixed IgG antibody or complement, *Immunology,* 16, 107, 1969.
54. **Messner, R. P. and Jelinek, J.,** Receptors for human G globulin on human neutrophils, *J. Clin. Invest.,* 49, 2165, 1970.
55. **Wong, L. and Wilson, J. D.,** The identification of Fc and C3 receptors on human neutrophils, *J. Immunol. Meth.,* 7, 69, 1970.
56. **Williams, L. T., Synderman R., Pike, M. C. et al.,** Specific receptor sites for chemotactic peptides on human polymorphonuclear leucocytes, Proc. Natl.Acad. Sci. U.S.A.), 74, 1206, 1975.
57. **Malech, H. L., Roof, F. K., and Gallin, J. I.,** Structural analysis of human neutrophil migration: centriole, microtubule and microfilament orientation and function during chemotaxis, *J. Cell. Biol.,* 75, 606, 1977.
58. **Stossal, T. P. and Pollard, T. D.,** Myosin in polymorphonculear leucocyte, *J. Biol. Chem.* 248, 8228, 1973.
59. **Altman, A. J. and Stossel, T. P.,** Functional immaturity of bone marrow bands and polymorphonuclear leucocytes, *Br. J. Haematol.,* 27, 241, 1974.
60. **Cronkite, E. P., Fliedner, T. M., Rubini, J. R., et al.,** Dynamics of proliferating cell systems of man studied with tritiated thymidine, *J. Clin. Invest.,* 37, 887, 1958.
61. **Cronkite, E. P., Fliedner, T. M., Bond, V. P., et al.,** Dynamics of hemopoietic proliferation in man and mice studied by H^3Thymidine incorporation in DNA, in *Progress in Nuclear Energy,* series VI, Vol. 2, Biological Sciences, Pergamon Press, London, 1959.
62. **Cronkite, E. P., Bond, V. P., Fliedner, T. M., and Killman, S. A.,** The use of tritiated thymidine in the study of haemopoietic cell proliferation, in *Ciba Foundation Symposium on Haematopoiesis,* Wolstenholme, G.E.W. and O'Connor, M., Eds., Churchill, London, 1960.
63. **Mauer, A. M., Athens, V. W., Warner, H. R. et al.,** An analysis of leukocyte radioactivity curves obtained with radioactive diisopropylfluoro phosphate (DEP^{32}), in *The Kinetics of Cellular Proliferation,* Stohlman, F., Jr., Ed., Grune and Stratton, New York, 1959.
64. **Mauer, A. M., Athens, J. W., Aschenbrucker, H., et al.,** Leukokinetic studies, II. A method for labeling granulocytes in vitro with radioactive diisopropylfluorophate, *J. Clin. Invest.,* 39, 1481, 1960.

65. **McMillan, R. and Scott, J. L.,** Leucocyte labeling with ^{51}chromium. I. Technic and results in normal subjects, *Blood,* 32, 738, 1968.
66. **Dresch, D., Najean, Y., and Bauchet, J.,** *In vitro* ^{51}Ct and ^{32}P-DFP labeling of granulocytes in man, *J. Nucl. Med.,* 12, 774, 1971.
67. **Dresch, C., Najean, Y., and Bauchet, J.,** Kinetics studies of ^{51}Cr and ^{32}P-DFP labeled granulocytes, *Br. J. Haematol.,* 29, 67, 1972.
68. **Uchida, T. and Vincent, P. C.,** *In vitro* studies of leucocyte labeling with technecium 99m, *J. Nucl. Med.,* 17, 730, 1976.
69. **Uchida, T.,** Leukokinetics studies of peripheral blood, I. Neutrophilic granulocyte kinetics in normal man, *Acta Haematol. Jpn.,* 35, 164, 1971.
70. **McAffe, J. G. and Thakur, M. L.,** Survey of radioactive agents for *in vitro* labeling of phagocytic leukocytes, I. Soluble agents, *J. Nucl. Med.,* 17, 488, 1976.
71. **McAffe, J. G. and Thakur, M. L.,** Survey of radioactive agents for *in vitro* labeling of phagocytic leukocytes, II. Particles, *J. Nucl. Med.,* 17, 488, 1976.
72. **Pluznik, D. H. and Sachs, L.,** The cloning of normal "mast cells" in tissue culture, *J. Cell. Comp. Physiol.,* 66, 319, 1965.
73. **Bradley, T. H. and Metcalf, D.,** The growth of mouse bone marrow cells *in vitro, Aust. J. Exp. Biol. Med. Sci.,* 44, 287, 1966.
74. **Robinson, W. A. and Pike, B. L.,** Colony growth of human bone marrow cells *in vitro,* in *Hematopoietic Cellular Proliferation,* Stohlman, E., Jr., Ed., Grune and Stratton, New York, 1970.
75. **Bøyum, A. and Borgstrom, R.,** The concentration of granulocytic stem cells in mouse bone marrow, determined with diffusion chamber technique, *Scand. J. Haematol.,* 7, 294, 1970.
76. **Squires, D. J. P.,** The growth of human bone marrow in diffusion chambers, *Br. J. Haematol.,* 29, 89, 1975.
77. **Metcalf, D.,** Recent results in cancer research, in *Hematopoietic Colonies,* Springer-Verlag, New York, 1977.
78. **Till, J. E. and McCulloch, E. A.,** A direct measurement of the radiation sensitivity of normal mouse bone marrow cells, *Radiat. Res.,* 14, 213, 1961.
79. **McCulloch, E. A.,** Granulopoiesis in cell culture, *Clin. Haematol.,* 4, 509, 1975.
80. **Cronkite, E. P. and Vincent, P. C.,** Granulocytopoiesis, *Semin. Haematol.,* 4, 3, 1969.
81. **Wintrobe, M. M., Lee, R. E., Boggs, D. K., et al.,** *Clinical Hematology,* 7th ed., Lea & Febiger, Philadelphia, 1974.
82. **Donohue, D. M., Rieff, R. H., Hawson, M. L., et al.,** Quantitative measurement of the erthrocytic and granulocytic cells of the marrow and blood, *J. Clin. Invest.,* 37, 1571, 1958.
83. **Deubelbeiss, K. A., Dancey, J. T., Harker, L. A., and Finch, C. A,** Neutrophil kinetics of the dog, *J. Clin. Invest.,* 55, 833, 1975.
84. **Deubelbeiss, K. A., Dancey, J. T., Harker, L. A. et al.,** Marrow erythroid and neutrophil cellularity in the dog, *J. Clin. Invest.,* 55, 825, 1975.
85. **Dancey, J. T., Deubelbeiss, K. A., Harker, L. A., and Finch, C. A.,** Neutrophil kinetics in man, *J. Clin. Invest.,* 58, 705, 1976.
86. **Vincent, P. C.,** Granulocyte kinetics in health and disease, *Clin. Haematol.,* 6, 695, 1977.
87. **Finch, C. A., Harker, L. A., and Cook, J. D.,** Kinetics of the formed elements of human blood, *Blood,* 50, 699, 1977.
88. **Athens, J. W., Haab. O. P., Raab, S. O. et al.,** Leukokinetic studies, IV. The total blood circulating and marginal granulocyte pools and the granulocyte turnover rate on normal subjects, *J. Clin. Invest.,* 40, 989, 1961.
89. **Dale, D. C., Fauci, A. S., and Wolff, S. M.,** Alternate day prednisone leukocyte kinetics and susceptibility to infection, *N. Engl. J. Med.,* 291, 1154, 1974.
90. **Godwin, H. A., Zimmerman, T. S., Kimball, H. Y., et al.,** Effect of etiocholanolone on entry of granulocytes into peripheral blood, *Blood,* 31, 461, 1968.
91. **Vogel, J. M., Kimball, H. R., Wolff, S. M., and Perry, S.,** Etiocholanolone in the evaluation of marrow reserves in patients receiving cytotoxic agents, *Ann. Intern. Med.,* 67, 1226, 1967.
92. **Paulus, H. E., Okun, R., and Calabro, J. J.,** Immunosuppressive therapy, guidelines for drug dosage. Depression of bone marrow granulocyte reserves in systemic lupus erythrematous, *Arthritis Rhem.,* 15, 29, 1972.
93. **Fink, M. E. and Calabresi, P.,** The granulocyte response to endotoxin (pyrexal) as a measure of functional marrow reserve in cancer chemotherapy, *Ann. Intern. Med.,* 57, 732, 1962.
94. **Dale, D. C. and Wolff, S. M.,** Studies of the neutropenia of acute malaria, *Blood,* 41, 197, 1973.
95. **Dale, D. C., Fauci, A. S., Guerry, D. IV, and Wolff, S. M.,** Comparison of agents producing a neutrophilic leucocytosis in man, *J. Clin. Invest.,* 56, 808, 1975.

96. **Orfonakis, N. G., Ostland, R. G., Bishop, C. R., and Adams, J. W.,** Normal blood leukocyte concentration values, *Am. J. Clin. Pathol.*, 53, 647, 1970.
97. **Boggs, D. R.,** Physiology of neutrophil proliferation, maturation and circulation, *Clin. Haematol.*, 4, 535, 1975.
98. **Cartwright, G. E., Athens, J. E., and Wintrobe, M. M.,** The kinetics of granulopoiesis in normal man, *Blood,* 24, 78, 1964.
99. **Uchida, R.,** Leukokinetic studies in peripheral blood. I. Neutrophilic granulocyte kinetics in normal man, *Acta Haematol. Jpn.*, 34, 2, 1970.
100. **Uchida, T. and Kariyone, S.,** Organ distribution of the 99m Tc-labeled white cells, *Acta Haematol. Jpn.*, 36, 78, 1973.
101. **Vincent, P. C., Chanann, A. P., Cronkite, E. P., and Joel, D. D.,** The intravascular survival of neutrophils labeled *in vivo, Blood,* 43, 371, 1974.
102. **Naegeli, O.,** *Blutkrankheiten und Blutdiagnostic,* Springer-Verlag, Berlin, 1923, 217.
103. **Rebuck, J. W. and Crowley, J. H.,** A method of studying leukocyte function *in vivo, Ann. N.Y. Acad. Sci.*, 59, 757, 1955.
104. **Cronkite, E. P.,** Granulocytes and their production and role in defense against bacterial infection, in *Best and Taylor's Physiological Basic of Medical Practice,* 10th ed., Brobeck J., Ed., Williams and Wilkins, Baltimore, 1979.
105. **Cronkite, E. P.,** Kinetics of granulocytopoiesis, *Clin. Haematol.*, 8, 351, 1979.
106. **Januar, M. and Cronkite, E. P.,** Do granulocytes normally enter tissues in pathogen-free animals? *Clin. Haematol.*, 8, 367, 1979.
107. **Keller, H. U., Hess, M. W., and Cotter, H.,** Physiology of chemotaxis and random motility, *Semin. Hematol.*, 12, 47, 1975.
108. **O'Flaherty, J. T. and Ward, P. A.,** Chemotaxis factors and the neutrophil, *Semin. Hematol.*, 16, 163, 1979.
109. **Allison, A. C. and Davies, P.,** Mechanisms of endocytosis and exocytosis, *Proc. Soc. Exp. Biol. Med.*, 28, 419, 1974.
110. **Stossel, T. P. and Hartwig, J. H.,** Interaction of myosin and a new actin binding protein of rabbit pulmonary macrophages, II. Role in cytoplasmic movement and phagocytosis, *J. Cell. Biol.*, 68, 602, 1978.
111. **Berlin, R. D. and Oliver, J. M.,** Analogous ultrastructure and surface properties during capping and phagocytosis in leukocytes, *J. Cell. Biol.*, 77, 789, 1978.
112. **Oliver, J. M., Krawjec, J. A., and Becker, E. L.,** The distribution of actin during chemotaxis in rabbit polymorphonuclear leucocytes, *J. Reticuloendothel Soc.*, 24, 694, 1978.
113, **Borisy, G. G., Olmsted, J. B., Marcum, J. M., and Allen, C.,** Microtubule assembly *in vitro, Fed. Proc.*, 33, 167, 1974.
114. **Olmsted, J. B. and Borisy, G. G.,** Microtubules, *Annu. Rev. Biochem.*, 42, 507, 1973.
115. **Stephens, R. E. and Edds, K. T.,** Microtubules, structure, chemistry and function, *Physiol. Rev.*, 56, 709, 1976.
116. **Pollard, T. D. and Weiling, B. H.,** Actin and myosin and cell movement, *CRC Crit. Rev. Biochem.*, 21, 1, 1974.
117. **Clarke, M. and Spucich, J. A.,** Non-muscle contractile proteins, the role of actin and myosin in cell motility and shape determination, *Annu. Rev. Biochem.*, 46, 792, 1977.
118. **Borgers, M. and de Brabander, M.,** *Microtubule Inhibitors,* North-Holland, Amsterdam, 1975.
119. **Hartwig, J. H. and Stossel, T. P.,** Interaction of actin, myosin, and actin binding protein of rabbit pulmonary macrophage, III. Effect of cytochalasin B, *J. Cell. Biol.*, 71, 295, 1976.
120. **Albertini, D. F., Berlin, R. D., and Oliver, J. M.,** The mechanisms of concavalin A cap formation in leukocytes, *J. Cell. Sci.*, 26, 57, 1977.
121. **Ward, P. A. and Becker, E. L.,** Biology of leukotaxis, *Rev. Physiol. Biochem. Pharmacol.*, 17, 125, 1977.
122. **Zigmond, S. H.,** Chemotaxis by polymorphonuclear leucocytes, *J. Cell. Biol.*, 77, 269, 1978.
123. **Zucker-Franklin, D. and Hirsch, J. G.,** Electron microscopic studies on the degranulation of rabbit peritoneal leukocytes during phagocytosis, *J. Exp. Med.*, 120, 569, 1964.
124. **Jensen, M. S. and Bainton, D. F.,** Temporal changes in pH within the phagocytic vacuole of the polymorphonuclear leukocyte, *J. Cell. Biol.*, 56, 379, 1973.
125. **Babior, B. M.,** Oxygen-dependent microbial killing by phagocytes, *N. Engl. J. Med.*, 298, 659, 1978.
126. **Cheson, B. D., Curnutte, J. T., and Babior, B.,** The oxidative killing mechanisms of the neutrophil, *Prog. Clin. Immunol.*, 3, 1, 1977.
127. **Klebanoff, S. J.,** Antimicrobial mechanism in neutrophilic polymorphonculear leukocytes, *Semin, Hematol.*, 12, 117, 1975.

128. **Masson. P. L., Heremans, J. F., and Schunne, E.,** Lactoferrin, an iron binding protein in neutrophil leukocytes, *J. Exp. Med.*, 130, 643, 1969.
129. **Mandell, G. L.,** Bactericidal activity of aerobic and anaerobic polymorphonuclear leukocytes, *Infect. Immunol.*, 9, 337, 1974.
130. **Spitznagel, J. K.,** Bactericidal mechanisms of the granulocyte, *Prog. Clin. Bio. Res.*, 13, 103, 1977.
131. **Douglas, S. D.,** Disorder of phagocyte function: ultrastructural aspects, *Prog. Clin. Biol. Res.*, 13, 141, 1977.
132. **Oliver, J. M.,** Cell biology of leukocyte abnormalities—membrane and cytoskeletal function in normal and defective cells, *Am. J. Pathol.*, 93, 221, 1978.
133. **Gabig, T. G.,** Leukocyte abnormalities, *Med. Clin. N. A.*, 64, 647, 1980.
134. **Price, T. H. and Dale, D. C.,** The selective neutropenia, *Clin. Haematol.*, 7, 501, 1978.
135. **Davidson, W. M.,** Inherited variation in leukocytes, *Br. Med. Bull.*, 17, 190, 1961.
136. **Davidson, W. M.,** Inherited variation of leukocytes, *Semin. Hematol.*, 5, 258, 1968.
137. **Undritz, E.,** Morphology and genetics in hereditary constitutional anomalies of leucocytes, *Acta Haematol.*, 24, 59, 1960.
138. **Dorr, A. D. and Moloney, W. C.,** Acquired pseudo-pelger anomaly of granulocytic leukocytes, *N. Engl. J. Med.*, 261, 742, 1959.
139. **Undritz, E.,** Eine neue Sippe mit erheblish-konstitutioneller Hochsegmentierung der Neutrophilen Kerne, *Schweiz. Med. Wochenschr.*, 88, 1000, 1958.
140. **Davidson, W. M. and Smith, D. R.,** in *Die Intersexualitat,* Overzier, C., Ed., Thieme, Stuttgart, 1960, 74.
141. **May, R.,** Leukocyteneinschlusse, *Dtsch. Arch. Klin, Med.*, 96, 1, 1909.
142. **Heggelin, R.,** Gleichzeitige konstitutionelle Veranderundgen an Neutrophilen und Thrombozyten, *Helv. Med. Acta,* 12, 439, 1945.
143. **Petz, A., Smith, I. and Nelson, N.,** The May-Heggelin Anomaly: a study of three cases, *Clin. Res.*, 8, 215, 1960.
144. **Wassmuth, D. R., De Groote, J. W., Hamilton, H. E., and Sheets, R. F.,** An anomaly of granulocytes and platelets: a newly established hereditary entity, *J. Lab. Clin. Med.*, 58, 969, 1961.
145. **Oski, F. A., Naiman, J. L., Allen, D., and Diamond, L. K.,** Leukocyte inclusions—Döhle bodies-associated with platelet abnormality (The May-Heggelin Anomaly); report of a family and review of the literature, *Blood,* 20, 657, 1962.
146. **Jordan, S. W. and Larsen W. R.,** Ultrastructural studies of the May Hegglin anomaly, *Blood,* 25, 921, 1965.
147. **Jenis, E. H., Takeuchi, A., Dillion, D. E., et al.,** The May-Heggelin Anomaly; ultrastructure of the granulocyte inclusion, *Am. J. Clin. Pathol.*, 55, 181, 1971.
148. **Bessis, M.,** *Living Blood Cells and Their Ultrastructure,* Springer-Verlag, New York, 1973, 339.
149. **Najean, Y., Schaison, G., Binet, J. L., et al.,** Le syndrome de May-Heggelin, *Presse Med.*, 74, 1649, 1966.
150. **Lechner, K., Breddin, K., Mober, K., et al.,** May-Heggelinsche anomalie, *Acta Haematol.*, 42, 303, 1969.
151. **Döhle, H.,** Leukocyteneinschlusse bei Scharlach, *Zbl. Bakt., (Abst. 1),* 61, 63, 1912.
152. **Weiner, W. and Topley, E.,** Döhle bodies in the leucocytes of patients with burns, *J. Clin. Pathol.*, 8, 324, 1955.
153. **Itoga, T. and Laszlo, J.,** Döhle bodies and other granulocytic alterations during chemotherapy and cyclophosphamide, *Blood,* 20, 668, 1962.
154. **Chediak, M.,** Nouvelle anomale leucocytaire de caractere constitutionnel et familial, *Rev. Hematol.*, 7, 362, 1952.
155. **Higashi, O.,** Congenital gigantism of peroxidase granules—first case ever reported of qualitative abnormality of peroxidase, *Tohoku J. Exp. Med.*, 59, 315, 1954.
156. **Blume, R. S., Bennet, J. M., Yankee, R. A., and Wolff, S. M.,** Defective granulocyte regulation in the Chediak-Higashi syndrome, *N. Engl. J. Med.*, 279, 1009, 1968.
157. **Page, A. R., Berendes, H., Warner, J., and Good, R. A.,** The Chediak-Higashi syndrome, *Blood,* 20, 330, 1962.
158. **Blume, R. S. and Wolff, S. M.,** The Chediak-Higashi syndrome. Studies in four patients and a review of the literature, *Medicine,* 51, 247, 1972.
159. **Davis, W. C., Spicer, S. S., Greene, W. B., and Padgett, G. A.,** Ultrastructure of bone marrow granulocytes in normal mink and mink with the homolog of the Chediak-Higashi trait of humans. I. Origin of the abnormal granules present in the neutrophils of mink with the C-HS trait, *Lab. Invest.*, 24, 303, 1971.
160. **Renshaw, H. W., Davis, W. C., Fudenberg, H. H., et al.,** Leukocyte dysfunction in the bovine homologue of the Chediak-Higashi syndrome of humans, *Infect. Immun.*, 10, 928, 1974.

161. **Bennet, J. M., Blume, R. S., and Wolff, S. M.,** Characterization and significance of leucocyte granules in the beige mouse: a possible homologue for Chediak-Higashi aleutian trait, *J. Lab. Clin. Med.*, 73, 235, 1969.
162. **Taylor, R. F. and Farrell, R. K.,** Light and electron microscopy of peripheral blood neutrophils in a killer whale affected with Chediak-Higashi syndrome, *Fed. Proc. (Abstr.),* 32, 822, 1973.
163. **Kramer, J. W., Davis, W. C., and Prieur, D. J.,** The Chediak-Higashi syndrome of cats, *Lab. Invest.*, 36, 554, 1977.
164. **White, J. G.,** The Chediak-Higashi syndrome: a possible lysosomal disease, *Blood,* 28, 143, 1966.
165. **White, J. G.,** The Chediak-Higashi syndrome: cytoplasmic sequestration in circulating leucocytes, *Blood,* 29, 435, 1967.
166. **Douglas, S. D., Blume, R. S., and Wolff, S. M.,** Fine structural studies of leukocytes from patients with the Chediak-Higashi syndrome, *Blood,* 33, 527, 1969.
167. **White, J. G.,** The Chediak-Higashi syndrome: fine structure of giant inclusions in freeze-fractured neutrophils, *Am. J. Pathol.*, 72, 503, 1973.
168. **Gallin, J. I., Klimerman, J. A., Paugett, G. A., and Wolff, S. M.,** Defective mononuclear leukocyte chemotaxis in the Chediak-Higashi syndrome of humans, mink and cattle, *Blood,* 45, 863, 1975.
169. **Root, R. K., Rosenthal, A. S., Balestra, D. J.,** Abnormal bactericidal, metabolic, and lysosomal function of Chediak-Higashi syndrome leukocytes, *J. Clin. Invest.*, 51, 649, 1972.
170. **Oliver, J. M., Zurier, R. B., and Berlin, R. D.,** Concavalin A cap formation on polymorphonuclear leucocytes of normal and beige (Chediak-Higashi) mice, *Nature,* 253, 471, 1975.
171. **Oliver, J. M. and Zurier, R. B.,** Correction of characteristic abnormalities of microtubule function and granule morphology in Chediak-Higashi syndrome with cholinergic agents. Studies *in vitro* in man and *in vivo* in the beige mouse, *J. Clin. Invest.*, 57, 1239, 1976.
172. **Boxer, L. A., Watanabe, A. M., Rister, M. et al.,** Correction of leukocyte function in Chediak-Higashi syndrome by ascorbate, *N. Engl. J. Med.*, 295, 1041, 1976.
173. **Check, W. A.,** Cell organelle defects associated with genetic disease, *JAMA,* 238, 461, 1977.
174. **Sandler, J. A., Gallin, J. I., and Vaughan, M.,** Effect of serotonin; carbamylcholine and ascorbic acid on leukocyte cyclic GMP and chemotaxis, *J. Cell. Biol.*, 67, 480, 1975.
175. **Miller, M. E., Oski, F. A., and Harris, M. R.,** Lazy leukocyte syndrome. A new disorder of leukocyte function, *Lancet,* 1, 665, 1971.
176. **Pinkerton, P. H., Robinson, J. B., and Senn, J. S.,** Lazy leukocyte syndrome. Disorder of the granulocyte membrane? *J. Clin. Pathol.*, 31, 300, 1978.
177. **Boxer, L. A., Hedley-White, E. T., and Stossel, T. P.,** Neutrophil actin dysfunction and abnormal neutrophil behavior, *N. Engl. J. Med.*, 291, 1093, 1974.
178. **Gallin, J. L., Malech, H. L., Wright, D. G. et al.,** Recurrent severe infection in a child with abnormal leukocyte function. Possible relationship to increased microtubule assembly, *Blood,* 51, 919, 1978.
179. **Grignaschi, V. J., Sperperato, A. M., Etchverry, M. J., and Marcario, A. J.,** Un nuevo cuadro citoquimico, negatividad de peroxidase, oxidases y lipido en la progenie neutrofilia y en los monocitos de los hermanos, *Rev. Assoc. Med. Argent.*, 77, 218, 1963.
180. **Undritz, E.,** Die Allius-Grignaschi anomalie der erblichkonstitutionelle Peroxydasedefect der Neutrophilen und Monzyten, *Blut,* 14, 29, 1966.
181. **Lehrer, R. I. and Cline, M. J.,** Leukocyte myeloperoxidase deficiency and disseminated candidiasis: the role of myeloperoxidase in resistance to candida infection, *J. Clin. Invest.*, 48, 1478, 1969.
182. **Arakawa, T., Wada, Y., Hayashi, T., et al.,** Uracil refractory anemia with peroxidase negative neutrophils, *Tohoko, J. Exp. Med.*, 87, 52, 1965.
183. **Higashi, O., Katsuyama, N., and Satudate, R. A.,** A case of hematologic abnormality characterized by the absence of peroxidase activity in blood polymorphonuclear leukocytes, *Tohoko, J. Exp. Med.*, 87, 77, 1965.
184. **Lehrer, R. I., Goldberg, L. S., Apple, M. A., and Rosenthal, N. P.,** Refractory megaloglastic anemia with myeloperoxidase deficient neutrophils, *Ann. Int. Med.*, 76, 447, 1972.
185. **Breton-Gorius, J., Houssay, D., and Dreyfus, B.,** Partial myeloperoxidase deficiency in a case of preleukemia. I. Studies of fine structure of peroxidase synthesis of promyelocytes, *Br. J. Haematol.*, 30, 1975.
186. **Strauss, B. G., Boue, K. E., Jones, J. F., et al.,** An anomaly of neutrophil morphology with impaired function, *N. Engl. J. Med.*, 290, 478, 1974.
187. **Komiyama, A., Morosawa, H., Nakahatak, T., et al.,** Abnormal neutrophil maturation in a neutrophilic defect with morphologic abnormality and impaired function, *J. Pediat.*, 94, 19, 1979.
188. **Spitznagel, J. K., Cooper, M. R., McCall, A. E., et al.,** Selective deficiency of granules associated with lysozyme and lactoferrin in human polymorphs (PMN) with reduced microbicidal capacity, *J. Clin. Invest.*, (*Abstr.*), 93, 51, 1972.

189. **Parmely, R. T., Ogawa, M., Darbey, C. P., Jr., and Spicer, S. S.,** Congenital neutropenia in neutrophil proliferation with abnormal maturation, *Blood,* 46, 723, 1975.
190. **Breton-Gorius, J., Mason, D. Y., Buriot, D., et al.,** Lactoferrin deficiency as a consequence of a lack of specific granules in neutrophils from a patient with recurrent infections, *Am. J. Pathol.,* 99, 413, 1980.
191. **Windhurst, D. S., Page, A. B., Holmes, B., et al.,** The patterns of genetic transmission of the leukocyte defect in fatal granulomatous disease of childhood, *J. Clin. Invest.,* 47, 1026, 1968.
192. **Azinci, P. H., Bodenheimer, J. H., Hintz, R. L., et al.,** Chronic granulmatous disease in three females siblings, *JAMA,* 206, 65, 1968.
193. **Holmes, B., Quie, P. G., Windhorst, D. A., and Good, R. A.,** Fatal granulomatous disease of childhood. An inborn abnormality phagocytic function, *Lancet,* 1, 1225, 1966.
194. **Quie, P. G., White, J. G., Homes, B., and Good, R. A.,** *In vitro* bactericidal capacity of human polymorphonuclear leucocytes. Diminished activity in chronic granulomatous disease of childhood, *J. Clin. Invest.,* 46, 668, 1967.
195. **Baehner, R. I. and Nathan, D. G.,** Leukocyte oxidase. Defective activity in chronic granulomatous disease, *Science,* 155, 835, 1967.
196. **Holmes, B., Page, A. B., and Good, R. A.,** Studies of the metabolic activity of leucocytes from patients with a genetic abnormality of phagocytic function, *J. Clin. Invest.,* 46, 422, 1967.
197. **Klebanoff, S. J.,** Oxygen metabolism and the toxic properties of phagocytes, *Ann. Intern. Med.,* 93, 480, 1980.
198. **Curnutte, J. T., Kipnes, R. S., and Babior, B. M.,** Defect in pyridine nucleotide dependent superoxide production by a particulate fraction from the granulocytes of patients with chronic granulomatous disease, *N. Engl. J. Med.,* 293, 628, 1975.
199. **Weening, R. S., Roos, D., Weemaes, C. M. R., et al.,** Defective initiation of the metabolic stimulation in phagocytozing granulocytes. A new congenital defect, *J. Lab. Clin. Med.,* 88. 757, 1976.
200. **Baehner, R. L., Johnston, R. B., and Nathan, D. G.,** Comparative study of the metabolic and bactericidal characteristics of severely glucose-6-phosphate dehyrogenase deficient polymorphonuclear leucocytes and leucocytes from children with chronic granulomatous disease, *J. Reticuloendothel Soc.,* 12, 150, 1972.
201. **Gray, G. R., Klebanoff, S. J., Stamaloyannapoulos, G., et al.,** Neutrophil dysfunction, chronic granulomatous disease and non-spherocytic hemolytic anemia caused by complete deficiency of glucose-6-phosphate dehydrogenase, *Lancet,* 2, 530, 1973.
202. **Baehner, R. L., Boxer, L. A., and Davis, J.,** The biochemical basis of nitroblue tetrazolium reduction in normal human and chronic granulomatous disease polymorphonuclear leukocytes, *Blood,* 48, 309, 1976.
203. **Cooper, M. R., DeChatelet, L. R., McCall, C. E., et al.,** Complete deficiency of glucose-6-phosphate dehydrogenase with defective bactericidal activity, *J. Clin. Invest.,* 51, 769, 1972.
204. **Hagler, L., Pasture, P. A., and Bergin, J. J.,** Aplastic anemia following viral hepatitis: report of two fatal cases and a review of the literature, *Medicine,* 54, 139, 1975.
205. **Kauder, E. and Mauer, A. M.,** Neutropenia of childhood, *J. Pediat.,* 68, 147, 1966.
206. **Kostmann, R. R. O.,** Infantile genetic agranulocytosis. A new recessive lethal disease in man, *Acta Paediat. Scand.,* (Suppl.), 105, 1956.
207. **Kostmann, R.,** Infantile genetic agranulocytosis. A review with presentation of ten new cases, *Acta Paediatr. Scand.,* 64, 362, 1975.
208. **L'Esperance, P., Brunning, R., and Good, R. A.,** Congenital neutropenia. *In vitro* growth of colonies mimicking the disease, *Proc. Natl. Acad. Sci. (USA),* 70, 669, 1973.
209. **Falk, P. M., Rich, K., Feig, S., et al.,** Evaluation of congenital neutropenic disorders by *in vitro* bone marrow culture, *Pediatrics,* 59, 739, 1977.
210. **Rich, K., Falk, P. M., Steiham, E. R., et al.,** Abnormal *in vitro* granulopoiesis in phenotypically normal parents of some children with congenital neutropenia, *Pediatrics,* 59, 346, 1977.
211. **Barak, Y., Paran, M., Levin, S., and Sach, L.,** *In vitro* induction of myeloid proliferation and maturation in infantile genetic agranulocytosis, *Blood,* 38, 74, 1971.
212. **Gansslen, M.,** Konstitutionelle familiare Leukpenie (Neutropenie), *Klin. Wochenschr.,* 20, 922, 1941.
213. **Hitzig, W. H.,** Familiare Neutropenie mit dominanten Erbgang and Hypogamma globulinaemia, *Helv. Med. Acta,* 26, 779, 1959.
214. **Schwachman, H., Diamond, L. K., Oski, F. A., and Khan, K. T.,** The syndrome of pancreatic insuffiency and bone marrow dysfunction, *J. Pediatr.,* 65, 645, 1964.
215. **Finch, S. C.,** Granulocytopenia, in *Hematology,* 2nd ed., Williams, W. I., Beutler, E., Erslev, A. J., and Rundles, R. W., Eds., McGraw Hill, New York, 1977, 717.
216. **Pincus, S. H., Boxer, L. A., and Stossel, T. P.,** Chronic neutropenias in childhood. Analysis of 16 cases and review of the literature, *Am. J. Med.,* 61, 849, 1976.

217. **Dale, D. C., DuPont, G., IV, Wewerka, J., et al.,** Chronic neutropenia, *Medicine,* 58. 128, 1979.
218. **Boxer, L. A., Greenberg, M. S., Boxer, G.J., and Stossel, T. P.,** Autoimmune neutropenia *N. Engl. J. Med.,* 293, 748, 1975.
219. **Amato, D., Freedman, M. H., and Saunders, E. F.,** Granulopoiesis in severe congenital neutropenia, *Blood,* 47, 531, 1976.
220. **Petz, L. D. and Fudenberg, H. H.,** Immunologic mechanisms in drug induced cytopenias, *Prog. Hematol.,* 9, 185, 1975.
221. **Schultz, W. and Jacobowitz, L.,** Die Agranulozytosen, *Med. Klin.,* 12, 1642, 1925.
222. **Evans, R. S. and Ford, W. P.,** Studies of the bone marrow in immunological granulocytopenia, *Arch. Intern. Med.,* 101, 244, 1958.
223. **Pisciotta, A.,** Immune and toxic mechanisms of drug-induced agranulocytosis, *Semin. Heamtol.,* 10, 279, 1973.
224. **Lalezari, D. and Radel, E.,** Neutrophil specific antigens: immunology and clinical significance, *Semin, Hematol.,* 11, 281, 1974.
225. **Lalezari, P.,** Neutrophil antigens: immunologic and clinical significance, *Prog. Clin. Biol. Res.,* 13, 209, 1977.
226. **Boxer, L. A., Yokoyama, M., and Lalezari, P.,** Isoimmune neonatal neutropenia, *J. Pediatr.,* 80, 783, 1972.
227. **Rosenthal, F. D., Beeley, J. M., Gelsthrope, K., and Doughty, R. W.,** White cell antibodies and the aetiology and Felty's syndrome, *Q. J. Med.,* 43, 187, 1974.
228. **Logue, G.,** Felty's syndrome: granulocyte bound immunoglobulin G and splenectomy, *Ann. Intern. Med.,* 85, 437, 1976.
229. **Page, A. R. and Good, R. A.,** Studies on cyclic neutropenia: a clinical and experimental investigation, *Am. J. Dis. Child.,* 94, 623, 1975.
230. **Morley, A. A., Carew, J. P., and Baikie, A. G.,** Familial cyclic neutropenia, *Br. J. Haematol.,* 13, 719, 1967.
231. **Guerry, D. IV, Dale, D. C., Omine, M., et al.,** Periodic hematopoiesis in human cyclic neutropenia, *J. Clin. Invest.,* 52, 3220, 1973.
232. **Morley, A. A.,** A neutrophil cycle in healthy individuals, *Lancet,* 2, 1220, 1966.
233. **King-Smith, E. A. and Morley, A. A.,** Computer simulation of granulopoiesis, normal and impaired granulopoiesis, *Blood,* 36, 254, 1970.
234. **Morley, A. A. and Stohlman, F., Jr.,** Cyclophosphamide induced cyclical neutropenia, *N. Engl. J. Med.,*282, 643, 1970.
235. **Vodopick, H., Rupp, E. M., Edwards, C. L., et al.,** Spontaneous cyclic leukocytosis and thrombocytosis in chronic granulocytic leukemia, *N. Engl. J. Med.,* 286, 1284, 1972.
236. **Lund, J. E., Padgett, G. A., and Ott, R. L.,** Cyclic neutropenia in grey collie dogs, *Blood,* 29, 452, 1971.
237. **Dale, D. C., Alling, D. N., and Wolff, S. M.,** Cyclic hematopoiesis: the mechanism of cyclic neutropenia in grey collie dogs, *J. Clin. Invest.,* 51, 2197, 1972.
238. **Dale, D. C., Kimball, H. R., and Wolff, S. M.,** Studies of cyclic neutropenia in grey collie dogs, *Clin. Res.,* 18, 402, 1970.
239. **Dale, D. C., Ward, S. B., Kimball, H. R., and Wolff, S. M.,** Studies of neutrophil production and turnover in grey collie dogs with cyclic neutropenia, *J. Clin. Invest.,* 51, 2190, 1972.
240. **Dale, D. C. and Graw, R. G.,** Transplantation of allogeneic bone marrow in canine cyclic neutropenia, *Science,* 183, 83, 1974.
241. **Weiden, P. L., Robinett, B., Graham, R. C., et al.,** Canine cyclic neutropenia: a stem cell defect, *J. Clin. Invest.,* 53, 950, 1974.
242. **Scott, R. E., Dale, D. C., Rosenthal, A. S., and Wolff, S. M.,** Cyclic neutropenia in grey collie dogs, *Lab. Invest.,* 28, 514, 1973.
243. **Finch, S. C.,** Granulocytosis, in *Hematology,* 2nd ed., Williams, W. J., Beutler, E., Erslev, A., and Rundles, R. W., Eds., McGraw Hill, New York, 1977, 746.
244. **Wintrobe, M. M.,** *Clinical Hematology,* 7th ed., Lea & Febiger, Philadelphia, 1974, 1301.
245. **Broxmeyer, H. E. and Moore, M.A.S.,** Communications between white cells and the abnormalities of this in leukemia, *Biochim. Biophys. Arch.,* 516, 129, 1978.
246. **Robinson, W. A. and Mangalik, A.,** The kinetics and regulation of granulopoiesis, *Semin. Hematol.,* 12, 7, 1975.
247. **Golde, D. W. and Cline, M. J.,** Regulation of granulopoiesis, *N. Engl. J. Med.,* 291, 1388, 1974.
248. **Mechanic, R. C., Frei, E., III, Landy, M., et al.,** Quantitative studies of human leukocytic and febrile response to single and repeated doses of purified bacterial endotoxin, *J. Clin. Invest.* 41, 163, 1962.
249. **Boggs, D. R., Chervenick, P. A., Marsh, J. C., et al.,** Neutrophil releasing activity in plasma of dogs injected with endotoxin, *J. Lab. Clin. Med.,* 72, 177, 1968.

250. **Gordon, A. S., Handler, E. S., Siegel, C. D., et al.,** Plasma factors influencing leukocyte release in rats, *Ann. N.Y. Acad.Sci.,* 113, 766, 1964.
251. **Chervenick, P. A.,** Relationship between neutrophil releasing factor (NRF) and colony stimulating factor (CSF), *Blood,* 40, 949, 1972.
252. **Broxmeyer, H., Van Zant, G., Zucali, G. R., et al.,** Mechanisms of leucocyte production and release. XII. A comparative assay of leukocytosis inducing factor, (LIF) and the colony stimulating factor (CSF), *Proc. Soc. Exp. Biol. Med.,* 145, 1262, 1974.
253. **Quesenberry, P., Morley, A., Miller, M., et al.,** Effect of endotoxin on granulopoiesis and the *in vitro* colony forming cells, *Blood,* 41, 391, 1973.
254. **Krumbhaar, E. B.,** Leukemoid blood pictures in various clinical conditions, *Am. J. Med. Sci.,* 172, 519, 1929.
255. **Hilts, S. U. and Shaw, C. C.,** Leukemoid blood reactions, *N. Engl. J. Med.,* 249, 434, 1953.
256. **Holland, P. and Mauer, A. M.,** Myeloid leukemoid reaction in children, *Am. J. Dis. Child.,* 105, 568, 1963.
257. **Fahey, R. J.,** Unusual leukocyte responses in primary carcinoma of the lung, *Cancer,* 4, 930, 1951.
258. **Hensler, L.,** Hohe Leukocytose durch Karzinom, *Schweiz. Med. Wochenschr.,* 83, 1032, 1953.
259. **Chen, H. and Walz, D. V.,** Leukemoid reactions in the bone marrow associated with malignant neoplasm, *Am. J. Clin. Pathol.,* 29, 345, 1958.
260. **Colman, R. W. and Shein, H. M.,** Leukemoid reaction hyperuricemia and severe hyperpyrexia complicating a fatal case of acute fatty liver in the alcoholic, *Ann. Int. Med.,* 57, 110, 1962.
261. **Twomey, J. J. and Leavell, B. S.,** Leukemoid reactions to tuberculosis, *Arch. Intern. Med.,* 116, 21, 1965.
262. **Skerberg, K. O., Lagerlof, B., and Reizenstein, P.,** Leukemia, leukemoid reactions and tuberculosis, *Acta Med. Scand.,* 182, 427, 1967.
263. **Retieff, F. P.,** Leucoerythroblastosis in the adult, *Lancet,* 1, 639, 1964.
264. **Burkett, L. L., Cox, M. L., and Fields, M. L.,** Leukoerythroblastosis in the adult, *Am. J. Clin. Pathol.,* 44, 494, 1965.
265. **Herring, W. B., Smith, L. G., Walker, R. E., and Herrion, J. C.,** Hereditary neutrophilia, *Am. J. Med.,* 56, 729, 1974.
266. **Dignan, P. S., Mauer, A. M., and Frantz, C.,** Phocomelia with congenital hypoplastic thrombocytopenia and myeloid leukemoid reaction, *J. Pediatr.,* 70, 561, 1967.
267. **Randall, D. L., Reiquam, C. N., Githens, J. H., and Robinson, A.,** Familial myeloproliferative disease, *Am. J. Dis. Child.,* 110, 479, 1965.
268. **Editorial,** An Odd-leukaemia-like disease, *Br. Med. J.,* 2, 376, 1966.
269. **Spencer, R. R., McPhedran, P., Finch, S. C., and Morgan, W. S.,** Persistant neutrophilic leucocytosis associated with idiopathic functional asplenia, *J. Nucl. Med.,* 13, 224, 1972.
270. **Ward, N. N. and Reinhard, E. H.,** Chronic idiopathic leucocytosis, *Ann. Intern. Med.,* 75, 193, 1971.
271. **Athens, J. W., Haab, O. P., and Raab, S. O.,** Leukokinetics studies. XI. Blood granulocyte kinetics in polycythemia vera, infection and myelofibrosis, *J. Clin. Invest.,* 44, 778, 1965.
272. **Ward, H. P. and Block, M. H.,** The natural histology of agnogenic myeloid methaplasia (AMM). A critical evaluation of its relationship with the myeloproliferative syndrome, *Medicine,* 50, 357, 1971.
273. **Gilbert, H. S.,** The spectrum of myeloproliferative disorders, *Med. Clin. N. A.,* 57, 355, 1973.
274. **Takacsi-Nagy, L. and Fraf, F.,** Definition, clinical features and diagnosis of myelofibrosis, *Clin. Haematol.,* 4, 291, 1975.
275. **Bernard, S. and Saab, O.,** *Dahlem workshop on Myelofibrosis, Osteosclerotic Syndrome, Advances in Biosciences No. 16,* Pergamon Press, Oxford, 1976.
276. **Cheng, D. S.,** Idiopathic myelofibrosis without splenomegaly, *Cancer,* 43, 1761, 1979,
277. **Tavassoli, M. and Weiss, L.,** An electron microscopic study of spleen in myelofibrosis with myeloid metaplasia, *Blood,* 42, 267, 1973.
278. **Soderstrom, N., Bandmann, U., and Lundh, B.,** Patho-anatomical features of the spleen and liver, *Clin. Hematol.,* 4, 309, 1975.
279. **Koler, R. D., Seaman, A. J., Osgood, E. E., and Vanbellinghen, P.,** Myeloproliferative disease, diagnostic value of the leukocyte alkaline phosphatase test, *Am. J. Clin. Pathol.,* 30, 295, 1958.
280. **Mitus, W. J., Bergna, L. J., Mednikoff, I. B., and Damashek, W.,** Alkaline phosphatase of mature neutrophils in chronic forms of the myeloproliferative syndrome, *Am. J. Clin. Pathol.,* 30, 85, 1958.
281. **Mitus, W. J., Gherardi, G. J., Mednicoff, I. B., and Damashek, W.,** Cytochemistry of myelofibrosis with myeloid metaplasia in relation to spleen changes, *Arch. Pathol.,* 67, 188, 1959.

282. **Nakai, G. S., Craddock, C. G., and Figueroa, W. G.,** Agnogenic myeloid methplasia, *Ann. Intern. Med.*, 57, 419, 1962.
283. **Anderson, R. E., Hoshino, T., and Yamamoto, T.,** Myelofibrosis with myeloid metaplasia in survivors of the atomic bomb, *Ann. Intern. Med.*, 60, 1, 1964.
284. **Rawson, R., Parker, E., Jr., and Jackson, H., Jr.,** Industrial solvents as possible etiologic agents in myeloid metaplasia, *Science*, 93, 541, 1941.
285. **Kiely, J. M. and Silverstein, M. N.,** Metastatic carcinoma simulating myeloid metaplasia and myelofibrosis, *Cancer*, 24, 1041, 1969.
286. **Viola, M. V., Kovi, J., and Nukhopadbyay, M.,** Reversal of myelofibrosis in Hodgkin's diseae, *JAMA*, 223, 1145, 1973.
287. **Clough, V., Geary, C. G., Hashmi, K., et al.,** Myelofibrosis in chronic granulocyte leukemia, *Br. J. Haematol.*, 42, 519, 1979.
288. **Kundel, D. W., Brecher, G., Bodey, G. P., and Brittin, G. M.,** Reticulum fibrosis and bone infarction in acute leukemia. Implications for prognosis, *Blood*, 23, 526, 1964.
289. **Hann, I. M., Evans, D. I. K., Marsden, H. B., et al.,** Bone marrow fibrosis in acute lymphoblastic leukemia of childhood, *J. Clin. Pathol.*, 31, 313, 1978.
290. **Jacobson, K. J., Salo, A., and Fialkow, R. J.,** Agnogenic myeloid metaplasia, a clonal proliferation of hemapoietic stem cells with secondary myelofibrosis, *Blood*, 51, 180, 1978.
291. **Greenberg, B., Wilson, F., Woo, L., and Jenks, H.,** Cytogenetic of fibroblastic colonies in Ph positive chronic myelocytic leukemia, *Blood*, 51, 1039, 1978.
292. **Hoshi, J. and Weiss, L.,** Rabbit bone marrow after administration of saponin, *Lab. Invest.*, 38, 67, 1978.
293. **Lewis, C. M. and Pegrum, C. D.,** Immune complexes in myeloproliferative disorder, *Lancet*, 2, 1151, 1977.
294. **Demmler, K.,** Die Histopatholgie des Gefassystems in spongiosen Knochen, in *Klinische und funktionelle Bedeuting bei Osteopathien und Myelopathien, Habilitationschrift*, Munich, 1974.
295. **Buyssens, N. and Bourgeois, N.H.,** Chronic myelocytic leukemia versus idiopathic myelofibrosis, *Cancer*, 40, 1548, 1977.
296. **Duhamel, G.,** *Histopathologie Clinique de la Moelle Osseuse*, Masson et cie, Paris, 1974.
297. **Lennert, K., Nagai, K., and Schwarze, E. W.,** Patho-anatomical features of the bone marrow, *Clin. Haematol.*, 4, 331, 1975.
298. **Silverstein, M. N. and Linman, J. W.,** Causes of death in agnogenic myeloid metaplasia, *Mayo Clin. Proc.*, 44, 36, 1969.
299. **Embarger, J. M., Wagner, A., and Izarn, P.,** La terminaison en leucemie aigue de l'osteomyelofibrose avec metaplasie myeloide hepatosplenique, *Nouv. Rev. Fr. Hematol.*, 9, 375, 1969.
300. **Glew, R. H., Haese, W. A., and McIntyre, T. A.,** Myeloid metaplasia with myelofibrosis. The clinical spectrum of extramedullary hematopoiesis and tumor formation, *John Hopkins Med. J.*, 132, 253, 1973.
301. **Lewis, S. M. and Szur, M.,** Malignant myelosclerosis, *Br. Med. J.*, 1, 472, 1963.
302. **Bergsman, K. L. and Van Slyck, E. J.,** Acute meylofibrosis. An accelerated variant of agnogenic myeloid metaplasia, *Ann. Intern. Med.*, 74, 232, 1971.
303. **Fabich, D. R. and Raich, P. C.,** Acute myelofibrosis. A report of three cases, *Am. J. Clin. Pathol.*, 67, 334, 1977.
304. **Weisenburger, D. D.,** Acute myelofibrosis terminating as acute myeloblastic leukemia, *Am. J. Clin. Pathol.*, 73, 128, 1980.
305. **Bird, T. and Proctor, S. J.,** Malignant myelosclerosis. Myeloproliferative disorder or leukemia? *Am. J. Clin. Pathol.*, 76, 512, 1977.
306. **Lobin, J., Rozen, S., and Rywlin, A. M.,** Malignant myelosclerosis, *Arch. Intern. Med.*, 136, 141, 1976.
307. **Bearman, R. M., Pangalis, G. A., and Rappaport, H.,** Acute (Malignant) myelosclerosis, *Cancer*, 43, 279, 1979.
308. **Bain, B., Catovsky, D., O'Brien, M. et al.,** Megakaryoblastic transformation of chronic granulocytic leukemia. An electron microscopic and cytochemical study, *J. Clin. Pathol.*, 30, 35, 1977.
309. **Breton-Gorius, J., Reyes, F., Vernant, J. B. et al.,** The blast crisis of chronic granulocytic leukemia: megakaryoblastic nature of cells as revealed by the presence of platelet peroxidase—a cytochemical ultrastructural study, *Br. J. Haematol.*, 39, 95, 1978.
310. **Efrati, P., Nir, E., Yaari, A. et al.,** Myeloproliferative disorders terminating in acute micromegakaryoblastic leukemia, *Br. J. Haematol.*, 43, 79, 1979.
311. **Lee, R. E., and Ellis, L. D.,** The storage cells in chronic myelocytic leukemia, *Lab. Invest.*, 24, 261, 1971.

312. **Gralnick, H. R., Harbor, J., and Vogel, C.,** Myelofibrosis in chronic granulocytic leukemia, *Blood,* 37, 152, 1971.
313. **McCaffrey, R., Harrison, T. A., Parkman, R., and Baltimore, D.,** Terminal deoxynucleotidyl transferase activity in human leukemic cells and normal thymocytes, *N. Engl. J. Med.,* 292, 775, 1975.
314. **Spiers, A. S. D.,** Anotation—Metamorphosis of chronic granulocytic leukemia: diagnosis classification and management, *Br. J. Haematol.,* 41, 1, 1979.
315. **Editorial.** Philadelphia chromosome positive leukemias, *Lancet,* 1, 857, 1979.
316. **Spiers, A. S. D.,** The clinical features of chronic granulocytic leukemia, *Clin. Haematol.,* 6, 77, 1977.
317. **Gailbraith, P. R.,** Granulocyte kinetics studies in chronic myelocytic leukemia, *Natl. Cancer Inst. Mongr.,* 30, 121, 1969.
318. **Gailbraith, P. R., and Abu-Zahra, H. T.,** Granulopoiesis in chronic granulocytic leukemia, *Br. J. Haematol.,* 22, 135, 1972.
319. **Stryckmans, P. A., Debusscher, L., and Collard, E.,** Cell kinetics in chronic granulocytic leukemia, *Clin. Haematol.,* 6, 21, 1977.
320. **Bessis, M.,** *Living Blood Cells and their Ultrastructure,* Springer-Verlag, New York, 1973, 569.
321. **Bottomley, R. H., Lovig, C. A., Holt, R., and Griffin, M. J.,** Comparison of alkaline phosphatase from human normal and leukemic leucocytes, *Cancer Res.,* 29, 1866, 1969.
322. **Chikkapa, G., Brecher, G., Borner, A. L., et al.,** Return of alkaline phsophatase in chronic myelogeneous leukemia cells in diffusion chamber cultures, *Proc. Soc. Exp. Biol Med.,* 143, 212, 1973.
323. **Trubowitz, S., Feldman, S., Benate, C., and Hunt, W. M.,** The alkaline phosphatase content of the human polymorphonuclear leucocyte in blood and marrow, *Am. J. Clin. Pathol.,* 31, 481, 1959.
324. **Hook, E. A. and Engel, R. R.,** Leukocyte life span, leukocyte alkaline phosphatase and the 21st chromosome, *Lancet,* 1, 112, 1964.
325. **Kelemen, E.,** Granulocyte alkaline phosphatase activity: a measure of the emergence time of the mature neutrophils? *Acta Haematol.,* 50, 19, 1973.
326. **Pederson, B. and Hayhoe, R. G. J.,** Relation between phagocytic activity and alkaline phosphatase content of neutrophils in chronic myeloid leukemia, *Br. J. Haematol.,* 21, 257, 1971.
327. **Williams, D. M., Lampert, I. A., and Evans, D. J.,** A comparison using quantitative enzyme cytochemistry between leucocyte alkaline phosphatase levels in the bone marrow and blood of the rats, *Br. J. Haematol.,* 40, 119, 1978.
328. **Paris, Conference,** Standardization in human cytogenetics, Birth defects, in *Original Article Series VII,* The National Foundation, New York, 7, 172, 1972.
329. **Rowley, J. D.,** A new consistent abnormality in chronic myelogenous leukemia identified by quinacrine fluorescence and Giemsa staining, *Nature,* 243, 290, 1973.
330. **Lawlor, S. D.,** The cytogenetics of chronic granulocytic leukemia, *Clin. Haematol.,* 6, 55, 1977.
331. **McCulloch, E. A., Howatson, A. F., Buick, R. V., et al.,** Acute myeloblastic leukemia considered as a conal hemopathy, *Blood Cells,* 5, 261, 1979.
332. **Nichos, T. M.,** An electron microscopic investigation of Auer bodies in acute myeloblastic leukemia, *Cancer Med. Assoc. J.,* 102, 865, 1970.
333. **Bessis, M. and Breton-Gorius, J.,** Pathologie et asynchronisme de development des organelles cellulaires an cours des leucemies aigues granulocytaires (etude an microscope electronique), *Nouv. Rev. Fr. Hematol.,* 9, 245, 1969.
334. **Bainton, D. F., Friedlander, L. M., and Shohet, S. B.,** Abnormalities in granule formation in acute myelogenous leukemia, *Blood,* 49, 693, 1977.
335. **Marchal, G., Bessi, M., and Thiery, J. P.,** Ultrastructure des corps d'Auer, *Rev. Hematol.,* 4, 413, 1959.
336. **MacDuffie, N. G.,** Crystalline patterns in Auer bodies and specific granules of human leucocytes, *J. Micro. (Paris),* 6, 321, 1967.
337. **White, J. G.,** Fine structural demonstration of acid phosphatase in Auer bodies, *Blood,* 29, 667, 1967.
338. **Tulliez, M. and Breton-Gorius, J.,** Three types of Auer bodies in acute leukemia, *Lab. Invest.,* 41, 419, 1979.
339. **Mintz, U., Djaldetti, M., Rozenszajn, L., et al.,** Giant lysosome like structures in promyelocytic leukemia: ultrastructural and cytochemical observations, *Biomedicine,* 10, 428, 1973.
340. **Ogawa, T.,** An electron microscopic investigation of acute promyelocytic leukemia, *Keio J. Med.,* 18, 163, 1969.
341. **Sultan, C., Heilmann-Gouault, M., and Tulliez, M.,** Relationship between blast cells morphology and the occurrence of a syndrome of disseminated intravascular coagulation, *Br. J. Haematol.,* 24, 255, 1973.

342. **Hanker, J. S. and Romanovicz, D. K.,** Phi bodies: peroxidase particles that produce crystalliodal cellular inclusions, *Science,* 197, 895, 1977.
343. **Hanker, J. D., Ambrose, W. W., James, C. J., et al.,** Facilitated light microscopic cytochemical diagnosis of acute myelogeneous leukemia, *Cancer Res.,* 39, 1635, 1979.
344. **Flandrin, G. and Bernard, J.,** Cytological classification of acute leukemia, *Blood Cells,* 1, 7, 1975.
345. **Bennett, J. M., Catovsky, D., Daniel, M. T., et al.,** Proposals for the classification of the acute leukemias, *Br. J. Haematol.,* 33, 431, 1976.
346. **Collins, R. D., Leech, J. H., Waldron, J. A., et al.,** Diagnosis of hematopoietic mononuclear and lymphoid cell neoplasms, *Manual of Clinical Immunology,* Rose, N. R., and Friedman, H., Eds., American Society of Microbiology, Washington, D.C., 1976, 718.
347. **Glick, A. D., Paniker, K., Flexner, J. M., et al.,** Acute leukemia of adults, *Am. J. Clin. Pathol.,* 73, 459, 1980.
348. **Valdivieso, M., Rodriguiez, V., Drewinko, B., et al.,** Clinical and pathological corrections in acute promyelocytic leukemia, *Med. Pediatr. Oncol.,* 1, 37, 1975.
349. **Golomb, H. M., Rowley, J. D., Vardiman, J. W., et al.,** Partial deletion of long arm of chromosome 17: a specific abnormality in acute promyelocytic leukemia? *Arch. Intern. Med.,* 136, 825, 1976.
350. **Rowley, J. D., Golomb, H. M., Vardiman, J. W., et al.,** Further evidence for a consistent chromosomal abnormality in acute promyelocytic leukemia, *Intern. J. Cancer,* 20, 869, 1977.
351. **First International Workshop on Chromosomes in Leukemia,** *Br. J. Haematol.,* 39, 311, 1978.
352. **Rowley, J. D.,** Chromosome changes in acute leukemia, *Br. J. Haematol.,* 44, 339, 1980.
353. **Van Den Berghe, H., Louwagie, A., Broeckaert-Van Orshoven A., et al.,** Chromosome abnormalities in acute promyelocytic leukemia, (APL), *Cancer,* 43, 558, 1979.
354. **Teerenhovi, L., Brogstrom, G. N., Mitelman, F., et al.,** Uneven geographical distribution of 15, 17, translocation in acute promyelocytic leukemia, *Lancet,* 2, 797, 1978.
355. **Golomb, H. M., Rowley, J. D., Vardiman, J. W., et al.,** ''Microgranular'' acute promyelocytic leukemia: a distinct clinical ultrastructural and cytogenetic entity, *Blood,* 55, 253, 1980.
356. **Berger, R., Bernheim, A., Daniel, M. T., et al.,** Une nouvelle variete de leucoemie aigue non promyelocytaire aves translocation (15:17), *Compt. Rend. Acad. Sci., Paris,* 288, 117, 1979.
357. **Bennett, J. M., Catovsky, D., Daniel, M. T., et al.,** A variant form of hypergranular promyelocytic leukemia, (M_3), *Br. J. Haematol.,* 44, 169, 1980.
358. **Liso, V., Troccoli, G., and Graude, M.,** Cytochemical study of acute promyelocytic leukemia, *Blut,* 30, 6, 1975.
359. **Rovera, G., O'Brien, T. G., and Diamond, L.,** Induction and differentiation in human promyelocytic leukemia cells by tumor promotors, *Science,* 204, 868, 1979.
360. **Beckstead, J. H. and Bainton, D. F.,** Enzyme histochemistry of bone marrow biopsies, reactions useful in the differential diagnosis of leukemia and lymphoma applied to 2 micron plastic sections, *Blood,* 55, 386, 1980.
361. **Hayhoe, F. G. and Cawley, J. C.,** Acute leukemia: cellular morphology, cytochemistry and fine structure, *Clin. Haematol.,* 1, 49, 1972.
362. **Perugini, S. and Soldati, M.,** Richerche citochimiche sulla componente protein delle cellule ematiche, *Rich. Istochim. Norm. Pat.,* 1, 217, 1954.
363. **Chervenick, P. A. and Boggs, D. R.,** *In vitro* growth of granulocytic and mononuclear cell colonies from blood of normal individuals, *Blood,* 37, 131, 1971.
364. **Kurnick, J. E. and Robinson, W. A.,** Colony growth of human peripheral white blood cells *in vitro, Blood,* 37, 136, 1971.
365. **McCredie, K. G., Hirsch, E. M., and Freireich, E. J.,** Cells capable of colony formation in the peripheral blood of man, *Science,* 171, 293, 1971.
366. **Zucker-Franklin, D. and Grusky, G.,** Ultrastructural analysis of hemopoietic colonies derived from human peripheral blood, a newly developed method, *J. Cell. Biol.,* 63, 855, 1974.
367. **Zucker-Franklin, D.,** Electron microscopic studies of human granulocytes: structural variations related to function, *Semin. Hematol.,* 5, 109, 1968.
368. **Sparrevohn, W. and Wulff, H. R.,** The nuclear segmentation of the nucleus under normal and pathological conditions, *Acta Haematol.,* 37, 120, 1967.
369. **Zucker-Franklin, D.,** Eosinophil disorders, *Adv. Intern Med.,* 19, 1, 1974.
370. **Polliack, A. and Douglas, S. D.,** Surface features of human eosinophils: a scanning and transmission EM study of a case of eosinophilia, *Br. J. Haematol.,* 30, 303, 1975.
371. **Miller, F., De Harven, E., and Palade, C.,** The structure of eosinophilic leukocyte granules in rodents and in man, *J. Cell. Biol.,* 31, 349, 1966.
372. **Behrens, M. and Marti, H. R.,** Gewinnung der eosinophilien Sobstanz aus isolierten eosinophilien Granulocyten des Pferdesblutes, *Biochim. Biophys. Acta,* 65, 551, 1962.

373. **Gleich, G. J., Loegering, D. A., Mann, K. G., et al.,** Comparative properties of the Charcot-Leyden crystal protein and the major and basic protein from human eosinophils, *J. Clin. Invest.*, 57, 633, 1976.
374. **Parmely, R. T. and Spicer, S. S.,** Cytochemical and ultrastructural identification of a small type granule in human late eosinophils, *Lab. Invest.*, 30, 557, 1974.
375. **Ross, R. and Klebanoff, S. J.,** The eosinophil leucocyte. Fine structure studies of changes in the uterus during the osestrus cycle, *J. Exp. Med.*, 124, 653, 1966.
376. **Bainton, D. F. and Farquhar, M. G.,** Segregation and packaging of granule enzymes in eosinophilic leucocytes, *J. Cell. Biol.*, 45, 54, 1970.
377. **Hardin, J. H. and Spicer, S. S.,** Ultrastructural study of human eosinophil granules: maturational stages and pyrantimonate reactive cation, *Am. J. Anat.*, 128, 283, 1970.
378. **Parmely, R. T. and Spicer, S. S.,** Cytochemical and ultrastructural identification of a small type granule in human late eosinophils, *Lab. Invest.*, 30, 557, 1974.
379. **Bentfield, M. E., Nichols, B. A., and Bainton, D. F.,** Ultrastructural identification of peroxidase in leucocytes of rat bone marrow and blood, *Anat. Res.*, 187, 219, 1977.
380. **Archer, G. T. and Hirsch, J. G.,** Isolation of granules from eosinophil leucocytes and study of their enzyme content, *J. Exp. Med.*, 118, 270, 1963.
381. **Archer, G. T., Air, G., Jakas, M., and Morell, D. B.,** Studies on rat eosinophil peroxidase, *Biochim. Biophys. Acta,* 99, 96, 1965.
382. **Lehrer, R. I., Hanifin, J., and Cline, M. J.,** Defective bactericidal activity in myeloperoxidase-deficient human neutrophils, *Nature,* 223, 78, 1969.
383. **Undritz, E.,** Die alius-Grignaschi anomale der erblich-konstiutionelle peroxidasedefekt der Neutrophilen und Monozyten, *Blut,* 14, 129, 1966.
384. **Presentey, B. Z.,** A new anomaly of eosinophilic granulocytes, *Am. J. Clin. Pathol.*, 49, 887, 1968.
385. **Presentey, B. and Szapiro, L.,** Hereditary deficiency of peroxidase and phospholipids in eosinophilic granulocytes, *Acta Haematol.*, 41, 359, 1969.
386. **West, B. C., Gelb, N. A., and Rosenthal, A. S.,** Isolation and partial characterization of human eosinophil granules, *Am. J. Pathol.*, 81, 575, 1975.
387. **Williams, D. M., Linder, J. E., Hill, M. W., and Gillett, R.,** Ultrastructural localization of alkaline phosphatase in rat eosinophil leucocytes, *J. Histochem. Cytochem.*, 26, 862, 1978.
388. **Borgers, M., Thone, F., DeCree, J., and De Cock, W.,** Alkaline phosphatase activity in human polymorphonuclear leucocytes, *Histochem. J.*, 10, 31, 1978.
389. **Ottesen, E. A. and Cohen, S. G.,** The eosinophil, eosinophilia, and eosinophil related disorders in *Allergy, Principles and Practice,* Vol. 2, Middleton, E., Jr., Reed, C. E., and Ellis, E. F., Eds., C. V. Mosby, St. Louis, 1975, 587.
390. **Kater, L. A., Goetzl, E. J., and, Austen, K. F.,** Isolation of human eosinophil phospholipase D., *J. Clin. Invest.*, 57, 1173, 1976.
391. **Gaidoni, J. J. and Goldberg, A. F.,** Light and electron microscopic localization of acid phosphatase activity in human eosinophil, *Am. J. Clin. Pathol.*, 45, 402, 1966.
392. **Mahmoud, A. A. F., Warren, K. S., and Buros, D. L.,** Production of a rabbit antimouse eosinophil serum with no cross reactivity to neutrophils, *J. Exp. Med.*, 137, 1526, 1973.
393. **Gleich, G. J., Loegering, D. A., and Olson, G. M.,** Reactivity of rabbit antiserum to guinea pig eosinophils, *J. Immunol.*, 115, 950, 1975.
394. **Butterworth, A. E., Coombs, R. R. A., Gurner, B. W., et al.,** Receptors for antibody opsonic adherence on the eosinophils of guniea pigs, *Int. Arch. Allergy Appl. Immunol.*, 51, 368, 1976.
395. **Gupta, S., Ross, G. D., Good, R. A., et al.,** Surface markers of human eosinophils, *Blood,* 48, 757, 1976.
396. **Sher, R. and Glover, A.,** Isolation of human eosinophils and their lymphocyte like rosetting properties, *Immunology,* 31, 337, 1976.
397. **Hudson, G.,** Quantitative study of eosinophil granulocytes, *Sem. Hematol.*, 5, 166, 1968.
398. **Mickenberg, I. D., Root, R. K., and Wolff, S. M.,** Bacericidal and metabolic properties of human eosinophils, *Blood,* 39, 67, 1972.
399. **Baehner, R. and Johnston, R. B.,** Metabolic and bactericidal activities of human eosinophils, *Br. J. Haematol.*, 20, 277, 1971.
400. **Zucker-Franklin, D., Grusky, G., and L'Esperance, P.,** Granulocytic colonies derived from lymphocyte fractions of human peripheral blood, *Proc. Natl. Acad. Sci. (U.S.A.)*, 71, 2711, 1976.
401. **Hudson, G.,** Marrow reserve pool of eosinophils: effect of cortical hormones of foreign protein response, *Br. J. Haematol.*, 10, 122, 1964.
402. **Alexander. P., Monette, F. L., LeBue, J. et al.,** Mechanisms of leukocyte production and release. X. Eosinophil proliferation in rats of different ages, *Scand. J. Haematol.*, 6, 319, 1969.

403. **Spry, C. J. F.,** Mechanisms of eosinophilia, V. Kinetics of normal and accelerated eosinopoiesis, *Cell Tissue Kinet.,* 4, 351, 1971.
404. **Herion, J. C., Glasser, R. M., Walker, R. I., et al.,** Eosinophil kinetics in two patients with eosinophilia, *Blood,* 36, 361, 1970.
405. **Parwaresch, M. R., Walle, A. F., and Arndt, D.,** The peripheral kinetics of human radiolabeled eosinophilia, *Virchows Arch., (Cell Pathol.),* 21, 57, 1976.
406. **Dale, D. C., Hubert, R. T., and Fauci, A.,** Eosinophil kinetics in hypereosinophilia syndrome, *J. Lab. Clin. Med.,* 87, 487, 1976.
407. **Athens, J. W., Haab, O. P., Raab, S. O., et al.,** Leukokinetics studies, IV. The total blood, circulating and marginal granulocyte pools and the granulocyte turnover rate in normal subjects, *J. Clin. Invest.,* 40, 989, 1961.
408. **Zucker-Franklin, D.,** The ultrastructure of cells in human thoracic duct lymph, *J. Ultrastruct. Res.,* 9, 325, 1963.
409. **Spry, C. J. F.,** Mechanisms of eosinophilia. VI. Eosinophil mobilization, *Cell Tissue Kinet.,* 4, 365, 1971.
410. **Hirsch, J. G.,** Neutrophil and eosinophil leukocytes, in *The Inflammatory Process,* Zweifach, B. W., Grant, L., and McCluskey, T. I., Eds., Academic Press, New York, 1965, 245.
411. **Stryckmans, P. A., Cronkite, E. P., Greenberg, M. L., and Schiffer, L. M.,** Kinetics of eosinophil leukocyte proliferation in man, in *Proceedings of the Twelfth Congress of the International Society of Hematology,* New York, 1968, 312 (abstract).
412. **Cohen, N. S., LoBue, B., and Gordon, A. S.,** Mechanisms of leukocyte production and release. VIII. Eosinophil and neutrophil kinetics in rats, *Scand. J. Haematol.,* 4, 339, 1967.
413. **Speirs, R. S. and Osanda, Y.,** Chemotactic activity and phagocytosis and eosinophils, *Proc. Soc. Exp. Biol. Med.,* 109, 929, 1962.
414. **Archer, R. K.,** The eosinophilic leucocytes, *Semin. Hematol.,* 1, 3, 1968.
415. **Teir, H., Rytomaa, T., Cederberg, A., et al.,** Studies on elimination of granulocytes in the intestinal rat, *Acta Patho. Scand.,* 59, 311, 1964.
416. **Rohr, K.,** *Das Menschliche Knochenmarke,* Georg Theme Verlag, Stuttgart, 1960, 316.
417. **McGarry, M. P., Miller, A. M., and Colley, D. G.,** Humoral regulation of eosinophil granulocytopoiesis, in *Experimental Hematology Today,* Baum J. J. and Ledney, D. E., Eds., Springer-Verlag, New York, 1977, 64.
418. **Basten, A. and Baeson, P. B.,** Mechanisms of eosinophilia. II. Role of the lymphocyte, *J. Exp. Med.,* 131, 1288, 1970.
419. **Walls, R. S., Bass, D. A., and Beeson, P. B.,** Mechanisms of eosinophils. X. Evidence for immunologic specificity of the stimulus, *Proc. Soc. Exp. Bio. Med.,* 145, 1240, 1974.
420. **McGarry, M. P., Speirs, R. S., Jenkins, V. K., and Trentin, J. J.,** Lymphoid cell dependence of eosinophil response to antigen, *J. Exp. Med.,* 134, 801, 1971.
421. **Speirs, R. S., Gallagher, M. T., Rauschwerster, J., et al.,** Lymphoid cell dependence of eosinophil response to antigen. II. Location of memory cells and their dependence of thymic influence, *Exp. Hematol.,* 1, 150, 1973.
422. **Cohen, N. S., LeBue, J., and Gordon, A. S.,** Humoral regulation of eosinophil production and release, in *Humoral Control of Growth and Differentiation,* Vol. 1, LoBue, J., and Gordon, A. S., Eds., Academic Press, New York, 1971, 69.
423. **Benvenisti, D. S. and Ultmann, J. E.,** Eosinophilic leukemia. Report of five cases and review of the literature, *Ann. Intern. Med.,* 71, 73, 1969.
424. **Flannery, E. P.,** Eosinophilic leukemia with fibrosing endocarditis and short Y chromosome, *Ann. Intern. Med.,* 77, 232, 1972.
425. **Chusid, M. J., Dale, D. C., West, B. C., and Wolff, S. M.,** The hypereosinophilic syndrome: analysis of fourteen cases with review of the literature, *Medicine,* 54, 1, 1975.
426. **Bitran, J. D., Rowley, J. D., Plapp, F., et al.,** Chromosomal aneuploidy in a patient with hypereosinophilic syndrome evidence for malignant disease, *Am. J. Med.,* 63, 1010, 1977.
427. **Butterworth, A. E., Wasom, D. L., Gleich, G. J., et al.,** Damage to schistomula of *Schistosoma mansoni* induced directly by eosinophil major basic protein, *J. Immunol.,* 122, 221, 1979.
428. **Bassom, D. L. and Gleich, G. J.,** Damage to *Trichinella spiralis* new born larvae by eosinophilic basic protein, *Am. J. Trop. Med. Hyg.,* 28, 860, 1979.
429. **Gleich, G. J., Frigas, E., Loegering, D. A., et al.,** Cytotoxic properties of the eosinophil major basic protein, *J. Immunol.,* 123, 2925, 1979.
430. **Durack, D. T., Sumi, S. M., and Klebanoff, S. J.,** Neurotoxicity of human eosinophils, *Proc. Natl. Acad. Sci.,* 76, 1443, 1979.
431. **Juhlin, L.,** Basophil leucocyte diffferential in blood and bone marrow, *Acta Haematol.,* 29, 89, 1963.

432. **Cooper, J. R. and Cruickshank, C. N. D.,** Improved method for direct counting of basophil leucocytes, *J. Clin. Patho.*, 19, 402, 1966.
433. **Michaels, N. A.,** The mast cells, reprinted from *Handbook of Hematology*, Downey, H., 1938, in *Ann. N. Y. Acad. Sci.*, 103, 1, 1963 (appendix).
434. **Hastie, R.,** A study of the ultrastructure of human basophilic leucocytes, *Lab. Invest.*, 31, 223, 1974.
435. **Zucker-Franklin, D.,** Electron microscopic study of human basophils, *Blood*, 29, 878, 1967.
436. **Dvorak, A. M., Dvorak, H. F., and Karnovsky, M. J.,** Uptake of horse radish peroxidase by guinea pig basophilic leucocytes, *Lab. Invest.*, 26, 27, 1972.
437. **Barker, B. E., Farnes, P., and Harrison, P. E.,** *In vitro* differentation of basophilic granulocytes from human blood CFU-C, *J. Cell. Biol.*, 701, (Abstr.), 100, 1976.
438. **Burgess, A. W., Metcalf, D., and Russel, S.,** Regulation of hematopoietic differentiation and proliferation by colony stimulating factors, in *Cold Spring Harbor Symposium on Differentiation of Normal and Neoplastic Hematopoietic Cells.*, Cold Spring, Harbor, N.Y., Sept. 6–11, 1977, Abstr. 21.
439. **Kerry, R. W., Bainton, D. F., and Farquhar, M. G.,** Formation and structure of specific granules in basophilic leukocytes of the guinea pig, *Lab. Invest.*, 21, 65, 1969.
440. **Ackerman, G. A.,** Cytochemical properties of the blood basophilic granulocyte, *Ann. N.Y. Acad. Sci.*, 103, 376, 1963.
441. **Benveniste, J.,** Platelet activating factor, a new mediator of anaphylaxis and immune complex deposition from rabbit and human basophils, *Nature*, 249, 581, 1974.
442. **Dvorak, H. F. and Dvorak, A. M.,** Basophilic leukocytes: structure, function and role in disease, *Clin. Haematol.*, 4, 651, 1975.
443. **Dvorak, A. M. and Dvorak, H. F.,** The basophil, *Arch. Pathol. Lab. Med.*, 103, 551, 1979.
444. **Hatanaka, K., Kitamura, Y., and Nishimune, Y.,** Local development of mast cells from bone marrow derived precursors in the skin of mice, *Blood*, 53, 142, 1979.
445. **Kitamura, Y., Shimada, M., Go S., et al.,** Distribution of mast cell precursors in hematopoietic tissues of mice, *J. Exp. Med.*, 150, 452, 1979.
446. **Zucker-Franklin, D.,** Ultrastructrual evidence for the common origin of human mast cells and basophils, *Blood*, 56, 534, 1980.
447. **Denburg, J., Davison, M., and Bienenstock, J.,** Basophil production, *J. Clin. Invest.*, 65, 390, 1980.
448. **Dvorak, H. F., Selvaggio, S. S., Dvorak, A. M. et al.,** Purification of basophilic leukocytes from guinea pig blood and bone marrow, *J. Immunol.*, 113, 1694, 1974.
449. **Rebuck, J. W., Hudson, J. M., Priest, B. J., and Barth, C. L.,** Basophilic granulocytes in inflammatory tissues of man, *Ann. N.Y. Acad. Sci.*, 103, 409, 1963.
450. **Dvorak, A. M., Dickerson, G. R., Connell, A. et al.,** Degranulation mechanisms in human leukemic basophils, *Clin. Immuno. Immunopathol.*, 5, 235, 1976.

Chapter 11

PATHOPHYSIOLOGY OF THE MONOCYTE-MACROPHAGE SYSTEM

Sidney Trubowitz and Stephen Davis

TABLE OF CONTENTS

I. INTRODUCTION

Almost 100 years ago, Metchnikoff[1] identified highly phagocytic cells in the vicinity of experimentally induced inflammation and named these cells macrophages. His studies led him to conclude that the macrophages were widely distributed in animal tissues and that in their aggregate they constitute a system of a particular cell type. He championed a central role for the macrophages in the animal's defense against invading microorganisms.[2] Kiyono,[3] in his studies on inflammation, showed that intravenously administered carmine appeared not only in cells which had accumulated in the inflammatory site, but also in cells widely distributed throughout the organism and far from the inflammatory area. Aschoff[4] utilized the findings of his collaborator, Kiyono,[3] to define a system of cells, the reticuloendothelial system (RES), whose common property was the ability to store intravitally administered dyes. The RES in its widest sense, included all cells with strong uptake of dye and which were found principally in the spleen, lymph nodes, bone marrow, Peyer's patches, adrenals, hypophysis, Kupffer cells, connective tissue histiocytes, and blood monocytes. The endothelial cells and fibroblasts showed weak uptake of dye and only under the extraordinary conditions of high dye dosage which raised some doubt about their relationship to the RES.[4]

In more recent years incisive studies on marrow transplantation into irradiated mice led to the unequivocal recognition of the bone marrow as the source of the circulating monocytes and the tissue macrophages.[5] By the application of appropriate markers, it was shown that the peritoneal macrophages, the alveolar macrophages, the Kupffer cells as well as the macrophages of spleen, lymph nodes, and bone marrow originate from the marrow cells of the donor.[6–8] More precise identification of the monocytes and macrophages was made possible by the elucidation of more specific morphological,[9] cytochemical,[10] and functional characteristics of these cells.[11,12]

About a decade ago the accumulated data on the monocytes and macrophages made it necessary to reorder and modify the concept of the RES and a new classification—the monocyte-macrophage system was introduced. The scheme derived the circulating monocyte from bone marrow percursors and through the monocyte the free and fixed macrophages in the lung, pleura, peritoneum, liver, spleen, bone marrow, lymphatic tissue, microglia of the nervous system, and the histiocytes of the connective tissue. Fibroblasts and endothelial cells were excluded from membership of the monocyte macrophage system.[14–17]

II. MONOCYTOPOIESIS

A. Morphology

Evidence from a variety of sources, both clinical[18] and experimental,[10,19–21] suggests a common progenitor cell for both monocytic and granulocytic proliferation. The exact level of maturation at which irrevocable commitment to either cell line of differentiation takes place is not known but is generally presumed to be at the level of the myeloblast or the committed cells immediately before it.

The monoblast cannot be reliably identified by current techniques. Those cells identified as monoblasts in acute monocytic leukemia display minimal if any functional activity usually associated with monocytes. Such cells show little motility, adhesiveness to glass, and are rarely phagocytic. Thus, the recognizable cells of monocyte differentiation in the marrow are limited essentially to two compartments, the promonocytes and monocytes.

The promonocytes and monocytes constitute 1.4 to 8.8% of the marrow cells obtained by needle aspiration of normal human subjects.[9] The mean value is 5.3% ± 2.0%, of which 1.0% ± 0.8% are promonocytes. The ratio of promonocytes: monocytes is about 1:3.5 to 4. The ratio of monocytes to segmented polymorphonuclear leucocytes in the marrow is about three times larger than the ratio of these cells in the blood.[10]

The promonocyte, the earliest identifiable cell of the monocyte lineage, is a large cell, about 10 to 15 μm in diameter with a large nuclear/cytoplasmic ratio. The cytoplasm is basophilic and has some peroxidase activity. The cells are identified by their ability to stick to glass and incorporate ^3H-thymidine. The cells show modest phagocytic ability. The nucleus is large, contains prominent nucleoli, is generally round, but may begin to show evidence of elongation. No granules are visible in the cytoplasm. On phase microscopy, the cell outline is irregular and some ruffling of the cell membrane is evident.[22–26]

On electron microscopic examination the promonocyte compartment consists of cells of varying degrees of maturity. The earliest promonocyte has a large nucleus with minimally condensed chromatin and large nucleoli; the nucleus occupies most of the cell volume. Peroxidase reaction product is present in the cisternae of the rough endocytoplasmic reticulum and of the Golgi complex and in mature and immature granules. In a slightly more mature promonocyte the nuclear cytoplasmic ratio is smaller. This is a result of an increase in cytoplasmic volume due to the expansion of rough endocytoplasmic reticulum, a more developed Golgi complex, and the newly generated granules. The peroxidase reaction product is seen throughout the cisternae of the rough endoplasmic reticulum and in the large, paranuclear Golgi complex. Increased numbers of more mature granules are present, all peroxidase positive.[27,28]

The process of granule formation is strikingly similar to that described for the neutrophilic cells. Small vesicles arise from the Golgi cisternes. The small vesicles fuse to form larger immature granules which by condensation form the mature granules. The immature granules are spherical, large, up to 500 nm in diameter, and contain dense clumps of peroxidase reaction product. The mature granules are smaller, 400 to 500 nm, and are homogeneously dense. The mature granules elongate and may show central constrictions.[29,30]

The monocyte of the human marrow is morphologically indistinguishable from the circulating monocyte. The cells range from 8 to 12 μm in diameter and possess an abundant gray blue cytoplasm with a modest content of fine azurophilic granules. The nucleus is elongated, indented, or horseshoe-shaped with a small barely noticeable nucleolus, and although the chromatin is more condensed than in the promonocytes, it still retains a more lacy structure and is much less condensed than the nucleus of the mature granulocyte. On phase microscopic observation, the monocyte is an actively motile cell forming large undulating ruffles.

In summary, the cells in the early stage of monocyte differentiation have high nuclear cytoplasmic ratio, fine chromatin pattern, nucleoli, and blue cytoplasm. The promonocytes are identified ultrastructurally by the initiation of granule formation and can be distinguished from promyelocytes by morphological criteria. The granules formed during the promonocyte level of maturation are lysosomal in character and contain peroxidase. With further maturation the cytoplasmic basophilia diminishes, azurophilic granules appear, and the nuclear chromatin becomes more compact. At this stage the formation of the primary lysosomal granules stops and a second population of peroxidase negative granules are formed.[27,28] The marrow monocyte is indistinguishable from its circulating counterpart and has on an average about 60 granules per thin section of which about half may be peroxidase positive.

The monocyte granules contain acid hydrolases, a monospecific lipase, lysozyme, and peroxidase.[29,30] Detailed information on the contents of the monocyte granules is not available, hindered in great measure by the small population of monocytes in blood and marrow making the application of analytic biochemical techniques difficult. With advancing maturation, the monocytic cells show, in addition to the predominant morphological features outlined, increasing adhesiveness to glass, enhanced phagocytic ability, heavier concentration of surface receptors for the Fc fragment of IgG and C_3, and more abundant membrane ruffles.

B. Kinetics

The application of tritiated thymidine or tritiated diisopropylfluorophosphate as kinetic markers and microautoradiography for evaluation of cells identified as monocytes by cytochemical means enabled Meuret and Hoffman[17,31] to obtain some basic information on monocyte kinetics in man. They enumerated the relative number of promonocytes in the human marrow at 3% and calculated a total medullary pool of promonocytes at 6×10^8 cells per kg body weight. Only about 40% of the promonocytes were actively proliferating with a mean cell cycle time of about 30 hr and a mean DNA synthesis time of about 10 hr. The remaining promonocytes were thought to be either out of cell cycle or had cell cycle time considerably longer than could be detected by their pulse labeling technique.

The transit time from stem cell to blood monocyte was estimated at about 55 hr. The rapidly proliferating monocytes divided twice in this period and achieved a monocyte production rate of about 7×10^5 monocytes per kg body weight per hr.[17] The nonproliferative promonocytes, in the schema proposed by Meuret and Hoffman, constituted a reserve pool that could be rapidly mobilized into the proliferative pool and designed to meet an increased demand for monocytes. The increased demand for monocytes by the organism could thus be met by the rapid recruitment of the nonproliferating promonocytes and a reduction of cell cycle time as well as by an increased inflow of precursor cells into the recognizable pool. The two processes were thought to be independent of each other.

The majority of the monocytes left the marrow after their normal maturation time of 55 to 60 hr. The cells, however, departed from the marrow at random and were almost all in a nonproliferative, G_1 phase. An increase in monocyte demand not only stimulated more marrow promonocytes into active cell proliferation but also shifted the release of earlier, less mature monocytes.

The monocytes on leaving the marrow circulated in the peripheral blood with a half disappearance time ($T\frac{1}{2}$) of 8.4 hr and formed, like the neutrophils, two pools, a circulating monocyte pool of about 18×10^6 cells per kg body weight and a marginated pool of 63×10^6 cells per kg. The total blood monocyte pool was 81×10^6 monocytes per kg body weight with a circulating to marginal monocyte pool ratio of 1:3.5. The circulating monocytes left the circulating pool in an exponential fashion and the monocyte turnover rate averaged 7×10^6 cells per kg body weight per hr. The monocyte turnover rate seen has been found to correspond to monocyte production rates in the marrow and the clearance of peripheral tissue macrophages.[32,33] The blood monocyte count showed a positive correlation with the total blood monocyte pool or the monocyte turnover rate.

In a more recent study, Van Furth et al.[34] examined the human mononuclear phagocytes from the bone marrow, the peripheral blood, the skin, and the peritoneal cavity. They emphasized the similarities between the mononuclear phagocytes of the different body sites with respect to their cytochemical reactions (esterase and peroxidase), the presence of surface receptors (IgG, C), and their pinocytotic and phagocytic activity. They estimated the monocyte content of the bone marrow at 0.99% ± 0.43% (SD) of the marrow nucleated cells, of which about 5.0% were promonocytes. Assuming a total bone marrow nucleated cell content of 10.5×10^9 cells per kg body weight, Van Furth et al.[34] estimated the total number of promonocytes for a 70-kg man at 0.4×10^9, cells/kg and monocytes at 1.7×10^9 cells/kg. Following incubation with ^{3}H-thymidine, 78.8% ± 7.7% of the promonocytes were labeled, indicative of an actively proliferating compartment. Conversely, only 0.196% of the marrow monocytes, were labeled—a nondividing compartment. They further estimated the cell cycle time of the promonocyte at 48.2 hr and a DNA synthesis time of 37.5 hr.

Van Furth et al.[34] estimated the number of circulating monocytes at $1.7 \times 10.^9$ They argued that the short half-life of 8.4 hr found for 32-DFP labeled monocytes was probably artifact due to cell damage incident to the handling of the cells. They accepted a half-life of 71 hr for the monocyte in circulation and argued against the existence of a marginating pool, as proposed by Meuret.[31] Assuming, then, a half-life of 71 hr for the human monocyte in circulation, Van Furth et al.[34] calculated the number of circulating monocytes exiting the circulation at 16.6×10^9 monocytes/hr and, hence, a daily blood monocyte turnover of 0.4×10^9 cells.

The mean circulation time of the monocyte in healthy men has been estimated at about 6 days,[34] and about 3 days in patients with monocytic leukemia.[35,36] Like the neutrophils, monocytes probably do not reenter the circulating blood following their migration into the tissues.

III. THE CIRCULATING MONOCYTE

The circulating blood monocyte is morphologically and cytochemically indistinguishable from the mature monocyte of the marrow. Monocytes are distinguishable from other large circulating mononuclear cells by their cell surface receptors and the presence of certain esterases. The monocyte has mitochondria, a Golgi complex, lamellae of endocytoplasmic reticulum and polyribosomes, and bundles of filaments,[25] which may be involved in cell movement, endocytosis, and phagocytosis.[37–40] The monocyte is thus well equipped to carry out its functional activities of adherence, ingestion, locomotion, and granule formation. These properties are enhanced on incubation of the monocytes with various stimulating factors, such as latex particles or Ig-coated red blood cells. Such stimuli may induce the monocyte to take on the morphological features of macrophages.[41]

A. Monocyte Blood Count

The absolute monocyte count for healthy adults is generally given as 300 to 450/mm^3 and 1000 to 1200/mm^3 in the first 2 weeks of postnatal life. There is a gradual decline of the monocyte count from childhood to adult life. The upper level of normal for the adult has been set by some authorities at 500 monocytes per mm^3 and 750 cells/mm^3 for children.[43] Bessis,[44] however, puts the normal monocyte count in blood at 1000 cells/mm^3 and the upper limit of normal at 2000 cells/mm^3. Transient monocytopenia has been reported to follow the administration of endotoxin[45] and antibody-coated red cells.[46] Glucocorticoids induce a monocytopenia possibly by inhibiting the release of monocytes from the bone marrow.[47] Monocytosis most commonly accompanies the chronic inflammatory states such as sarcoidosis, Hodgkin's disease, tuberculosis, and the collagen vascular diseases and malignancy. Monocytopenia, in a clinical setting, has not thus far achieved significance or relevance.

B. Monocyte-Macrophage Transformation

The monocytes under steady state conditions spend a relatively brief period of their life span in the blood stream. They leave the intravascular compartment in a random fashion throughout all the capillary beds by migrating between the endothelial cells.

Once in the tissues, the cells do not reenter the intravascular compartment and in response to stimuli as yet unknown undergo further maturation and are transformed into functionally more active cells, the tissue macrophages. The tissue macrophages are ubiquitous, present in all parenchymatous tissues, but most abundantly in the lungs as the alveolar macrophages; in the liver as the Kupffer cells; in lymph nodes, spleen, and bone marrow where they are often referred to as histiocytes; and in the pleural and peritoneal spaces. The macrophages are distributed most prominently about the blood vessels and sinusoids.[12,84,49] The tissue macrophages thus formed under steady state conditions have a fairly long life span, greater than 60 days, with a very low order of replication. However, the capacity to replicate is retained.

Monocytes accumulate at sites of both acute and chronic inflammation whether provoked by endogenous or experimentally introduced exogeneous agents, and promote monocyte macrophage transformation.[50,51] Monocytes also transform readily into macrophages in tissue culture and can be maintained as a primary culture for study.[48,52–54] Macrophages arising in response to inflammation, lymphokines, and chemotactic agents may show enhanced pinocytosis, phagocytosis, augmented numbers of cytoplasmic granules, and a greater capacity for microbial and tumor cell destruction. Such cells have been loosely termed activated macrophages. The study of macrophages from different anatomical sites and under different experimental conditions has led to considerable confusion in nomenclature.[55]

Spicer et al.[56] view the transformation of the monocyte to macrophage as the conversion of the cytoplasmic granules from a population of primary lysosomes into one of secondary lysosomes of heterophage nature. The process begins with the pinocytotic uptake of macromolecules or small particles, or the formation of phagosomes following the phagocytosis of large particulate material. The vesicles or phagosomes fuse with the primary lysosomes to form the heterophagic dense bodies. The endocytic activity causes increase in the lysosomal enzymes.[57]

C. Multinucleated Giant Cells

Macrophages, under appropriate influence, are capable of forming multinucleated giant cells, a characteristic feature of many of the specific granulomata. It is now generally agreed that the macrophage-giant cell transformation is achieved principally through cell fusion, rather than by endomitosis.[58] More recent evidence suggests that the formation of the multinucleated giant cell is mediated by T cells,[59,60] via a lymphokine (mol wt 6000 D), the macrophage fusion factor.[61,62] The surface ultrastructure of multinucleated giant cells produced by macrophage fusion factor from BCG-treated lymphocytes was shown to be similar to that of a macrophage.[63] The function of the multinucleated giant cell is not quite clear. Is it simply a beefed-up macrophage or a cell with newly acquired talents? Sutton and Weiss[54] concluded from their anatomical studies that active transport may be the primary role of the multinucleated giant cell. For them, the function of the monocyte appears to be the synthesis and storage of lysosomes, the formation of the macrophage, and the formation of secondary lysosomes and phagosomes, whereas, the function of the multinucleated giant cell is active transport in addition to the sequestration of foreign particles.

IV. MONOCYTE AND MACROPHAGE HETEROGENEITY

Recent studies purport to show heterogeneity for both monocytes and macrophages. Utilizing peroxidase, acid phosphatase, and nonspecific esterase stains, Kaplow[64] demonstrated variability in reaction, particularly in nonspecific esterase and peroxidase. The significance of the cytochemical heterogeneity is not clear. Arenson et al.[65] separated the human blood monocytes by volume. They found three populations of cells with approximate volumes of 150, 250, and 480 μm^3. The large cells of group 3 were considerably more responsive to a chemotactic stimulus than the smaller cells in the two remaining groups. The macrophage was recognized quite early as a much more heterogeneous cell in terms of its structural characteristics than the monocyte.[66] The heterogeneity of macrophages exists not only between macrophages isolated from different anatomical sites such as between alveolar macrophages and Kupffer cells, but also among the macrophages isolated from a single source, as for example, the cells isolated from the peritoneum or lung. Heterogeneity of the macrophages may result from local, environmental factors of specific tissues, for example, lung vs. marrow vs. liver; or, arise from differences in the degree of differentiation or maturation within a given population of cells, or possibly by their origin from distinctly different monocyte lines. Important determinants of heterogeneity at any local site are recruitment and turnover, influenced greatly by the intensity, and the nature of the stimulus at that site. Different stimuli may affect different subpopulations of monocytes and macrophages.[9,67]

Some basic strategies have been devised in the pursuit of well-defined marcrophage subsets. Macrophages can be cultivated from the bone marrow, peritoneal exudates, or liver[68–70] to give populations of different anatomical origin. Cells can be separated by appropriate antisera or by virtue of size. Support for the approach by cell size is based on the knowledge that monocyte macrophage transformation is accompanied by a three-fold increase in cell volume without cell division,[70,71] and indeed functionally distinct subpopulations of macrophages at various stages of differentation have been separated according to size.[65]

Morphologic and cytochemical heterogeneity of macrophages obtained from the peritoneal cavity of guinea pigs led Daems and Brederou[72] to question whether all of the macrophages are monocyte derived. In their study, structural and cytochemical differences distinguished the resident macrophages from the exudate (induced by sterile physiological saline) macrophages. The exudate macrophages retained the peroxidase activity characteristic of the monocyte and it was therefore concluded that the exudate macrophages are derived directly from monocytes and that the tissue macrophages are resident cells from a selfsustaining population. In a follow up, study Daems et al.[73] showed that monocytes in diffusion chambers implanted in the peritoneal cavity of guinea pigs became macrophages but did not acquire the characteristics of tissue macrophages, and they, therefore, concluded that the tissue macrophages arose from a source other than the bone marrow, most likely from local precursors in the tissue. The authors cited studies[74–76] which showed that an increase in liver macrophages is dependent on the proliferation of Kupffer cells rather than on the migration of monocytes, in support of their argument. They also referred in this connection to the observations of Golde et al.[77] that the alveolar macrophage population persisted and is selfsustaining in patients with severe monocytopenia. On the other hand, evidence has been provided to support the contention that all macrophages arise from monocytes and that the heterogeneity observed is a reflection of differentiation and maturation. Cline and Sumner[78] studied monocytes and macrophages in tissue culture and described a series of stages of differentation beginning with an undifferentiated blast cell which was characterized by active DNA synthesis and positive peroxidase activity but lacking the properties of glass adherence, phagocytosis, or receptor binding of IgG. This stage was followed by a promonocyte, monocyte, immature macrophage, and finally the mature macrophage. A steady increase in the monocytic characteristics of glass adhesiveness, phagocytosis, and receptors for IgG paralleled the advancing maturation of the cell. DNA synthetic and mitotic activity and peroxidase activity declined in the sequence of increasing maturation.

Bodel et al.[79] cautioned against the use of peroxidase localization as a basis for advocating the existence of two separate lines of macrophages. They were able to show that the free peritoneal macrophages, elicited into the peritoneal cavity by various stimulants, lacked peroxidase activity in the rough endocytoplasmic reticulum and perinuclear cisternae, unlike the resident peritoneal macrophages which contain the enzyme. The cells, however, acquired peroxidatic activity in their rough endocytoplasmic reticulum and perinuclear cisternae following their adherence to fibrin-coated or plastic surfaces in culture. They concluded that the macrophages, like the blood monocytes, may rapidly acquire peroxidase activity in response to the plasma membrane/external surface interaction. The confusion implied in Bloch's descriptive appellation for the macrophages as the motley phagocytes had not yet been lifted.[80]

In Romanowsky stained material the macrophage is recognized by its large size, some 20 to 50 μm in diameter, and an eccentrically placed elongated or lobulated nucleus whose chromatin is often clumped. The cells tend to be oval with an abundant faintly acidophilic cytoplasmic mass that contains numerous vacuoles. The cell margins may be indistinct. On phase microscopy, the macrophages are slowly motile with intense ruffling of their membranes. Phase-dense granules are present in the central zones of the cytoplasm and absent from the outer peripheral zones where many refractile lipid droplets can be seen. The ultrastructural features include a large Golgi complex, lysosomal granules, and an irregular surface from which many small marrow projections protrude.

V. FUNCTIONS OF MONOCYTE-MACROPHAGE SYSTEM

The monocyte-macrophage system has long been considered one of the central pillars in the normal host's defense system, by virtue of its extraordinary capacity to ingest and digest microorganisms, and damaged tissue components, and to remove and dispose of a variety of foreign materials.[1,2] In recent years the catalog of functions ascribed to the monocyte-macrophage systems has grown considerably. In addition to their predominant phagocytic role these cells are capable of synthesizing and secreting a number of biologic molecules such as collagenase, elastase,[81,82] plasminogen activators,[83] interferons,[84] lysozyme,[85] prostaglandin,[86] certain complement components,[87] chemotactic factors, and pyrogen. Monocytes and macrophages also secrete colony stimulating activity, a glycoprotein, which stimulates the growth of granulocyte precursors cells in vitro and which may be an important regulatory arm of stem cell proliferation in the marrow[88–94] (see previous chapters).

Monocytes and macrophages are significantly involved in the initiation and regulation of the immune response. Macrophages play an important role in the induction of the immune response by their ingestion and localization of the antigen which the cell can handle in two ways:

1. The elimination of the bulk of the antigenic material by digestion
2. The retention of a small amount of antigenic fragments associated with RNA which is highly immunogenic and critical for the initiation of the immune response by the lymphocyte [95]

The monocytes interact with both T and B cells by direct contact and by the secretion of regulatory molecules. The processed immunogen is transferred by the macrophage to the appropriate lymphocyte. T-cell proliferation requires interaction with antigen bearing macrophages. The macrophage is a principal control site of the immune response gene and is intimately involved in both the humoral and cellular immune response. The macrophages can amplify the immune response through its action on the helper T cells and conversely suppress the reaction, possibly by direct action on the B cell or indirectly through its action on the suppressive T cells. The macrophage in turn are affected by lymphokines secreted by T cells. Macrophage activity and macrophage secretions in the immune reaction are responsible for many of the clinical and pathological manifestations of the allergic and inflammatory diseases. The details of macrophage interaction with the lymphocytic system and the immune response have been covered in great detail in recent reviews and the reader is referred to them for a comprehensive account.[96–105]

The realization of the active involvement of the monocyte macrophage system in cellular immunity has directed attention to the antitumor activity of these cells. Under experimental conditions, mononuclear phagocytes can inhibit the growth or even kill tumor cells. Suggestive evidence for the involvement of the macrophages in tumor immunity came with the early demonstration by Old et al.[106] that BCG infection can render mice resistant to a tumor graft. The methods, for the most part, by which macrophage-mediated antitumor activity was demonstrated, were based on cytotoxicity. Peritoneal macrophages were convincingly shown to be capable of rejecting tumor cells.[107–111] The mechanism of macrophage cytotoxicity has not been clearly defined and can apparently be mediated by both specific and nonspecific means. Thus, peritoneal macrophages obtained from animals infected with parasites were found to be nonspecifically cytotoxic for tumor cells.[110] Specific cytotoxicity is probably mediated by sensitized lymphocytes. Macrophage phagocytosis and lysosomal triggering are the most likely direct mechanisms in tumor cell killing. Macrophages may also play an indirect role in tumor rejection by their stimulation of T and B cell lymphocytes. For reviews of macrophage function in malignant disease see References 112–114.

The catalog of functions and secretory products attributed to the monocyte-macrophage system has indeed become prodigious. Macrophages are thought to interact with fibroblasts and play an important role in wound healing. The macrophage is the principal phagocytic cell in wound repair and responsible for wound healing both in terms of onset and rate of proliferation of fibroblasts. The macrophages may also be involved in the fibrotic reaction encountered in certain inflammatory states as in the pneumoconioses.[14,115,116] The macrophages secrete, in addition to their lysosomal enzymes, chemical mediators such as the prostaglandins, cytolytic factors, complement factors, fibronectin,[117] procoagulant activity,[118] colony stimulating factor, etc.[119–121]

VI. THE BONE MARROW MACROPHAGES

Macrophages are widely distributed throughout the body and their general functions may be modified to subserve the more specific requirements of the organs or tissues of residence. The marrow macrophages may be derived from the circulating monocytes which reenter the marrow or from the promonocytes and monocytes of the marrow. The question of a nonmonocyte origin of the marrow macrophages is moot.

The marrow macrophage is a large cell, up to 30 μm in diameter on smears with an abundant light grey cytoplasm containing scarce to small numbers of azurophilic granules and variable amounts of debris. The nucleus is eccentric, oval or round. The cells are found in association with the sinusoids, erythrocyte precursors, granulocytic precursors, lymphocytes, and plasma cells.

The macrophages of the bone marrow appear to be part of the three dimensional syncytium of stromal cells, the so-called reticulum cells, which constitute the basic cellular matrix of the hemopoietic microenvironment. This network of cells extends throughout the entire marrow parenchyma and consists of phagocytic and nonphagocytic reticulum cells.[122] The two cell populations can be distinguished cytochemically. The nonphagocytic cells are rich in alkaline phosphatase.[123,124] The phagocytic reticular cell or macrophage displays considerable acid phosphatase activity.[125,126] The latter cells have long been associated with the proliferating red cell precursors in the so-called erythroblastic island.[127] Westen and Bainton[128] in a combined cytochemical and ultrastructural study of rodent marrows found alkaline phosphatase-rich reticulum cells concentrated near the endosteum and in close association with the myeloblasts and the neutrophilic promyelocytes. The acid phosphatase-containing macrophage type of reticulum cell was distributed uniformly throughout the marrow and was associated mainly with the red cell precursors.

Reticular cells have also been observed in close association with lymphocytes as lymphocytic islands,[129] and with plasma cells, the plasmocytic islands.[130–132] It is of interest that Undritz,[133] who first called attention to the blood cell nests, identified the central, regional cell as a monocyte. Whether all of the marrow reticular cells are derivatives of a single cell lineage modified by local environmental circumstances or are differentiated cells of different cell lines is not known. It is, however, clear that the entire gamut of reticular cells play a fundamentally important role in the different functions of the bone marrow: in the regulation of hematopoiesis, in the removal of the debris resulting from cell proliferation, and in the large immune capacity of the marrow.

The monocyte-macrophage system is a widely distributed continuum of cells throughout the body with a particularly heavy concentration in the liver, spleen, lymph nodes, and marrow. The bone marrow occupies a unique position in this constellation of cells for it serves not only as the organ of origin of the cells of the mononuclear phagocyte system but also as an integral and important member of the system in the host's defense against infection and tumor. Further, through its participation in iron and lipid metabolism and its secretion of regulatory molecules, the marrow macrophages serve the marrow in its primary task of hematopoiesis.

VII. MARROW MACROPHAGES IN DISEASES

It is clear from what has been described above that the monocyte-macrophage system with its highly complex assortment of varied morphological and functional attributes and its interlocking directorate with multilineal cell systems would present in its disordered state an intricate display of clinical manifestations. Some attempts have been made to bring order into this maze. Territo and Cline[134] and Cline and Golde[135–137] classified the malignant disorders of the macrophage system according to the level of cell differentation. The acute and more malignant disorders arise, according to this scheme, from the monoblasts and promonocytes and the more chronic and less aggressive diseases from the mature "B" macrophage. They further subdivided the disorders of the monocyte-macrophage system into the storage cell disease arising from metabolic abnormalities of the macrophage; dysfunction syndromes due to disorders of impaired bone marrow function; and the reactive hyperplasias due to the secondary response of the mononuclear phagocyte system to some systemic disorder.

Meuret[138] advanced a somewhat similar grouping of the disorders of the monocyte-macrophage system. He divided the macrophage disorders into four basic groups:

1. Those diseases arising from alterations in the association of the monocyte-macrophage system with hematopoiesis and which included the acute and chronic nonlymphocytic leukemias, the preleukemic states, aplastic anemia, and myelofibrosis.
2. The disorders arising from alterations in the association of the monocyte-macrophage system and granulocytopoiesis which include chronic granulomatous disease, mye-

loperoxidase deficiency, Chediak-Higashi syndrome, and the congenital neutropenias

3. The disorders due to alterations of macrophage function and include the lipid storage diseases and the idiopathic histiocytoses
4. The disorders arising from alterations of the association of the monocyte-macrophage system and the lymphocytes and encompass the various inflammatory, infectious, immune, and malignant diseases

A. Monocytosis and Reactive Hyperplasia

Hyperplasia of the monocyte-macrophage system is a well-recognized phenomenon in the response of the host to certain chronic infections, such as tuberculosis,[139] subacute bacterial endocarditis, syphilis, etc;[43] chronic inflammatory disorders such as sprue and ulcerative colitis; collagen vascular disease such as rheumatoid arthritis, subacute lupus erythematosus, and periarteritis nodosa. Macrophage hyperplasia may also accompany the pneumoconioses (silica, beryllium) and those disorders characterized by a rapid turnover of cells, e.g., hemolytic anemias, idiopathic thrombocytopenia purpura, and the solid tumors.[140,141] The increased demand for macrophages is met by an increased recruitment of monocytes from the blood, stimulating therefore increased monocytopoiesis in the bone marrow. The peripheral blood may reflect this demand by monocytosis, with monocyte counts greater than 500 cells/mm^3 in the adult.[4]

The increased demand for macrophages imposed by the inflammatory state is met by increased replication of the monoblasts and promonocytes in the marrow, more rapid cell differentiation, a decreased marrow transit time, and an earlier release of the marrow monocytes.[142] Meuret et al.[143] describe the following regularly occurring blood monocyte responses and the marrow manifestations of increased monocytopoiesis stimulated by both acute and chronic inflammatory disorders, infection, immune mediated diseases and malignancy:

1. An increase in the mononuclear phagocytes, i.e., all cells recognized by the sodium fluoride-sensitive Naphthol-AS-D acetate esterase reaction
2. A shift from the recognizable monocyte population toward both large and small cells with round or oval nuclei
3. An increase in DNA synthetic activity
4. An increase in the percentage of DNA synthesizing blood monocytes
5. An increase in the nonlobulated blood monocytes at the expense of the lobulated forms
6. An increase in the esterase activity of the blood monocytes
7. An increase in blood monocyte count

Meuret et al.[143] assessed the monocytopoietic activity of the bone marrow from an index determined from the mononuclear phagocyte population (MNP) of the marrow and the ^{3}H-labeled thymidine uptake (TdR-^{3}H):

$$\text{Monocytopoietic activity index} = \frac{\text{MNP} \times \text{TdR-}^3\text{H of test subject}}{\text{MNP} \times \text{TdR-}^3\text{H of normal median control}}$$

They reported that the monocytopoietic activity index varied considerably in different disease states. It was barely elevated in sarcoidosis and increased slightly to a little less than twice normal in other disorders, in the following order: psoriasis, ulcerative colitis, and Crohn's disease. The index rose to 3.5 to 4 times normal in patients with gastric and duodenal ulcers, chronic eczematoid skin disease, and tuberculosis.

Spector[144,145] described two types of chronic inflammation with respect to the macrophage turnover. The high turnover granulomata were characterized by increased recruitment of blood monocytes and increased marrow proliferation. In the low turnover granulomata blood monocyte recruitment was only minimally increased and the macrophage requirement was satisfied by the local accumulation of long lived macrophages. In this context, then, sarcoidosis is the prototype of a low turnover granuloma and tuberculosis of the high turnover type.

As was pointed out in the discussion of the heterogeneity of the monocytes, the origin of the tissue macrophage is still under question. The majority view holds that the tissue macrophages are derived from marrow precursor cells.[146] The minority view claims that a variety of inflammatory agents can stimulate monocytopoiesis and monocytosis.[148,149] Other studies have emphasized the variability of response to the different inflammatory stimuli and the differences, morphologic and functional, between the population of the induced macrophages from the resident macrophages.[150] Resolution of this question is necessary before an explanation of the variability of bone marrow response to the varied stimuli of inflammation, infection, and tumor can be provided.

In the clinical situation, the appreciation of an hyperplastic reaction of the monocyte-macrophage system in the bone marrow is difficult to assess from the morphologic findings elicited from examination of the smears of the bone marrow aspirate. The marrow population of mononuclear phagocytes is small, estimated by Meuret[31] at 2.8% of the total marrow cell population. The highest increases in the marrow mononuclear phagocyte population associated with the high turnover states did not exceed much beyond twice normal, about 6% of the total marrow population of cells. Hence modest increases in the monocyte-macrophage cells of the marrow may be readily overlooked.

Attention to an increase in marrow macrophages may be directed by the presence of plasmocytosis and an increase in mast cells. The plasmocytic islands—nests of plasma cells surrounding macrophages should suggest a chronic inflammatory state particularly in those conditions where the serum gamma globulin levels are elevated.

The diagnosis of specific infectious processes can occasionally be made from the presence of organisms within the macrophage. On rare occasions, the presence of subacute bacterial endocarditis can be suspected by the presence of cocci in the macrophage. Leprae bacilli may be revealed by the use of the Fite stain[151] and tubercle bacilli by the Ziehl-Nielsen stain. The Leishmann-Donovan bodies of kala-azar may fill the cytoplasm of the marrow macrophage as does the fungus *Histoplasma capsulatum*. Culture of the marrow aspirate may be helpful in the further characterization of the organism.

The histologic section of a bone marrow biopsy affords better opportunity for the diagnosis of a specific infection. The characteristic tubercle composed of lymphocytes, histiocytes, and the Langhans giant cell is the morphologic signature of tuberculosis. A similar granuloma is seen in leprosy, but the giant cell, the Virchow cell, has a foamy vacuolated appearance and may contain the Leprae bacilli. Typical granuloma of sarcoidosis are found rather frequently in patients with sarcoidosis. Bone marrow microgranuloma are associated with brucellosis, infectious mononucleosis, and on rare occasions with rheumatoid arthritis. The end stage of granulomatous disease of the marrow is fibrosis and the clinical picture of myelofibrosis has been observed as a consequence of miliary tuberculosis.

B. Inflammation, the Mononuclear Phagocyte, and Metal Metabolism

The anemia accompanying chronic infection, inflammation, or malignancy is the most commonly encountered anemia. The anemia is usually mild; rarely does the hemoglobin level fall below 8.0 grams percent. Varying degrees of hypochromia and modest decreases in the mean corpuscular volume of the red cell may appear in the more severe and prolonged anemias, complicating the chronic disorders.[152] The serum iron and total iron binding capacity are usually low, the plasma zinc levels fall,[153] and plasma copper levels rise.[154] Red cell free protoporphyrin and red cell free coproporphyrin increase, suggesting lack of available iron for heme synthesis. The bone marrow generally reveals increased quantities of storage iron, best visualized in the macrophages by the Prussian blue reaction. Low serum iron, decreased plasma transferrin, and increased macrophage iron in the marrow constitute a unique triad diagnostic of this form of anemia. The pathophysiology of this disorder and the role of iron in its relationship to the monocyte macrophage system have been extensively reviewed.[155,156]

During the early phase of chronic infection, inflammation or neoplasia, reutilization of iron from catabolized hemoglobin is impaired and this impairment in iron turnover has been proposed by some as the central mechanism for the anemia.[155] Evidence, however, has been presented to suggest that the inhibition of iron reutilization is lifted in the more chronic stages of these disorders and hence its central role in the production of the anemia is questioned.[157] Decreased red cell survival and marrow failure, presumably due to erythropoietin lack[158] or possibly lack of available iron[152] or stem cell competition,[159] have been invoked as possible pathogenetic mechanisms of the anemia of chronic disease.

An endogenous factor, the leukocyte endogenous mediator (LEM) secreted by activated mononuclear macrophage, has been proposed as the agent responsible for the inhibition of iron transport in infection, inflammation, or malignancy.[160] Activation of the monocyte-macrophages system by bacteria, viruses, endotoxin, or lymphokines causes release of a low molecular weight factor, about 12 to 15,000 daltons. On injection into an experimental animal LEM produces a rapid drop in the plasma concentration of zinc and iron and a slow increase in plasma concentration of copper. LEM also stimulates the production and release of neutrophils from the marrow; it is pyrogenic and alters the rate of synthesis of a variety of acute phase proteins.[161]

The hypoferremia of the anemia of the chronic inflammatory states, infection and malignancy, mediated by the monocyte-macrophage system has been considered part of the host's defense against invading organisms and possibly against tumor cells as well,[162–164] by denying the invader the iron it requires for its own growth. Bacteria are known to manufacture potent iron chelators, siderophores, by which they can extract iron from the host's transferrin if the latter is saturated at 30% or more with iron.[165]

The monocyte-macrophage system has the capacity to synthesize apo-transferrin and to take up and degrade transferrin,[166–169] thus adding another dimension to its role in the distribution of iron. The significance and importance of the role of the monocyte-macrophage system in metal metabolism in host resistance has yet to be fully elucidated: it promises to be interesting.

C. Mononuclear Phagocyte and Blood Cell Destruction

The monocyte-macrophage cells of spleen, liver, and bone marrow remove the old or damaged red cells from the circulation, catabolize the hemoglobin to amino acids and bilirubin, remove the iron, and return it to the proliferating red cell precursors for reutilization.[155] Although damaged or antibody-coated red cells can be ingested and catabolized by all cells of the monocyte-macrophage system, the cells of the peritoneum[170] or lung behave differently in this regard from the cells of the spleen, liver, and bone marrow.[171]

Under normal daily conditions of destruction of aged erythrocytes, the bone marrow in man is probably the main erythroclastic organ. In the hemolytic anemias, whether congenital (such as the thalassemias, spherocytic hemolytic anemia, etc.) or acquired, whether of immune (antibody-coated red cells) or nonimmune (Heinz body anemia, PNH, etc.) origin, the spleen and to a lesser extent the liver become the primary sites of destruction. Thus, in long-standing hemolytic anemias, hypertrophy of the macrophage elements of the spleen, liver, and to some extent lymph nodes takes place to produce the splenomegaly, so frequently appreciated as a clinical finding in these states.

The bone marrow clearly displays the anticipated hemopoietic responses to an increased red cell demand associated with hemolysis. The marrow is hyperplastic and the M/E ratio shifts much in favor of the red cell precursor population, and there is a marked increase in the number of erythroblastic islands. The central macrophages of the erythroblastic islands are large and frequently stuffed with hemosiderin. The Romanowsky stain often imparts a dirty green color to the macrophage: a result of the yellow hemosiderin and the absorbed blue color of the dye.

The high turnover of red cell membrane which accompanies the hemolytic anemias may overwhelm the enzymatic apparatus of the macrophage and lead to the formation of Gaucher-like foam cells. This phenomenon has been described in Cooley's disease[172] and in congenital dyserythropoietic anemia, type II (HEMPAS).[173]

In similar fashion, the accelerated production and excessive destruction of granulocytes in chronic myelocytic leukemia or platelets in thrombocytopenic purpura stimulate hyperplasia of the elements of the monocyte-macrophage system. Again, the excessive membrane turnover provide alterations in the macrophages which are remarkably similar to the histiocytes of Gaucher's disease or sea-blue histiocytosis.[174–176]

D. Dust Inhalation Disorders

Some foreign inorganic materials, notably beryllium, silica, and asbestos can, on inhalation, stimulate a chronic inflammatory reaction which bears much resemblance to the inflammatory reaction of sarcoidosis and tuberculosis, namely granuloma formation with reactive hyperplasia of the mononuclear phagocytes and lymphocytes. The effect of the different dusts on the macrophages appears to be different. Silica reacts with the phagosomal membrane of the macrophage and exerts a cytotoxic effect on the cell.[177] The damaging effect of silica has been attributed to its electron structure which can induce catalytic activation of membrane lipids or membrane enzymes on contact.[178] Asbestos is thought to activate the macrophage rather than damage it.[179]

The response of the marrow monocyte-macrophage system to the dust-induced inflammatory states has not been studied systematically. Diseases such as asbestosis have been characterized as inflammatory states with a slow macrophage turnover.[179] One would therefore anticipate only modest changes similar to those changes which have been described in sarcoidosis.

VIII. LYSOZYME AND THE MONOCYTE-MACROPHAGE SYSTEM

Lysozyme (mucopeptide-acetyl-muramyl hydrolase) is elevated in chronic granulomatous diseases such as sarcoidosis,[180,181] tuberculosis,[182] leprosy,[183] Crohn's disease,[184,185] and in malignant proliferative disorders, monocytic leukemia, and the myeloproliferative disorders.[85,186]

The cells of the monocyte-macrophage system are the major sites of lysozyme synthesis and secretion.[187,188] Osserman[190] has drawn a parallel between lysozyme as a mediator of certain affector functions of the macrophage with immunoglobins as mediators in the effector function of plasma cells and raised the possibility that the plasma cell immunoglobulin system may have evolved from the more primitive macrophage-lysozyme system.[189,190] Lysozyme is continuously produced and secreted by the macrophages; activation of the macrophage is not required.[85] The presumption, then, is that lysozyme is involved in basic and major functions of the monocyte-macrophage system.

The bacteriolytic action of lysozyme through its cleavage of complex polysaccharides is the most clearly defined function of the enzyme. However, evidence has accumulated to suggest that the significance of lysozyme in the host defense mechanisms may extend beyond its bacteriolytic action and may be involved in the host's reaction to tumor.[191]

The suggestion has been made that the serum concentration of lysozyme may reflect the macrophage mass and may serve as a marker of its activity[188,189] and thus may have clinical diagnostic value in preleukemia and monocytic leukemia. The assay of serum lysozyme concentration may find potential application in both clinical and experimental studies as an index of macrophage mass and function.[192]

IX. PROLIFERATIVE DISEASE OF MONOCYTE-MACROPHAGE SYSTEM

A. Leukemia

Historically acute monocytic leukemia was divided into two types: the acute myelomonocytic leukemia of Naegeli which was presumed to arise from a bone marrow myeloblast precursor common to the granulocyte and monocyte, and the pure monocytic leukemia of Schilling believed to originate from a distinct monoblast precursor of reticuloendothelial origin and offered as evidence to support the trinitarian origin of the blood cell elements.[193] The distinction between these two types of monocytic leukemia was blurred early by the morphological and cytochemical findings,[194,195] and declared arbitrary. The present day concepts of the bone marrow origin of the monocyte-macrophage cells and their origin from a common progenitor cell with the granulocytic cells support Naegeli's hypothesis of a single category of monocytic leukemia with varying proportions of granulocytic and monocytic elements.[190–198]

The polymorphic appearance of monocytic leukemia produced by varying admixtures of granulocytic elements and by the degree of differentation of the monocyte precursors has been used by the FAB cooperative group in its classification and subdivision of acute monocytic leukemia.[198] Depending on the percent admixture of granulocytic elements, monocytic leukemia is divided into an acute myelomonocytic form (M_4) and a monocytic type (M_5). In the acute myelomonocytic leukemia the proportion of promonocytes and monocytes exceeds 20% of the total nucleated cell population of the marrow or in the blood or in both. The percent of myeloblasts and promyelocytes generally exceeds 20% of the marrow cells and thus the picture may be difficult to distinguish from acute myeloblastic leukemia (M_2). As the percentage of promonocytes and monocytes increases, the morphologic appearance of the marrow sample resembles the monocytic leukemia (M_5).

Monocytic leukemia (M_5) is subdivided into poorly differentiated and differentiated cell types. In the poorly differentiated type large blast cells replace the marrow and may also be present in the blood. These blast cells have a high nuclear cytoplasmic ratio, delicate lacy chromatin, and one, occasionally up to three, prominent vesicular nucleoli. A small number of promonocytes may be present. In the differentiated form of acute monocytic leukemia monoblasts, promonocytes and monocytes are present in the marrow. The predominant marrow cell is the promonocyte which has more abundant cytoplasm than the blast cell and a large cerebriform nucleus. The cytoplasm is blue-grey in color and contains fine azurophilic granules. The percent of monocytes in the marrow is smaller than the percent of monocytes in the peripheral blood. In both subtypes of acute monocytic leukemia there is almost total replacement of the marrow by leukemic cells. The content of granulocytic cells is generally less than 10 to 15%. A few may contain Auer rods. The diagnosis of acute monocytic leukemia, both M_4 and M_5, must be confirmed by the fluoride-inhibited esterase reaction.

The clinical features of acute monocytic leukemia are similar to those of acute myeloblastic leukemia. Anemia, granulocytopenia, and thrombocytopenia with infection and bleeding are common. Tissue infiltration is more common in acute monocytic leukemia and related to the degree of maturation of the monocytic cells. Lichtman and Weed[195,199] presented evidence to suggest that cytoplasmic differentiation may be the important factor in the infiltration of the extravascular tissues by leukemic monocytes; that maturation may equip the monocyte for its entry into tissue. High levels of serum and urinary lysozyme may be present and may be a useful marker for diagnosis and treatment.

A chronic form of myelomonocytic leukemia has been described and is now grouped with the preleukemic syndromes.[200] Anemia, monocytosis, an increase in the marrow myelocytes and promyleocytes, and a prolonged clinical course characterize this illness.

B. Malignant Histiocytosis

Originally defined by Scott and Robb-Smith,[201] malignant histiocytosis is a systemic, progressive, invasive proliferative disease of atypical histiocytes. Malignant histiocytosis is characterized clinically by fever, wasting, generalized lymphadenopathy associated with splenic and hepatic enlargement, and in the final stages, jaundice, purpura, and anemia with profound leucopenia. The diagnosis is established by the demonstration of a focal or diffuse proliferation of atypical histiocytes in the lymph nodes, spleen, liver, or bone marrow. In general, material obtained by aspiration of the marrow or by touch imprint of the surgically extirpated lymph node affords better appreciation of the structural characteristics of the abnormal histiocytes than the histological preparations of these tissues. The histiocytes show varying level of differentiation, but are morphologically and cytochemically distinctive.

The marrow is usually intensely infiltrated with varying proportions of poorly and well-differentiated histiocytes. The poorly differentiated histiocytes tend to be round or oval with a large nucleus whose chromatin is diffuse and which contains several nucleoli. The cytoplasm is basophilic, and frequently filled with small vesicles. Mitoses are frequent. The acid phosphatase and naphthol-AS-acetate esterase reactions are faintly positive. On electron microscopy the nuclei are indented and contain large, occasionally multiple nuceoli. The Golgi complex varies in size, being large in the more differentiated cells, and is associated with vesicles. Many polyribosomes, lipid droplets, and vacuoles fill the cytoplasm.

The well-differentiated histiocyte is large, its shape irregular. The cytoplasm is grey, abundant, with many azurophilic granules, vesicles, phagocytosed material and debris. The cell margins are irregular and blurred. The acid phosphatase and nonspecific asterase show strong reactivity. On electron microscopy the nuclei are usually lobulated with prominent folds. Nucleoli may be present. The Golgi complex is large with many surrounding vesicles. Active phagocytosis of red cells or other nucleated cells is a regular and striking feature of this disease. The Sudan black stain often reveals fat droplets in the vacuoles.[202–210]

Malignant histiocytosis has shown a striking preference for Chinese and Africans, particularly Ugandans, and has been seen as a terminal event in acute leukemia.[210] A leukemic phase, with cell counts up to 170,000 blasts/mm^3 during the course of malignant histiocytosis has been reported.[211] The cells showed the cytochemical characteristics of monocytes.

C. Leukemic Reticuloendotheliosis

Hairy cell leukemia is now a well-established entity characterized clinically by its chronic course, marked splenomegaly most often associated with pancytopenia, absence of lymphadenopathy and bone marrow and splenic infiltration by large abnormal mononuclear cells with filamentous projections. It is these hair-like projections from the cell's surface, best appreciated in phase microscopy, that have given the cell and the disease its pilose designation.

The precise nature of the cell is uncertain and has attracted a considerable amount of attention and engendered considerable difference of opinion on its origin. The cell is readily recognized in the usual Romanowsky stained preparations or by phase microscopy.[211–213] Cytochemically, the hairy cells are characterized by a specific tartrate-resistant acid phosphatase reaction.[214,215] A cytoplasmic inclusion, the ribosome-lamella complex, has been found in about half of the patients with hairy leukemia on ultrastructural examination of the hairy cells.[218] The surface characteristics, as demonstrated by scanning electron microscopy, consist of prominent and broad based ruffled membranes, resembling more closely the surface morphology of the monocyte.[217]

Definitive classification of this cell and disease has not yet been made. Some regard the cell as of monocytic origin,[218,219] and others as an unequivocal B-cell derivative.[220] Burns and Cawley[222] have recently summarized the evidence pro and con and conclude that the so-called monocytic features of the hairy cells are compatible with the current view that hairy cell leukemia is a form of B-cell lymphoproliferation. Jansen et al.[223] recently reexamined the phagocytic potential of the hairy cells of leukemic reticuloendotheliosis and found that the particles and bacteria seemingly ingested by the cell were actually extracellular; and that the cells showed no increased oxygen consumption on exposure to the bacteria, no lysozyme or peroxidase activity, and a very weak nonspecific esterase activity. They concluded that the hairy cells of leukemic reticuloendotheliosis are not of monocytic origin. The consensus at present considers hairy cell leukemia a lymphoproliferative disease, and more appropriately included in the section on lymphocytes.

The bone marrow in hairy cell leukemia is often tightly infiltrated and dry taps are frequent. The histopathologic features on both light and electron microscopy have been described by Vykoupil et al.[224] Light microscopy revealed diffuse or patchy dense infiltrations of mononuclear cells with characteristics loose and spongy arrangement of the cells. This reticulum-like arrangement of the hairy cells, particularly conspicuous on thin section, enables ready differentiation from other infiltrations of the bone marrow with neoplastic cells. A felt-like network of thin reticulin fibers is generally present early in the illness and is associated with collagen in the later stages.

The electron microscopic examination confirms the light microscopic findings of a loose arrangement of villous, mononuclear cells in and around the sinuses. The cells show a continuous line of maturation from large blastic cells with high nuclear-cytoplasmic ratio to the typical hairy cell with numerous cytoplasmic processes.[225]

Other interesting features of hairy cell leukemia are the peripheral blood monocytopenia[226] and an elevated leukocyte alkaline phosphatase.[227,228] The significance of these findings is not clear. The monocytopenia may contribute to the increased risk of infection in these patients. The high leukocyte alkaline phosphatase activity has been thought to be an expression of an impaired granulocyte reserve compartment.[228] Impaired marrow granulocyte reserve and leukocyte mobilization has been reported in patients with leukemic reticuloendotheliosis.[229]

D. Idiopathic Histiocytosis

Idiopathic histiocytosis (histiocytosis, reticuloendotheliosis) refers to a group of disorders of unknown etiology, not associated with any known infectious agent or metabolic abnormality, and characterized by the proliferation and accumulation of sheets of well-differentiated macrophages. The major clinical entities included among the histiocytosis are eosinophilic granuloma, solitary or multiple (equivalent to the Hand-Schuller-Christian disease) and Letterer-Siwe disease.

Understanding of the histiocytosis has been blurred by problems of nomenclature and the uncertainty of the identity and the relationships of the syndromes to each other. Lichtenstein[230] concluded from his observations on eosinophilic granuloma, Hand-Schuller-Christian disease, and Letterer-Siwe disease that the three syndromes were different clinical presentations of a single nosologic entity which he titled ''histiocytosis X.'' This view was subsequently challenged by Lieberman et al.[231] who saw Hand-Schuller-Christian disease as the equivalent of multifocal eosinophilic granuloma and separated Letterer-Siwe disease as a distinct entity. Zinkman,[232] in his editorial on the subject, cautioned against the absolute acceptance of the doctrine at this time and felt that more study was necessary to establish with certainty the identity of multifocal eosinophilic granuloma and Hand-Schuller-Christian disease. Cline and Golde[135] in their review and reevaluation of the histiocytic disorders supported the concept that multifocal eosinophilic granuloma and Hand-Schuller Christian disease are equivalent.

Danenshbod and Kissane[233] divided the histiocytic disorders into two groups: disseminated visceral histiocytosis (or Letterer-Siwe disease) involving more than two organ systems, and histiocytosis confined to one or more bones. Disseminated visceral histiocytosis is a fulminating illness afflicting children in infancy or early childhood and characterized by hepatosplenomegaly, moderately enlarged nontender, discrete lymphadenopathy, extensive skin involvement by a maculopapular purpuric eruption, low grade fever, localized bone defects, and generalized histiocytic hyperplasia of spleen, liver, lymph nodes, skin, bone marrow, and thymus.

The histiocytosis confined to bones is a chronic affliction usually of children and young adults. The prognosis is generally good and when it is limited to a single bone is asymptomatic. The multifocal disease is characterized by well-circumscribed bone lesions ususally in the skull, ribs, or other flat bones. The disease appears to be more common in men than women and more common in the white population than the black.[134,234,235] The triad of membranous bone involvement, diabetes insipidus, and exopathalmos represent the classic constellation of Hand-Schuller-Christian disease but is rarely seen in its entirety.

The histologic picture is suggestive of an inflammatory rather than a neoplastic disorder. The lesions consist of mixtures of benign appearing histocytes, eosinophils, giant cells, and necrosis. Bone marrow function is usually not disturbed. On further progression of the lesion, the eosinophils and giant cells regress and fibrosis follows. The histiocytes become large and foamy and cholesterol accumulates in the necrotic areas.

Marrow aspirates of affected bone reveals many eosinophils with the occasional presence of Charot-Leyden crystals as well as many large macrophages, often multinucleated with highly vacuolated cytoplasm. In polarized light the macrophages display the anisotropic lipid droplets typical of foam cells. The aspirate may suggest the diagnosis, but bone marrow biopsy and histologic examination is required for confirmation.

Letterer-Siwe disease has been reported in several family members and has been listed with a variety of other rare histiocytic disorders of presumed familial occurrence such as familial lipochrome histiocytosis, familial histiocytic (or hemophagocytic) reticulosis, and X-linked reticuloendotheliosis.[236] The role of genetics in the etiology of Letterer-Siwe disease has yet to be determined.

X. STORAGE DISEASE

The storage diseases are conveniently divided into the primary abnormalities in sphingolipid metabolism and the secondary storage states due to the overtaxing of the normal enzymatic machinary of sphingolipid metabolism by excess substrate. The congenital abnormalities of sphingolipid metabolism include Tay-Sachs disease, Niemann-Pick disease, Gaucher's disease, GM1 gangliosidosis, metachromatic leukodystrophy, Fabry's disease, and Krabbe's disease (all extensively reviewed in reference 237). Of these disorders Gaucher's disease, Niemann-Pick disease, and Fabry disease are the principal lipidoses in which the lipid-laden macrophages accumulate in the bone marrow.

A. Gaucher's Disease

Gaucher's disease is the most commonly encountered sphingolipid storage disorder, in which the underlying defect appears to be a deficiency of a β-glucosidase[238] and hence an inability to cleave the glucose from the glucosyl ceramides. The glucosyl-ceramides accumulate in the macrophages of the marrow, spleen, lungs, and liver converting the macrophages into the highly characteristic and diagnostic Gaucher cells. The disease included two or more hereditary disorders of glucosyl-ceramide metabolism and, although clinically diverse, all share the common manifestations of hepatosplenomegaly, Gaucher cells in the bone marrow, and elevated concentrations of serum acid phosphatase.

The Gaucher cell is a large cell, about 40 μm in diameter, readily obtained by marrow aspiration, and best visualized by phase microscopy. The cells may be isolated or exist in clumps or sheets. The nucleus is pycnotic and eccentrically placed, pushed to the cell margin by the massive accumulation of lipid. A dense network of cytoplasmic fibrils of varying lengths can be dramatically visualized by phase contrast microscopy. The fibrils are birefringent and their recognition is highly diagnostic of Gaucher's disease and readily differentiates the Gaucher cell from other storage cells. In the usual Romanowsky stain the cytoplasm appears pale, almost colorless and has a rather wrinkled appearance. Fibrils are present but more difficult to appreciate than in the supravital preparations examined by phase microscopy. The cells contain large concentrations of nonglycogen polysaccharides which stain intensely with the periodic acid-Schiff stain. The Mallory trichrome stain is useful in bringing out the cytoplasmic features of the Gaucher cells. The cells also contain considerable amounts of iron and give a strong acid phosphatase reaction.[239] On ultrastructural examination the cells show cytoplasmic residual bodies or secondary lysosomes, which are filled with tubular structures.[240,241] Similar tubules have been formed in vitro from glucosyl-ceramide. The origin of the glucosyl-ceramide in the Gaucher cell is not certain but the evidence would favor the erythrocyte membranes as the principal source of the cerebroside, and phagocytosis or pinocytosis as the principle mechanism.[242]

B. Niemann-Pick Disease

An hereditary deficiency of sphingomyelinase causes sphingomyelin (phosphoryl choline ceramide) to accumulate in the macrophages of the tissues of children afflicted with Niemann-Pick disease.[243] At least four different phenotypes have been defined. Hepatosplenomegaly is always present. The spleen, bone marrow, and lymphatic tissues are heavily infiltrated with foam cells.

In phase microscopy the foam cells of Niemann-Pick disease are large cells with an eccentric nucleus whose cytoplasm is filled with many droplets and particles and hence easily distinguished from the fibrillar Gaucher cells. The droplets are birefringent and fluoresce greenish-yellow in ultraviolet light. The cells stain strongly for lipid (Sudan black B, oil red-O).[237]

On electron microscopic examination residual bodies are present, scattered throughout the cytoplasm. Myelin figures may be present. The presence of a foam cell is not diagnostic of Niemann-Pick disease and chemical demonstration of sphingomyelin accumulation is required for the definitive diagnosis.

C. Fabry's Disease

This glycosphingolipid disease is a sex-linked disorder characterized by the accumulation of galactosyl-galactosyl-glucosyl ceramide in most tissues of the body. A deficiency of an galactosyl hydrolase has been shown to be responsible for the metabolic abnormality and the accumulation of the glycosphingolipid in all varieties of cells and tissues of the body. The deposits of the glycosphingolipids are responsible for the clinical manifestations of the illness: the typical angiectatic lesions of the skin particularly about the buttock and genitalia, designated as angiokeratoma corposis diffuseum; vascular lesions of conjunctiva and oral mucosa; azotemia and progressive renal failure; and corneal opticites, bone pain, and fever. The heart, the kidney, and the nervous system are frequently involved.

Involvement of macrophages of the bone marrow has been reported. Foam cells are nearly always present in the urine. The lipid laden foam cells contain birefringents lipid droplets with maltese crosses. Lipid bodies have been revealed by electron microscopy. Diagnosis should be established by chemical analysis for the trihexoside ceramide.[237] The striking enlargement of liver, spleen, and lymph nodes seen in Gaucher's disease is not found in Fabry's disease.

D. Sea-Blue Histiocytosis

The primary syndrome of the sea-blue histiocyte is an ill-defined entity which derives its name from its most outstanding feature, the presence of numerous marrow histiocytes which take on a sea-blue color with Romanowsky stains. The criteria proposed for diagnosis include: an enlarged spleen in which large numbers of sea-blue histiocytes are present; large numbers of sea-blue histiocytes in the marrow aspirate; sea-blue histiocytes in the liver biopsy and in the biopsies of nervous system, lung and gastrointestinal (GI) tract; and/or the presence of a foveal ring in the ocular fundus.

The metabolic and genetic aspects of the primary, presumably hereditary, sea-blue syndrome have not been clearly established. Excessive quantities of phosphosphingolipids, glycosphingolipids, and ceroid have been identified in the liver, spleen, and other organs. An additional error in mucopolysaccharide metabolism is suspected.[244,245]

The sea-blue histiocyte is a large cell 20 to 60 μm in diameter with an eccentrally placed nucleus. The chromatin is condensed but a nucleolus may be discerned. The cytoplasm contains variable quantities of sea-blue or blue-green staining granules of variable size, shape, and staining intensity. The cells may exist singly or in groups.[245]

E. Acquired Lipidosis

Cells which, on Romanowsky stain, resemble sea-blue histiocytes and Gaucher cells have been observed in chronic myelocytic leukemia,[174] HEMPAS,[173] idiopathic thrombocytopenic purpura,[175] and a variety of diverse clinical situations such as hyperlipoproteinemia,[246] nutritional abnormalities and as a complication of a drug administration. The sea-blue histiocyte has been found in association with low serum cholesterol.[247] Light-green crystals, up to 20 μm in length, have been observed in the marrow macrophages of patients with both acute and chronic myeloid leukemia, but not in the lymphocytic leukemias.[248]

Significant morphologic differences have been noted between the ultrastructural morphology of Gaucher cells and Gaucher-like cells of chronic myelocytic leukemia. The tubules of Gaucher cells are approximately twice the diameter of tubules in the Gaucher-like cells, whose cytoplasm is often filled with myelin bodies rather than sacs of tubules.

Acid phosphatase and periodic acid silver stains are positive in both Gaucher and Gaucher-like cells. However, the non-Gaucher cells showed no glucoceramide on thin layer chromatography.[249,250]

Hayhoe et al.[251] describe three varieties of compound lipid inclusions in the marrow macrophages of acquired lipidosis, detectable and distinguishable by Romanowsky staining, ultraviolet fluorescence, and polarized light. Blue lanceolate crystals 6 to 12 μm in length may fill a macrophage and endow it with the striations reminiscent of a Gaucher cell. The crystals are birefringent and often not appreciated on Romanowsky-stained smears. The Gaucher-like cell is generally smaller than the Gaucher cell and has fewer and less densely packed crystals under polarized light than the true Gaucher cell. Hayhoe et al.[251] find however that under the electron miscroscope the microtubular arrangement in the crystals is similar in both the Gaucher and Gaucher-like cell.

Hayhoe et al.[251] describe the sea-blue granules as small rounded bodies 1 to 3 μm in diameter which are not birefringent but show a pink-colored autofluorescence. They stain variably with Sudan black. On electron microscopic examination rounded osmophilic inclusions are found.

The third type of lipid inclusion recognized by Hayhoe et al. consists of large grey-green crystals, usually thicker and longer than the birefringent blue crystals. The crystals are not birefringent and do not autofluoresce. Like Stavem et al.[248] Hayhoe et al.[251] found the grey-green crystals almost exclusively in patients with myeloid leukemia.

Thus, a range of inclusions have been identified in the macrophages of acquired lipidosis seen most frequently in states of abnormal myelopoiesis and attributed to an excessive turnover of sphingomyelin. The factors determining the variable morphologic forms from sea-blue histiocyte, to grey-green crystals, and to Gaucher-like cells have yet to be determined.

XI. MONOCYTOPENIA AND THE MACROPHAGE DYSFUNCTION SYNDROMES

The clinical significance of a decreased blood monocyte count has not received much attention. Twomey et al.[252] found a clinically significant relationship between the total polymorphonuclear cell (including band cells) counts and the total monocyte count in healthy individuals and in patients with aplastic anemia and speculated on the contribution of the monocytopenia to the increased suseptibility to infection in aplastic anemia. Studies on patients with benign neutropenia also suggest a compensatory and protective role of the monocytes.[253] Baehner and Johnson,[254] on the other hand, studied the monocytes of children with congenital neutropenia, cyclic neutropenia, and chronic infections and found them to be similar in all three disease states but displayed much lower phagoyctic, metabolic, and bactericidal function, than the polymorphonuclear leucocytes. The bactericidal capacity of the monocyte of the normal individual is said to be equal to that of the neutrophil.[255] Baehner and Johnson[254] concluded that the severity and extent of infection in neutropenia is most likely due to the deficiency of the polymorphonuclear leukocytes, ''the superior phagocyte of the peripheral blood.''

Monocyte and macrophage function can be assessed in a manner similar to that of the polymorphonuclear leukocyte. The major activities of the monocyte-macrophage system in man involve antigen processing and presentation to the lymphocytes, phagocytosis, and effective bactericidal activity. Like the neutrophil, the monocyte must be able to move and respond to various chemotactic factors to be fully effective.

Delay in the development of immunocompetence of neonatal and newborn animals has been attributed to macrophage immaturity. The newborn animal is endowed with a limited repertoire of antigen responses, which becomes broader and more heterogeneous with the maturation of the animal. The defect in antigen response of the newborn can be overcome by the administration of adult macrophages with the antigen.[256] The survival of newborn mice infected with *Listeria monocytogenes* can be markedly improved by the administration of adult macrophages. In like manner the survival of mice infected with cytomegalovirus can be favorably influenced.[257] A defect in the antigen presenting function of macrophages from neonatal mice has been reported and has been attributed to a decrease in the number of macrophages bearing Ia antigens.[258] Thus, both immaturity of the macrophages and a deficiency of the number of specific macrophage populations have been invoked to explain the defective immune responses of the newborn.

The macrophage of the human newborn is said to be immature with respect to antigen-processing chemotaxis, and possibly bactericidal function. The clinical significance of this macrophage immaturity of the newborn has not been determined, but the susceptibility of newborn infants to listeria infection is well known.[259] Little information is available on the bone marrow events relative to monocyte and macrophage production in the human neonate and infant.

The macrophages in chronic granulomatous disease possess the same metabolic defect as the neutrophils.[260] The same structural and functional abnormalities are found in both macrophages and neutrophils in Chediak-Higashi syndrome.[261–263] The monocytes of chronic mucocutaneous candidiasis show failure of migration in vitro toward two chemotactic stimuli: lymphocyte derived chemotactic factor in C5A.[264]

Monocytes and macrophages are considered critical in the destruction of malignant cells in both animals and man. With progressive tumor formation macrophage function may be altered. Monocyte chemotaxis, to lymphocyte derived chemotactic factor and C5A, has been found to be deficient in a variety of cancers, including melanoma, lung, breast, and gastrointestinal.[265] In animals, tumors have been shown to produce a factor which inhibits chemotaxis in vivo.[266]

Significant inhibition of monocyte chemotaxis has been demonstrated in acute lymphoblastic leukemia and chronic lymphocytic leukemia but not in chronic or acute myelocytic leukemia. The monocytes were quantitatively sufficient suggesting that lack of chemotaxis may be due to lack of lymphocyte chemotactic factor in the lymphocytic leukemias.[267]

Patients with Hodgkin's disease are highly susceptible to herpes simplex infection, with a very high incidence of dissemination. Patients with stage III and IV disease have defective monocyte chemotaxis and bactericidal activity. Antibody-dependent cellular toxicity of monocytes and macrophages was found to be low at time of diagnosis as was the natural killer cytotoxicity. No impairment of lymphocyte natural killer cytotoxicity of antibody-dependent cellular toxicity was found.[268] The monocyte-macrophage defects are consistent with the high risk of viral infection. Herpes simplex virus is apparently capable of diminishing monocyte chemotaxis,[269] which raises the question whether the described monocyte abnormalities in Hodgkin's disease are due to Hodgkin's disease or to a concommitant herpes infection.

Enhanced susceptibility to opportunistic infection following corticosteroid administration is well recognized. Small doses of steroids have been shown to depress monocyte chemotaxis in vitro and large doses in vivo diminished the bactericidal capacity of the monocyte.[270] Leukocyte mobilization into areas of inflammation was impaired by corticosteroid administration.[271]

Macrophage dysfunction has been proposed as a mechanism for the failure of intracellular killing of bacteria or fungi in the chronic granulomatous illnesses such as miliary tuberculosis, disseminated fungal infections, or lepromatous leprosy.[272] The details of the mechanisms, whether maturational abnormalities in the bone marrow or environmental factors, which are responsible for the depressed monocyte-macrophage function have yet to be elucidated.

REFERENCES

1. **Metchnikoff, E.,** Phagocytic cells of the lymphoid tissue take up particulate material and foreign protein, *Ann. Rev. Inst. Pateur.,* 13, 47, 1899.
2. **Metchnikoff, E.,** *Leçons sur la Pathologie Comparée de l'Inflammation,* Masson et cie, Paris, 1892.
3. **Kiyono, K.,** *Die Vitale Karminspeicherung,* Ein Beitrag sur Lehre von der vitalen Farbung mit besonderer Berucksichtigung der Zelldifferenzierunge in entzundlichen Gewebe, G. Fischer, Jena, 1914.
4. **Aschoff, L.,** Daz reticulo-endotheliale system, *Ergebenisse d'Inn. Med.,* 26, 2, 1924.
5. **Blaner, H.,** Identification of peritoneal macrophages in mouse radiation chimeras, *Transplantation,* 1, 217, 1963.
6. **Virolainen, M.,** Hemopoietic origin of macrophages as studied by chromosome markers in mice, *J. Exp. Med.,* 127, 943, 1968.
7. **Van Furth, R. and Cohn, Z. A.,** The origin and kinetics of mononuclear phagocytes, *J. Exp. Med.,* 128, 415, 1965.
8. **Volkman, A. and Gowans, J. L.,** The origin of macrophages from the bone marrow, *Br. J. Pathol.,* 46, 62, 1965.
9. **Cohn, Z. A.,** The structure and function of monocytes and macrophages, *Adv. Immunol.,* 9, 163, 1968.
10. **Leder, L. D.,** Die Herkunft der Blutmonozyten und ihre Beziehungen zu den sog, Histiozyten, *Haematol. Bluttransfus.,* 8, 10, 1969.
11. **Cline, M. J., Lehrer, R. I., Territo, M. C., and Golde, D. W.,** Monocytes and macrophages: function and disease, *Ann. Int. Med.,* 88, 78, 1978.
12. **Van Furth, R.,** Ed., *Mononuclear Phagocytes in Immunity, Infection and Pathology,* Blackwell, Oxford, 1975.
13. **Van Furth, R., Cohn, A. Z., Hirsch, J. G. et al.,** The mononuclear phagocyte system: a new classification of macrophages, monocytes, and their precursor cells, *Bull. WHO,* 46, 845, 1972.
14. **Leibovich, S. J., and Ross, R.,** The macrophage and the fibroblast, in *Mononuclear Phagocytes in Immunity, Infection and Pathology,* Van Furth, R., Ed., Blackwell, Oxford, 1975, 347.
15. **Spector, W. G., Walter, M. N. C., and Willoughby, D. A.,** The origin of mononuclear cells in inflammatory exudates induced by fibrinogen, *J. Pathol. Bacteriol.,* 9, 181, 1965.
16. **Stuart, A. E.,** *The Reticuloendothelial System,* E. S. Livingstone, Edinburgh, 1970.
17. **Meuret, G.,** Origin, ontogeny and kinetics of mononuclear phagocytes, *Adv. Med. Biol.,* 73, 71, 1976.
18. **Brandt, L., Levan, G., Mitelman, F., et al.,** Trisomy G-21 in adult myelomonocytic leukemia, *Scand. J. Haematol.,* 12, 117, 1974.
19. **Bradley, T. R., and Metcalf, D.,** The growth of mouse bone marrow cells *in vitro, Aust. J. Exp. Biol. Med. Sci.,* 44, 287, 1966.
20. **Ichikawa, Y., Pluznik, D. H., and Sachs, L.,** *In vitro* control of the development of macrophage and granulocyte colonies, *Proc. Natl. Acad. Sci. (U.S.A.),* 56, 488, 1966.
21. **Leder, L. D.,** Fermentcytochemische Untersuchungen zur Herkunft der Blutmonocyten, *Klin Wochenschr.,* 44, 25, 1966.
22. **Territo, M. C. and Cline, M. J.,** Mononuclear phagocyte proliferation, maturation and function, *Clin. Haematol.,* 4, 685, 1975.
23. **Zucker-Franklin, D.,** Physiological and pathological variations in the ultrastructure of neutrophils and monocytes, *Clin. Haematol.,* 4, 485, 1975.
24. **Lessin, L. S., Bessis, M., and Douglas, S. D.,** Morphology of monocytes and macrophages in *Hematology,* 2nd ed., Williams, W. S., Beutler, E., Erslev, A. S., et al., Eds., McGraw Hill, New York, 1977, 881.
25. **Fedorko, M. E. and Hirsch, J. G.,** Structure of monocytes and macrophages, *Sem. Hematol.,* 7, 109, 1970.
26. **Cline, M. J.,** *The White Cell,* Harvard University Press, Cambridge, 1975, 459.

27. **Nichols, B. A., Bainton, D. F., and Farquhar, M. G.,** Differentiation of monocytes, origin, nature, and fate of their azurophilic granules, *J. Cell. Biol.,* 50, 498, 1971.
28. **Nichols, B. A. and Bainton, D. F.,** Differentiation of human monocytes in bone marrow and blood. Sequential formation of two granule populations, *Lab. Invest.,* 29, 27, 1973.
29. **Braunsteiner, H. and Schmalzl, F.,** Cytochemistry of monocytes and macrophages in, *Mononuclear Phagocytes,* Van Furth, R., Ed., F. A. Davis, Philadelphia, 1970, 62.
30. **Briggs, R. S., Perillie, P. E., and Finch, S. C.,** Lysozyme in bone marrow and peripheral blood cells, *J. Histochem. Cytochem.,* 14, 167, 1966.
31. **Meuret, G. and Hoffman, G.,** Monocyte kinetics studies in normal and disease states, *Br. J. Haematol.,* 24, 273, 1973.
32. **Roser, G.,** The origin, kinetics and fate of macrophage populations, *J. Reticuloendothel. Soc.,* 8, 139, 1970.
33. **Spritzer, A. A., Watson, J. A., and Huld, J. A., Guettnoff, H.,** Pulmonary macrophages clearance, the hourly rates of transfer of pulmonary macrophages to the oropharynx of the rat, *Arch. Environ. Health,* 17, 726, 1968.
34. **Van Furth, R., Raeburn, J. A., and Van Zwet, T. L.,** Characteristics of human mononuclear phagocytes, *Blood,* 54, 485, 1979.
35. **Killmann, S. A., Cronkite, E. P., Bond, U. P., and Fliedner, T. M.,** Proliferation of human leukemic cells studied with tritiated thymidine *in vivo,* in *Proc. of the 8th Congress of the European Society of Hematology,* S. Karger, Basel, 1962, 63.
36. **Osgood, E. E., Tivey, H., Davison, K. B. et al.,** The relative rates of formation of new leukocytes in patients with acute and chronic leukemias, measured by the uptake of radioactive phosphorus in the isolated deoxyribosenucleic acid, *Cancer,* 5, 331, 1952.
37. **Allison, A. C., Davies, P., and De Petris, S.,** Role of contractive microfilaments in macrophage movement and endocytosis, *Nature, (New Biol.),* 232, 153, 1971.
38. **Reaven, E. P. and Axline, S. G.,** Subplasmalemmal microfilaments and microtubules in resting and phagocytosing cultivated macrophages, *J. Cell. Biol.,* 59, 12, 1973.
39. **Breton-Gorius, J. and Reyes, F.,** Ultrastructure of human bone marrow cell maturation, *Int. Rev. Cytol.,* 46, 251, 1976.
40. **Cline, M. J. and Lehrer, R. L.,** Phagocytosis by human monocytes, *Blood,* 32, 423, 1968.
41. **BoBoglio, A. F., Contran, R. S., and Jandl, J. H.,** Red cells coated with immunoglobulin G: binding and sphering by mononuclear cells in man, *Science,* 158, 1582, 1967.
42. **Reyes, F., Le Go, A., Delrieu, F., and Bach, J. F.,** Ultrastructure of cell binding immunoglobulin-coated erythrocytes in rheumatoid arthritis, *Clin. Exp. Immunol.,* 17, 533, 1974.
43. **Cassileth, P. A.,** Monocytosis in, *Hematology,* 2nd ed., Williams, W. J., Beutler, E., Erslev, A., et al., Eds., McGraw Hill, New York.
44. **Bessis, M.,** *Living Blood Cells and Their Ultrastructure,* Springer-Verlag, New York, 1973, 500.
45. **Scully, E. J.,** The reaction after intravenous injections of foreign protein, *JAMA,* 69, 20, 1917.
46. **Jandl, J. H., and Tomlinson, A. S.,** The destruction of red cells by antibodies in man. II. Pyrogenic, leukeocytic and dermal response to immune hemolysis, *J. Clin. Invest.,* 37, 1202, 1958.
47. **Thompson, J. and Van Furth, R.,** The effect of glucocorticosteroids on the proliferation and kinetics of promonocytes and monocytes of the bone marrow, *J. Exp. Med.,* 137, 10, 1973.
48. **Gordon, S. and Cohn, Z. A.,** The macrophage, *Int. Rev. Cytol.,* 36, 171, 1973.
49. **Sannes, P. L., Eguchi, M., and Spicer, S. S.,** Ultrastructural localization of a complex carbohydrate in rat monocytes and peritoneal and alveolar macrophages, *Lab. Invest.,* 41, 135, 1979.
50. **Ebert, R. H. and Florey, H. W.,** Extravascular development of monocytes observed *in vivo, Br. J. Exp. Pathol.,* 20, 342, 1939.
51. **Van Furth, R.,** Origin and kinetics of monocytes and macrophages, *Sem. Hematol.,* 7, 125, 1970.
52. **Lewis, M. R. and Lewis, W. H.,** Transformation of mononuclear blood cells into macrophages, epitheloid cells and giant cells in hanging drop cultures of lower vertebrates, Carnegie Inst. Washington, Pub. No. 96, *Contrib. Embryol.,* 18, 95, 1926.
53. **Hetherington, D. C. and Pierce, E. J.,** The transformation of monocytes into macrophages and epithelioid cells in tissue cultures of buffy coats, *Arch. Exp. Zellforsch.,* 12, 1, 1931.
54. **Sutton, J. S. and Weiss, L.,** Transformation of monocytes in tissue culture into macrophages, epithelioid cells and multinucleated giant cells. An electron microscopic study, *J. Cell. Biol.,* 28, 303, 1968.
55. Editorial, Macrophage nomenclature: Where are we going? *J. Reticuloendothel. Soc.,* 27, 223, 1980.
56. **Spicer, S. S., Sannes, P. L., Eguchi, M., and McKeever, P. E.,** Fine structural and cytochemical aspects of the development of macrophages and of their endocytic secretory activities, *J. Reticuloendothel Soc.,* 26, 49, 1979.

57. **Cohn, A. Z. and Fedorko, M.,** in *Lysosomes in Biology and Pathology,* Dingle, J. T. and Fell, H. B., Eds., North Holland, Amsterdam 1969, 43.
58. **Spector, W. G.,** The granulomatous inflammation exudate, *Int. Rec. Exp. Pathol.,* 8, 1, 1969.
59. **Sher, N. A., Chaparas, S. D., Greenberg, L. E., et al.,** Response of congenitally athymic (nude) mice to infection with mycobacteria bovis (strain BCG), *J. Natl. Cancer Inst.,* 54, 1419, 1975.
60. **Ueda, K., Yamazaki, S., and Someya, S.,** Experimental mycobacterial infection in congenitally athymic "nude" mice, *J. Reticuloendothel Soc.,* 19, 77, 1976.
61. **Galindo, B.,** Antigen mediated fusion of specifically sensitized rabbit alveolar macrophages, *Infect. Immunity,* 5, 583, 1972.
62. **Galinda, B., Lazdins, J., and Castillo, R.,** Fusion of normal rabbit alveolar macrophages induced by supernatant fluids from BCG sensitized lymph node cells after elicitation by antigen, *Infect. Immunity,* 9, 212, 1974.
63. **Warfel, A. H.,** Macrophage fusion and multinucleated giant cell formation, surface morphology, *Exp. Mol. Pathol.,* 28, 163, 1978.
64. **Kaplow, L. S.,** Cytochemical heterogeneity of human circulating monocytes, *Acta Cytol.,* 19, 358, 1975.
65. **Arenson, E. B., Jr., Epstein, M. B., and Seeger, R. C.,** Volumetric and functional heterogeneity of human monocytes, *J. Clin. Invest.,* 65, 613, 1980.
66. **Bennett, W. E. and Cohn, Z. A.,** The isolation and selected properties of blood monocytes, *J. Exp. Med.,* 123, 145, 1966.
67. **Hopper, K. E., Wood, P. R., and Nelson, D. S.,** Macrophage heterogeneity review, *Vox. Sang.,* 36, 257, 1979.
68. **Pulford, K. and Souhami, R. L.,** Cell division and giant cell formation in Kupffer cell cultures, *Clin. Exp. Immunol.,* 42, 67, 1980.
69. **Van Furth, R., Diesselhoff-En-Dulk, M. M. C., and Mattie, H.,** Quantitative study on the production and kinetics of mononuclear phagocytes during an acute inflammatory reaction, *J. Exp. Med.,* 138, 1314, 1973.
70. **Lee, K-C, Kay, J., and Wong, M.,** Separation of functionally distinct subpopulations of corynebacterium parvum-activated macrophages with predominantly stimulatory or suppressive effects on cell mediated cytotoxic T cell response, *Cell. Immunol.,* 42, 28, 1979.
71. **Lee, K-C.,** On the origin and mode of action of functionally distinct macrophage subpopulations, *Mol. Cell. Biochem.,* 30, 39, 1980.
72. **Daems, W. Th. and Brederou, P.,** Electron microscopical studies on the structure, phagocytic properties and peroxidatic activity of the resident and exudate peritoneal macrophages in the guinea pig, *Z. Zellforsch.,* 144, 247, 1973.
73. **Deams, W. Th., Koerten, H. K., and Soranzo, M. R.,** Differences between monocyte derived and tissue macrophages, *Adv. Exp. Biol. Med.,* 75, 27, 1978.
74. **North, R. J.,** The relative importance of blood monocytes and fixed macrophages to the expression of cell-mediated immunity, *J. Exp. Med.,* 132, 521, 1970.
75. **Widman, J. J., Cotran, R. S., and Fahimi, H. D.,** Mononuclear phagocytes (Kupffer cells) and endothelial cells: identification of two functional cell types in rat liver sinusoids by endogenous peroxidase activity, *J. Cell. Biol.,* 52, 159, 1972.
76. **Wisse, E.,** Observations on the fine structure and peroxidase cytochemistry of normal rat liver Kupffer cells, *J. Ultrastruct. Res.,* 46, 393, 1974.
77. **Golde, D. W., Finely, T. N., and Cline, M. J.,** The pulmonary macrophages in acute leukemia, *N. Engl. J. Med.,* 290, 875, 1974.
78. **Cline, M. J. and Sumner, M. A.,** Bone macrophage precursors: I. Some functional characteristics of the early cells of the mouse macrophage series, *Blood,* 40, 62, 1972.
79. **Bodel, P. T., Nichols, B. A., and Bainton, D. F.,** Differences in peroxidase localization of rabbit peritoneal macrophages after surface adherence, *Am. J. Pathol.,* 91, 107, 1978.
80. **Bloch, H.,** The motley phagocytes, *N. Engl. J. Med.,* 264, 914, 1961.
81. **Werb, Z. and Gordon, S.,** Secretion of a specific collagenase by stimulated macrophages, *J. Exp. Med.,* 142, 346, 1975.
82. **Werb, Z. and Gordon, S.,** Elastase secretion by stimulated macrophages, *J. Exp. Med.,* 142, 361, 1975.
83. **Gordon, S., Ukeless, J., and Cohn, A. Z.,** Induction of plasminogen activator by endotoxin stimulation and phagocytosis: evidence for a two stage process, *J. Exp. Med.,* 104, 995, 1974.
84. **Smith, T. J. and Wagner, R. R.,** Rabbit macrophage interferons: I. Conditions for biosynthesis by virus infected uninfected cells, *J. Exp. Med.,* 125, 159, 1967.
85. **Gordon, S., Todd, J., and Cohn, Z. A.,** *In vitro* synthesis and secretion of lysozyme by mononuclear phagocytes, *J. Exp. Med.,* 139, 1228, 1974.

86. **Humes, J. L., Bonney, R. J., Pelus, L., et al.,** Macrophages synthesize and release of prostaglandins in response to inflammatory stimuli, *Nature,* 269, 149, 1977.
87. **Colten, H. R.,** Biosynthesis of serum complement in *Progress in Immunology,* Vol. 2, Brent, L. and Holborrow, J., Eds., North Holland, Amsterdam, 1974, 183.
88. **Eaves, A. C. and Bruce, W. R.,** *In vitro* production of colony-stimulating activity: I. Exposure of mouse peritoneal cells to endotoxin, *Cell. Tissue Kinet.,* 7, 19, 1974.
89. **Metcalf, D.,** Acute antigen-induced elevation of serum colony stimulating factor (CSF) levels, *Immunology,* 21, 427, 1971.
90. **Chervenick, P. A.,** Effects of endotoxin and plasma on *in vitro* granulopoiesis, *J. Lab. Clin. Med.,* 79, 1014, 1972.
91. **Quesenberry, P. J., Morley, A., Stohlman, F., Jr., et al.,** Effect of endotoxin on granulopoiesis and colony stimulating factor, *N. Engl. J. Med.,* 286, 227, 1972.
92. **Stanley, E. R., Hansen, C., Woodcock, J., and Metcalf, D.,** Colony stimulating factor, and the regulation of granulopoiesis and macrophage production, Fed. Proc., Fed. Am. Soc. Exp. Biol., 34, 2272, 1975.
93. **Deimann, W. and Fahimi, H. D.,** Induction of focal hemopoiesis in adult rat liver by glucan, a macrophage activator: a cytochemical and ultrastructure study, *Lab. Invest.,* 42, 217, 1980.
94. **Apte, R. W., Heller, E., Hertogs, C. F., and Pluznik, D. H.,** Macrophages as regulators of granulopoiesis, *Adv. Exp. Med. Biol.,* 121A, 433, 1979.
95. **Unanue, E. R. and Cerottini, J-C.,** The function of macrophages in the immune response, *Sem. Hematol.,* 7, 225, 1970.
96. **Rosenthal, A. S., Lipsky, P. E., and Shevach, E. M.,** Macrophage-lymphocyte interaction and antigen recognition, *Fed. Proc.,* 34, 1743, 1975.
97. **Basten, A. and Mitchell, J.,** Role of macrophages in T cell, B cell collaboration in antibody production in *Immunobiology of the Macrophage,* Nelson, D. S., Ed., Academic Press, New York, 1978, 45.
98. **Rosenthal, A. C.,** Regulation of the immune response-role of macrophage, *N. Engl. J. Med.,* 303, 1152, 1980.
99. **Unanue, E. R.,** Cooperation between mononuclear phagocytes and lymphocytes in immunity, *N. Engl. J. Med.,* 303, 977, 1980.
100. **Unanue, E. R.,** The regulatory role of the macrophate in antigenic stimulation, *Adv. Immunol.,* 15, 95, 1975.
101. **Rosenthal, A. S.,** Determinant selection and macrophage function in genetic control of immune response, *Immunol. Rev.,* 40, 136, 1978.
102. **Zuckerman, R. H. and Douglas, S. D.,** Dynamics of the macrophage plasma membrane, *Ann. Rev. Microbiol.,* 33, 287, 1979.
103. **Feldman, M. and Rosenthal, A.,** Macrophage-lymphocyte interactions in immune induction, *Int. Rev. Cytol.,* 60, 149, 1979.
104. **Rinehart, J. J., Orser, M., and Kaplan, M. E.,** Human monocyte and macrophage modulation of lymphocyte proliferation, *Cell. Immunol.,* 44, 131, 1979.
105. **Schecter, G. P., Wahl, L. M., and Oppenheim, J. J.,** Suppressor monocytes in human disease, a review, *Adv. Exp. Med. Biol.,* 121B, 283, 1979.
106. **Old, L. J., Clarke, D. A., and Benacerraf, B.,** Effect of bacillus Calmette-Guerin infection on transplanted tumors in the mouse, *Nature,* 184, 291, 1959.
107. **Den Otter, W., Evans, R., and Alexander, P.,** Cytotoxicity of murine peritoneal macrophages in tumor allograft immunity, *Transplantation,* 14, 220, 1972.
108. **Lohmann-Mattes, M. L., Schipper, H., and Fischer, H.,** Macrophage-mediated cytotoxicity against allogeneic target cells in vitro, *Eur. J. Immunol.,* 2, 45, 1972.
109. **Evans, R. and Alexander, P.,** Mechanism of immunologically specific killing of tumor cells by macrophages, *Nature,* 236, 615, 1972.
110. **Hibbs, J. B., Lambert, L. H., and Remington, J. S.,** Possible role of macrophage mediated nonspecific cytotoxicity in tumour resistance, *Nat. New Biol.,* 235, 48, 1972.
111. **James, J., McBridge, B., and Stuart, A.,** Proceedings EURES symposium on the macrophage in cancer published by the organizers and editors, 1977.
112. **Alexander, P.,** The function of the macrophage in malignant disease, *Annu. Rev. Med.,* 27, 207, 1976.
113. **Samak, R., Israel, L., and Edelstein, R.,** Influence of tumor burden, tumor removal, immune stimulation, plasmapheresis on monocyte moblization in cancer patients, *Adv. Exp. Med. Biol.,* 121B, 411, 1979.
114. **Lejeune, F. J.,** Role of macrophages in immunity with special reference to tumor immunology, a review, *Biomedicine,* 22, 25, 1975.

115. **Leibovich, S. J. and Ross, R.,** The role of the macrophage in wound repair: A study with hydrocortisone and anti-macrophage serum, *Am. J. Pathol.,* 78, 71, 1975.
116. **Leibovich, S. J.,** Production of macrophage-dependent fibroblast-stimulating activity (M-FSA) by immune macrophages: effects on BALBc 3T3 fibroblasts, *Exp. Cell. Res.,* 113, 47, 1978.
117. **Alitalo, K., Hovi, T., and Vaheri, A.,** Fibronectin is produced by human macrophages, *J. Exp. Med.,* 151, 602, 1980.
118. **Levy, G. A. and Eding, T. S.,** Lymphocyte cooperation is required for amplification of macrophage procoagulant activity, *J. Exp. Med.,* 151, 1232, 1980.
119. **Page, R. C., Davies, P., and Allison, A. C.,** The macrophage as secretory cell, *Int. Rev. Cytol.,* 52, 119, 1978.
120. **Davies, P. and Bonney, R. J.,** Secretory products of mononuclear phagocytes: a brief review, *J. Reticuloendothel Soc.,* 28, 37, 1979.
121. **Legeune, F. J. and Vercammen-Grandjean, A.,** Secretory activity of macrophages in relation to cytotoxicity and modulation of cell function, *Frontiers Biol.,* 48, 425, 1979.
122. **Weiss, L.,** The hematopoietic microenvironment of the bone marrow: ultrastructural study of the stroma in rats, *Anat. Rec.,* 186, 161, 1976.
123. **Loffler, H.,** Untersuchungen uber die Activitat der alkalischen Phosphatase und der unspezifische esterase in den, Reticulumzellen des Knochenmarkes, aln Vergleich zwischen Knochenmark und Lymphknoten, *Folia. Haematol., (Leipz),* 6, 164, 1961.
124. **Trubowitz, S. and Masek, B.,** A histochemical study of the reticuloendothelial system of human marrow—its possible transport role, *Blood,* 32, 610, 1968.
125. **Wetzel, B. K., Spicer, S. S., and Horn, R. G.,** Fine structural localization of acid and alkaline phosphatase in cells of rabbit blood and bone marrow, *J. Histochem. Cytochem.,* 15, 311, 1967.
126. **Marton, P. F.,** Ultrastructural study of erythrophagocytosis in the rat bone marrow, *Scand. J. Haematol.,* Suppl., 23, 1, 1975.
127. **Bessis, M.,** L'ilot erythroblastique, unite functionelle de la moella osseuse, *Rev. Hematol.,* 13, 8, 1958.
128. **Westen, H. and Bainton, D.,** Association of alkaline phosphatase, positive reticulum cells in bone marrow with granulocytic precursors, *J. Exp. Med.,* 150, 919, 1979.
129. **Nossal, G. J. U., Ada, S. L., and Austin, C. M.,** Antigens in immunity: IV. Cellular localization of ^{125}labelled and ^{13}I-labelled flagellae in lymph nodes, *Austr. J. Exp. Biol. Med. Sci.,* 42, 311, 1964.
130. **Thiery, J. P.,** Etude au microscope electronique de l'ilot plasmacytaire, *J. Microscopie,* 1, 275, 1962.
131. **Blom, J.,** The ultrastructure of contact zones between plasma cells and macrophages in the bone marrow of patients with multiple myeloma, *Acta Pathol. Microbiol. Scand. Sect. A,* 85, 345, 1977.
132. **Shanmugathas, M., Sobel, H., Marquet, E., and Trubowitz, S.,** Plasma cells with inclusions containing iron, *Arch. Pathol. Lab. Med.,* 103, 577, 1979.
133. **Undritz, E.,** Die regionaren Monozyten der blutkorperchen Nesten, *Fol. Haematol.,* 70, 32, 1950.
134. **Territo, M. and Cline, M. J.,** Macrophages and their disorders in man, in *Immunobiology of the Macrophage,* Nelson, D. S., Ed., Academic Press, New York, 1976, 593.
135. **Cline, M. and Golde, D. W.,** A review and re-evaluation of the histiocyte disorders, *Am. J. Med.,* 55, 49, 1973.
136. **Golde, D. W.,** Disorders of mononuclear phagocyte proliferation, maturation and function, *Clin. Haematol.,* 4, 705, 1975.
137. **Groopman, J. E. and Golde, D. W.,** The histiocyte disorders: a pathophysiologic analysis, *Ann. Int. Med.,* 94, 95, 1981.
138. **Meuret, G.,** Disorders of the mononuclear phagocytic system: an analytic review, *Blut,* 34, 317, 1977.
139. **Ando, M. and Dannenberg, A. M., Jr.,** Macrophage accumulation, division, maturation and digestive and microbicidal capacities in tubercuolous lesions, IV. Macrophage turnover, lysosomal enzymes, and division in healing lesions, *Lab. Invest.,* 27, 466, 1972.
140. **Evans, R.,** Macrophages and the tumour bearing host, *Br. J. Cancer,* 28, 19, 1973.
141. **Husby, G., Hoagland, D. M., Strickland, R. D., and Williams, R. C., Jr.,** Tissue T and B cell infiltration of primary and metastic cancer, *J. Clin. Invest.,* 57, 1471, 1976.
142. **Neuret, G., Detel, U., Kolz, H. P. et al.,** Human monocytopoiesis in acute and chronic inflammation, *Acta Haematol.,* 54, 328, 1975.
143. **Meuret, G., Schmitt, E., Senn, H. J., and Hoffman, G.,** Monozytopoese, Makrophagenumsatz bei entzündlichen und malignen Erkrankungen, *Haematol. Bluttransfus.,* 21, 353, 1978.
144. **Spector, W. G.,** The macrophage in inflammation, *Ser. Haematol.,* 3, 132, 1970.
145. **Spector, W. G. and Mariano, M.,** Macrophage behavior in experimental granulomas, in *Mononuclear Phagocyte in Immunity, Infection, and Pathology,* Van Furth, R., Ed., Blackwell, Oxford, 1975, 927.

146. **Van Furth, R.**, Origin and kinetics of mononuclear phagocytes, *Ann. N.Y. Acad. Sci.*, 278, 161, 1976.
147. **Volkman, A.**, Disparity in origin of mononuclear phagocyte population, *J. Reticuloendothel Soc.*, 19, 249, 1976.
148. **Wolmark, N. and Fisher, B.**, The effect of a single and repeated administration of corynebacterium parvum on bone marrow macrophage colony production in syngenetic tumor-bearing mice, *Cancer Res.*, 34, 2869, 1974.
149. **Karnovsky, M. L., Lazdins, J., Drath, D., and Harpier, A.**, Biochemical characteristics of activated macrophages, *Ann. N.Y. Acad. Sci.*, 256, 266, 1975.
150. **Bursuker, I. and Goldman, R.**, Quantitative and function differences induced in bone marrow derived mononuclear phagocytes by inflammatory stimuli, *J. Reticuloendothel Soc.*, 25, 533, 1979.
151. **Lawrence, W. and Schreiber, A. J.**, Leprosy's footprints in bone marrow histiocytes, *N. Engl. J. Med.*, 300, 834, 1979.
152. **Cartwright, G. E.**, The anemia of chronic disorders, *Semin. Haematol.*, 3, 351, 1966.
153. **Kampschmidt, R. F. and Upchurch, H. F.**, The effect of endogenous pyrogen on the plasma zinc concentration of the rat, *Proc. Soc. Exp. Biol. Med.*, 134, 1150, 1974.
154. **Pekarek, R. S., Powanda, M. C., and Wannemacher, R. W., Jr.**, The effect of leukocytic endogenous mediator (LEM) on serum copper and ceruloplasmin concentrations in the rat, *Proc. Soc. Exp. Biol. Med.*, 141, 1029, 1972.
155. **Haurani, F. I. and Meyer, A.**, Iron and the reticuloendothelial system, *Adv. Exp. Med. Biol.*, 73. 171. 1976.
156. **Lynch, S. R., Lipschitz, D. A., Bothwell, T. F., and Charlton, R. W.**, Iron and the reticuloendothelial system, in *Iron in Biochemistry and Medicine*, Jacobs, A. and Worwood, M., Eds., Academic Press, New York, 1974, 563.
157. **Zarrabi, M. H., Lysik, R., Di Stafano, J., and Zucker, S.**, The anaemia of chronic disorders: studies of iron reutilization in the anemia of experimental malignancy and chronic inflammation, *Br. J. Haematol.*, 35, 647, 1977.
158. **Douglas, S. W. and Adamson, J. W.**, The anemia of chronic disorders: studies of marrow regulation and iron metabolism, *Blood*, 45, 55, 1975.
159. **Steinberg, H. N., Handler, E. S., and Handler, E. E.**, Assessment of erythrocytic and granulocytic colony formation of in an *in vivo* plasma clot diffusion chamber culture system, *Blood*, 47, 1041, 1976.
160. **Kampschmidt, R. F.**, Leukocyte endogenous mediator, *J. Reticuloendothel. Soc.*, 23, 287, 1978.
161. **Kampschmidt, R. F.**, Role of RES and leukocyte endogenous mediator in iron, zinc and copper metabolism, *Adv. Exp. Med. Biol.*, 121A, 403, 1979.
162. **Kochan, I.**, The role of iron in bacterial infections with special consideration of host-tubercle bacillus interaction, *Curr. Top. Microbiol. Immunol.*, 60, 1, 1973.
163. **Weinberg, E. D.**, Iron and susceptibility to infectious disease, *Science*, 184, 952, 1973.
164. **Sobocinski, P. Z., Canterbury, W. J., Jr., and Powanda, M. C.**, Differential effect of parenteral zinc on the course of various bacterial infections, *Proc. Soc. Exp. Biol.*, 156, 334, 1977.
165. **Sussman, M.**, In *Iron Biochemistry and Medicine*, Jacobs, A. and Worwood, M., Eds., Academic Press, New York, 1974, 649.
166. **MacSween, R. W. M. and MacDonald, R. A.**, Iron metabolism by reticulendothelial cells: *in vitro* uptake of transferrin-bound iron by rat and rabbit cell, *Lab. Invest.*, 21, 230, 1969.
167. **MacDonald, R. A., MacSween, R. W. M., and Pechet, G. A.**, Iron metabolism by reticuloendothelial cells *in vitro:* physical and chemical conditions, lipotrope deficiency, and acute inflammation, *Lab. Invest.*, 21, 236, 1969.
168. **Hemmaplardh, D. and Morgan, E. H.**, Transferrin and iron uptake by human cells in culture, *Exp. Cell. Res.*, 87, 207, 1974.
169. **O'Shea, M. J., Kershenobich, D., and Tavill, A. S.**, Effects of inflammation on iron and transferrin metabolism, *Br. J. Haematol.*, 25, 707, 1973.
170. **Kleber, E. E., Lynch, S. R., Skikne, B., et al.**, Erthrocyte catabolism in the inflammatory peritoneal monocyte, *Br. J. Haematol.*, 39, 42, 1978.
171. **Marton, P. F.**, Erthrophagocytosis in the human bone marrow, *Scand. J. Haematol.*, 7, 177, 1970.
172. **Beltrami, C. A., Bearzi, I., and Fabris, G.**, Storage cells of spleen and bone marrow in thalassemia, an ultra structure study, *Blood*, 41, 901, 1973.
173. **Van Dorpe, A., Broeckaert-Van Orshoven, A., Desmet, V., and Verwilghen, R. L.**, Gaucher-like cells and congenital dyserythropoietic anaemia type II (HEMPAS), *Br. J. Haematol.*, 25, 165, 1973.
174. **Dosik, H., Rosner, F., and Sawitsky, A.**, Acquired Gaucher-cells and sea blue histiocytes in chronic granulocytic leukemia, and other disorders, *Semin. Hematol.*, 9, 3, 1972.

175. **Rywlin, A. M., Hernandex, J. A., Chastain, D. E., and Pardo, V.,** Ceroid histiocytosis of spleen and bone marrow in idiopathic thrombocytopenia purpura (ITP): a contribution to the understanding of the sea blue histiocyte, *Blood,* 37, 587, 1971.
176. **Lee, R. E. and Ellis, L. D.,** The storage cells of chronic myelogenous leukemia, *Lab. Invest.,* 24, 281, 1971.
177. **Allison, A. C. and Davies, P.,** Increased biochemical and biological activities of mononuclear phagocytes exposed to various stimuli, with special reference to secretion of lysosomal enzymes, in *Mononuclear Phagocytes in Immunity, Infection and Pathology,* Van Furth, R., Ed., Blackwell Scientific, Oxford, 1975, Chap. 32.
178. **Robock, K.,** A new concept of the pathogenesis of silicosis: luminescence measurements and biochemical cell experiments with SiO_2 dust, *Staub,* 28, 15, 1968.
179. **Miller, K.,** The effects of asbestos on macrophages, *CRC Rev. Toxicol.,* 5, 319, 1978.
180. **Ota, H. and Yasuma, A.,** Lysozyme activity in hematologic and non-hematologic disorders with special reference to reactive monocytosis associated with chronic infections and inflammatory reactions, *Tohoku J. Exp. Med.,* 114, 15, 1974.
181. **Pascual, R. S., Gee, J. B., and Finch, S. C.,** Usefulness of serum lysozyme measurement in diagnosis and evaluation of sarcoidosis, *N. Engl. J. Med.,* 289, 1076, 1973.
182. **Klockars, M., Pettersson, T., and Riska, H.,** Pleural fluid lysozyme in tuberculous and non-tuberculous pleurisy, *Br. Med. J.,* 1, 1381, 1976.
183. **Rea, T. H. and Taylor, C. R.,** Serum and tissue lysozyme in leprosy, *Infect. Immun.,* 18, 847, 1977.
184. **Dobbins, J. W., Binder, H. J., Spriro, M. H., and Finch, S. C.,** Serum lysozyme in inflammatory bowel disease, *Gastroenterology,* 70, 469, 1976.
185. **Nugent, F. W., Mallari, R., George, H., and Ridley, N.,** Serum lysozyme in inflammatory bowel disease, *Gastroenterology,* 70, 1014, 1976.
186. **Osserman, E. F. and Lawlor, D. O.,** Serum and urinary lysozyme (muramidase) in monocytic and myelomonocytic leukemia, *J. Exp. Med.,* 124, 921, 1966.
187. **McClellan, D. B. L. and Van Furth, R.,** *in vitro* synthesis of lysozyme by human and mouse tissues and leucocytes, *Immunology,* 28, 1099, 1975.
188. **Osserman, E. F. and Canfield, R. E., and Bechok, S.,** *Lysozyme,* Academic Press, New York, 1974.
189. **Osserman, E. F.,** Postulated relationships between lysozyme and immunoglobulins as mediators of macrophage and plasma cell function, *Adv. Pathol.,* 4, 98, 1976.
190. **Osserman, E. F.,** Lysozyme, *N. Engl. J. Med.,* 292, 424, 1975.
191. **Currie, G. A. and Accles, S. A.,** Serum lysozyme as a marker of host resistance. I. Production by macrophages resident in rat sarcomata, *Br. J. Cancer,* 33, 51, 1976.
192. **DiLuzio, N. R.,** Lysozyme activity: an index of macrophage functional status, *Frontiers Biol.,* 61, 447, 1979.
193. **Rohr, K.,** *Das Menschliche Knockenmark,* Georg Thieme Verlag, Stuttgart, 1960, 410.
194. **Hayhoe, F. G. J., Quaglino, D., and Doll, R.,** The cytology and cytochemistry of acute leukemias, a study of 140 cases, MRC Spec. Rep. Ser., Her Majesty's Stationary Office, London, 1964.
195. **Lichtman, M. A. and Weed, R. I.,** Peripheral cytoplasmic characteristics of leukocytes in monocytic leukemia: relationship to clinical manifestations, *Blood,* 40, 52, 1972.
196. **Hayhoe, E. F. J. and Cawley, J. C.,** Acute leukaemia: cellular morphology, cytochemistry and fine structure, *Clin. Haematol.,* 1, 49, 1972.
197. **Cawley, J. C., Burns, G. F., Workman, C. P., et al.,** Morphological and immunological similarity of the monocytes from pure and mixed monocytic leukaemias, *Scand. J. Haematol.,* 21, 233, 1978.
198. **Bennett, J. M., Catovsky, D., Daniel, M. T., et al.,** Proposals for the classification of the acute leukaemias, French-American British (FAB) cooperative group, *Br. J. Haematol.,* 33, 452, 1976.
199. **Lichtman, M. A. and Weed, R. I.,** Alteration of the cell periphery during granulocyte maturation relationship to cell function, *Blood,* 39, 301, 1972.
200. **Miescher, P. and Farquet, J. J.,** Chronic myelomonocytic leukemia in adults, *Sem. Hematol.,* 11, 129, 1974.
201. **Scott, R. B. and Robb-Smith, A. H. T.,** Histiocyte medullary reticulosis, *Lancet II,* 194, 1939.
202. **Rappaport, H.,** Tumors of the hematopoietic system, in *Atlas of Tumor Pathology,* Armed Forces Institute of Pathology, Washington, D.C., 1966, 49.
203. **Byrne, G. E., Jr. and Rappaport, H.,** Malignant histiocytosis, *Gann Monogr. Cancer Res.,* 15, 145, 1973.
204. **Huhn, D. and Meister, P.,** Malignant histiocytosis: morphologic and cytochemical findings, *Cancer,* 42, 1341, 1978.

205. **Lampert, I. A., Catovsky, D., and Bergier, N.,** Malignant histiocytosis: a clinicopathological study of 12 cases, *Br. J. Haematol.,* 40, 65, 1978.
206. **Warnke, R. W., Kim, H., and Dorfman, R. F.,** Malignant histiocytosis (histiocytic medullary reticulosis) I. Clinico pathological study of 29 cases, *Cancer,* 35, 215, 1975.
207. **Vilpo, J. A., Klemi, P., Lassila, O., et al.,** Cytological and functional characterization of three cases of malignant histiocytosis, *Cancer,* 46, 1795, 1980.
208. Editorial: Proliferation and phagocytic histiocytes, *Lancet,* ii, 937, 1974.
209. **Trubowitz, S., Sobel, H., Davis, S.,** Null cell (Non T and Non B) acute lymphoblastic leukemia terminating as malignant histiocytosis, *Am. J. Clin. Pathol.,* 73, 725, 1980.
210. **Harousseau, J. L., Degos, L., Daniel, M. T., and Flandrin, G.,** Leukemic phase of malignant histiocytosis (arguments in favor of the histiomonocytic origin of the abnormal cells), *Med. Ped. Oncol.,* 6, 339, 1979.
211. **Schrek, R. and Donnelly, W. J.,** Hairy cells in blood in lymphoreticular neoplastic disease and ''flagellated'' cells of normal lymph nodes, *Blood,* 27, 199, 1966.
212. **Burke, J. S., Byrne, G. E., and Rappaport, H.,** Hairy cell leukemia (leukemic reticuloendotheliosis). II. A clinico-pathological study of 21 patients, *Cancer,* 33, 1399, 1974.
213. **Mubius, W., Hennekeuser, H. H., Westerhausen, M., et al.,** Haarzelle Leukemia, *Acta Haematol.,* 53, 1, 1975.
214. **Katayama, L., Li, C. Y., and Yam, L. T.,** Histochemical study of acid phosphatase isoenzyme in leukemic reticuloendotheliosis, *Cancer,* 29, 157, 1972.
215. **Yam, L. T., Li, C. Y., and Finkel, H. E.,** Leukemic reticuloendotheliosis: the role of tartrate-resistant acid phosphatase in diagnosis and splenectorm in treatment, *Arch. Int. Med.,* 130, 248, 1972.
216. **Rosner, M. C. and Golomb, H. M.,** Ribosomelamella complex in hairy cell leukemia, ultrastructure and distribution, *Lab. Invest.,* 42, 236, 1980.
217. **Golomb, H. M., Braylan, R., and Polliack, A.,** Hairy cell leukaemia (leukemic reticuloendotheliosis): a scanning electron microscopic study of eight cases, *Br. J. Haematol.,* 29, 455, 1975.
218. **Jaffe, E. S., Shevach, E. M., Frank, M. M., and Green, I.,** Leukemic reticuloendotheliosis: presence of receptor for cytophilic antibody, *Am. J. Med.,* 57, 108, 1974.
219. **Delsol, G., Pellegrin, M., Corbedand, J., et al.,** Hairy cell leukemia: a disease of the mononuclear phagocytes? in *Kupffer Cells and Other Liver Sinusoidal Cells,* Wisse, E. and Knock, D. L., Eds, Elsevier/North Holland, Amsterdam, 1977, 191.
220. **Burns, G. F., Cawley, J. C., Workman, C. P., et al.,** Multiple heavy chain isotypes on the surface of the cells of hairy cell leukemia, *Blood,* 52, 1132, 1978.
221. **Burns, G. F. and Cawley, J. C.,** A reexamination of the alledged monocytic features of hairy cell leukemia, *Scand. J. Haematol.,* 22, 386, 1979.
222. **Gordon, J. and Smith, J. L.,** Free immunoglobulin light chain synthesis by neoplastic cells in leukemic reticuloendotheliosis, *Clin. Exp. Immunol.,* 31, 244, 1978.
223. **Jansen, J., Meijer, C. J. L. M., Van der Walk, P., et al.,** Phagocytic potential of hairy cells, *Scand. J. Haematol.,* 23, 69, 1979.
224. **Vykoupil, K. F., Thiele, J., and Georgii, A.,** Hairy cell leukemia: bone marrow findings in 24 patients, *Virchows Arch. Pathol. Anat. Histol.,* 370, 273, 1976.
225. **Burke, J. S.,** The value of bone marrow biopsy in the diagnosis of hairy cell leukemia, *Am. J. Clin. Pathol.,* 70, 876, 1978.
226. **Seshadri, R. S., Brown, E. J., and Zipursky, A.,** Leukemia reticuloendotheliosis: a failure of monocyte production, *N. Engl. J. Med.,* 295, 181, 1976.
227. **Zeya, H. I., Keku, E., Richards, F., II, and Spurr, C. L.,** Absence of neutral protease and alkaline phosphatase in neutrophils of a case of hairy cell leukemia, *Am. J. Pathol.,* 95, 55, 1979.
228. **Aiba, M., Raffa, P. P., and Katayama, I.,** Significance of leukocyte alkaline phosphatase in hairy cell leukemia, *Am. J. Clin. Pathol.,* 74, 297, 1980.
229. **Yam, L. T., Chaudhry, A. A., and Janckila, A. J.,** Impaired marrow granulocyte reserve and leukocyte moblization in leukemic reticuloendotheliosis, *Ann. Int. Med.,* 87, 744, 1977.
230. **Lichtenstein, L.,** Histiocytosis X. Integration of eosinophilic granuloma of bone, ''Letterer-Siwe disease'' and ''Schuller-Christian disease'' as related manifestations of a single nosologic entity, *Arch. Pathol.,* 56, 64, 1953.
231. **Lieberman, P. H., Jones, C. R., Dergeon, H. W. K., and Begg, C. F.,** A reappraisal of eosinophilic granuloma of bone, Hand-Schuller-Christian syndrome and Letterer-Siwe syndrome, *Medicine,* 48, 375, 1969.
232. **Zinkham, W. H.,** Editorial—Multifocal eosinophilic granuloma, natural history, etiology, management, *Am. J. Med.,* 60, 457, 1976.
233. **Daneshbod, K. and Kissane, J. M.,** Idiopathic differentiated histiocytosis, *Am. J. Clin. Pathol.,* 70, 381, 1978.

234. **Kaufman, A., Bukberg, P. R., Werlin, S., and Young, F. S.,** Multifocal eosinophilic granuloma (Hand-Schuller-Christian disease), report illustrating HSC chronic and diagnostic challenge, *Am. J. Med.,* 60, 541, 1976.
235. **Vogel, J. M. and Vogel, P.,** Idiopathic histiocytosis: a discussion of eosinophilic granuloma, the Hand-Schuller-Christian syndrome and the Letterer-Siwe syndrome, *Semin. Hematol.,* 9, 149, 1972.
236. **McKusick, V. A.,** *Mendelian Inheritance in Man,* 4th ed., John Hopkins University Press, Baltimore, 1975.
237. **Stanbury, J. B. and Wyngaarden, J. B.,** *The Metabolic Basis of Inherited Disease,* 3rd ed., Frederickson, D. S., Ed., McGraw-Hill, New York, 615.
238. **Brady, R. O., Kanfer, J. N., and Shapiro, D.,** Metabolism of glucocerebrosides, II. Evidence of an enzymatic deficiency in Gaucher's disease, *Biochem. Biophys. Res. Commun.,* 18, 221, 1965.
239. **Volk, B. W., Adachi, M., and Schneck, L.,** The pathology of the sphingolipidoses, *Semin. Hematol.,* 9, 317, 1972.
240. **Djaldetti, M., Fishman, P., and Bessler, H.,** The surface ultrastructure of Gaucher cells, *Am. J. Clin. Pathol.,* 71, 146, 1979.
241. **Lee, R. E., Balczerzak, S. P., and Westerman, M. P.,** Gaucher's disease: a morphologic study and measurement of iron metabolism, *Am. J. Med.,* 42, 841, 1967.
242. **Lee, R. E.,** The fine structure of the cerebroside occurring in Gaucher's disease, *Proc. Natl. Acad. Sci. (U.S.A.),* 61, 454, 1968.
243. **Sloan, H. R., Uhlendorf, B. W., Kanfer, J. W., et al.,** Deficiency of sphingomyelincleaving enzyme activity in tissue culture derived from patients with Niemann-Pick disease, *Biochem. Biophys. Res. Commun.,* 34, 582, 1969.
244. **Silverstein, M. N. and Eliefson, R. D.,** The syndrome of the sea-blue histiocyte, *Semin. Hematol.,* 9, 299, 1972.
245. **Sawitsky, A., Rosner, F., and Chodsky, S.,** The sea blue syndrome, a review: genetic and biochemical studies, *Semin. Hematol.,* 9, 285, 1972.
246. **Yamamoto, A., Adachi, S., Ishibe, T., et al.,** Accumulation of acidic phospholipids in a case of hyperlipidemia with hepatosplenomegaly, *Lipids,* 5, 566, 1970.
247. **Maranoff, R., Fite, F. K., and Frumin, A. M.,** Greenish-blue granular marrow histiocytes associated with low serum cholesterol, *Am. J. Clin. Pathol.,* 57, 103, 1972.
248. **Stavem, P., Ly, B., and Bjrnecklett, A.,** Light green crystals in May-Grundwald and Giemsa-stained bone marrow macrophages in patients with myeloid leukaemia, *Scand. J. Haematol.,* 18, 62, 1977.
249. **Kirchen, M. E. and Marshall, G. J.,** Marrow storage cells: an ultrastructural study, *J. Reticuloendothel Soc.,* 19, 109, 1976.
250. **Takahashi, K., Terashima, K., Kojima, M., et al.,** Pathological histiochemical and ultrastructural studies on sea blue histiocytes and Gaucher-like cells in acquired lipidosis occurring in leukemia, *Acta Pathol. Jpn.,* 27, 775, 1977.
251. **Hayhoe, F. G. J., Flemans, R. J., and Cowling, D. C.,** Acquired lipidosis of marrow macrophages, *J. Clin. Pathol.,* 32, 420, 1979.
252. **Twomey, J. J., Douglass, C. C., and Sharkey, O., Jr.,** The monocytopenia of aplastic anemia, *Blood,* 41, 187, 1973.
253. **Kay, A., White, A., Barclay, G., et al.,** Monocyte function in chronic benign neutropenia, *Lancet,* i, 391, 1975.
254. **Baehner, R. L. and Johnson, R. B., Jr.,** Monocyte function in children with neutropenia and chronic infections, *Blood,* 40, 31, 1972.
255. **Rodey, G. E., Park, B. H., Winhorst, D. B., and Good, R. A.,** Defective bactericidal activity of monocytes in fatal granulomatous disease, *Blood,* 33, 813, 1969.
256. **Blaesse, R.,** Macrophages and the development of immunocompetence, in *The Phagocytic Cell in Host Resistance,* Belanti, J. and Dayton, D., Eds., Raven Press, New York, 1971, 309.
257. **Segrade, M. and Osborn, J.,** Role of macrophages in resistance to murine cytomagalovirus, *Infect. Immunol.,* 10, 1383, 1974.
258. **Lu, C. Y., Calmai, E. G., and Unanue, F. R.,** A defect in the antigen presenting function of macrophages from neonatal mice, *Nature,* 282, 327, 1979.
259. **Albrecht, R. M. and Hong, R.,** Basic and clinical considerations of the monocyte-macrophage system in man, *J. Pediatr.,* 88, 751, 1976.
260. **Good, R., Quie, P., Windhorst, D., et al.,** Fatal (chronic) granulomatous disease of childhood: a hereditary defect of leukocyte function, *Semin. Hematol.,* 5, 215, 1968.
261. **Oliver, C. and Essner, E.,** Formation of anomalous lysosomes in monocytes, neutrophils, and eosinophils from bone marrow of mice, with Chediak-Higashi syndrome, *Lab. Invest.,* 32, 17, 1975.
262. **White, J. and Clawson, C. C.,** The Chediak-Higashi syndrome, microtubules in monocytes and lymphocytes, *Am. J. Hematol.,* 7, 349, 1979.

263. **Gallin, J., Klimerman, J., Padgett, G., and Wolf, S.,** Defective mononuclear leukocyte chemotaxis in the Chediak-Higashi syndrome of humans, mink and cattle, *Blood,* 45, 863, 1975.
264. **Snyderman, R., Altman, L., Frankel, A., and Blaes, R.,** Defective mononuclear leucocyte chemotaxis, a previously unrecognized immune dysfunction, *Ann. Int. Med.,* 78, 509, 1973.
265. **Boetcher, D. and Leonard, E.,** Abnormal monocyte chemotactic response in cancer patients, *J. Natl. Cancer Inst.,* 52, 1091, 1974.
266. **Snyderman, R. and Pike, M. C.,** Macrophage migratory disturbance in cancer, *Am. J. Pathol.,* 88, 727, 1977.
267. **Norris, D., Weston, W. L., Tubergen, D. G., et al.,** Monocyte chemotaxis in leukemia patients, *J. Lab. Clin. Med.,* 95, 609, 1980.
268. **Kohl, S., Pickering, L. K., Sullivan, M. P., and Walters, D. L.,** Impaired monocyte-macrophage cytotoxicity in patients with Hodgkin's disease, *Clin. Immunol. Immunopathol.,* 15, 577, 1980.
269. **Kleinerman, E., Snyderman, R., and Daniels, C.,** Depression of monocyte chemotaxis by herpes simplex and influenza virus, *Fed. Proc.,* 33, (Abstr.), 788, 1976.
270. **Rinehart, J., Sagone, A., Balczerak, S., et al.,** Effects of corticosteroid therapy on human monocyte function, *N. Engl. J. Med.,* 292, 236, 1975.
271. **Dale, D. C., Fauci, A. A., and Wolff, S. M.,** Alternate-day predinisone, leukocyte kinetics and susceptibility to infection, *N. Engl. J. Med.,* 291, 1154, 1974.
272. **Drutz, D. J., Cline, M. J., and Levy, L.,** Leukocyte antimicrobial function in leprosy, *J. Clin. Invest.,* 53, 380, 1974.

Chapter 12

THROMBOPOIESIS

Sidney Trubowitz and Stephen Davis

TABLE OF CONTENTS

I. INTRODUCTION

In their fundamental studies on the bone marrow in 1869, both Bizzozero[1] and Neumann[2] clearly described the giant cell which we now recognize as the megakaryocyte. Bizzozero[3,4] further established the blood platelet as a structural and functional entity and appreciated its role in blood coagulation and thrombus formation. However, the relationship between the platelet and the magakaryocyte had to await the insightful observations, some 35 years later, of James Homer Wright[5] who was struck by the similarity in appearance of the platelet granulomere and the azurophilic granulation of the cytoplasm of the mature megakaryocyte. In in vitro studies of megakaryocytes, Wright[5] observed the formation of cytoplasmic protrusions which projected into the sinusoids and appeared to separate from the cell body. He concluded and proposed that platelets arise from megakaryocytes by a process of cytoplasmic fragmentation. Although Wright's hypothesis of platelet histogenesis was widely accepted, considerable dispute arose among investigators on the details of platelet formation, principally between the group[6–9] who favored a strictly cytoplasmic origin and their opponents[10–12] who centered on the large nuclear mass of the megakaryocyte as the principal site of platelet formation. Pisciotta et al.[13] were unable to detect pseudopodia and platelet formation in their studies of living human megakryocytes by phase microscopy in vitro. Thiery and Bessis,[14] on the other hand, noted cytoplasmic protrusions in their phase contrast cinematographic observations of human megakaryocytes. They[14] described octopus-like megakaryocytes whose long extensions underwent violent movements which they believed to be the initial and preparatory events of platelet release.

Howell[15] coined the term megakaryocyte, to distinguish those giant cells which possessed one giant nucleus from the giant cells, the polykaryocytes which were essentially multinucleated. Subsequent investigations on the giant cells of the marrow led to sharp differences of opinion concerning the structure and formation of the megakaryocyte nucleus. Proposed mechanisms for the production of the large megakaryocyte nucleus included nuclear fragmentation,[16] multipolar division,[17–19] nuclear overgrowth,[20] and cell fusion.[21,22]

Japa,[23] in a classic study on the development of the human megakaryocyte, recognized five classes of megakaryocytes distinguished by the number of nuclei in multiples from two to 32. He found two to five megakaryocytes per thousand marrow cells and distributed by class as follows: 2.5% for cells with 2 nuclei, 25.5% for cells with 4 nuclei, 5.3% with 8, 18% with 16, and 1% with 32 nuclei. He further concluded that the megakaryocytes arose by repeated mitotic division of the nuclei and that all the nuclei divided synchronously. He estimated the mitotic index at about 17 per thousand. Schwartz,[24] in his studies of human megakaryocytes obtained from patients with polycythemia vera and thrombocytopenic purpura, classified the megakaryocytes by the appearance of the cytoplasm and the degree of granule formation. The megakaryoblast was defined by its deep blue cytoplasm. The initiation of granulopoiesis morphologically identifiable as a reddish granular area, the "functional area" at the side of the nuclear indentation corresponding to what Schwartz speculated might be the site of the archoplasm of the Golgi apparatus, marked the transition from megakaryoblast to the promegakaryocyte, and the maturing megakaryocytes. The "functional area" expanded to involve more and more of the cytoplasmic volume and ultimately converted the entire cytoplasm into an azurophilic mass. Thus by 1950 the two principal features of megakaryocyte development, namely, nuclear polyploidy and cytoplasmic granulopoiesis, were well established. The 30 years that followed witnessed enormous expansion of our appreciation of megakaryocyte morphology, megakaryocytopoiesis, the relationship between cytoplasmic maturation and nuclear polyploidy, and of platelet structure and function.

II. MEGAKARYOCYTOPOIESIS

The megakaryocytes constitute a minor population of the nucleated cells of the human bone marrow, but their large size and multilobed nuclei permit ready recognition even under moderate magnification. An estimate of the megakaryocyte number can be made from the Romanowsky stained squash preparations of marrow particles where the megakaryocytes are found to constitute about 0.05% of the nucleated cells. Like other elements of hemopoiesis, megakaryocytes make their debut in the yolk sac, appear later in the fetal liver and spleen, and at 3 months of prenatal life begin their residence in the bone marrow.[25–27] In the adult the megakaryocytes are essentially confined to the bone marrow, though small numbers are present in circulating blood and in the pulmonary circuit.[28,29]

Megakaryocytes, like the other hemopoietic cell lines, presumably originate from the pluripotential stem cell from which a diploid committed stem cell compartment is created. The cells of the diploid committed stem cell compartment are in cycle or capable of entering into cell cycle in response to appropriate stimulation and thus constitute a pool of dividing megakaryocytic precursors. Cultures of murine marrow cells have demonstrated the presence of colony forming megakaryocyte precursors, CFU-M, presumably members of the proliferative committed stem cell pool.[30–34]

A. Ploidy

Polyploidy is a unique feature of megakaryocytopoiesis and it is the cellular enlargement associated with polyploidy that characterizes the megakaryocyte in the recognizable compartment.[23] Cells of the precursor-committed cell compartment in preparation for maturation, on arriving at a tetraploid state, cease dividing, but continue their DNA synthesis and synchronous nuclear doubling. The endomitosis results in populations of megakaryocytes at varying levels of polyploidy. The megakaryocytes can thus be classified by their polyploidy level, and their relative distribution among the ploidy classes is similar in the different animals studied: 1 to 2% for 4N, 10 to 25% for 8N, 46 to 76%, 16N; 15 to 32%, 32N; and 1% for 64N.[35–37] The nuclei of the polyploid megakaryocytes form irregular lobes connected by strands of DNA. The lobes do not contain precise 2N quantities of DNA, and the total nuclear DNA may not always fall evenly within a ploidy class.[38–40] Levine et al.[40] found, in their analysis of megakaryocyte ploidy of guinea pig and monkey marrow, that 8N was the predominant class and that the distribution of the megakaryocyte among the different ploidy classes was shifted by platelet demand. Thrombocytopenia was associated with a shift to higher ploidy levels, increased megakaryocyte size, and the delivery of more platelets per magakaryocyte. Thrombocytosis, on the other hand, was associated with a shift to the lower ploidy classes and a smaller megakaryocyte. Similar shifts in megakaryocyte ploidy were previously observed by Pennington et al.[41] in rats.[42]

The significance of polyploidy in megakaryocytopoiesis is not fully understood, but it has been suggested that polyploidy is the mechanism by which the cell can increase or modify its cytoplasmic volume,[41,42] which is presumed to be an index of the capacity of the megakaryocytes for platelet production. Thus, depending on its ploidy the megakaryocyte can produce an average of 4000 to 8000 platelets[42–44] which would require some 12 to 13 cell divisions if platelets were produced in a fashion similar to the other hemopoietic cell lines. Since the bulk of the megakaryocytes are distributed in the 8N and 16N ploidy classes, the process of platelet production, under normal circumstances, is accomplished with three to four endomitotic divisions, a remarkable savings of time and space.

Levine[45] isolated human megakaryocytes from the marrow obtained from ribs resected at operation. The megakaryocytes averaged 0.37% of the nucleated marrow cells. He determined 8N to be the predominant ploidy class, similar to his findings in guinea pigs and monkeys[40] but contrary to previous reports which placed the peak value at 16N.[29,46,47] The mean diameter of the isolated megakaryocytes was found to be 24 μm with a range of 12 to 45 μm. A minimum cell diameter of 11.5 μm was offered as a threshold value for the separation of megakaryocytes from nonmegakaryocytic cells in suspensions of human marrow cells and as an objective criterion for the identification of the megakaryocyte.

Early investigators[48] held to the view that nuclear polyploidy and cytoplasmic maturation were simultaneous events. The evidence, however, suggests that polyploidy develops prior to cytoplasmic maturation and that most megakaryocytes cease DNA synthesis at the 8N, 16N, or 32N ploidy level.[39,49] There is some overlap between nuclear polyploidy and cytoplasmic maturation, which begins somewhat before the end of DNA synthesis.[50,51] The speculation has been made that the synthesis of thrombosthenin in the cytoplasm signals the termination of DNA synthesis, regardless of the level of ploidy.[52]

In summary, those tetraploid cells of the committed stem cell compartments embarking on their journey to maturation cease to divide but continue to double their DNA content to become polyploid cells. Cell size increases with polyploidy formation and the megakaryocytes become easily recognizable, by virtue of size and nuclear structure, at the 8N level of ploidy. Ploidy formation can cease at any ploidy level, but the mechanisms for the termination of DNA synthesis are not understood. The large majority of the megakaryocytes of the marrow are distributed in the 8N and 16N classes where for the most part DNA synthesis stops. Cell size is proportional to nuclear ploidy. Cytoplasmic differentiation begins before and continues uninterruptedly toward its termination after cessation of DNA synthesis. For a brief and concise discussion of polyploidy of the blood cells see Reference 53.

B. Cytoplasmic Maturation

Maturation is a cytoplasmic process and since maturation of the megakaryocyte can begin at different levels of ploidy the stages of maturation are best defined by the cytoplasmic changes rather than by changes in size or by ploidy class. The megakaryocytes have been defined, on basis of the characteristics discerned by examination of the Romanowsky stained preparations of marrow, as megakaryoblasts, promegakaryocytes, and granular megakaryocytes.[54]

1. Morphological Characteristics—Light Microscopy

The megakaryoblasts vary considerably in size, depending on the degree of ploidy, but can be recognized on smear only when they attain a diameter of 30 μm or greater. The small rim of cytoplasm is intensely basophilic and contains no granules. The nucleus is round, and the chromatin, in which small barely visible nucleoli are imbedded, is compact. The megakaryoblasts represent but a small percentage of the marrow megakaryocytes and are indeed difficult to find in the normal marrow.

The promegakaryocyte or basophilic megakaryocyte marks the subsequent stage of maturation. The nuclear-cytoplasmic ratio has decreased; the nucleus is lobulated; and the chromatin is more compact. The cytoplasm is basophilic, most prominently in its peripheral dimensions. A pink area surrounded by small azurophilic granules is now discernible adjacent to the nucleus in the area of the Golgi complex. With further maturation, the pink area, the functional area of Schwartz,[24] spreads peripherally, becomes increasingly granular, and finally transforms the cell into the acidophilic mature megakaryocyte.

The acidophilic granular megakaryocyte displays a highly lobulated nucleus with highly compact chromatin. The lobules vary in size and are often separated by fine chromatin bridges. The lobulation is quite irregular and individual lobules do not correspond to individual nuclei. The cytoplasm is abundant and the nuclear cytoplasmic ratio considerably smaller than in the earlier forms. The cytoplasm becomes increasingly acidophilic and granular. The mature, acidophilic megakaryocytes make up about two thirds of the total megakaryocyte population of the marrow.

This basic description of megakaryocyte maturation is widely employed, though some prefer to refer to these maturation steps as stages I, II, and III, respectively. Because of the difficulty in assigning the ultrastructural images to the comparable maturation stages recognizable in the Romanowsky smears, the megakaryocyte maturation sequence has been divided into the broader categories of immature, maturing, and mature stages of differentiation.[50]

Following the complete sequestration of the megakaryocyte's cytoplasmic mass into platelets, the highly condensed, pyknotic, lobulated nucleus is left behind as the naked, megakaryocytic nucleus. These nuclei, devoid of cytoplasm and readily recognizable, are probably removed, like the extruded nuclei of the normoblasts, by the reticular macrophages of the marrow or possibly following entry into blood by the alveolar macrophages of the lung. The incidence of naked megakaryocytic nuclei in human bone marrow smears was estimated to be about 12% in a group of hospitalized patients.[55]

2. *Ultrastructural Characteristics of Megakaryocyte Maturation*

The electron microscope has provided the means for the appreciation of the ultrastructural details of the megakaryocyte and of their development during the cytoplasmic differentiation of the cell in man[26,27,56–62] and other mammals.[53,63–68] The electron microscope has generally confirmed the early morphological impression of the similarity of the megakaryocyte in the different mammalian species.

The platelet bears an evolutionary kinship with the granulocytic cells. In invertebrates the hemostatic function of the platelet and the antibacterial function of the leucocyte reside in a single specific cell, the hemocyte. In the lower vertebrates (fish, reptiles, and birds) the dual functions of the hemocyte are passed on to two separate cell lines, the granulocytes and the nucleated thrombocytes, each derived from successive divisions of their precursor cells.[69] In the mammal, further refinement of the process led to the creation of the megakaryocyte which can produce thousands of platelets, the hemostatic equivalent of the hemocyte and the nucleated thrombocyte, by sequestration of its cytoplasm. Phylogenetically, a relationship exists between the granulocyte and the platelet, and indeed the formation of granules and the elaboration of a demarcation membrane system are the most conspicuous morphological events of cytoplasmic maturation of the megakaryocyte.[70,71]

The megakaryoblasts and promegakaryocytes are fairly uncommon in normal human marrow and make up less than 5% of the total megakaryocyte population. Megakaryoblasts are indeed rare. Only 8.7% of megakaryocytes in the rat bone marrow are labeled 1 hr after injection of tritiated thymidine, and of the labeled cells only 20% are immature.[51] They are recognized by virtue of their large size. The cells are richly endowed with polyribosomes and contain a prominent Golgi complex in association with numerous small vesicles. The centrioles and their satellites are situated in the center of the Golgi complex, from which the microtubules radiate peripherally to the cell membrane. Early membranes of the demarcation membrane system are observed in continuity with the plasma membrane. One or more nucleoli are usually present in the nucleus.

The acidophilic, mature megakaryocyte has a lobulated nucleus with numerous nuclear pores.[72] The cytoplasm has increased considerably and can be conveniently divided into three zones: a perinuclear zone rich in ribosomes; a central zone, which includes the Golgi apparatus, and is conspicuous for its content of granules and demarcation membranes; and the peripheral zone which contain the microtubles, microfibrils, and glycogen granules.[73–75]

3. *The α Granules*

a. Origin

The granules of the megakaryocyte are formed by the Golgi complex.[76] They arise from small complexes consisting of three to four cisterns. In the immature cells the complexes are present between the nuclear lobes, the area corresponding to Schwartz's functional area. In the more mature megakaryocytes the granules become more numerous in the central zone of the cells but are rare in the peripheral zone. The vesicles may be homogeneous or present with the characteristic, electron-dense nucleoid of the granules (bull's-eye granules). The role of the Golgi complex in the formation of the granules is supported by the demonstration that the bulk of administered ^{32}S appears in mucopolysaccharides in the Golgi complex. A small proportion of the ^{32}S is found in the demarcation membranes and in the membrane of the platelets.[77]

b. Content

The main constituents of the α granules are the platelet-specific proteins, the cationic proteins, and some coagulation factors. The α granules contain platelet factor 4, a small polypeptide of 1800 daltons which is bound to a 59,000-dalton proteoglycan. The complex is secreted intact by the platelet. It is dissociated by heparin, which then binds with the polypeptide for which it has a high affinity. Platelet factor 4 neutralizes heparin activity. Beta thromboglobulin consists of four identical chains (each 80,000 daltons) which show great homology to platelet factor 4. This protein has a short half-life in the circulation and a lower binding affinity for heparin. The α granules contain in addition to the cationic proteins: growth mitogenic factor, a permeability factor, a chemotactic factor which can activate C_5, a bacterial factor (B-lysin), fibrinogen, factor V, and a glycoprotein of 147 to 185,000 daltons. These proteins are presumably synthesized by the megakaryocyte and packaged by the Golgi complex.[82] The α granules are spherical and measure 300 to 500 nm in diameter.[78]

4. *Dense Granules*

The very dense granules are present in human platelets in small numbers and are rich in serotonin. They are 250 to 300 nm in diameter, highly osmophilic, generally spherical, but may be elongated. The serotonin of the dense granule is not synthesized by the megakaryocyte but is absorbed by the platelet from the plasma. Megakaryocytes are capable of absorbing serotonin and storing it in a dense granule, but dense granules are normally quite rare in the megakaryocyte. In addition to serotonin the dense granule in the platelet contains a high concentration of calcium (60 to 70% of the total calcium of the platelet), ATP, and ADP. About two thirds of the platelet nucleotides are stored in the dense granules in a ratio of ATP/ADP equal to 2:3 and are metabolically inert.[78,79] The origin of the dense granule in the platelet is not known for certain, but in vitro investigations led White[80] to suggest that they are the principal secretory organelles of the platelet. He also further cited his findings on a child with the Hermansky-Pudlak syndrome whose platelets showed a marked reduction in the number of dense bodies and reduced levels of serotonin as clinical support for the hypothesis that the dense granules are centrally involved in the secretory function of the platelet. Depletion of the platelet serotonin by reserpine does not affect the hemostatic function of the cell.

5. Lysosomes

Human platelets contain lysosomal, acid hydrolases such as acid phosphatase, glucoronidase, galactosidase, cathepsin, β-glycerophosphatase, etc. The acid hydrolases are stored neither in the α granules nor in the dense granules, but are secreted by the platelet when activated by thrombin or collagen. In the rat, the primary lysosomes of the megakaryocyte and of the platelet are small vesicles derived from the Golgi complex and endoplasmic reticulum and can be identified only by cytochemical staining. The vesicles are distinct from both the α granules and dense granules. The lysosomal vesicles in the immature and maturing megakaryocytes are small, and with increasing maturation, fuse to form larger vesicles, about 175 to 250 nm, which are dispersed throughout the cytoplasm and are ultimately found in the platelet.[81]

C. The Demarcation Membrane System

The development of an extensive system of membranes, the demarcation membrane system, is a conspicuous and highly specific ultrastructural feature of the cytoplasmic maturation of the megakaryocyte. The demarcation system defines the borders of the cytoplasmic territories of the megakaryocyte destined ultimately for delivery as individual platelets. The membranes of the demarcation system which partition the cytoplasm also serve to form the cell membranes of the platelets. The development of the demarcation membranes begins in the immature megakaryocytes and grows rapidly into an extensive network of membrane-limited cisternae in the late granular megakaryocyte.[82]

The origin of the demarcation membrane is still under dispute. Some favor the endocytoplasmic reticulum, smooth or rough,[65,67] others the Golgi complex[59,62,67] as the source of the demarcation membranes. However, the bulk of current evidence supports the suggestion that the demarcation membranes are formed by the formation of membrane-bound tubules arising from the cell membrane of the megakaryocyte. Tracers, such as thorotrast, horseradish peroxidase, ferritin, or ruthenium red injected intravenously enter the cisternae of the demarcation system, but no other cellular organelle, including the Golgi complex.[63,74,83–85] These studies indicate that a communication exists between the demarcation membrane system and the extracellular environment and supports the argument that the membranes arise from the cell membrane of the megakaryocyte.

Further support for the cell membrane origin of the demarcation membranes has come from the visualization of acetyl cholinesterase activity which has been shown to be present almost exclusively in the megakaryocytes of the cat, guinea pig, and rat bone marrow.[86] The enzyme is localized in the cell membrane of the megakaryocyte and in the membranes of the demarcation system.[87] Further, both platelets and megakaryocytes possess a similar surface coat of acid mucopolysaccharides. The surface coat of the platelet and the megakaryocyte and the membranes of the demarcation system stain with alcian blue, ruthenium red, and lanthanum salts.[64,88–90]

The demarcation membrane system is thought to arise initially from one or several sites of the cell membrane as membrane bound sacs or tubules. The tubules remain in open connection with the extracellular space. Later, the tubules extend from the periphery toward the central zone and, with further maturation of the cell, the tubules take on a lamellar appearance. Dense compartments, consisting of four or five stacked lamellae, have been described.[74] The demarcation membrane system ultimately forms an anastomosing network that involves the entire cytoplasm.

D. Microtubules and Microfilaments

Bundles of microfibrils are often present between the intermediate and marginal zones of the megakaryocyte. The fibrils are about 80 to 120 Å in diameter and can also be found surrounding the demarcation membranes.[62] The megakaryocytic microfilaments are abundant when visualized by prior glycerination before fixation and become more abundant as the cell matures. The thinner filaments behave as actin and form typical "arrow head" complexes with meromyosin isolated from muscle.[90] The thicker microfilaments are thought to be aggregates of myosin.[91,92]

Nachman et al.[92] have shown that cultured guinea pig megakaryocytes can synthesize abundant quantities of actin, molecular weight 42,000 daltons. These molecules probably exist in monomeric, rather than in polymerized filamentous forms in the normal megakaryocyte, as they do in the platelet.[93,94]

The microtubles are found in all stages of maturation; they increase with maturation, but do not assume prominent proportions. As a cytoplasmic component, the microtubules may play a role in the projection of the cytoplasmic pseudopod into the sinusoid: the microtubules are found oriented parallel to the long axis of the cytoplasmic projection.[63]

The megakaryocyte, in its maturation, synthesizes a variety of substances which are also present in the platelets. Cultured guinea pig megakaryocytes synthesize actin,[92] factor VIII antigen,[94] and platelet-derived growth factor.[95] A single megakaryocyte contains a quantity of growth factor equivalent to the content of 1000 to 5000 platelets—a value approximately equal to the number of platelets shed from a single megakaryocyte.[96] Growth factor is released by the platelet along with the α granules following its stimulation by thrombin, arachidonic acid, or collagen.[96] By use of a ferritin-conjugated antibody for factor VIII antigen, Piovella et al.[97] localized the factor VIII antigen in the canalicular system of human megakaryocyte and platelet, and in endothelial cells. Factor VIII antigen was found in the granules. They suggested that the platelet may derive its factor VIII antigen not only from its megakaryocytic precursor but from the serum as well. Fibrinogen[98] and factor XIII[99] may be synthesized by the megakaryocytes. The rich glycogen content of both the platelets and the megakaryocytes is readily appreciated by the intense red color of these cells following their exposure to the periodic acid-Schiff stain. This reaction may be of value in the differentiation of the megakaryocyte from other giant cells in the marrow, e.g., the Reed-Sternberg cell. Glycogen is not present in the promegakaryocytes, but increases rapidly with increasing maturation of the megakaryocytes and ultimately exists as small aggregates in the acidophilic megakaryocyte.[100–103]

Under appropriate conditions of fixation and incubation, peroxidase activity can be localized in the dense tubular system of the platelets[104] and in the endoplasmic reticulum and perinuclear space of the megakaryocyte. The reaction is seen only in mature cells having granules and demarcation membranes. Reaction product is also present in the perinuclear space and may be found in the thin rim of cytoplasm surrounding naked megakaryocyte nuclei. No peroxidase activity is seen in the Golgi complex. The function of this enzyme in the megakaryocyte of platelet is unknown, but it has served as a marker for the identification of the megakaryocyte.[104]

Megakaryocytes, during their maturation, synthesize surface antigens which they share in common with the platelets.[105,106] The commonly shared antigenic determinants (procoagulants, chemical composition, and enzymatic activity) between megakaryocyte and platelet in addition to their ultrastructural similarities lend strong support to the argument that the platelets arise from the megakaryocyte.

Megakaryocytes in normal human marrow may on occasion contain one or several bone marrow cells such as the nucleated red cells or granulocytes.[107,108] The enclosed cells appear normal and unaltered. The cells presumably gain access to the megakaryocyte cytoplasm by emperipolesis,[109] a proposal supported in part by the demonstration of free-moving granulocytes within the megakaryocyte cytoplasm. An alternate hypothesis suggests that the foreign cells gain access to the megakaryocyte's interior via the canalicular system of the demarcation membranes. In a retrospective study, marrow cell uptake by megakaryocytes was encountered in 13% of routine bone marrow aspirates. Bleeding and carcinoma were most commonly associated with this phenomenon.[110,111] Most normal cells, except the lymphocyte, obey contact inhibition. An early property of malignant cells is the loss of contact inhibition and the display of tumor cell emperipolesis. The significance of megakaryocyte emperipolesis remains to be clarified.

III. CYTOPLASMIC SEQUESTRATION AND PLATELET RELEASE

Consensus has it that the demarcation membrane system of the megakaryocyte partitions the cytoplasmic mass into the individual platelets. The demarcation system consists of tubular structures which in some fashion must convert to flat membranes to enclose the platelet zones. MacPherson[51] postulated that the demarcation membranes proceed from a single site on the cell membrane and by continuous concentric infolding of the cell membrane produce a system of flat sheets. Evidence obtained from the application of the freeze fracture technique to the study of thrombopoiesis does not support the concepts proposed by MacPherson and have led Shaklai and Tavassoli[84,112] to propose that the demarcation system arises by the formation of tubules from multiple sites on the cell membrane of the megakaryocytes. The tubules connect and branch to ultimately form a continuous network of tubules lying side by side and oriented in the same direction. Multiple points of fusion bind the tubules and fission of the fenestrations between fused tubules gives rise to two flat membranes with a canal between. The two membranes now border two contiguous platelet zones.

Geographically, megakaryocytes assume positions in the bone marrow adjacent to the sinusodal lumen.[113–116] The mature megakaryocyte produces about six cytoplasmic projections, each about 2.5 $\times$ 120 μm, known as proplatelets.[116] Each proplatelet is probably fragmented within the sinusoidal lumen to deliver some 1000 platelets. The intimate details of platelet separation are still unknown. Platelet formation has been studied principally by the in vitro observation of isolated megakaryocytes[14,116–121] and by electron microscopy. The details of the in vivo birth of platelets; their delivery from megakaryocytes in their normal anatomical location have yet to be determined. There are minority voices[122,123] which oppose the widely held view that the demarcation membrane system is involved in the liberation of platelets from the megakaryocyte cytoplasm and propose bleb formation as the major mechanism.[123] The relationship of the demarcation membrane to bleb and/or pseudopod formation to platelet release has yet to be clarified.

IV. CIRCULATING AND PULMONARY MEGAKARYOCYTES

The presence of megakaryocytes in the pulmonary capillaries of patients with pneumonia and in the lungs of dogs with experimentally produced pneumonia was reported by Aschoff.[124] He theorized that an intense chemotactic stimulus led to the release of the megakaryocytes from the marrow and their subsequent transport to the lungs. A few years later Foa[125] suggested that the migration of megakaryocytes from the marrow to the lung was a normal phenomenon which was exaggerated by pathological events. Abundant evidence has been presented to confirm the presence of megakaryocytes in both the peripheral venous blood bed and the capillaries of the pulmonary venous blood of man, and their origin from the bone marrow.[126–134] The number of megakaryocytes per ml of blood varies with the sampling site: the highest values are in the inferior vena cava, intermediate values in the cubital vein, and the lowest in the arterial blood.[131] The megakaryocytes recovered from the peripheral venous blood consist almost exclusively of naked nuclei; only 0.5 to 1.0% have an associated cytoplasmic mass.[135–141] The number of circulating megakaryocytes appears to increase after bleeding,[142] surgery,[143] and infection.[142–144] Megakaryocytes are thought to be released continually under normal circumstances; they are trapped in the pulmonary circulation where they release their platelets. Stimulation of marrow megakaryocytopoiesis increases the concentration of circulating megakaryocytes. It is not clear whether the entrance of megakaryocytes into the blood from the marrow is purely accidental or part of the programmed physiologic process of platelet formation. The contribution of the circulating megakaryocyte to platelet production has been variously estimated from a low of 7%[135] to a high of 70%.[139]

V. THROMBOKINETICS

The best estimate of the normal megakaryocyte number in man is 6.1×10^6 cells per kg.[43] Measurements on 15 normal subjects gave a mean platelet count of 250,000 platelets per μl ± 35,000 and mean platelet survival of ^{51}Cr-labeled cells of 9.9 days ± 0.6. The immediate recovery of the labeled platelets was 64.6% ± 4.1 of the injected platelets, reflecting largely the quantity of platelets sequestered by the spleen. The platelet turnover, calculated from the above data was 35,000 platelets per μℓ per day ± 4300. The total megakaryocyte mass in the normal subject was $2.8 \times 10^{10} \mu m^3/kg$ ± 0.3. Sixty five percent of the megakaryocytes of the normal marrow contained eight nuclei, 23% 16, and 12% four nuclei. From their thrombokinetics measurements of normal subjects and of patients with thrombocytopenia and thrombocytosis, Harker and Finch[43] concluded that thrombopoiesis was regulated by alterations in megakaryocyte number and volume.

Megakaryocytopoiesis can be stimulated or suppressed in the experimental animal by perturbation of the platelet count. Acute thrombocytopenia induced by exchange transfusion with platelet-poor blood,[145–147] injection of antiplatelet serum,[148–150] or irradiation[151,152] causes an increase in size, number, nuclear lobes, and more rapid maturation. A delay of 15 to 20 hr between induction of the thrombocytopenia and the increase in the number of megakaryocytes in the marrow suggests that the stimulus for the increased megakaryocytopoiesis acts on a precursor cell antecedent to the recognizable cell compartment. An increase in ploidy, maximum at 48 hr, suggests an extra replication of DNA.[39] Conversely, thrombocytosis, induced by transfusion of freshly collected platelets, suppresses megakaryocytopoiesis[153] manifested by a reduction in megakaryocyte number, a shift toward lower ploidy levels, and a decrease in megakaryocyte size. Human megakaryocytopoiesis, in its response to thrombocytopenia appears to behave in a fashion similar to the experimental animal as described above.[154] Acute thrombocytopenia induced by thrombopheresis in man is followed by a steady rise in the platelet count over the ensuing 84 hr; a rise in the number of young megakaryocytes at 24 hr; and an increase in the lobulation of the megakaryocyte nucleus and a peak level of the response at 72 hr after the thrombopheresis. The ploidy state returns to normal after 6 days.[42] In idiopathic thrombocytopenic purpura, the megakaryocytes are increased in both number and size (volume) to about twice normal. The maturation time is decreased and the platelet turnover increased.[155–157]

The regulation of megakaryocytopoiesis, namely its response to alterations in the platelet count, is mediated in part by a humoral poietin, the thrombopoietic stimulating factor (TSF).[158–160] Bioassays have shown that plasma from thrombocytopenic donors stimulates thrombopoiesis and that plasma from thrombocytotic donors does not. The origin of the TSF has not been determined, but the material has been partially purified from the plasma of thromocytopenic rabbits.[161,162]

The evidence suggests that thrombocytopenia induces the production of the TSF in the experimental animal and in man. The reinfusion of plasma from human subjects made platelet poor by thrombocytopheresis after their recovery from the thrombocytopenia resulted in an increase in the immature megakaryocytes and a rise in the platelet count.[163] It was also shown that the plasma of thrombocytopenic donors stimulated the maturation of the mouse megakaryocytes in culture.[34]

The site or sites of TSF action are not completely understood but the suggestion was made that TSF acts by stimulating megakaryocyte endomitosis.[164,165] The injection of plasma from thrombocytopenic rats into mice stimulates an increase in the endomitotic index 32 hr after the injection and a subsequent rise in the platelet count.[165] Further, TSF can apparently be transferred between species. Regeneration following acute thrombocytopenia was also shown to be enhanced by hypertransfusion and the effect could be reversed by the administration of erythropoietin.[166]

Factors other than the platelet count may affect thrombocytopoiesis. Thrombocytosis may be seen clinically in inflammatory disorders, iron deficiency, and hemolytic anemia.[167] How these conditions stimulate thrombopoiesis is not clear and the details of regulation and autoregulation of megakaryocytopoiesis have yet to be elucidated.[168]

VI. PLATELET AND MEGAKARYOCYTE HETEROGENEITY

Platelet heterogeneity with respect to size,[169,170] buoyant density,[171] reactivity to ADP and collagen,[171,173] and metabolic function[174,175] has been well established. It has been argued that the younger platelets are larger and show greater bouyant density, greater activity for protein synthesis increased glycogen synthesis and glycolytic activity than the older platelets.[171,174,175,177,180,181] However, though the platelets released from the marrow during recovery from thrombocytopenia are large and show increased protein synthesis, increased platelet factor 3, etc., such young platelets do not show the increased buoyant density so characteristic of the dense, putative, young platelets.[176] The functional significance and mechanism of platelet heterogeneity have yet to be determined. Paulus[177] pointed out that the heterogeneity of the platelet with respect to size takes on a log normal distribution which should be anticipated when particles are produced by fragmentation of growing tissues. Evidence has been presented to show that labeled platelets of different species do not change their buoyant densities throughout their life span in the peripheral blood.[178–180]

Pennington et al.[181] reinvestigated the problem of platelet heterogenity and found that the dense, intermediate, and the light platelets are released simultaneously from the marrow. Subsequently, Pennington and his co-workers[182] demonstrated a decreasing concentration of granules and mitochondria in the cytoplasm of the megakaryocytes with increasing ploidy and cell volume. The light platelets were thus found to correspond morphometrically with the 32N megakaryocyte and the dense platelet with the 8N. These studies demonstrate that the heterogeneity of megakaryocytes may be a major source of the heterogeneity of the platelets. Again, the functional significance of megakaryocyte heterogeneity with respect to granule concentration is not understood.

In summary, thrombopoiesis is currently conceived as a sequence which begins with commitment of the pluripotential stem cell to megakaryocyte differentiation. Amplification is achieved through division of the diploid committed stem cells which at some point are triggered into a polyploid state. Most cells cease their DNA synthesis at 8N, 16N, or 32N, and cell size increases proportionally to the ploidy class. The cytoplasmic differentiation begins before complete cessation of DNA synthesis and represents the earliest form of the recognizable megakaryocytes. The megakaryocytes of the recognizable compartment are nonproliferative cells and can be subdivided into immature megakaryoblasts and promegakaryocytes, and mature megakaryocytes. Maturation is characterized by the formation of granules, the development of an intricate demarcation membrane system, and a continuous disintegration of cytoplasmic RNA. The time required for maturation of the recognizable megakaryocytes in man is not known precisely but has been estimated at about 5 days in one subject.[183] Platelet release is achieved, presumably, by the shedding of cytoplasm or through the sequestration of cytoplasmic projections through the sinusoidal endothelium. Heterogeneity of platelets with respect to size, buoyant density, and function has been established and has been related to platelet senescence and to the heterogeneity of the megakaryocytes. The regulation of thrombopoiesis has not been elucidated but evidence suggests that megakaryocytopoiesis is regulated in part by a thrombopoiesis-stimulating factor and by the platelet mass.

It is apparent that the clinical hematologists are handicapped by the limitations imposed by the minor population of megakaryocytes in the marrow (less than 1.0%) and the limits of resolution of the light microscope in their attempt to assess the adequecy or abnormalities of megakaryocytopoiesis from the meager morphological data that can be derived from the examination of the smears of the marrow aspirate or from the histologic sections of the marrow biopsy.

Normally there are about 20 megakaryocytes per square millimeter of bone marrow, a fact best appreciated in the sections of marrow biopsies. Enumeration of megakaryocytes in smears is most inaccurate because of the tendency of the spreader to push the large megakaryocytes to the feather edge of the smear. A reasonable qualitative guess can be made by examining many areas of a squash preparation under the low power objective, where, on average, 1 to 3 megakaryocytes per field are found. Megakaryoblasts are indeed scarce and are rarely found in the normal human marrow. Thus, for the most part the normal human marrow presents two morphological forms, the promegakaryocyte and the mature granular megakaryocyte in a ratio of about 1:3. The granular acidophilic megakaryocytes make up 2/3 to 3/4 of the total number of megakaryocytes in the marrow. A small percentage about 5 to 6%, of naked megakaryocytic nuclei are present in the normal marrow.

Different polyploidy classes are found at every level of cytoplasmic maturation of the megakaryocytes. Principally three ploidy classes, 8N, 16N, and 32N, are observed, with peak value at 8N. About 2/3 of the megakaryocytes in the normal bone marrow smear belong to this ploidy class.

VII. ABNORMALITIES OF MEGAKARYOCYTOPOIESIS

Aberrations of platelet production can be divided conveniently into the quantitative disorders characterized by an over- or under-production of platelets, whether absolute or relative, or disorders characterized by the production of qualitatively abnormal, functionally deficient platelets.

A. Thrombocytosis

Thrombocytosis, defined as a platelet count greater than 400,000 platelets/mm^3, is a frequently encountered reactive phenomenon in a wide variety of clinical situations. Elevated platelet counts are seen in chronic inflammatory states such as rheumatoid arthritis, periarteritis nodosa, ulcerative colitis, sarcoidosis, etc.; following an acute hemorrhage; in the hemolytic anemias, iron deficiency anemia; in malignant disease as in carcinomatosis, lymphoma, and Hodgkin's disease; and in postoperative states, regardless of their nature and postsplenectomy.[167,184,185]

The platelet count is used as an index of disease activity in Hodgkin's disease and the increased megakaryocytes in the marrow have been confused morphologically with the Reed-Sternberg cells. Such confusion can be readily resolved by a PAS stain which endows the megakaryocyte cytoplasm with a deep red color, but does not affect the cytoplasm of the Reed-Sternberg cells.

1. Reactive Thrombocytosis

In reactive thrombocytosis, the platelet life span is normal but megakaryocytopoiesis is increased as evidenced by an increase in the number and size of the megakaryocytes in the marrow, and an increase in megakaryocyte ploidy. The stimulus for the increased platelet production is not known. The reactive thrombocytosis of iron deficiency anemia has been investigated experimentally in the laboratory animal.[185] The nature of megakaryocytopoiesis was found to differ with the severity of the iron deficiency anemia. In moderate anemia, thrombocytosis was invariably present and the marrow showed an increase in the labeling index and an increase in the proportion of immature megakaryocytes. No change in the concentration, size, or mitotic index of the megakaryocytes was observed, and these findings were thought to suggest an increase in the rate of in flow of precursor cells and a shortened marrow transit time. In severe anemia the platelet count was lower, closer to normal values, but never thrombocytopenic. Again the labeling index and the percentage of immature megakaryocytes in the marrow were increased, but now, megakaryocyte size and mitotic index were significantly increased in the face of some decrease in megakaryocyte concentration. It was concluded that the platelet count was maintained by the higher ploidy and increased platelet output per megakaryocyte. The mechanism for these changes in megakaryocytopoiesis is not understood, but the speculation was made that the stem cells, stimulated by the demand for erythropoiesis but blocked in their maturation by the iron deficiency, are diverted into other pathways of hematopoiesis, namely, granulopoiesis and megakaryopoiesis.

2. Primary Thrombocytosis

In contrast to reactive thrombocytosis, autonomous or primary thrombocytosis is seen in the so-called myeloproliferative disorders, polycythemia rubra vera, myelofibrosis with myeloid metaplasia, primary or essential thrombocythemia, chronic granulocytic leukemia, and megakaryocytic leukemia.

a. Polycythemia Rubra Vera

Polycythemia rubra vera is characteristically a panmyelosis with an increase in the concentration of all of the circulating blood elements. Thrombocytosis is a regular feature of this disease and although the disease is believed to be of clonal stem cell origin[186] megakaryocytopoiesis is not totally autonomous.[187] The bone marrow biopsy of polycythemia vera shows a marked and striking increase in cellularity of all of the hemopoietic elements and almost complete disappearance of the marrow fat. The M/E ratio is decreased to between 2 to 1:1; red cell maturation is shifted toward the mature forms with an increase in the marrow reticulocyte number. Granulopoiesis is shifted toward the younger forms with an increase in the myelocyte compartment. The megakaryocytes are increased in number with particular increase of the mature, granular acidophilic cells. Especially impressive is the appearance of extraordinarily large megakaryocytes though they comprise but a small percentage of the total population of megakaryocytes.[188] There is considerable heterogeneity with respect to size among the megakaryocytes in polycythemia vera. Abnormal or asynchronous maturation in polycythemia vera is not discernible by light microscopy, though the increase in platelet size[189] and abnormalities of in vitro platelet function [190] suggest abnormality of cytoplasmic maturation. The described ultrastructural differences between the megakaryocytes from patients with polycythemia vera and megakaryocytes from normal individuals consisted essentially of an increase in nuclear and cytoplasmic size and in increase in ribosomal content. About 10% of the polycythemia vera megakaryocytes were decidedly abnormal in their total absence of differentiation despite an abundant cytoplasmic mass.[191] The distribution of megakaryocyte ploidy in polycythemia vera is similar to, and occasionally somewhat higher than normal.[47,192]

b. Myelofibrosis, Leukemia

Myelofibrosis with myeloid metaplasia presents classically with splenomegaly, fibrosis of the marrow, and a leukemoid blood picture. Thrombocytosis is often present. The bone marrow is slowly replaced by fibrous tissue leaving foci of hyperplastic marrow in which many megakaryocytes are found. Extramedullary hematopoiesis with active megakaryocytopoiesis is found in the liver and spleen.

Platelet production in myelofibrosis is increased and the platelets are macrocytic.[193] Maldonado et al.[194] call attention to the dual population of small and large platelets in a group of patients with variant forms of myelofibrosis and to two particular forms seen on the Romanowsky stained smears—the "blue platelet," a huge cell 3.0 to 13.0 μm in diameter, with a clear blue agranular aspect, and the giant granular forms. The blue platelets are spherical when viewed by phase or interference microscopy, and on electron microscopy the microtubules are disorganized and poorly developed; the granules are scarce or absent and the canalicular system is hypertrophied. The dysplastic platelets are thought to reflect a defect in the megakaryocyte maturation. These patients also have small lymphoblast-like cells in their peripheral blood. These cells are 8 to 25 μm in diameter; their cytoplasm is light blue and appears to release fragments with features of the so-called "blue" platelets. On electron microscopy the cells are readily identified as megakaryocytes by their "bull's-eye" granules, demarcation membrane system, and the open canalicular system.[194] It is of interest that Minot[195] called attention to the presence of small megakaryocytes in the circulating blood of patients with myeloproliferative disease. Such micromegaloblasts may be found in the marrow of myeloid metaplasia, preleukemia, and in large numbers in both marrow and blood in what has been ascribed to an accelerated phase of myelofibrosis and in megakaryocytic myelosis.[196–201] Acute micromegakaryoblastic leukemia has also been described as a terminal event in chronic granulocytic leukemia[202–206] and as a feature of acute myeloblastic leukemia.[207] Identification of the micromyeloblast may be difficult without the aid of electron microscopy and appropriate cytochemical techniques. The marrow fibrosis characteristic of the disease may be a secondary response to mediators released by megakaryocytes.

In essential thrombocythemia, the marrow is hypercellular with a marked increase in number, size, and lobulation of the megakaryocytes. The megakaryocytes often exist in groups or clusters. The granulocytic precursor compartment is enlarged with peaking of cells at promyelocyte and early myelocyte level. The spleen is enlarged and rich in megakaryocytes. The recognizable megakaryocytes are considerably expanded; their number per mm^2 exceed the normal by five-fold. The megakaryocyte area is 1.4 times normal and the megakaryocyte volume about seven times normal. Platelet production is six times normal and the megakaryocyte lobe count is increased.[208] In addition to their large size, the megakaryocytes of essential thrombocythemia have been shown to contain abnormal amounts of enzymes.[209]

c. *Essential Thrombocythemia*

The nature of essential thrombocythemia and its relationship to myeloid metaplasia on one hand and chronic myelocytic leukemia on the other are incompletely understood. For some the disorder is a distinct entity, proliferative in character,[210] for others,[211] a phase in the development of polycythemia vera, myeloid metaplasia, or chronic myelogeneous leukemia. Some have challenged the malignant nature of anogenic myeloid metaplasia and its variants[212] and others[214] have presented ultrastructural evidence of asynchronism of megakaryocyte maturation in support of its malignant character.

Thrombocytosis is a regularly observed finding in chronic myelocytic leukemia. The megakaryocytes in chronic myelogenous leukemia tend to be smaller than normal and shifted toward lower ploidy levels, but with an overall increase in numbers.[192,194,208] Cytoplasmic abnormalities of differentiation have been detected in small numbers of megakaryocytes by electron microscopy in chronic granulocytic leukemia.[192] The megakaryocytes on light microscopy are small, often no larger than myelocytes, but fully mature and granular.[215] An underlying stem cell disorder was considered to be responsible for the small cell size. The cells appear responsive to feedback regulation.[216] The presence of micromegakaryocytes in the peripheral blood of patients with chronic myelocytic leukemia may signal the onset of the blast transformation.[205,217] In some cases of preleukemia the megakaryocytes are small mono- and binucleated,[208,218,219] and are similar to the megakaryocytes seen in acute myeloblastic leukemia.[220]

B. Thrombocytopenia

Thrombocytopenia is the result of either inadequate platelet production or decreased platelet survival or sequestration. Marrow production of platelets may be compromised by a quantitatively deficient stem cell population or by qualitative abnormalities of megakaryocyte maturation and inefficient thrombopoiesis.

1. Congenital

Thrombocytopenia in the newborn due to congenital deficiency of megakaryocytes has been observed in association with a variety of skeletal, cardiac, or renal malformations. Bilateral aplasia of the radii is the most commonly associated skeletal abnormality. The marrow is almost completely devoid of megakaryocytes and the few remaining megakaryocytes are small and immature.[221,222] A leukemoid blood picture has been described in some patients with this disorder. The disturbance probably occurs at 6 to 8 weeks of intrauterine life when the megakaryocytes, the heart, and the radii are developing and has been linked to rubella infection in some reports. Qualitative abnormalities of the platelets have also been reported and suggest maturational adnormalities in addition to the quantitative deficiency of megakaryocytes. Thrombocytopenia and megakaryocytopenia may also occur in constitutional aplastic states, as in the Fanconi syndrome.[221–233]

Thrombocytopenia of the newborn may be seen in the newborn infected with rubella[234,235] and cytomegalovirus.[236] The megakaryocytes are often reduced in number and the pathogenesis of the thrombocytopenia associated with viral disease has been investigated in the experimental animal infected with the murine leukemia viruses. Thrombocytopenia was found to be a most sensitive index of early infection with both

Friend and Rauscher viruses,[237,238] and ultrastructural studies demonstrated the presence of the murine leukemia viruses in the cytoplasm of both megakaryocytes and platelets.[239,240] The marrow response to Rauscher virus infection is reported to be diphasic. In early infection the marrow is hypercellular with an increase in the number of megakaryocytes which appear morphologically normal. Late in the infection the marrow is normally cellular, but a sharp drop in the megakaryocyte count ensues.[241]

Thrombocytopenia is an infrequent complication of varicella and a fatal case of thrombocytopenic purpura during a course of viral illness believed to be malignant chicken pox has been reported. A high percent of the megakaryocytes were found to be infected with a virus whose ultrastructural features resembled the herpes group.[242]

Hereditary thrombocytopenias associated with functional or morphological platelet abnormalities are most commonly associated with other hereditary anomalies though rare isolated forms may exist.[243,244] Familial thrombocytopathic thrombocytopenia is a rare autosomal dominant hereditary disorder characterized by abnormal platelet morphology and a deficiency of platelet factor 3.[245–247] The number of megakaryocytes in the marrow is normal with an increase in the basophilic promegakaryocytes having apparently normal ploidy levels. The number and form of the dense granules are said to show striking differences from the normal. These findings, admittedly sketchy, have been interpreted to represent a disturbance in megakaryocyte maturation. In a study of a family afflicted with thrombocytopathic thrombocytopenia, the platelets were found to show an extremely low number of dense granules. The megakaryocyte development was asynchronous as manifested by a severe defect in the maturation of specific granules and by a retardation and abnormality of the demarcation membranes.[248]

The Wiskott-Aldrich syndrome is a sex-linked disorder characterized by eczema, thrombocytopenia, and susceptibility to infection related to an immunological abnormality. The platelets are smaller than normal, contain fewer granules, and have a shorter life span. The marrow megakaryocytes are normal or somewhat increased in number and show ultrastructural abnormalities.[249,250] Bone marrow transplantation corrects both the platelet and lymphocyte abnormalities suggesting a common genetic abnormality.[251] Lymphokines from mitogen-activated lymphocytes exert a stimulating effect on the growth of murine megakaryocytes colonies in vitro, suggesting a regulatory role for the lymphocyte in megakaryocytopoiesis.[252,253]

The May-Heggelin anomaly is transmitted as an autosomal dominant trait and is characterized by the presence of bizarre giant platelets and basophilic inclusions in the neutrophils. About one third of the patients are thrombocytopenic[254] but the total platelet mass is normal[255] and the hemorrhagic manifestations, if any, are generally mild. Platelet survival, function, and ultrastructure are reported to be normal.[256,257] Some observers have found small, scarce granules in the platelets of the May-Hegglin anomaly,[257] suggesting some variability in platelet morphology. The megakaryocytes and the circulating giant platelets were found to contain a giant membrane complex in a single patient with May-Hegglin anomaly.[258] However, similar structures have been found in normal subjects and in the megakaryocytes of hereditary giant platelet syndrome,[259] preleukemia,[260] and in the myeloproliferative disorders. The significance of the giant membrane complex in the mature megakaryocytes in normal and pathological states has not been determined but Breton-Gorius[258] suggested an association with ineffective thrombopoiesis. Polyploidization of the megakaryocytes in the May-Hegglin anomaly has been shown to be different from normal. There was considerable increase in 8N cells among the immature cells; a relative increase in the size of the promegakaryocyte compartment, and a corresponding decrease in the mature megakaryocyte compartment, with almost a complete reversal of the ratio between the two compartments. These findings suggested an increased influx of precursor cells into the recognizable population of megakaryocytes coupled with a decreased maturation capacity of the promegakaryocytes.[261] Cytochemical studies have revealed abnormalities which were presumed to reflect as well disturbances in the metabolism of the May-Hegglin megakaryocyte.[262]

A medley of disorders has been grouped into the so-called giant platelet syndrome, defined by the presence of thrombocytopenia, macrothrombocytes, and functional platelet defects.[263–266] The giant platelet syndrome has been observed in association with nephrosis and deafness and as a benign morphological variant, Mediterranean macrothrombocytopenia. A cytochemical and ultrastructural study of the megakaryocyte of a single patient with the giant platelet syndrome revealed changes indicative of disturbances in RNA and arginine-rich histone metabolism, and abnormalities in the glycolytic enzymes. On electron microscopy the megakaryocytes exhibited a decrease in glycogen and ribosomes.[266]

2. Acquired

Megakaryocytopenia and thrombocytopenia are seen in both the idiopathic and secondary aplastic anemias and in the myelopthisic states of marrow infiltration by tumor, storage disease cells, granuloma, etc. Ionizing radiation and the myelosuppressive agents commonly used in the treatment of malignant disease regularly induce thrombocytopenia by suppression probably of the committed stem cells. Thiazides,[267] estrogen,[268] and alcohol[269,270] are capable of inducing thrombocytopenia, presumably by direct action on the megakaryocyte by mechanisms as yet unknown. These agents produce a decrease in the number of megakaryocytes in the marrow, which however appear morphologically normal. The possibility of an immune mechanism in the thiazide-induced thrombocytopenia has been raised.[271]

The platelet count is often reduced in the megaloblastic anemia of folate and B_{12} deficiency. The pathogenetic mechanisms for the thrombocytopenia parallel the mechanisms involved in the production of the anemia, namely shortened survival of the platelet and ineffective thrombopoiesis.[147] The megakaryocytes are large and appear hyperlobulated, and DNA synthesis is abnormal.[46] In iron deficiency too, low platelet counts may be observed which return to normal after the administration of iron.[272,273] Iron may play a role as a regulator of thrombopoiesis.[274]

C. Qualitative Platelet Abnormalities

The term thrombocytopathy encompasses those bleeding disorders in which functionally abnormal platelets are present, but the platelet counts are normal. Glanzmann's thrombasthenia is a recessive autosomal disorder characterized by onset in early life of mucosal and cutaneous bleeding. The platelets do not aggregate spontaneously or on exposure to ADP. Two groups of patients are encountered: Group I exhibits low platelet fibrinogen, low surface contractile protein, and normal ADP content and represents about 80% of all cases. In Group II, platelet ADP is low. Platelet ultrastructure is generally normal but abnormal dense granules and a significant increase in "bull's-eye" granules, vesicles, and mitochondria have been described, particularly in Group II.[275] In an electron microscopic study of the megakaryocytes of Type I disease, the maturation sequence appeared normal and no dense bodies or vesicles, as seen in the platelets, were seen. However, morphological changes in the rough endocytoplasmic reticulum were observed and thought to be responsible for the abnormal platelet membrane.[276]

The storage pool deficiency syndromes are a heterogeneous group of disorders which may manifest mild to severe bleeding and deficient platelet bound ADP, with a greater than normal ATP/ADP ratio and deficiency of the platelet constituents.[78]

The human platelets contain two types of granules. The α granules, about 20 to 200 per platelet, are spherical with a diameter of 300 to 500 nm. The granules may show an eccentric zone of higher electron density, hence called "bull's-eye" granules. The dense bodies are very osmophilic, spherical, or elongated about 250 to 300 nm in diameter. They have the highest density of any of the platelet organelles. They are fewer in number and average about two to ten per platelet. In addition to the two granules, the platelet contains membrane-enclosed empty vesicles, about 175 to 200 μm in diameter, which store the acid hydrolases.[277] The main constituents of the α granules include the platelet-specific proteins, namely factor 4, β thromboglobulin and cationic proteins, growth factor (mitogenic factor), permeability factor, chemotactic factors, B lysin, glycoprotein, and the coagulation factors, fibrinogen, and factor V. The dense bodies store serotonin which they absorb from the plasma and additionally, calcium, ATP, and ADP in a ratio of 2:3 and pyrophosphate. The pool of granule-bound ATP and ADP does not exchange with the pool of cytoplasmic nucleotides. The lysosomal enzymes are stored in the membrane-bound vesicles.

There are several subgroups of the storage syndrome. One group, associated with oculocutaneous albinism, includes the Chediak-Higashi syndrome and the Hermansky-Pudlak syndrome in which there is a decrease both in number and contents of the dense bodies. In the Hermansky-Pudlak syndrome a ceroid-like substance is found in the bone marrow. The gray platelet syndrome is representative of a deficiency of α granules only; the dense bodies are normal in number and content. Other subgroups have been defined by their deficiency of the dense bodies with partial dimunition of the α granules and by their deficiency of both α granules and dense bodies.[278]

D. Idiopathic Thrombocytopenic Purpura

A decrease in platelet survival, whatever its mechanism, is responsible for the thrombocytopenia of a variety of clinical disorders such as immune neonatal thrombocytopenia, the Kasabach-Merritt syndrome, disseminated intravascular coagulation, renal transplant rejection, drug sensitivity, thrombotic thrombocytopenic purpura, acute idiopathic thrombocytopenia, and chronic idiopathic thrombocytopenic purpura.

Idiopathic thrombocytopenic purpura, an autoimmune disease in which the platelet[279] and possibly the megakaryocytes[280] are coated with antibody, serves as the prototype for the investigation of immune mechanisms in platelet destruction and the megakaryocytopoietic responses of the bone marrow to increased platelet demand.[281]

Chronic idiopathic thrombocytopenia purpura (ITP) has been described as an autoimmune disease characterized by a destructive thrombocytopenia caused by an antibody, produced by the patient, directed toward an antigen on the patients platelets.[281] Immune-mediated thrombocytopenia may be seen in association with other disorders, such as chronic lymphatic leukemia and lupus erythromatosis, and is separated from ITP etiologically, though the pathogeneic mechanisms are similar.

The peripheral blood smear of ITP shows diminution of the platelet number but an increase in platelet size. Of the platelets of patients with ITP, 38% were found to be greater than 2.5 μm in diameter compared to about 11% of control subjects.[282] Significant changes in platelet size are more likely to occur in severe thrombocytopenia and are uncommonly encountered in patients whose platelets counts exceed 50,000/ mm^2.[283] The bone marrow is normally cellular with a normal M/E ratio and normal maturation of the red cell and white cell precursors. The megakaryocytes are normal or increased in number with an increase in the promegakaryocyte compartment.

The platelet life span in ITP has been shown by most investigators to be shortened,[284–286] but the capacity of the normal bone marrow to respond to the increased requirement for platelets is in question. Evidence has been produced to indicate a reduction[149,287] in the marrow capacity to produce platelets presumed to be due to the inhibitory action on the marrow by the antiplatelet antibodies. Antigens common to both platelets and megakaryocytes have been demonstrated.[281,288,289] On the other hand, other measurements have shown that in ITP the marrow is capable of increasing platelet production some three- to five-fold[156,290,291] and that the production rate in ITP is similar to the increased platelet production found in man and laboratory animals made thrombocytopenic by nonimmunologic mechanisms.[148,291]

Megakaryocyte morphology in ITP was considered abnormal by the majority of earlier observers. Rohr,[292] in a review of his own experience and of the literature up to 1960, summarized the concensus as follows: ''The megakaryocytes are remarkably altered, often abnormally large and appear as giant forms. They contain a homogeneous blue, partially vacuolated plasma with well-defined markings, with or absent granulation and a young scarcely indented nucleus . . . normal platelet formation is absent; on the other hand pathological platelet formation . . . is seen. All the findings point to a profound disturbance in megakaryocyte maturation with inhibition of platelet formation.'' The maturation arrest was attributed to a splenic factor since megakaryocyte morphology returned to normal following splenectomy.

Bessis,[293] in a later review of the marrow findings in ITP, states that the megakaryocytes in ITP do not mature, are in a state of maturation arrest, and show signs of cytoplasmic degeneration (vacuolization) and the presence of large irregular clumps of glycogen.

A variety of changes in the ultrastructure of the megakaryocytes have been reported and considered to be morphologic evidence of a functional abnormality. In some studies vacuolization of the cytoplasm and deficient formation of the demarcation membranes were noted.[59,294] On the other hand, Paulus[295] found a shift in the megakaryocyte population toward the more immature cells with peak increase in the promegakaryocytes. They found no qualitative abnormalities of the organelles, except for the presence of large membrane complexes, and platelet production was evident. Ridell and Branehog,[296] in an ultrastructural and kinetic study of eight patients with ITP, found significantly increased platelet production which correlated with the increased number and volume of the megakaryocytes. They found no difference in the ultrastructural characteristics of ITP and normal megakaryocytes of similar levels of maturation. In a small percentage of megakaryocytes large membrane complexes were found. They concluded that the ultrastructure of the megakaryocytes in ITP is normal and that platelet production is increased.

The significance of the large membrane complexes is not clear. Breton-Gorius,[258] who described them in different pathological states and in young normal megakaryocytes, considered them to be the morphologic markers of a maturation arrest. In experimental thrombocytopenia induced by X-ray, MacPherson[297] found an increase in the demarcation system membranes during the recovery phase. Bentfield, Barker, and Bainton[298] studied the changes in ultrastructure of rat megakaryocytes after prolonged thrombocytopenia induced by plateletpheresis or multiple injections of antiplatelet serum. The number of megakaryocytes in the stimulated animals increased, as did the diameter of the mature megakaryocytes, by about one third. The proportion of immature megakaryocytes increased but the cells were only slightly larger than comparable cells of the controls. The fine structural changes were confined to a greater development of the rough endocytoplasmic reticulum in the maturing cells, large areas of hypertrophied membranes of the demarcation system, less nucleus chromatin condensation, and an increase in the number, size, and persistance of nucleoli. The most striking change, the hypertrophy of the demarcation membrane system with formation of dense compartments was thought possibly to reflect the expanded cell size and the accelerated maturation—changes presumably mediated by thrombopoietin.

Thus, whether the morphological changes observed in the megakaryocytes in ITP reflect pathological alterations in maturation or represent the normal structural responses to accelerated maturation cannot be resolved at present, but the available evidence would favor the latter.

REFERENCES

1. **Bizzozero, G.,** Sul midollo delle ossa, Morgagni, Naples, 1869.
2. **Neumann, E.,** Ueber die Bedeutung des Knonchenmarkes fur die Blutbildung, Centralbl. Med. Wissensch., 689, 1868.
3. **Bizzozero, G.,** Ueber einen neuen Formbestandteil des Saugetierblutes und die Bedeutung desselben für die Thrombosis und die Blutgerinnung ueberhaupt, Centralbl. Med. Wissensch., 17, 1882.
4. **Bizzozero, G.,** Ueber einen neuen Formbestandteil des blutes und desser Rolle bei der Thrombose und die Blutgerinnung, *Arch. Pathol. Anat. Physiol.*, 90, 261, 1882.
5. **Wright, J. H.,** The origin and nature of the blood platelet, *Boston Med. Surg. J.*, 154, 643, 1906.
6. **Ogata, S.,** Megakaryozyten-embolie und Knochenmarkembolie, *Beitr. Pathol. Anat.*, 53, 120, 1912.
7. **Seeliger, S.,** Ueber Plättchenerzeugung und Phagozytose als Funkton der Knochenmarksriesenzellen, *Folia Haematol.*, 29, 23, 1923.
8. **Seeliger, S.,** Ueber Organ Befunde und ihre Bedeutung für die Pathogenese bei essentieller Thrombopoenia und Aleukie, *Klin. Wochenschr.*, 3, 731, 1924.
9. **Frank, E.,** Die haemorrhagischen diathesen, in *Handbuch der Krankheiten des Blutes und der blutbildenden Organe,* Vol. 2, Schittenhelm, A., Ed., Julius Springer, Berlin, 1925, 289.
10. **Willi, H.,** Ueber den Bau und die Funktion der Megakaryozyten und ihre Beziehungen zu thrombopenischen Purpura, *Folia Haematol.*, 53, 426, 1935.
11. **Rohr, K. and Koller, F.,** Ueber die Abstammung der Thrombozyten, *Klin. Wochenschr.*, 15, 1549, 1936.
12. **Downey, H.,** The origin of the blood platelets, *Folia Haematol.*, 15, 25, 1913.
13. **Pisciotta, A. V., Stefanini, M., and Damashek, W.,** Studies of platelets, X. Morphologic characteristics of megakaryocytes by phase contrast microscopy in normals and in patients with idiopathic thrombocytopenic purpura, *Blood,* 8, 703, 1953.
14. **Thiery, J. B. and Bessis, M.,** La genese des plaquettes a partir des megacaryocytes observes sur la cellule vivante, *C. R. Acad. Sci.*, 242, 290, 1956.
15. **Howell, W. H.,** Observations upon the occurrence, structure and function of the giant cells of the marrow, *J. Morph.*, 4, 117, 1894.
16. **Jordan, H. E.,** A contribution to the problems concerning the origin, structure, genetic relationship and function of the giant-cells of hemopoietic and osteolytic foci, *Am. J. Anat.*, 24, 225, 1918.
17. **Maximow, A.,** In *Handbuch der mikroskopischen Anatomie des Menschen,* Vol. 2, part 1, Mollendorf, W., Ed., Springer, Berlin, 1927.
18. **Downey, H., Palmer, M., and Powell, L.,** Origin of megakaryocytes in spleen and liver in case of atypical myelosis, *Folia Haematol.*, 41, 55, 1930.
19. **Potter, J. S. and Ward, E. N.,** Development of megakaryocyte in adult mice, *Anat. Rec.*, 77, 77, 1940.
20. **Rothermel, J.,** A note on the megakaryocyte of the normal cat's spleen, *Anat. Rec.*, 47, 251, 1930.
21. **DiGuglielmo, G.,** Sul sistema delle cellule giganti midollari, *Haematologica,* 6, 156, 1925.
22. **Baserga, A.,** Osservazione sulla genesi idelle cellule giganti midollari, *Arch. Ital. Anat. Embryol.*, 30, 215, 1932.
23. **Japa, J.,** A study of the morphology and development of the megakaryocytes, *Br. J. Exp. Pathol.*, 4, 73, 1943.
24. **Schwartz, E.,** Studies on the megakaryocyte. I. The normal granulopoiesis of the megakaryocyte, *Arch. Pathol.*, 45, 333, 1948.
25. **Gilmour, J. R.,** Normal haematopoiesis in intrauterine and neonatal life, *J. Pathol. Bact.*, 52, 25, 1941.
26. **Hoyes, A. D., Riches, D. J., and Martin, B. G. H.,** The fine structure of haemopoiesis in the human fetal liver. I. The haemopoietic precursor cells, *J. Anat.*, 115, 99, 1973.
27. **Hoyes, A. D., Riches, D. J., and Martin, B. G. H.,** The fine structure of haemopoiesis in the human fetal liver, II. Origin and differentiation of the megakaryocytes, *Haematologia,* 9, 179, 1975.

28. **Kaufman, R. M., Airo, R., Pollock, S., et al.,** Origin of pulmonary megakaryocytes, *Blood,* 25, 767, 1965.
29. **Kaufman, R. M., Airo, R., Pollock, S., et al.,** Circulating megakaryocytes and platelet release in the lung, *Blood,* 26, 720, 1965.
30. **Metcalf, D., MacDonald, H. R., Odartchenko, N., and Sordat, B.,** Growth of mouse megakaryocytes *in vitro, Proc. Natl. Acad. Sci., U.S.A.,* 72, 1744, 1975.
31. **McLeod, D. L., Shreue, M. M., and Axelrod, A. A.,** Induction of megakaryocyte colonies with platelet formation *in vitro, Nature,* 261, 492, 1976.
32. **Nakeff, A., Dicke, K. A., and Van Noord, M. J.,** Megakaryocytes in agar cultures of mouse bone marrow, *Ser. Haematol.,* 8, 4, 1975.
33. **Nakeff, A.,** Colony forming unit, megakaryocyte(CFU-m): its use in elucidating the kinetics and humoral control of the megakaryocytic committed progenitor cell compartment. In *Experimental Hematology Today.* Baum, S. J. and Ledney, M., Ed., Springer-Verlag, New York, 1977, 111.
34. **Williams, N., Jackson, H., Sheridan, A. P. C., et al.,** Regulation of megakaryopoiesis in long term murine bone marrow cultures, *Blood,* 51, 245, 1978.
35. **Garcia, A. M.,** Feulgen-DNA values in megakaryocytes, *J. Cell. Biol.,* 20, 342, 1964.
36. **Odell, T. T., Fr., Jackson, C. W., and Gossler, D. G.,** Maturation of rat megakaryocytes by microspectrophotometric measurements of DNA, *Proc. Soc. Exp. Biol. Med.,* 119, 1194, 1965.
37. **De Leval, M.,** Etude cytochimique quantitative des acides desoxyribonucleiques au cours de la maturation megakaryocytaire, *Nouv. Rev. Fr. Hematol.,* 8, 392, 1968.
38. **De Leval, M. and Paulus, J. M.,** Megakaryocytes, uninucleate, polyploid or plurinucleate cells? In *Platelet Kinetics,* Paulus, J. M., Ed., North-Holland, Amsterdam, 1971, 190.
39. **Odell, T. T., Jr.,** Megakaryocytopoiesis and its response to stimulation and suppression in *Platelets: Production, Function, Transfusion and Storage,* Baldini, M. G. and Ebbe, S., Eds., Grune and Stratton, New York, 1974, 11.
40. **Levine, R. F., Bunn, P. A., Jr., Hazzard, K. C., and Schlam, M. L.,** Flow cytometric analysis of megakaryocyte ploidy. Comparison with Feulgen microdensitometry and discovery that 8N is the predominant ploidy class in guinea pig and monkey marrow, *Blood,* 56, 210, 1980.
41. **Pennington, D. G., Stretfield, K., and Weste, S.,** Megakaryocyte ploidy and ultrastructure in stimulated thrombopoiesis in *Platelets: Production, Function, Transfusion and Storage,* Baldini, M. and Ebbe, S., Eds., Grune and Stratton, New York, 1974, 115.
42. **Harker, L. A.,** Kinetics of thrombopoiesis, *J. Clin. Invest.,* 47, 458, 1968.
43. **Harker, L. A. and Finch, S. A.,** Thrombokinetics in man, *J. Clin. Invest.,* 48, 963, 1969.
44. **Harker, L. A.,** Megakaryocyte quantitation, *J. Clin. Invest.,* 47, 452, 1968.
45. **Levine, R. F.,** Isolation and characterization of normal human megakaryocytes, *Br. J. Haematol.,* 45, 457, 1980.
46. **Queisser, U., Queisser, W., and Spiertz, B.,** Polyploidization of megakaryocytes in normal humans, in patients with idiopathic thrombocytopenia and with pernicious anemia, *Br. J. Haematol.,* 20, 489, 1951.
47. **Lagerlof, B.,** Cytophotometric study of megakaryocyte ploidy in polycythemia vera and chronic granulocytic leukemia, *Acta Cytol.,* 16, 240, 1972.
48. **Kinosita, R., Ohno, C., and Nakazawa, M.,** On the differentiation of the thrombocytic series of cells, *Proc. Am. Assoc. Cancer Res.,* 3, 33, 1959.
49. **Odell, T. T., Jr., Jackson, C. W., and Friday, T. J.,** Megakaryocytopoiesis in rats with special reference to ployploidy, *Blood,* 35, 775, 1970.
50. **Paulus, J. M.,** DNA metabolism and development of organelles in guinea pig megakaryocytes: a combined ultrastructural, autoradiographic and cytophotometric study, *Blood,* 35, 298, 1971.
51. **MacPherson, G. G.,** Development of megakaryocytes in bone marrow of the rat: an analysis by electron microscopy and high resolution autoradiography, *Proc. Royal Soc. London B,* 177, 265, 1971.
52. **Paulus, J. M.,** Multiple differentiation in megakaryocytes and platelets, *Blood,* 29, 407, 1967.
53. *Atlas of Haematology,* 2nd ed., rev., Sandoz LTD, Basel, Switzerland, 1973, 20.
54. **Bessis, M.,** *Living Blood Cells and their Ultrastructure,* Springer-Verlag, New York, 1973, 370.
55. **Spanos, G., Kaira, J., and Rosner, F.,** Naked megakaryocyte nuclei revisited, *Med. Pediatr., Oncol.,* 6, 215, 1979.
56. **Jean, G., Lambertenghi-Delilier, G., Ranzi, T., and Poitrier-Basetti, M.,** The human bone marrow megakaryocytes. An ultrastructural study, *Haematology,* 5, 253, 1971.
57. **Bussi, L., Jean, G., and Le Coultre, L.,** Ultrastructural aspects of platelets and megakaryocytes in a case of "primary" thrombocythaemia, *Acta Haematol.* (Basel), 35, 113, 1966.
58. **Falcao, L.,** La demarcation des plaquettes sanguines dans les megakaryocytes de la moelle osseuse humaine, *Coagulation,* 1, 229, 1968.

59. **Schulz, H.,** *Thrombozyten und Thrombose im elektronenmikroskopischen Bild,* Springer-Verlag, Berlin, 1968.
60. **Spicer, S. S., Green, W. B., and Hardin, J. H.,** Ultrastructural localization of acid muco-substances and antimonate precipitable cation in human and rabbit platelets and megakaryocytes, *J. Histochem. Cytochem.,* 17, 781, 1969.
61. **Zucker-Franklin, D.,** The ultrastructure of megakaryocytes and platelets. IIV. *Regulation of Hematopoiesis,* Vol. 2, Gordon, A. S., Ed., Appleton-Century, Crofts, New York, 1970, 1553.
62. **Breton-Gorius, J.,** Aspects ultrastructurals de la maturation des mégakaryocytes humains normaux, *Nouv. Rev. Fr. Hematol.,* 13, 504, 1975.
63. **Behnke, O.,** An electron microscope study of the megakaryocyte of the rat bone marrow. I. The development of the demarcation membrane system and the platelet surface coat, *J. Ultrastruct. Res.,* 24, 412, 1968.
64. **Behnke, O.,** An electron microscope study of the rat megakaryocyte. II. Some aspects of platelet release and microtubules, *J. Ultrastruct. Res.,* 26, 111, 1969.
65. **de Bruyn, P. P.,** The fine structure of the megakaryocytes of the bone marrow of the guinea pig, *Z. Zellforsch.,* 64, 111, 1964.
66. **Farago, S. and Olah, I.,** Electron microscopic investigation of the developing forms of megakaryocytes, *Haematology,* 4, 103, 1970.
67. **Han, S. S. and Baker, B. L.,** The ultrastructure of megakaryocytes and blood platelets in the rat spleen, *Anat. Rec.,* 149, 251, 1964.
68. **Yamada, E.,** The fine structure of the megakaryocyte of the mouse spleen, *Acta Anat.* (Basel), 29, 267, 1957.
69. **Deckhuyzen, M. C.,** Ueber die Thrombocyten (Blutplattchen), *Anat. Anz.,* 19, 529, 1901.
70. **Jordan, H. E. and Beans, H. W.,** Origin and proliferation of thrombocytes in splenectomized salamanders, *Proc. Soc. Exp. Biol. Med.,* 27, 67, 1929.
71. **Andrew, W.,** *Comparative Hematology,* Grune and Stratton, New York, 1965.
72. **Keyhani, E.,** Étude au microscope électronique de la structure des mégakaryocytes de cobaye par la technique de cryodécapage, Comparison avec la technique des coupes, *J. Microsc.,* 9, 63, 1970.
73. **Pennington, D. G. and Stretfield, K.,** Heterogeneity of megakaryocytes and platelets, *Sem. Haematol.,* 8, 1, 1975.
74. **Behnke, O., Tingaard, A., and Pedersen, W.,** Ultrastructural aspects of megakaryocyte maturation and platelet release, in *Platelets: Production, Function, Transfusion and Storage,* Baldini, M. G. and Ebbe, S., Eds., Grune and Stratton, New York, 1974, 21.
75. **Tranum-Jensen, J. and Behnke, O.,** Electron microscopic identification of the committed precursor cell of the megakaryocyte compartment, *Cell. Biol. Int. Rep.,* 1, 445, 1977.
76. **Jones, O. P.,** Origin of the megakaryocyte granules from Golgi vesicles, *Anat. Res.,* 138, 105, 1960.
77. **MacPherson, G. G.,** Synthesis and localization of sulphated mucopolysaccharide in megkaryocytes and platelets of rats. An analysis by electron microscope autoradiography, *J. Cell. Sci.,* 10, 705, 1972.
78. **Holmsen, H. and Weiss, H. J.,** Secretable storage pools in platelets, *Annu. Rev. Med.,* 30, 119, 1979.
79. **Tranzer, J. P., Da Prada, M., and Pletscher, A.,** Storage of 5-Hydroxytryptamine in megakaryocytes, *J. Cell. Biol.,* 52, 191, 1972.
80. **White, J. G.,** Origin and function of platelet dense bodies, *Semin. Hematol.,* 3, 4, 1970.
81. **Bentfield, M. E. and Bainton, D. F.,** Cytochemical localization of lysosomal enzymes in rat megakaryocytes and platelets, *J. Clin. Invest.,* 56, 1635, 1975.
82. **Geyer, G. and Schaaf, P.,** The megakaryocyte demarcation membrane (DM)—endo plasmic or superficial origin? *Acta. Histochem.,* 44, 137, 1972.
83. **French, J. E.,** Blood platelets, morphological studies on their properties and life cycle, *Br. J. Haematol.,* 13, 595, 1967.
84. **Shaklai, M. and Tavassoli, M.,** Demarcation system in rat megakaryocyte and mechanism of platelet formation, J. Ultrastruct. Res., 62, 270, 1978.
85. **Jackson, C. W.,** Some characteristics of rat megakaryocytes precursors identified by using cholinesterase as a marker, in *Platelet: Production, Function, Transfusion, and Storage,* Baldini, M. G. and Ebbe, S., Eds., Grune and Stratton, New York, 1974, 33.
86. **Lautenshclager, J., Borst, R. H., and Meusers, P. J.,** Elektronenemikroskopisc Untersuchungen zur Verteilung der Cholinesterasen in Megakaryocyten der Ratte, *Histochemie,* 26, 348, 1971.
87. **Nakao, K. and Angrist, A. A.,** Membrane surface specialization of blood platelets and megakaryocytes, *Nature,* 217, 960, 1968.
88. **Fedorko, M. E. and Levine, R. E.,** Tannic acid effect on membrane of cell surface origin in guinea pig megakaryocytes and platelets, *J. Histochem. Cytochem.,* 24, 601, 1976.

89. **Behnke, O. and Emmersen, J.**, Structural identification of thrombosthenin in rat megakaryocytes, *Scand. J. Haematol.*, 9, 130, 1972.
90. **Behnke, O., Kristensen, B. I., and Nielsen, L. E.**, Electron microscopical observations on actinoid and myosinoid filaments in blood platelets, *J. Ultrastruct. Res.*, 37, 351, 1971.
91. **Bettez-Galland, M., Luscher, E. F., and Weibel, E. R.**, Thrombosthenin-Electron microscopical studies on its localization in human blood platelets and some properties of its subunits, *Thromb. Diath. Hemmorh.*, 22, 431, 1969.
92. **Nachman, R., Levine, R., and Jaffe, E.**, Synthesis of actin by cultured guinea pig megakaryocytes, *Biochim, Biophys, Acta.*, 543, 91, 1978.
93. **Luscher, E. F. and Bettex-Galland, M.**, Thrombosthenin, the contractile protein of blood platelets. New facts and problems, *Pathol. Biol.*, *(Paris)*, 20, 89, 1972.
94. **Nachman, R., Levine, R., and Jaffe, E.**, Synthesis of factor VIII antigen by cultured guinea pig megakaryocyte, *J. Clin. Invest.*, 60, 914, 1977.
95. **Chernoff, A., Levine, A. F., and Goodwin, D. S.**, Origin of platelet derived growth factor in megakaryocytes of guinea pigs, *J. Clin. Invest.*, 65, 926, 1980.
96. **Ross, R. and Vogel, A.**, The platelet derived growth factor, *Cell*, 14, 203, 1978.
97. **Piovella, F., Nalli, G. D., Malamani, I., et al.**, The ultrastructural localization of factor VIII antigen in human platelets, megakaryocytes and endothelial cells utilizing a ferritin labeled antibody, *Br. J. Haematol.*, 32, 209, 1978.
98. **Castaldi, P. A. and Caen, J.**, Platelet fibrinogen, *J. Clin. Pathol.*, 18, 579, 1965.
99. **McDonagh, J., Kiesselbach, T. H., and Wagner, R. H.**, Origin of platelet factor XIII (fibrin stabilizing factor), *Fed. Proc.*, 28, 745, 1969.
100. **Thiery, J. P.**, Mise en evidence des polysaccharides sur coupes fines au microscope electronique, *J. Microsc.*, 6, 987, 1967.
101. **Cawley, J. C. and Hayhoe, F. G. J.**, The megakaryocyte series, in *Ultrastructure of Haemic Cells*, a cytological atlas of normal and leukemic blood and bone marrow, W. B. Saunders, Philadelphia, 1973, 122.
102. **Murata, F., Momose, Y., and Nagata, T.**, Demonstration of intracytoplasmic glycogen of megakaryocytes and blood platelets by means of periodic acid-thiocarbo-hydrazide-silver proteinate method, *Histochemistry*, 52, 307, 1977.
103. **Behnek, O.**, Electron microscopic observations on the membrane systems of the rat blood platelet, *Anat. Rec.*, 158, 121, 1967.
104. **Breton-Gorius, J. and Guichard, J.**, Ultrastructural localization of peroxidase activity in human platelets and megakaryocytes, *Am. J. Pathol.*, 68, 277, 1972.
105. **Vaquez, J. J. and Lewis, J. H.**, Immunocytochemical studies in platelets, the demonstration of a common antigen in human platelets and megakaryocytes, *Blood*, 16, 968, 1960.
106. **de Leval, M.**, Mise en evidence d' antigenes plaquetaires des anticorps fluorescents. Application a l etude de la maturation des megakaryocytes dans la moelle osseuse de cobaye, *C.R. Soc. Biol.*, *(Paris)*, 161, 978, 1967.
107. **Tanaka, Y. and Goodman, J. B.**, *Electron Microscopy of Human Blood Cells*, Harper and Row, New York, 1972.
108. **Humble, J. G., Jayne, W. H. W., and Pulvertaft, R. J. V.**, Biological interaction between lymphocytes and other cells, *Br. J. Haematol.*, 2, 283, 1956.
109. **Larsen, T. E.**, Emperipolesis of granular leukocytes within megakaryocytes in human hemopoietic bone marrow, *Am. J. Clin. Pathol.*, 53, 185, 1970.
110. **Sahebekhtiari, H. A. and Tavassoli, M.**, Marrow cell uptake by megakaryocytes in routine bone marrow smears during blood loss, *Scand. J. Haematol.*, 16, 13, 1976.
111. **Chenitz, J. and Bichel, P.**, Tumor cell emperipolesis, studies by transmission electron microscopy, *Exp. Cell. Res.*, 82, 319, 1973.
112. **Tavassoli, M.**, Megakaryocyte-platelet axis and the process of platelet formation and release, *Blood*, 55, 537, 1980.
113. **Lichtman, M. A., Chamberlain, J. K., Simon, W., and Santillo, P. A.**, Para sinusoidal location of megakaryocytes in the marrow, a determinant of platelet release, *Am. J. Hematol.*, 4, 303, 1978.
114. **Becker, R. P. and De Bruyn, P. P. H.**, The transmural passage of blood cells into myeloid sinusoids and the entry of platelets into sinusoids circulation. A scanning electron microscopic investigation, *Am. J. Anat.*, 145, 183, 1976.
115. **Crosby, W. H.**, Delivery of megakaryocytes by the marrow. The derivation of platelets in *Topics in Hematology*, Senos, D., Takako, F., and Irino, S., Eds., Excerpta Medica, Amsterdam, 1976, 416.
116. **Thiery, J. P. and Bessis, M.**, Mechanisms de la plaquettogenèse, étude *in vitro* par la microcinematographie, *Rev. Hematol.*, 2, 162, 1956.

117. **Albrecht, M.,** Studien zur Thrombocytenbildung an Megakaryocyten in menschlichen Knochenmarkskulturen, *Acta Haematol.*, 17, 160, 1957.
118. **Hiraki, K., Sunami, H., and Ogawara, K.,** Studies on the megakaryocytes. Platelet separation and degeneration, *Acta Med. Okayama,* 12, 187, 1958.
119. **Izak, G., Nelson, D., and Gurevitch, J.,** Studies on thrombopoiesis. I. Thrombopoiesis *in vitro:* experiments with animals and normal human materials, *Blood,* 12, 507, 1957.
120. **Kinosita, R. and Ohno, S.,** Biodynamics of thrombopoiesis, in *Blood Platelets,* Johnson, S. A., Monto, R. W., Rebuck, J. W., et al., Eds., Little, Brown, Boston, 1958.
121. **Murata, T.,** Mechanism of platelet liberation, Tohoku, *J. Exp. Med.,* 116, 67, 1975.
122. **Ihzumi, T., Hattori, A., and Sanada, M.,** Megakaryocyte and platelet formation. A scanning electron microscope study in mouse spleen, *Arch. Histol. Jpn.,* 40, 305, 1977.
123. **Djaldetti, M., Fishman, P., Bessler, H., and Notti, I.,** SEM observations on the mechanisms of platelet release from megakaryocytes, *Thrombos. Haemostas.,* (*Stuttgart*), 42, 611, 1979.
124. **Aschoff, L.,** Uber capillare Embolie von riesenhaltigen Zellen, *Arch. Pathol. Anat. Physiol.,* 134, 11, 1893.
125. **Foa, P.,** Beitrag zum Studium des Knochenmarks, *Ziegel. Beitrag,* 25, 376, 1899.
126. **Minot, G. R.,** Megakaryocytes in the peripheral circulation, *J. Exp. Med.,* 16, 1, 1922.
127. **Whitby, L.,** The significance of megakaryocytes in the peripheral circulation, *Blood,* 3, 934, 1948.
128. **Efrati, P. and Rozenszain, L.,** The morphology of buffy coat in normal human adults, *Blood,* 32, 393, 1960.
129. **Herbeuval, R., Herbeuval, H., and Duheille, J.,** Particularites cytolgiques des megakaryocytes observes dans le sang peripherique, *C.R. Soc. Biol.,* 155, 370, 1961.
130. **Scheinin, T. M. and Korvuniemi, A. P.,** Large benign cells in circulation and their significance in the identification of cancer cells, *Cancer,* 15, 972, 1962.
131. **Melamed, M. R., Clifton, E. E., Merler, C., and Koss, L. G.,** The megakaryocyte blood count, *Am. J. Med. Sci.,* 252, 301, 1966.
132. **Kaufman, R. M., Airo, R., Pollock, S., et al.,** Origin of Pulmonary megakaryocytes, *Blood,* 25, 767, 1967.
133. **Pedersen, N. T.,** The pulmonary vessels as a filter for circulating megakaryocytes in rats, *Scand, J. Haematol.,* 13, 225, 1974.
134. **Maniatis, A. K.,** Megakaryocytes and platelets in central venous and arterial blood, *Acta Haematol.,* 42, 330, 1969.
135. **Kaufman, R. M., Airo, R., Pollack, S., and Crosby, W. A.,** Circulating megakaryocytes and platelet release in the lung, *Blood,* 26, 720, 1965.
136. **Hansen, M. and Pedersen, N. T.,** Circulating megakaryocytes in blood from the antecubital vein in healthy adult humans, *Scand. J. Haematol.,* 20, 371, 1978.
137. **Aabo, K. and Hansen, K. B.,** Megakaryocytes in pulmonary blood vessels. I. Incidence at autopsy, clinico-pathological relations especially to disseminated intravascular coagulation, *Acta Pathol. Microbiol. Scand.,* 86, 285, 1978.
138. **Pedersen, N. T.,** Occurrence of megakaryocytes in various vessels and their retention in the pulmonary capillaries in man, *Scand. J. Haematol.,* 21, 369, 1978.
139. **Herbeuval, H., Dubeille, J., Cuny, G., and Guerci, O.,** La megacaryocytemie physiologique, *C.R. Soc. Biol.,* 156, 172, 1962.
140. **Kallinokos-Maniatis, A.,** Megakaryocytes and platelets in central venous and arterial blood, *Acta Haematol.,* 42, 330, 1969.
141. **Airo, R.,** Pulmonary megakaryocyte increase after phlebotomy in rabbits, *Haematologica,* 63, 548, 1978.
142. **Hansen, M. S. and Pedersen, N. T.,** Circulating megakaryocytes in patients with pulmonary inflammation and patients subjected to cholecystectomy, *Scand. J. Haematol.,* 23, 211, 1979.
143. **Breslow, A., Kaufman, R. M., and Lawsky, A. R.,** The effect of surgery on the concentration of circulating megakaryocytes and platelets, *Blood,* 32, 393, 1968.
144. **Smith, E. B. and Butcher, J.,** The incidence distribution and significance of megakaryocytes in normal and disease human tissue, *Blood,* 7, 214, 1952.
145. **Ebbe, S., Stohlman, F., Jr., Overcash, J., et al.,** Megakaryocyte size in thrombocytopenic and normal rats, *Blood,* 12, 383, 1968.
146. **Odell, T. T., Jr., Jackson, C. W., Friday, T. J., and Du, K. Y.,** Assay of megakaryocytopoiesis in thrombocytopenic rats, *Br. J. Haematol.,* 21, 233, 1971.
147. **Odell, T. T., Jr., Jackson, C. W., Friday, T. J., and Charsha, D. E.,** Effect of thrombocytopenia in megakaryocytopenic rats, *Br. J. Haematol.,* 21, 233, 1971.
148. **Rolovic, Z., Baldini, M., and Damashek, W.,** Megakaryocytopoiesis in experimentally induced immune thrombocytopenia, *Blood,* 35, 173, 1970.

149. **Harker, L. A. and Finch, S. A.,** Thrombokinetics in man, *J. Clin. Invest.*, 48, 963, 1969.
150. **Odell, T. T., Murphy, J. R., and Jackson, C. W.,** Stimulation of megakaryocytopoiesis by acute thrombocytopenia in rats, *Blood,* 48, 765, 1976.
151. **Ebbe, S. and Stohlman, F., Jr.,** Stimulation of thrombocytopenia in irradiated mice, *Blood,* 35, 783, 1970.
152. **Odell, T. T., Jr., Jackson, C. W., and Friday, T. J.,** Effects of radiation on the thrombocytopoietic system of mice, *Radiat. Res.*, 48, 107, 1971.
153. **Pennington, D. G. and Olsen, T. E.,** Megakaryocytes in states of altered platelet production, cell numbers, size and DNA content, *Br. J. Haematol.*, 18, 447, 1970.
154. **Sullivan, L. W., Adams, W. H., and Liv, Y. K.,** Induction of thrombocytopenia by thrombopheresis in man, patterns of recovery in normal subjects during ethanol ingestion and abstinence, *Blood,* 49, 197, 1977.
155. **Harker, L. A.,** Thrombokinetics in idiopathic thrombocytopenic purpura, *Br. J. Haematol.*, 19, 95, 1970.
156. **Branehog, I., Kutti, J., and Weinfeld, A.,** Platelet survival and platelet production in idiopathic thrombocytopenia purpura (ITP), *Br. J. Haematol.*, 27, 127, 1974.
157. **Branhog, I., Kutti, J., Ridell, B., et al.,** The relation of thrombokinetics to bone marrow megakaryocytes in idiopathic thrombocytopenic purpura (ITP), *Blood,* 45, 551, 1975.
158. **Abildgaard, C. F. and Simone, J. B.,** Thrombopoiesis, *Am. J. Physiol.*, 218, 1376, 1970.
159. **Ebbe, S.,** Megakaryocytopoiesis in *Regulation of Hematopoiesis,* Vol. 2, Gordon, A. S., Ed., Appleton-Century-Crofts, New York, 1970, 1587.
160. **Levin, J.,** Humoral control of thrombopoiesis, in *Formation and Destruction of Blood Cells,* Greenwalt, T. J. and Jamieson, G. A., Eds., Lippincott, Philadelphia, 1970, 141.
161. **Harker, L. A.,** Regulation of thrombopoiesis, *Am. J. Physiol.*, 218, 1376, 1970.
162. **Evatt, B. I., Levin, J., and Alagazy, K. M.,** Partial purification of thrombopoietin from the plasma of thrombocytopenic rabbits, *Blood,* 54, 377, 1979.
163. **MacDonald, R. P.,** Assays for thrombopoietin, *Scand. J. Hematol.*, 18, 5, 1977.
164. **Adams, W. H., Liu, Y. K., and Sullivan, L. N.,** Humoral regulation of thrombopoiesis in man, *J. Lab. Clin. Med.*, 91, 141, 1978.
165. **Odell, T. T. and Boran, D. A.,** The mitotic index of megakaryocytes after acute thrombocytopenia, *Proc. Soc. Exp. Biol. Med.*, 155, 149, 1977.
166. **Odell, T. T., McDonald, T. P., Shelton, C., and Clifton, R.,** Stimulation of mouse megakaryocyte endomitosis by plasma from thrombocytopenia rats, *Proc. Soc. Exp. Biol. Med.*, 160, 263, 1979.
167. **Smith, P. J., Jackson, C. W., Whidden, M. A., and Edwards, C. C.,** Effect of hypertransfusion on bone marrow regeneration sublethally irradiated mice, enhanced recovery, *Blood,* 56, 58, 1980.
168. **Tranum, B. L. and Haut, A.,** Thrombocytosis: platelet kinetics in neoplasia, *J. Lab. Clin. Med.*, 84, 615, 1974.
169. **Ebbe, S. and Phalen, E.,** Does autoregulation of megakaryocytopoiesis occur? *Blood Cells,* 5, 123, 1979.
170. **McDonald, T. P., Odell, T. T., Jr., and Gosslee, P. G.,** Platelet size in relation to platelet age, *Proc. Soc. Exp. Biol. Med.*, 115, 684, 1964.
171. **Karpatkin, S.,** Heterogeneity of human platelets. I. Metabolic evidence suggestive of young and old platelets, *J. Clin. Invest.*, 48, 1073, 1969.
172. **Karpatkin, S.,** Heterogeneity of human platelets. II. Functional evidence suggestive of young and old platelets, *J. Clin. Invest.*, 48, 1083, 1969.
173. **Mannucci, P. M. and Sharp, A. A.,** Platelet volume and shape in relation to aggregation and adhesion, *Br. J. Haematol.*, 26, 105, 1967.
174. **Hirsh, J., Glynn, M. F., and Mustard, J. F.,** The effect of platelet age on platelet adherence to collagens, *J. Clin. Invest.*, 47, 466, 1968.
175. **Karpatkin, S.,** Human platelet senescence, *Annu. Rev. Med.*, 23, 101, 1972.
176. **Ginsberg, A. D. and Aster, R. H.,** Changes, associated with platelet aging, *Thromb. Diath. Hemmorrh.*, 27, 407, 1972.
177. **Paulus, J. M.,** Platelet size in man, *Blood,* 46, 321, 1975.
178. **Boneu, B., Boneu, A., Raisson, C. L., et al.,** Kinetics of platelet populations in the stationary state, *Thromb. Res.*, 3, 605, 1973.
179. **Boneu, B., Pris, J., Raisson, C. L., et al.,** Kinetics of platelets of various densities in five thrombocytopenic patients, *Pathologie-Biologie,* 22(Suppl.), 22, 1974.
180. **Busch, C. and Olsen, P. S.,** Density distribution of 51-Cr labeled platelets within the circulating dog platelet population, *Thromb. Res.*, 3, 1, 1973.
181. **Pennington, D. G., Lee, N. Y. T., Roxburgh, A. E., and McGready, J. E.,** Platelet density and size. The interpretation of heterogeneity, *Br. J. Haematol.*, 34, 365, 1976.

182. **Pennington, D. G., Streatfield, K., and Roxburgh, A. E.,** Megakaryocytes and the heterogeneity of circulating platelets, *Br. J. Haematol.*, 34, 639, 1976.
183. **Cronkite, E. P., Bond, U. P., Fliedner, T. M., et al.,** Studies on origin, production and destruction of platelets, in *Blood Platelets*, Johnson, S. A., Monto, R. W., Rebuck, J. W., and Horn, R. C., Jr., Eds., Little Brown, Boston, 1960, 595.
184. *Hematology*, 2nd ed., Williams, W. J., Beutler, E., Erslev, A. J., and Rundles, R. W., McGraw Hill, New York, 1977, 1364.
185. **Choi, S. I., Simone, J. V., and Jackson, C. W.,** Megakaryocytopoiesis in experimental iron deficiency anemia, *Blood*, 43, 111, 1974.
186. **Adamson, I. W., Fialkow, P. J., Murphy, S., et al.,** Polycythemia vera: stem cell and probable clonal origin of the disease, *N. Engl. J. Med.*, 292, 913, 1976.
187. **Morley, A.,** Blood cell cycles in polycythemia vera, *Austr. Ann. Med.*, 18, 124, 1969.
188. **Albrecht, M. and Fulle, H. H.,** Morphologie der Megakaryozyten bei Blutkrankheiten, *Blut*, 28, 109, 1974.
189. **Weinfeld, A., Branehog, I., and Kutti, J.,** Platelets in the myeloproliferative syndrome, *Clin. Haematol.*, 4, 373, 1975.
190. **Berger, S., Aledort, L. M., Gilbert, H. S., et al.,** Abnormalities of platelet function in patients with polycythemia vera, *Cancer Res.*, 33, 2683, 1973.
191. **Lagerlof, B. and Franzen, S.,** The ultrastructure of megakaryocyte in polycythemia vera and chronic granulocytic leukemia, *Acta Pathol. Microbiol. Scand. (Section A)*, 80, 71, 1972.
192. **Pennington, D. G.,** Megakaryocyte ploidy measurement in thrombocytosis in *Platelet Kinetics*, Paulus, J. M., Ed., North Holland, Amsterdam, 1971, 311.
193. **Maldonado, J. E., Pintado, T., and Pierre, R. O.,** Dysplastic platelets and circulating megakaryocytes in chronic myeloproliferative disease. I. The platelets: ultrastructure and peroxidase reaction, *Blood*, 43, 797, 1974.
194. **Maldonado, J. E., Pintado, T., and Pierre, R. O.,** Dysplastic platelets and circulating megakaryocytes in chronic myeloproliferative disease. II. Ultrastructure of circulating megakaryocytes, *Blood*, 43, 811, 1974.
195. **Minot, G. R.,** Megakaryocytes in the peripheral circulation, *Exp. Med.*, 36, 1, 1922.
196. **Breton-Gorius, J., Daniel, M. T., Flandrin, G., and Denoel, G. K.,** Fine structure and peroxidase activity of circulating micro-megakaryoblasts and platelets in a case of acute myelofibrosis, *Br. J. Haematol.*, 25, 331, 1973.
197. **den Ottolander, G. J., te Velde, J., Brederoo, P., et al.,** Megakaryoblastic leukemia (acute myelofibrosis): a report of three cases, *Br. J. Haematol.*, 42, 9, 1979.
198. **Fabich, D. R. and Raich, P. C.,** Acute myelofibrosis. A report of three cases, *Am. J. Clin. Pathol.*, 67, 334, 1977.
199. **Lubin, J., Rozen, S., and Rywlin, A. M.,** Malignant myelosclerosis, *Arch. Intern. Med.*, 136, 141, 1976.
200. **Bergsman, K. L. and Van Slyck, E. J.,** Acute myelofibrosis, *Ann. Intern. Med.*, 74, 232, 1971.
201. **Efrati, P., Nir, E., Yaari, A., et al.,** Myeloproliferative disorders terminating in acute micromegakaryoblastic leukemia, *Br. J. Haematol.*, 43, 79, 1979.
202. **Bernstein, R., Katz, J., Bezwoda, W., and Lynch, S. R.,** Acute blastic transformation in patients with chronic granulocytic leukemia and myelofibrosis, *S. Afr. Med. J.*, 50, 616, 1976.
203. **Bain, B., Catovsky, D., and O'Brien, M.,** Megakaryoblastic transformation of chronic granulocytic leukemia. An electron microscopy and cytochemical study, *J. Clin. Pathol.*, 30, 235, 1977.
204. **Armenta, D., Long, L. A., Pretty, H. M., et al.,** Crise blastique d'un leucémie myeloide chronique-leucémie mégakaryoblastique? *L'Union Med. Can.*, 105, 1339, 1976.
205. **Breton-Gorius, J., Reyes, F., Vernant, J. P., et al.,** The blast crisis of chronic granulocytic leukemia: megakaryoblastic nature of cells as revealed by the presence of platelet peroxidase a cytochemical ultrastructural study, *Br. J. Haematol.*, 39, 295, 1978.
206. **Hossfeld, D. K., Tormey, D., and Ellison, R. R.,** Phi-positive megakaryoblastic leukemia, *Cancer*, 36, 576, 1975.
207. **Nigro, M., Ascari, E., Compagnonoi, A., and Menestrina, F.,** Leucemia myeloide aigue a predominance megakaryocytaire et proliferation megakaryocytaires malignes, *Ann. d'Anat. Pathol., (Paris)*, 24, 171, 1979.
208. **Branehog, I., Ridell, B., Swolin, B., and Weinfeld, A.,** Megakaryocyte quantifications in relation to thrombokinetics in primary thrombocythemia and allied disease, *Scan. J. Haematol.*, 15, 321, 1975.
209. **Kass, L.,** Enzymatic abnormalities in megakaryocytes, *Acta Haematol.*, 49, 193, 1973.
210. **Frick, P. G.,** Primary thrombocythemia. Clinical, hematological and chromosomal studies in patients, *Helv. Med. Acta*, 35, 20, 1971.

211. **Hardisty, R. M. and Wolf, H. H.,** Haemorrhagic thrombocythemia: a clinical and laboratory study, *Br. J. Haematol.,* 1, 390, 1955.
212. **Ward, H. P. and Block, H. M.,** The natural history of agnogenic myeloid metaplastic (AMM) and a critical evaluation of its relationship with myeloproliferative syndrome, *Medicine,* 50, 357, 1971.
213. **Thiele, J., Ballard, A-C, and Georgii, A.,** Freeze fracture of the normal and pathological megakaryocyte lineage in chronic megakaryocyte-granulocytic myelosis, *Virchows Arch. B. Cell. Pathol.,* 23, 33, 1977.
214. **Thiele, J., Ballard, A. C., Georgii, A., and Vykoupil, K. F.,** Chronic megakaryocytic-granulocytic myelosis, an electron microscopic study. I. Megakaryocytes and thrombocytes, *Virchows Arch, A. Pathol. Anat. Histol.,* 373, 191, 1977.
215. **Brecher, G.,** Atypical megakaryocytes—a reflection of a stem cell disorder, in *Platelets: production, Function, Transfusion and Storage,* Baldini, M. G. and Ebbe, S., Eds., Grune and Stratton, New York, 1974, 93.
216. **Chikkappa, G., Borner, G., Burlington, H., et al.,** Periodic oscillation of blood leucocytes, platelets and reticulocytes in a patient with chronic granulocytic leukemia, *Blood,* 47, 1023, 1976.
217. **Udomratin, T., Steinberg, M. H., Dreiling, B. J., and Lockhard, U.,** Circulating micromegakaryocytes signaling blast transformation of chronic myeloid leukemia, *Scand. J. Haematol.,* 16, 394, 1976.
218. **Smith, W. B., Ablin, A., Goodman, J. R., and Brecher, G.,** Atypical megakaryocytes in preleukemic phase of acute leukemia, *Blood,* 42, 535, 1973.
219. **Queisser, W., Queisser, U., Ansmann, M., et al.,** Megakaryocyte polyploidization in acute leukemia and preleukemia, *Br. J. Haematol.,* 25, 261, 1974.
220. **Brandt, L., Levan, G., Mitelman, F., and Sjugren, U.,** Defective differentiation of megakaryocytes in acute myeloid leukemia, *Acta Med. Scand.,* 196, 227, 1974.
221. **Greenwald, H. M. and Sherman, I.,** Congenital essential thrombocytopenia, neonatal thrombopenia, *Am. J. Dis. Child.,* 38, 1245, 1925.
222. **Landolt, R. F.,** Kongenitale (neonatale) Thrombopenien, *Helvet. Paediatr. Acta,* 3, 13, 1948.
223. **Dignan, P. S. J., Mauer, A. M., and Frantz, C.,** Phocomelia with congenital hypoplastic thrombocytopenia and myeloid leukemoid reaction, *J. Pediatr.,* 70, 561, 1967.
224. **Hall, J. G., Levin, J., Kuhn, J. P., et al.,** Thrombocytopenia with absent radii (TAR), *Medicine,* 48, 411, 1969.
225. **Eisenstein, E. M.,** Congenital amegakaryocytic thrombocytopenic purpura, *Clin. Pediatr.,* 5, 143, 1966.
226. **Matoth, Y. and Mundel, G.,** Isolated megakaryocytopenia, *Acta Haematol.,* 13, 209, 1954.
227. **Emery, J. L., Gordon, R. R., Rendle-Short, J., et al.,** Congenital amegakaryocytic thrombocytopenia with congenital deformities and a leukemoid blood picture in the new born, *Blood,* 12, 567, 1957.
228. **Fruhling, L., Roger, S., and Tobard, P.,** L'hematologie normale (tissus et organes hemopoietiques sang circulant) de l'embryon et du nouveau ne humains, *Sang,* 20, 313, 1949.
229. **Berge, T., Brunhage, F., and Nilsson, L. R.,** Congenital thrombocytopenia in rubella embryopathy, *Acta Paediatr., Scand.,* 52, 349, 1963.
230. **Sultan, Y., Scrobohaci, M. L., Rendu, F., and Caen, J. P.,** Abnormal platelet function, population and survival time in a boy with congenital absent radii and thrombocytopenia, *Lancet,* 2, 653, 1972.
231. **Day, H. J. and Holmsen, H.,** Platelet adenine nucleotide storage pool deficiency in the thrombocytopenic absent radii syndrome, *JAMA,* 221, 1053, 1972.
232. **Armitage, J. P., Hoak, J. C., Elliott, T. E., and Fry, G. L.,** Syndrome of the thrombocytopenia and absent radii: qualitatively normal platelets with remission following splenectomy, *Scand. J. Haematol.,* 20, 25, 1978.
233. **Bernard, J., Boivin, P., and Caen, J.,** Les cytopenies hypoplatiques congenitales dissociees: purpura thrombopenique congenital avec megakaryocytopenie, neutropenie congenitale, *Sem. Hop. Paris.,* 32, 1597, 1956.
234. **Cooper, L. Z., Green, R. H., Krugman, S., et al.,** Neonatal thrombocytopenia purpura and other manifestations of rubella contracted in utero, *Am. J. Dis. Child.,* 110, 416k 1966.
235. **Vossaugh, P., Leikin, S., Avery, G., et al.,** Neonatal thrombocytopenia in association with rubella, *Acta Haematol.,* 35, 158, 1966.
236. **Hanshaw, H. B.,** Congenital and acquired cytomegalovirus infection, *Pediatr. Clin. N. Am.,* 139, 179, 1966.
237. **Brodsky, I., Kahn, S. B., Ross, E. M., et al.,** Prelymphoid leukemia phase of Rauscher virus infection, *J. Natl. Cancer Inst.,* 38, 779, 1967.
238. **Dennis, L. and Brodsky, I.,** Thrombocytopenia induced by the Friend Leukemia virus, *J. Natl. Cancer Inst.,* 35, 993, 1965.

239. **De Harven, E.,** Further electron microscopic studies of a mouse leukemia induced by cell-free filtrates, *J. Biophys, Biochem. Cytol.*, 7, 747, 1960.
240. **Dalton, A. J., Law, L. W., Moloney, J. B., and Manaker, R. A.,** An electron microscopic study of a series of murine lymphoid neoplasm, *J. Natl. Cancer Inst.*, 27, 747, 1961.
241. **Brodsky, I., Ross, E. M., Kahn, S. B., and Petkov, G.,** The effect of leukemia virus on thrombopoiesis, *Cancer Res.*, 28, 2406, 1971.
242. **Espinoza, C. and Kohn, C.,** Viral infection of megakaryocytes in varicella with purpura, *Am. J. Clin. Pathol.*, 61, 203, 1971.
243. **Quick, A. J. and Hussey, C. U.,** Hereditary thrombopathic thrombocytopenia, *Am. J. Med. Sci.*, 245, 643, 1963.
244. **Krick, W., Jurgens, R., and Hiepler, E.,** Gerinnungsphysiologische Untersuchungen beim familiaren Morbus Werlhof, *Klin. Wochenschr.*, 37, 865, 1959.
245. **Cullum, C., Cooney, D. P., and Schrier, S. L.,** Familial thrombocytopenic thrombocytopathy, *Br. J. Haematol.*, 13, 147, 1967.
246. **Kurstjens, R., Bolt, C., Vossen, M., and Haanen, C.,** Familial thrombopathic thrombocytopenia, *Br. J. Haematol.*, 15, 305, 1968.
247. **Vossen, M. E. M. H., Stadhouders, A. M., Kurstjedns, R., and Haanen, C.,** Observations on platelet ultrastructure in familial thrombocytopathic thrombocytopenia, *Am. J. Pathol.*, 53, 1021, 1968.
248. **Libanska, J., Falcao, L., and Gautier, A.,** Thrombocytopenie thrombocytopathique hypogranulaire hereditaire, *Nouv. Rev. Fr. Hematol.*, 15, 165, 1975.
249. **Grottum, K. A., Hovig, T., Holmsen, H., et al.,** Wiskott-Aldrich syndrome: qualitative platelet defects and short platelet survival, *Br. J. Haematol.*, 17, 373, 1969.
250. **Kuramoto, H., Steiner, M., and Baldini, M.,** Lack of platelet response to stimulation in Wiscott-Aldrich syndrome, *N. Engl. J. Med.*, 282, 475, 1970.
251. **Parkman, R., Rappeport, J., Geha, R., et al.,** Complete correction of the Wiskott-Aldrich syndrome by allogeneic bone marrow transplantation, *N. Engl. J. Med.*, 298, 921, 1978.
252. **Metcalf, D.,** Hemopoietic colonies, in *In vitro Cloning of Normal and Leukemic Cells,* Springer-Verlag, New York, 1977.
253. **Ebbe, S.,** Experimental and clinical megakaryocytopoiesis, *Clin. Haematol.*, 8, 371, 1979.
254. **Oski, F. A., Naiman, J. L., Allen, D. M., and Diamond, L. K.,** Leukocyte inclusions. Dohle bodies-associated with platelet abnormalities (the May-Hegglin anomaly). Report of a case and review of the literature, *Blood,* 20, 652, 1962.
255. **Goodwin, H. A. and Ginsburg, A. D.,** May-Hegglin anamoly: a defect in megakaryocyte fragmentation? *Br. J. Haematol.*, 26, 117, 1974.
256. **Jordan, S. W. and Larson, W. E.,** Ultrastructural studies of the May-Hegglin anomaly, *Blood,* 25, 921, 1969.
257. **Volpe, E., Cuccurullo, L., Valenta, H., et al.,** The May-Hegglin anomaly, *Acta Haematol.*, 52, 238, 1974.
258. **Breton-Gorius, J.,** Development of two distinct membrane systems associated in giant complexes in pathological megakaryocytes, *Ser. Haematol.*, 8, 1, 1975.
259. **Epstein, C. J., Sahud, M. A., Piel, C. F., et al.,** Hereditary macrothrombocytopathia, nephritis and deafness, *Am. J. Med.*, 52, 299, 1972.
260. **Kinet-Denoel, C. and Breton-Gorius, J.,** Teneurs en ADN, ultrastructure et activite peroxidasique des megakaryocytes medullaires dans un cas d'anemie refractaire, *Nouv. Rev. Fr. Hematol.*, 13, 661, 1973.
261. **Mayer, M., Sperling, H., Schaeffer, J., and Queisser, W.,** Megakaryocyte polyploidization in May-Hegglin anomaly, *Acta Haematol.*, 60, 45, 1978.
262. **Kass, L.,** Megakaryocytes in the May-Hegglin anomaly, *Arch. Pathol.*, 98, 112, 1974.
263. **Niewiarowski, S., Poplawski, A., Prokopowiscz, J., et al.,** Abnormalities of platelet function and ultrastructure in macrothrombocytic thrombocytopathia, *Scand. J. Haematol.*, 6, 377, 1969.
264. **Eckstein, J. D., Filip, D. F., and Watts, J. C.,** Hereditary thrombocytopenia, deafness and renal disease, *Ann. Intern. Med.*, 82, 639, 1975.
265. **Von Behrens, W. E.,** Mediterranean macrothrombocytopenia, *Blood,* 46, 199, 1975.
266. **Kass, L., Lichtman, D. A., Beals, T., and Schnitzer, B.,** Megakaryocytes in the giant platelet syndrome. A cytochemical and ultrastructural study, *Thrombus. Haemostas.*, 38, 625, 1977.
267. **Kutti, J. and Weinfeld, A.,** The frequency of thrombocytopenia in patients with heart disease treated with oral diuretics, *Acta Med. Scand.*, 183, 245, 1968.
268. **Cooper, B. A. and Bigelow, E. S.,** Thrombocytopenia associated with the administration diethylstilbesterol in man, *Ann. Intern. Med.*, 52, 907, 1960.

269. **Sullivan, L. W.**, Effect of alcohol on platelet production, in *Platelet Kinetics*, Paulus, J. M., Ed., North Holland, Amsterdam, 1972, 247.
270. **Cowan, D. H. and Graham, R. C., Jr.**, Studies of the platelet defect in alcoholism, *Thromb. Diath. Haemorrh.*, 33, 310, 1975.
271. **Eisner, E. V. and Crowell, E. B.**, Hydrochlorothiazide-dependent thrombocytopenia due to IgM antibody, *JAMA*, 215, 480, 1971.
272. **Sonneborn, D.**, Thrombocytopenia and iron deficiency, *Ann. Intern. Med.*, 80, 111, 1974.
273. **Scher, H. and Silber, R.**, Iron responsive thrombocytopenia, *Ann. Intern. Med.*, 84, 572, 1976.
274. **Karpatkin, S., Garg, S. K., and Freedman, M. L.**, Role of iron as a regulator of thrombopoiesis, *Am. J. Med.*, 57, 521, 1974.
275. **Caen, J.**, Glanzmann thrombasthenia, *Clin. Haematol.*, 1, 383, 1972.
276. **Falcao, L.**, Étude ultrastructurale des megakaryocytes dans la thrombobasthenie Glasnzmann, *Blut*, 28, 337, 1974.
277. **Holmsen, H.**, The platelet: its membrane physiology and biochemistry, *Clin. Haematol.*, 1, 235, 1975.
278. **Weiss, H. J., Witte, L. D., Kaplan, K. L., et al.**, Heterogeneity in storage pool deficiency studies on granule-bound substances in 18 patients including variants deficient in α granules, platelet factor 4, β-thromboglobulin and platelet derived growth factor, *Blood*, 54, 1296, 1979.
279. **Dixon, R., Rosse, W., and Ebbert, L.**, Quantitative determination of antibody in idiopathic thrombocytopenic purpura, *N. Engl. J. Med.*, 292, 230, 1975.
280. **McKenna, R. and Pisciotta, A. V.**, Fluorescence of megakaryocytes in idiopathic thrombopenic purpura (ITP) stained with fluorescent antiglobulin serum, *Blood*, 19, 664, 1962.
281. **McMillan, R.**, The pathogenesis of immune thrombocytopenia purpura, *Crit. Rev. Clin. Lab. Sci.*, 8, 303, 1977.
282. **Garg, S. K., Amorosi, E. L., and Karpatkin, S.**, Use of megathrombocyte as an index of megakaryocyte number, *N. Engl. J. Med.*, 284, 11, 1971.
283. **Ziegler, Z., Murphy, S., and Gardner, F. H.**, Microscopic platelet size and morphology in various hematologic disorders, *Blood*, 48 (Abstr.), 1006, 1976.
284. **Aster, R. H. and Keene, W. R.**, Sites of platelet destruction in idiopathic thrombocytopenic purpura, *Br. J. Haematol.*, 16, 61, 1969.
285. **Najean, Y., Ardaillou, N., Caen, J., et al.**, Survival of radiochromium labeled platelets in thrombocytopenias, *Blood*, 22, 718, 1963.
286. **Baldini, M.**, Idiopathic thrombocytopenic purpura and the ITP syndrome, *Med. Clin. N. Am.*, 56, 47, 1972.
287. **Pizzi, F., Carrara, P. M., Aldeghi, A., and Eridani, S.**, Immunofluorescence of megakaryocytes in thrombocytopenic purpura, *Blood*, 27, 521, 1966.
288. **Joshi, B. C. and Jain, N. C.**, Detection of antiplatelet antibody in serum and megakaryocytes of dogs with autoimmune thrombocytopenia, *Am. J. Vet. Dis.*, 37, 613, 1976.
289. **McMillan, R., Luiken, G. A., and Levy, R.**, Antibody against megakaryocytes in idiopathic thrombocytopenia, *JAMA*, 239, 2460, 1978.
290. **Branehog, L., Kutti, J., and Weinfeld, A.**, Platelet survival and platelet production in idiopathic thrombocytopenic purpura (ITP), *Br. J. Haematol.*, 27, 127, 1974.
291. **Kraytman, M.**, Influence of repeated acute thrombocytopenias on the reappearance of circulating blood platelets, *Blood*, 37, 323, 1971.
292. **Rohr, K.**, *Das Menschliche Knochenmark*, 3rd ed., Georg Thieme Verlag, Stuttgart, 1960, 331.
293. **Bessis, M.**, *Living Blood Cells and Their Ultrastructure*, Springer-Verlag, Berlin, 1973, 399.
294. **Falcao, L., Caen, J., and Gautier, A.**, Etude evolutive de L'ultrastructure des megakaryocytes dans un cas de purpura thrombopenique idiopathique apres splenectomie, *Blut*, 19, 156, 1969.
295. **Paulus, J. M., Breton-Gorius, J., Kinet-Denoel, C., and Bonvier, J.**, Megakaryocyte ultrastructure and ploidy in human macrothrombocytosis, in *Platelets: Production, Function Transfusion and Storage*, Baldini, M. and Ebbe, S., Eds., Grune and Straton, New York, 1974, 131.
296. **Ridell, B. and Branehog, J.**, The ultrastructure of the megakaryocyte in idiopathic thrombocytopenic purpura (ITP) in relation to thrombokinetics, *Path. Eur.*, 11, 179, 1976.
297. **MacPherson, G. G.**, Changes in megakaryocyte development following thrombocytopenia, *Br. J. Haematol.*, 26, 105, 1974.
298. **Bentfield-Barker, M. E. and Bainton, D. F.**, Ultrastructure of rat megakaryocytes after prolonged thrombocytopenia, *J. Ultrastruct. Res.*, 61, 201, 1977.

Chapter 13

BONE MARROW LYMPHOPOIESIS AND LYMPHOPROLIFERATIVE DISORDERS

Stephen Davis, Pietro Rambotti, and Sidney Trubowitz

TABLE OF CONTENTS

I. INTRODUCTION

In the adult endothermic vertebrate the bone marrow is the central organ of hemopoiesis. It is the major source of all cellular elements that circulate in the blood. Only recently has it been established, however, that the majority of lymphocytes originate in the bone marrow and that, at least in rodents, the rate of production of small lymphocytes in the marrow exceeds that of any other lymphoid organ. In fact, there is reason now for regarding the bone marrow as the primary lymphoid organ.

II. THE LYMPHOCYTE IN A STEM CELL ROLE

The existence of a pluripotent hematopoietic stem cell has been adequately established by modifications of the spleen colony technique (see previous chapters). Many attempts have been made to classify these stem cells by morphologic criteria. Although several controversial points remain with regard to the identity of the stem cell the candidate supported by several, but not all lines of investigation, display the morphology of cells included in the lymphocyte-transitional cell population. The stem cell by this definition is a cell with no morphologic signs of differentiation but capable of differentiation into red cells, white cells, and platelets.

In this model developed primarily by Yoffey[1] the fully developed mammalian marrow does not contain a single specific stem cell but rather a stem cell compartment—the lymphocyte transitional cell (LT) compartment. The transitional cells comprise a spectrum of cells of varying sizes, proliferative capacities, and degrees of basophilia. Basophilic transitional cells are believed to be derived from pale transitional cells which themselves are capable of selfmaintenance. Implicit in this model is the fact that not all cells in the compartment function as stem cells.

In the LT compartment the most undifferentiated cells are the pale transitional cells (Figure 1). These cells may either undergo proliferation or leave the compartment. When pale transitionals proliferate, small transitional cells grow into large ones which then divide. When they leave the compartment they may develop basophilia and then become blast cells or they may divide into small lymphocytes, which can leave the marrow by traversing the sinusoids (Figure 1).

McCulloch[1a] feels that the search for a morphological identifiable stem cells "is a waste of time." His objections lie in the fact that morphology fails to identify a discrete class of cells. Despite McCulloch's cautions the LT hypothesis has been useful in evaluating bone marrow function.

A. Morphologic Comparison of Transitional Cells with Small Lymphocytes

On fixed smears of guinea pig and rodent bone marrow, small lymphocytes and transitional cells range in diameter from 5.5 to 14 μm.[2,3] Small lymphocytes are designated as cells sized 5.5 to 8.0 μm, whereas, the cells sized between 8.0 μm to 14 μm are termed transitional cells. These cells, similarly, fall into two categories with respect to their capacity to incorporate tritiated thymidine (TdR^3H). Cells with diameters of 8 μm or more (transitional) belong to a proliferating population, while small cells do not synthesize DNA. There is only minimal overlap. A similar distribution exists in the human fetal,[4] newborn, and infant marrow where about 60 to 80% of cells fall into the size range below 8 μm (small lymphocytes).[5]

Rosse and Yoffey[6] examined the nuclear structure of small lymphocytes and of transitional cells in marrow using fixed and living preparations. In transitional cells a considerable fraction of the nuclear chromatin was finely dispersed. The transitional cells had more leptochromatic nuclei, while small lymphocytes have pachychromatic

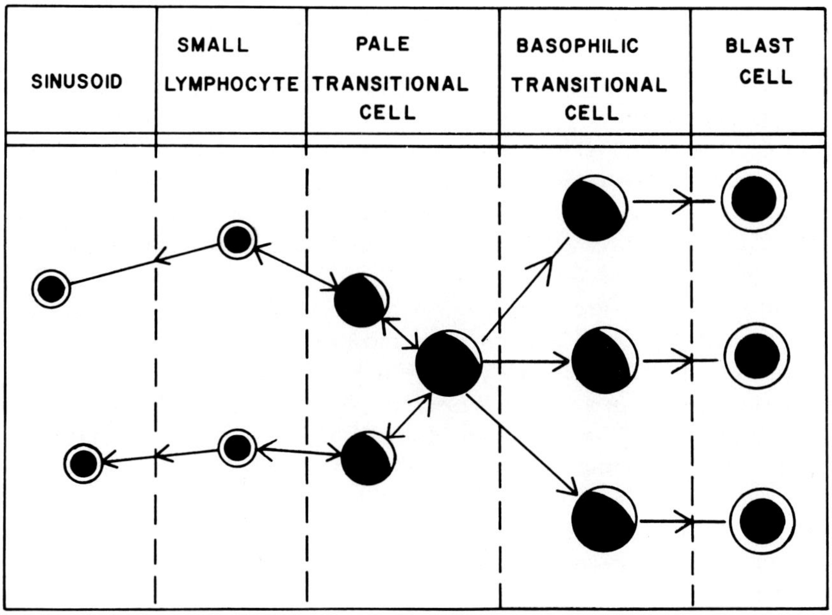

FIGURE 1. The lymphocyte transitional cell compartment (modified from Yoffey[1]). The pale transitional cells either undergo proliferation or leave the compartment. Small pale transitionals may become basophilic transitionals and then committed blast cells, or small pale transitionals may directly traverse the sinusoids as small lymphocytes. Pale transitionals may enter the bloodstream directly (path not shown).

nuclei.[7–10] Among all hemopoietic cells, the high degree of nuclear chromatin dispersion is a characteristic of transitional cells. Apart from a minimal amount of heterochromatin apparent as small discontinuous clumps to the inner laminar of nuclear envelope, the overwhelming bulk of chromatin is in the extended state. This nuclear morphology is a reflection of the high metabolic and proliferative activity that characterizes transitional cells. Likewise, increasing RNA content of lymphocyte nuclei is correlated not only with increasing cell size, but also with the greater degrees of diffuseness seen in the nuclear chromatin.[11] RNA synthesis as well as DNA synthesis is associated predominantly with extended chromatin.[12–14] Transitional cells are usually active in synthesizing DNA and the rate of RNA synthesis in these cells is paralleled in the marrow only by the rate of RNA synthesis found in proerythroblasts and basophilic erythroblasts.[15,16] With light microscopy, a direct correlation between the degree of chromatin dispersion and the capacity of transitional cells to incorporate TdR-^{3}H is seen. It was shown by in vitro microcinematographic studies that following a mitosis some transitional cells yielded daughter cells which, instead of growing, failed to enlarge and their nuclear chromatin became more condensed. These observations permit a dynamic interpretation of the variation in chromatin configuration and in cell size; at least in some of the transitional cells, chromatin undergoes a condensation phenomenon in the course of lymphocyte maturation.

Small lymphocytes in the marrow like small lymphocytes of lymph and blood possess nucleoli.[17–19] In transitional cells, similar in many respects to "blast cells," nucleolar complexes are not apparent on fixed smears.[20] Nucleoli are often difficult or impossible to detect in living cells as well as by phase contrast microscopy.[6] Staining with toluidine blue, however, does reveal some scanty nucelolar material in all transitional cells. In contrast to those in blast cells, the nucleoli in transitional cells are small and number only one to two per cell. In near equatorial sections of transitional cells nucleolar material can usually be demonstrated by the electron microscope. Only in the larger cells and only in those in which the cytoplasm contains numerous polyribosomes is the nucleolus of any significant size. In such cells an irregular nucleolar complex is usually apposed to the nuclear envelope, often at the side of an indentation. The nucleolema is complex and honeycomb-like, enclosing a considerable amount of intranuclear heterochromatin. Such nucleolar structure is characteristic of cells actively engaged in RNA and protein synthesis and is best seen in the marrow in the early identifiable members of the erythroid series; in smaller cells with more heterochromatin the nucleoli resemble more closely those seen in small lymphocytes.[20] In many sections no nucleolar material is evident at all, and this is true of most of the published illustrations of transitional cells.[7,9,21] In small lymphocytes the nucleolus consists of a small amorphous homogeneous core without any spaces or chromatin in the nucleolema. It is surrounded concentrically by dense fibrillar and/or granular material creating a ring-like appearance. A considerable amount of heterochromatin is associated with the nucleolar complex.

A small amount of cytoplasm is a distinct characteristic of small lymphocytes and transitional cells of the marrow. The majority of larger lymphoid cells elsewhere in the lymphoid complex possess considerably more cytoplasm and have a relatively high nuclear cytoplasmic ratio. In transitional cells, the cytoplasm may be visible only as a narrow rim embracing part of the nucleus. Cells with more abundant cytoplasm usually possess several nucleoli and are not included with transitional cells although they may be related to them.

Rosse and Yoffey[6] described variation of cytoplasmic basophilia among transitional cells. These cells were separated into basophilic and pale transitional cells. It was shown that the basophilia is due to the presence of RNA; mouse transitional cells treated with RNAase lose all the basophilic substance from the cytoplasm.[5] In basophilic transitional cells, the nuclei also stain darker with polychrome stains than the nuclei of pale transitional cells. While it may appear arbitrary to classify cells in terms of their cytoplasmic staining characteristics with polychromatic stains, several studies have confirmed that there are consistent differences between pale and basophilic transitional cells in terms of their proliferative behavior and in their responses to various hemopoietic stimuli.[3,6] Ultrastructurally these differences are reflected in the number of cytoplasmic ribosomes and ribosome clusters. The density of polyribosomes is greater in basophilic transitional cell populations.[21,22]

B. Morphologic Comparison of Transitional Cells with Large and Medium Lymphocytes

Large and medium lymphocytes of blood as well as lymph possess prominent nucleoli and considerably more heterochromatin than transitional cells. The blood and lymph node cells have cytoplasm that is more abundant and a Golgi apparatus that is developed to a greater degree than in transitional cells. By light microscopy thoracic duct lymphocytes exhibit a range of cytoplasmic basophilia similar to that of transitional cells.[6,23] This basophilia is due, in many large lymphocytes, to increasing amounts of rough-surfaced endoplasmic reticulum, although the number of free mono- and polyribsomes also shows considerable variation.[24,25] In transitional cells there is very little rough-surfaced endoplasmic reticulum.[5]

In contrast to lymphocytes of mammals, a number of lymphoid cells found in the bursae of newly hatched chicks are strikingly similar to transitional cells.[5,26] Further studies have corroborated this finding at the electron microscope level.[27,28]

Lymphoid cells similar to transitional cells may be found in the thymus among the more rapidly proliferative cells. This is particularly true in the neonatal guinea pig.[5] Transitional cells have been described in human fetal liver[29,30] and blood[31,32] as well as in the blood of newborn infants.[33] Some of the cells of acute lymphocytic leukemia and of stem cell leukemias also bear a close morphologic resemblance to transitional cells of marrow.[34]

C. Morphologic Comparison of Transitional Cells with Lymphocytes Transformed by Mitogens

Viewed with the light microscope, a large proportion of lymphocytes stimulated by phytohemagglutinin (PHA) acquire the characteristic morphology of transitional cells.[35] This observation has been viewed as evidence corroborating the origin of transitional cells from small lymphocytes in the bone marrow. The available evidence on the rate of turnover of transitional cells under physiological conditions does not lend support to this hypothesis.[3,36] The morphological similarity between transitional cells and lymphocytes transformed by mitogens may be a reflection of similar but unrelated metabolic and proliferative events. Comparison of the ultrastructure of transitional and transformed cells reveals several differences. Nuclear changes in PHA transformed lymphocytes include principally an increase in the number and size of nucleoli as early as 4 hr after stimulation. These nuclear structures are distinctly different from the morphology of transitional cells. Similarly, Tanaka[25] noted a significant increase in the volume of cytoplasm of lymphocytes 3 to 4 hr after stimulation. It is characteristic of transitional cells to possess only minimal cytoplasm although admittedly somewhat more than a small lymphocyte. On the whole transformed lymphocytes cannot be confused with transitional cells.[37,39]

D. Transitional Cells

1. Hemopoietic Progenitor Cells

Evidence is available that suggests that the progenitor cells of erythroblasts, granulocytes, and mononuclear phagocytes, as well as those of bone marrow small lymphocytes, may be among the cells in the marrow that are identified by morphological criteria as transitional cells.

Early studies showed that lymphoid progenitors were not present in spleen colonies (colony forming unit spleen—CFU-S) of lethally irradiated mice. These studies suggested that the CFU-S and lymphoid progenitors were derived from a common primitive stem cell.[40] Recent studies by Abramson[41] have clarified the relation between myeloid and lymphoid stem cells. These workers repopulated stem cell deficient W/W^v mice with limiting dilution levels of marrow containing irradiation-induced chromosomal markers. In some mice, the marrow, spleen and thymus cells, CFU-S and phytohemagglutinin and lypopolysaccharide-stimulated spleen cells contained large proportions of cells bearing the same chromosomal marker. Repopulation with hematopoietic and lymphopoietic cells had therefore resulted from a single primitive stem cell. In other mice only bone marrow and CFU-S contained a common chromosomal marker.

This result showed that a stem cell existed that could only differentiate into myelopoietic cells; this stem cell was presumed to be the classic CFU-S. Another pattern was characterized by chromosomal aberrations only in thymus cells; this pattern suggested the presence of a stem cell restricted to T lymphocyte differentiation. The majority of cells in this population are undoubtedly committed to lymphocyte production. The cells that progress along the lymphocytic line of differentiation retain the morphological features of transitional cells, whereas those that advance along the line of erythroid or granulocytic development are no longer included in this compartment in view of the morphologically evident changes such lines of differentiation bring about.

2. Progenitors of Erythroblasts

The erythroblast progenitors are not immigrant cells but are derived from a population within the marrow. That this population might be equated with basophilic transitional cells was suggested by the differences observed in this morphologically defined compartment in the marrow between normal, polycythemic, and erythropoietically stimulated guinea pigs.[42,43] In stimulated animals the fall in TdR^3-H labeled cells was disproportionately accelerated in basophilic transitional cells. During the first 48 hr following injection 80 to 90% of TdR^3-H activity was lost from this population, while in the normal and polycythemic animals it fell only 35 to 45% during the same period.

The observed fall in activity in transitional cells after erythropoiesis is stimulated represented a six- to seven-fold greater rate than the rate observed in the normal animal. In all three groups the behavior of pale transitional cells was quite distinct from that of basophilic cells, and no direct relationship was evident between the kinetics of pale cells and the state of erythropoiesis. The experiments do not directly identify erythroblast progenitor cells with basophilic transitional cells, although they do make a strong case for such an interpretation of the data. They do not exclude the possibility that another population of cells might also contribute to the erythroid increase.

When erythropoiesis was restimulated in polycythemic animals, hemoglobin synthesis was demonstrated in cells that were morphologically indistinguishable from basophilic transitional cells.[20] Proerythroblasts and basophilic erythroblasts were practically absent from the marrow of polycythemic animals, but 40 hr after erythropoietic stimulation both types of cells were detected and they synthesized and contained hemoglobin. At this stage, hemoglobin synthesis was also present in a small number of basophilic transitional cells. In summary, a proportion of basophilic transitional cells may fulfill the function of erythropoietic-responsive progenitors of erythroblasts.

3. Progenitors of Granulocytes and Macrophages

Evidence for the existence of a transitional cell progenitor pool for granulocytes and macrophages is based on an in vitro culture system in which colonies of granulocytes or macrophages develop in semisolid media if colony stimulating factor is also present. Several groups of investigators have looked into the question of the morphological identity of the cells from which the in vitro colonies are derived and there seems to be general agreement that they belong to a class of transitional cells. Moore et al.[44] achieved a high degree of enrichment of in vitro colony forming cells by a two-step density separation procedure of monkey bone marrow. They confirmed the clonal nature of the colonies by plating individual cells selected at a high magnification from the cell fraction enriched in progenitor cells. They obtained evidence that granulocytes and macrophages were derived from a single cell. The data obtained by the combined use of TdR-^{3}H suicide, radioautography, and morphological analysis reduced the number of possible candidates for the granulocyte macrophage progenitor to two types of cells. These were transitional cells and larger, undifferentiated blasts. However, in the fraction enriched in progenitor cells, the blasts were too few to be the only source of colony forming cells. On radioautographs after suicidal doses of TdR-^{3}H these investigators equated the granulocyte-macrophage progenitor with basophilic transitional cells which measured 9 to 11 μm in diameter and had a high TdR-^{3}H labeling index. Zucali et al.[45] demonstrated a similar correlation between granulocyte macrophage progenitor and transitional cells in rat bone marrow, and the report of Daniels[46] shows the same in the guinea pig.

III. SMALL LYMPHOCYTES IN THE BONE MARROW

A. Population Size

It has been adequately documented that in the rodent the small lymphocyte compartment of the bone marrow represents one of the largest pools of lymphocytes in the body.[22,53] Chicken bone marrow contains fewer lymphocytes than the marrow of rodents but still represent a large lymphocyte pool.[47,48] Rosse[5] found 7.11 ± 2.61% of cells to be small lymphocytes in the marrow of 4-week-old chicks. In 8- to 9-week-old birds the estimate ranges from 5 to 12.3%. The cells included in this estimation do not incorporate TdR-^{3}H and as expected they have detectable membrane immunoglobulins. Various estimates for the incidence of small lymphocytes in human marrow were reviewed by Yoffey[22] and were found to range in the adult from 5 to 20%. Burkart and Meuwissien[49] paid particular attention to the frequency of small lymphocytes in human marrow obtained by duplicate sampling, using curetting or aspiration. In six adult donors the two methods gave different values, 8 ± 3% in curettes and 13 ± 4% in aspirate analysis. In children, the marrow lymphocyte population is considerably larger. The values quoted by Yoffey[22] obtained from various investigators range from 14 to 57%. Using the same morphological criteria as rodents, Rosse[5] found that in the marrow of 40 black and 38 white normal American infants the percentage of small lymphocytes remained remarkable constant up to the age of 18 months. In serial biopsies aspirated between 1 and 18 months of age, the lowest value was 44 ± 11% and the highest 49.1 ± 9.7%. In 21 cases of acute lymphoblastic leukemia ranging in age from 5 to 48 years, Borella and Sen[50] found that marrow small lymphocytes varied from 25 to 60%. At the time of the biopsy the patients had been in continuous remission for 3 to 5 years and had received no treatment for 1 month to 5 years. This latter data must be interpreted cautiously as we have insufficient knowledge to state that these patients have been cured or that the lymphocytes observed are normal.

It is clear that there is a need for a more thorough understanding of the changes in the small lymphocyte population of human marrow. However, the age related changes in the lymphocyte population, in total cellularity, as well as in the compartment size of lymphocytes are well documented and consistant for rodent, guinea pig, and human marrow.

B. Turnover

The turnover of lymphocytes in mouse marrow has been analyzed by infusing ^{3}H-thymidine (TdR-^{3}H) in vivo to label all DNA-synthesizing cells and their progeny.[3,9,51–55]

The vast majority of small lymphocytes of the marrow (98%), like small lymphocytes elsewhere, do not synthesize DNA and consequently do not directly incorporate TdR-^{3}H. The small lymphocyte labeling index slowly increases indicating the presence of some renewed cells. Two groups of marrow small lymphocytes are defined on the basis of their renewal and origin.[56–58] The major population of rapidly renewed small lymphocytes are maximal in numbers and incidence in young animals. The turnover of this population exceeds the turnover of lymphocytes in any other lymphoid tissue, including the thymus. Selective ^{3}H-thymidine labeling of bone marrow in vivo has demonstrated that these cells are produced within the marrow itself from proliferating progenitors and that many of them soon migrate to the spleen and lymph nodes.[56,57] The existence of a long-lived marrow lymphocyte can be assumed from TdR-^{3}H studies as the second group of marrow small lymphocytes.[58] If TdR-^{3}H is administered over a prolonged period of time not only will the rapidly proliferating cells become labeled, but also a proportion of those cells that have a slow rate of turnover. After discontinuation of

TdR^3-H the concentration of the radioactive marker in proliferating cells will be reduced progressively to a level undetectable by radioautography. At the time when isotope reutilization can be excluded, only those cells will retain labels that were formed during the period of availability of TdR-^{3}H and survived for the time of sampling. Guinea pigs were injected with TdR-^{3}H for 14 days and were allowed to survive for a further 2 to 6 weeks.[58] During the first 2 weeks following the injection, the proportion of labeled erythroblasts and granulocytes suggested that label had not been completely eliminated from proliferating cells. Two weeks later, however, the labeling of such cells was not above background. Four weeks and 6 weeks after the completion of injections, 6.9 and 7.2%, respectively, of small lymphocytes were found to be significantly labeled in the marrow.

The experiments were repeated on mice by Ropke and Everett[59] with identical results. Their studies extended over a period of 9 weeks and confirmed the presence of a stable population of long-lived lymphocytes in the marrow. This minor population of slowly renewed small lymphocytes in the marrow increases in both incidence and absolute number with age.[60]

When the labeling was commenced in newborn guinea pigs, fewer labeled long-lived cells were found in the marrow than when labeling was started in adult animals.[58,61] In the latter group 86% of small lymphocytes were renewed in the marrow within 4 days and, of the remaining 14% with a longer life span 7% were generated during a 2-week course of TdR-^{3}H injections. Their life span exceeded 4 weeks. In the group of guinea pigs studied by Osmond the long-lived population was smaller. In 6-week-old BALB/C/mice 75% of marrow small lymphocytes were renewed within 3 days, but the life span in the remaining 25% ranged from weeks to months.[62] The origin of this minor population of long-lived small lymphocytes in the marrow remains largely unknown. Rosse feels that these probably are immigrants from the recirculating lymphocyte pools.[5] Contamination of experimental material by peripheral blood lymphocytes can not be excluded.

It has been established that B lymphocytes with a long-lived life span are generated by a bone marrow inoculum in suitable recipients.[63,64] Long-lived T lymphocytes may only account for a small fraction of the long-lived population in the marrow. In the guinea pig the long-lived population is not influenced significantly by neonatal thymectomy and lymphocytes with a long life span are present in the marrow of mice with congenital lack of a functioning thymus (nu/nu, nude).[65]

C. The Traffic of Lymphocytes to and from the Marrow

By various experimental approaches it has been possible to demonstrate that under relatively physiologic conditions both afferent and efferent streams of lymphocytes exist in the marrow.[52] The majority of lymphocytes discharged from the marrow are recently generated cells, and apparently only a negligible number of them if any, returns to the marrow. A second smaller compartment consisting of nonproliferating long-lived cells seem to circulate between the marrow and blood.[61] The marrow origin of this second compartment has not been proved.

When the circulation to an animal hindlimb is temporarily arrested and TdR-^{3}H is injected into the medullary cavity of a bone in that limb the uptake of the isotope can be confined to the marrow, but labeled lymphocytes make their appearance not only in the injected marrow but in blood and various lymphoid tissues; they are observed outside the marrow as soon as 12 hr after the injection and they evidently continue to seed from the marrow for several days.[66,67] Thus the lymphocytes may be presumed to have migrated through the sinusoidal endothelium.

Recent experiments in the mouse indicate that a large proportion of newly generated small lymphocytes discharged from the marrow function as precursors of B and T cells and complete their differentation in the spleen, thymus, and possibly in other lymphoid tissues. Although in lymph nodes and spleen T and B cells have been shown to localize preferentially in "thymus-dependent" and "thymus-independent" zones, respectively.[68–70] It is interesting to note that newly generated lymphocytes of guinea pigs discharged from the marrow initially seed more or less randomly in both these areas.[67] Further maturation is evidently necessary before they acquire the capacity to specifically home to known B-cell and T-cell dependent zones.

Lymphocytes discharged from the marrow enter the lymphoid tissues mainly through postcapillary vessels. Only a small proportion of them find their way into the thoracic duct. Their ability to recirculate from blood to lymph seem to be extremely limited. Nor do they reenter the bone marrow in significant numbers, if at all.

Back et al.[71] injected TdR-^{3}H into the bone marrow of chicks of three different ages. The presence of heavily labeled cells 48 hr later in the spleen, cecal tonsil, and thymus suggested that they originated in the injected marrow. In newly hatched chicks labeled cells were also seen in the bursa. The few cells that, after local TdR-^{3}H labeling of the marrow, immigrate to the thymus, are probably prethymic T lymphocytes.

The average span of time spent in the marrow by lymphocytes may be computed from radioautographic data. In the guinea pig this was originally estimated to be about three days.[56] A somewhat shorter value is implied by more recent data.[16] The compartment transit time for the so-called long-lived lymphocytes in the marrow is not known.

In guinea pigs, rats, and mice only a negligible number, if any, of lymphocytes that have recently emerged from a proliferating marrow progenitor pool reenter the bone marrow. The access of lymphocytes to the marrow is a critical question; very few of newly generated thymocytes can be found to home to the marrow in guinea pigs, hamsters, calves, rats, newborn mice, or chicks of various ages.[72–77] Thus, the bone marrow of rodents resembles the thymus in that it admits only a negligible number of newly generated lymphocytes whatever their origin might be in comparison with lymph nodes and spleen.[52,62,78]

A dissimilar relationship seems to exist between avian marrow and the bursa at the time of development, when the bursa is actively producing lymphocytes. Local labeling of the bursa with TdR-^{3}H indicates that newly generated bursal lymphocytes do migrate to the marrow directly, as they do to the spleen and cecal tonsil.[79]

D. Factors Controlling Lymphocyte Production in the Marrow

The thymus has been credited with the elaboration of substances that greatly influence the generation of mature thymic lymphocytes.[80] This influence is exerted mainly on one population of marrow lymphocytes, i.e., those of prethymic origin. Thymectomy in young rats however, has no influence on the number of lymphocytes present in the bone marrow.[81,82] The same was confirmed in guinea pigs thymectomized within 24 hr of birth and evaluated 6 to 8 weeks later. Coursa, however, observed a fall in bone marrow lymphocytes of guinea pigs after thymectomy, a decline that could be halted by the administration of thymic extracts.[83] Hays in neonatally thymectomized mice showed an initial decrease of bone marrow lymphocytes, and by 12 weeks none were present in the marrow.[84] Subcutaneous implantation of thymic epithelial tissue retarded the fall in marrow lymphocytes. The reasons for this apparent contradiction on the effect of the thymus on the absolute number of marrow small lymphocytes is unclear.

The avian bursa exerts a negligible influence on bone marrow lymphocytes production. The bone marrow of chicks in which the development of the bursa was prevented by the injection of testosterone proprionate into the egg during incubation, contained lymphocytes in normal proportions although the birds proved to be agammaglobulinemic or severely hypogammaglobulinemic.[5] More recent data (see below) suggest that although quantitatively the lymphocyte population in the marrow is not affected by thymectomy or bursectomy, T and B maturation is impaired.

While an encounter with antigens can augument the production of lymphocytes in peripheral lymphoid tissue, the available evidence indicates that antigens do not exert such an effect on the marrow. Recently, Claesson et al.[85] compared the population size and rate of turnover of bone marrow lymphocytes in germ-free and conventional mice. In the two animals the size of the population was not significantly different as were rates of lymphocyte turnover in the marrow. The data concur with those of Osmond and Nossal[86] who found similar proportions of lymphocytes in germ-free and conventional mice.

It is not known whether, through feedback mechanisms, the generation of bone marrow lymphocytes also depends on the size of certain lymphocytes subpopulations within or outside the marrow. Vaughn and McGregor[87] found, however, that the pool size of recirculating peripheral blood lymphocytes did not influence the rate of generation of marrow lymphocytes.

Corticosteroids have been shown to delete preferentially those lymphocytes that are renewed at a rapid rate.[88,89] There is evidence that the lymphocytes of some species such as the rat, rabbit, and mouse are more sensitive than others, for example, than man and the guinea pig.[90] It is evident from the work of Esteban[88] that in the rat the loss of lymphocytes in the marrow following glucocorticosteroid administration is due to preferential deletion of newly generated lymphocytes. In none of these experiments was the regeneration of marrow lymphocytes or the effect on the rate of lymphocyte production investigated following corticosteroid administration.

An increase in bone marrow lymphocyte pool has been brought about in three types of experiments. In the first, within 4 hr of injecting a "leukocyte promoting factor" into guinea pigs, a substantial increase was observed in marrow lymphocytes parallel with a fall in granulocytes.[91] In the second, splenectomy in both the guinea pig and the rat was reported to lead to an increase in marrow lymphocytes over a prolonged period of time.[9] The third type of study showed substantial increase in the size of the small lymphocyte compartment during a posthypoxic period induced in animals.[22] In these studies the number of small lymphocytes per unit volume or unit weight of marrow doubled or tripled; lymphocytes could account for up to 75% of all nucleated cells in the marrow. The increases took place over several days and was accounted for by newly generated lymphocytes.[36,92] The lymphocytes were generated by progenitors confined to the marrow and the increases in the compartment were not due to migration of lymphocytes into the marrow. The increase in the small lymphocyte population can be explained by an increase in transitional cells in posthypoxic marrow compared to the normal and that a larger proportion of these cells gave rise to more small lymphocytes than in normal nonhypoxic marrow.

Analysis of the above-mentioned kinetic behavior of transitional cells allows us to make the following hypothesis. A proportion of small lymphocytes in the marrow is generated as part of a mechanism that limits the size of the proliferating progenitor cell pool. The number of lymphocytes produced by this process varies inversely with the rate at which progenitor cells enter the erythroid, and possibly also granulocytic compartment. The small lymphocytes thus produced should also acquire characteristics of marrow B and pre-T cells. If the stimulus for proliferation is great a proportion of lymphocytes in the marrow and blood that appear may not show differentiation markers for either T or B cells (null cells).

E. Marrow Prethymic Lymphocytes

It is generally accepted that T lymphocytes, like other differentiated cells in the blood, arise ultimately from pluripotent hemopoietic stem cells. However, the differentiation stages between stem cells and thymocytes remain obscure. Few stem cells are found in the thymus itself, and this is true even in the thymus of a lethally irradiated mouse during repopulation from injected bone marrow.[93] El-Arini and Osoba[94] found evidence for the existence in bone marrow of a thymus-repopulating cell which, on the basis of density, was distinct both from stem cells and from mature thymocytes. Similar cells were identified by Basch and Kadish[95] who characterized them in greater detail. The repopulating cells were found to be cells of medium size, of fairly low buoyant density, nonadherent to glass wool but partially adherent to nylon fiber, sensitive to hydrocortisone cytolysis and of low mitotic activity under normal conditions, insensitive to antithymocyte antiserum, but sensitive to cytolysis by a rabbit antimouse brain serum. Kadish and Basch[95] found that the thymus-repopulating cells had physical and biological characteristics generally similar to stem cells but in addition they carried detectable quantities of the membrane antigen Thy 1. These cells were able to return to the thymus and proliferate within 4 days after transfer to irradiated animals, a capacity not shared by bone marrow progenitors or by the vast majority of cortical thymocytes. The bone marrow (and spleen) of congenitally athymic "nude" mice have been reported to contain up to 18% of weakly Thy 1-positive cells.[96] Additionally, the TL antigen (a surface marker of cortical thymocytes) was detectable on some of the cells. Weakly Thy 1-positive cells are also found in the thymus of 13 days, but not in 15- to 16-day embryo mice. It is suggested that these cells are "prethymocytes" and that their numbers in the bone marrow are under feedback control by the thymus, i.e., a functional thymus tending to suppress the development of the cells or at least their expression of Thy-1 and TL surface markers.

A limited amount of T-like differentiation however, may be possible in the absence of the thymus. It is not entirely possible to exclude in "nude" mice the possibility that T cell induction is not a function of the rudimentary thymic epithelium.[97,98] Furthermore, it has been repeatedly demonstrated that various agents not specifically associated with the thymus can induce T-cell surface characteristics in vitro by interacting with beta adrenergic receptors.[99] Bone marrow cells in which T-cell surface markers have been induced in vitro by the thymic oligopeptide thymopoietin have been reported to be efficient repopulators of previously irradiated thymus.[100] It seems probable that thymopoietin-induced bone marrow cells represent the early cortical thymocytes as identified by Basch and Kadish.[95]

The marrow is thus the source of prethymic T cells. It is believed these cells arise *in situ* from the yolk sac and/or fetal liver cells that immigrate to the marrow.[101] Prethymic T-cell precursors are large in size (10 to 15 μm) and are resistant to cytolysis by irradiation. Since prethymic T cells cannot be separated from transitional cells the relationship of these two cells remains to be explored. However, prethymic T cells are functionally distinguishable from transitional cells. Prethymic T cells can be induced to express mature thymocyte membrane antigens, i.e., Lys-1,2,3, with thymus hormones and have a positive reaction with antisera to mouse brain.

Terminal deoxynucleotidyl transferase (Tdt) is an enzyme with the ability to add mononucleotide to segments of DNA. It is normally found only in thymus and bone marrow. The enzyme may be concerned with B-cell programming in marrow. Baltimore has suggested that variable regions of immunoglobulins arise because single-stranded gaps are made in an inherited gene which encodes these regions and that during repair of these gaps Tdt inserts the wrong bases causing a mutation.[102] The high Tdt levels in thymus have suggested its role in T cell maturation. Among hemopoietic cells Tdt is restricted in distribution to mature thymocytes and marrow prethymocytes.[103] Bollum believes Tdt to be a somatic mutator for thymocyte diversification.[104] During fetal life Tdt positive cells are first detected in the thymus, but appear in bone marrow immediately in the neonatal period. They account for 4% of all nucleated marrow cells at this time. In the adult human marrow less than 1% of cells are Tdt positive. In contrast to the cytoplasmic location of Tdt in cortical thymocytes marrow pre-T lymphocytes have nuclear Tdt staining. Tdt-positive cells are smaller than Tdt-negative cells suggesting that positive cells are more mature, perhaps differentiating from Tdt-negative cells. Following administration of dexamethasone 75% of rat marrow lymphocytes are lysed. Reappearance of Tdt-containing lymphocytes appears to occur as a cohort. The regenerating cells at days 1 to 5 are characterized by the rapid proliferation of large, Tdt-negative lymphoid cells. By days 6 to 11, the cells divide less rapidly, are Tdt-positive in the nucleus, and morphologically classifiable as transitional lymphocytes. At day 15 the cells are small lymphocytes with 1% Tdt-positive cells. These data support the hypothesis that marrow prethymocytes are derived from the transitional cell pool.[105] TdT-positive cells appear in the marrow in normal percentages even in the absence of and independent of a thymus. TdT-positive cells in mouse marrow are prethymic T cells.[106] Their differentiation, however, advances up to a point which falls short of expressing thymus-dependent immunocompetence. Upon exposure to thymic hormones Tdt-positive mouse pre T cells express Ly-1,2,3, antigens. Although the exact nature of Tdt-positive marrow cells is not as yet defined, it appears that in postnatal life, marrow Tdt-positive cells represent a mobilizable pool of T lymphocytes.[101] Since thymic hormone is believed to be produced by thymic epithelial remnants in adulthood the T lymphocyte in the mature mammal might well be replenished from marrow prethymic T cells.

F. Marrow B Lymphocyte Pool

When lethally irradiated mice received a transplant of bone marrow cells, the entire B-lymphocyte population, identified by Ig and complement surface receptors, is reconstituted quantitatively in lymph nodes and spleen, within the space of 8 to 12 weeks.[107,108] Over a similar period of time, the same population of lymphocytes is regenerated in lethally irradiated hosts if, instead of bone marrow, mouse yolk sac cells or 10- to 14-day-old fetal liver cells are transplanted.[109] These tissues are known to contain the pluripotent stem cells which are essentially devoid of surface Ig-bearing lymphocytes. The fact that, in lethally irradiated mice, the reconstitution of mature lymphocyte functions such as the ability to bind surface antigen and antibody production can be effected by the progeny of as few as 4 to 13 stem cells derived from bone marrow[11] or by the progeny of a single or very few stem cells derived from fetal liver[111] makes it evident that B lymphocytes, like erythroblasts and granulocytes, are derived from pluripotent stem cells.

Only in the chick has a privileged anatomical site other than marrow been demonstrated in which the generation of B lymphocytes occurs.[26,112–114] After hatching, however, this monopoly is relinquished by the bursa and is taken over increasingly by the marrow and the spleen.[115] Only bursal cells obtained from embryonic or young donors can effect full morphological and functional restoration of the bursa-dependent immune system in 3-day-old cyclophosphamide treated, immune deficient chicks. A functional reconstitution of humoral immunity can be brought about in the same test animal by the transplantation of bone marrow or spleen cells obtained from older donors in which the bursa is no longer functional.[116–118] This capacity is acquired by the marrow 4 to 5 weeks after hatching and is exhibited to a greater extent than by the spleen.[115]

Thus, although the bursa functions as a primary site from which B cell progenitors are dispersed; later in life, the bone marrow acquires a population of cells which has the capacity to generate B lymphocytes independently of bursal influence. In man, the ontogenic development of B lymphocytes is not complicated by a known bursal influence. One series of experiments for identifying the origin of B cells is that of Lafleur and associates.[119–121] In the bone marrow and spleen of the mouse, they distinguished two subpopulations of cells that bound fluorescence labeled anti-Ig-sera. One subpopulation that had the same velocity sedimentation profile as small lymphocytes was shown to consist of immunocompetent B cells. The second Ig-positive subpopulation, made up of larger cells, was immunoincompetent in the same assay. However, when transplanted, the larger cells generated immunocompetent B lymphocytes in the spleen of recipient mice, within the span of 7 days. These larger cells were designated precursor B cells.[119] Although precursor B cells can interact with antigen, it was revealed that in the marrow only 0.05% of the total Ig-positive precursor population gave rise to the immunocompetent B-cell progeny that eventually interacted with antigen.[121] The findings were interpreted to suggest that antigen specificity, known to be restricted to B cells, may already be attained in the precursor population. Such an interpretation implies that the Ig molecules on the surface of precursor B cells are specific receptors for the antigen to which their progeny will respond. In addition to functional immaturity and larger size, precursor B cells were different from immunocompetent B cells in that they possessed a lower density of Ig surface determinants and were absent from lymph nodes.[119–121]

The studies of Hayes and Claman[122] suggest that differences may exist between the marrow and spleen as far as their potential for B-cell generation is concerned. When mice were rendered immunoincompetent by 500-r whole-body irradiation, the ability of bone marrow to generate antibody-forming cells against sheep erythrocytes recovered to a normal level within 11 days, while in the spleen this recovery had reached only 3 to 4% of normal. It is not known, of course, whether the regeneration of B-cell activity was effected by stem cells or by surviving B-cell precursor. The findings fall well in line with the work of Osmond,[123] Stocker,[124] and Ryser and Vassalli.[125] These groups of investigators, who employ similar experimental approaches, present evidence on the presence of B-lymphocyte precursors in murine bone marrow. Their work suggests that B-cell precursors migrate via the blood from the marrow to the spleen.

Transitional cells are believed to be the morphologic progenitors of the small lymphocytes in the marrow. Most small lymphocytes in the marrow of the guinea pig turn over at a rapid rate and 40 to 50% display Ig receptors. Both pale and basophilic transitional cells specifically bind polyvalent ^{125}I-labeled rabbit antiguinea pig Ig antibody.[5] In all size categories, the percentage of labeling was found to be higher in the pale than in basophilic transitional cells. The smaller cells in the pale population had the largest proportion of Ig-positivity. This increase in antigen labeling, related inversely to cell size, correlated well with the proportion of small lymphocytes that displayed surface-bound Ig. The same correlation of size and labeling did not hold true for basophilic transitional cells.

It is thus suggested that in the process of marrow lymphocyte production cell transformation progresses from large to small cells, the data indicates that pale transitional cells are preferentially committed to generating small lymphocytes with detectable Ig molecules. The density of Ig receptors per cell was found to increase inversely with the change in cell size and was the highest in small lymphocytes. Small lymphocytes of the marrow are less densely labeled with anti-Ig than small lymphocytes in the spleen; the significance of this is unknown.

In the mouse, however, neither Osmond and Nossal[123] nor Ryser and Vassali[125] could demonstrate Ig on transitional cells. Both groups of investigators presented evidence that small lymphocytes of the marrow with demonstrable surface Ig were derived without cell division from small lymphocytes that carried neither T nor B cell markers (null cells). Ryser and Vassalli[125] showed that the same hold true for the appearance of the B-lymphocyte-specific-antigen. The small lymphocytes which, in the marrow, acquired Ig or other B-cell markers, were produced by proliferating transitional cells devoid of surface markers. The evidence was obtained by double radioautography with TdR-^{3}H and ^{125}I-labeled anti-Ig.[123] The immunoglobulin marker did not appear on small lymphocytes until 1-1/2 to 2 days after they had been produced by transitional cells which incorporated TdR-^{3}H. It is likely that in guinea pig marrow studies of Rosse[5] a proportion of small lymphocytes devoid of T- and B-cell markers fulfills the same function as in the mouse. However, in the guinea pig, surface Ig is already expressed in some of the proliferating progenitors of bone marrow small lymphocytes. It is possible that, in the course of the generative cycle, the membrane molecules that characterizes B cells appear sooner in the guinea pig than in the mouse.

The precursor B-cell population of guinea pig marrow resembles more closely the B-cell precursor found in the bursa of chicks than the case seems to be with mouse marrow. Practically all large lymphocytes of the bursa are Ig positive and presumably generate a progeny of Ig-positive small lymphocytes.[26]

The differentiation and functional maturation of B lymphocytes is a process that is accomplished step by step over a period of several days. It is appropriate to regard the B-cell progenitor pool as a heterogenous population which contains committed cells in various stages of differentiation.

The first recognizable member of the B-lymphocyte series (pre-B cells) can be found in the fetal liver and is characterized by the presence of small amounts of intracytoplasmic IgM but they, as mentioned previously, completely lack surface immunoglobulin. This fact has demonstrated as early as the 12th day of gestation in the mouse and in human fetuses 5 to 7 weeks.[126–128] At the time intracytoplasmic IgM is expressed in human lymphocytes the membrane receptor for mouse erythrocytes (MRBC rosette) appears.[129] Whether MRBC receptors or cytoplasmic immunoglobulin is expressed first is at present undetermined. Thus, the first identifiable stage of B-cell differentiation from transitional cells (pluripotent stem cells) probably involves MRBC receptor and/or cytoplasmic IgM expression. The MRBC receptors persist but cytoplasmic IgM is lost.[126,129] Surface Ig subsequently appears in the mouse within about 4 days.[130,131] The presence of some cells which show both intracytoplasmic and surface Ig suggests a maturation sequence.[132] The in vitro studies of Owen et al.[133] indicate that precursor cells carrying cytoplasmic IgM (cIgM) proliferate and give rise to small cIgM lymphocytes which simultaneously express IgM on their surface. Other markers of lymphocyte differentiation do not appear in the mouse until after birth. At this time there is a rapid rise in the percentage of B cells bearing Fc receptors. Gupta et al.[134] and Kagan et al.[129] demonstrated that the receptor for the Fc region of heat-aggregated IgG is an early B-cell marker and is expressed on human fetal liver lymphocytes as early as surface IgM. Surface IgG follows the appearance of surface IgM[126,132] and may be detected as early as 3 days after birth in mice,[135,136] and the percentage of IgD-positive cells rises steadily thereafter, until at 3 months it is quantitively the dominant cell surface immunoglobulin.[137]

The last of the well-established differentiation markers of the B-lymphocyte series to appear is the C3 receptor; C3R-positive B cells first appear in the mice on the 10th day of postnatal life and rise rapidly in number during the following few days.[138] The studies of Hammerling, Chin, and Abbott[139] suggest the existence of a maturation sequence in which Ig-negative, Ia-negative, C3R-negative cells acquire first Ig and finally C3R.

Melchers[140] employed an in vitro technique to calculate the frequency of "pre B cells" in mouse fetal liver. He found the frequency to be 1 in 106 at day 13 of gestation and this rose steadily to 1 in 30 on the 19th day. It is of interest that in vitro the maturation process only proceeded efficiently in the presence of adult thymus cells. Other authors have found that B lymphocytes from mouse fetuses or neonates produce antibody responses of restricted heterogeneity compared with B cells from animals 10 or more days old.[141] Subsequently they have suggested that the lack of heterogeneity is not due to any intrinsic lack of genetic information for the production of a heterogeneous response, but is due to the absence of maturational influence of thymus cells.[142,143] The capacity of thymus cells to provide this maturational influence only occurs 7 to 10 days after birth. These studies raise the possibility that the thymus has an influence on the maturation of B lymphocytes.

IV. IMMUNOLOGIC FUNCTIONS OF MARROW CELLS

As expanded on in previous sections the reticular macrophages form a loose and incomplete syncytium in the bone marrow. The cells are in direct contact with the sinusoidal lining cells as well as with islands of erythrocytes. These cells play a role in antibody formation. Evidence has accumulated to support the hypothesis that the reticular macrophage remove antigens and processes the antigen for transfer to the appropriate antibody producing cells.[144,145] Macrophages are in close proximity to plasma cells and lymphocytes; Thiery[146] demonstrated plasma cell islands surrounding macrophages. In addition, cytoplasmic interaction between the reticular macrophage and plasma cells has been demonstrated as well as transfer of particles through a connecting corridor of cytoplasm.[147,148] Azar et al.[149] in an electron microscopic study of syphilitic chancres found treponema in plasma cells and macrophages. Similarly, cytoplasmic bridges between macrophages as well as cytoplasmic flow in these bridges with transfer of bacilli has been demonstrated.[150] This proposed antigenic processing is believed to be the first step in antibody formation.

The important role of macrophages in lymphocyte induction is well documented.[151] Although the nature of the contribution made by macrophages is not fully defined, their role has been referred to as "accessory." In the last few years a number of antigen nonspecific macrophage-derived soluble factors with both positive and negative immunomodulating properties have been reported.[152,153] The requirement for macrophages is in the production of cytotoxic T cells; T-helper cell cultures also require macrophages for their continuous growth.[154] Additionally, macrophage factors are mitogenic for T cells although they are not capable of sustaining continuous growth themselves.[155]

Two macrophage factors have been identified:

1. Interleükin-1, which is characterized by a molecular weight of 12 to 18,000 daltons, isoelectric point of 6.5 to 7.5, pH2 insensitive, no Ia, unrestricted species activity, and whose distinguishing bioactivity is in the facilitation of the induction of cytotoxic T cell responses
2. Interleükin-2, which is characterized by a molecular weight of 30 to 35,000 daltons, an isoelectric point of 3.5 to 5.5, requires both T cells and macrophages for its production, and whose distinguishing bioactivity is the ability to promote and maintain long-term cytotoxic T cells in culture [156]

Unanue[157] demonstrated that marrow cells, which bind a specific antigen, will be differentiated specifically to respond to that antigen. Similarly, the antibody response to the antigen keyhole limpet hemocyanin (KLH) was markedly impaired in lethally irradiated mice that received bone marrow cells pretreated with a highly radioactive hemocyanin which was likely to kill cells that bound it. Specific binding of labeled antigen has been demonstrated in human marrow cells and human marrow cells have been shown to respond to several antigens.[158] It would appear that the bone marrow does contribute to the antibody response of the host. The magnitude and significance is unknown. The capacity of marrow cells to make antibodies has been correlated with the plasma cell content of the marrow.[159] However, antibodies are also secreted by other cells of varied morphology which include lymphocytes.[160–162] Presumably, it appears necessary that antibody forming cells and/or their precursors within the marrow cooperate with T cells. It is not known whether immunization with T-cell-dependent antigens brings about blood or lymph T-cell migration into the marrow (long-lived lymphocytes) or that the marrow prethymic T-cell pool interacts with the antibody forming cells.

Miller and Cudkowicz[163] demonstrated that marrow cells develop a secondary immune response three to five times greater than obtained with unprimed marrow cells. The secondary antibody response of rat marrow cells to tetanus toxoid is mediated by cells which are not eliminated by chronic thoracic duct drainage, i.e., T cells.[164] This does not imply that circulating T cells plays no role in immunologic memory of marrow cells but it does emphasize the necessity for considering the role of noncirculating cells, or cells that do not circulate via central lymph. At the present time we can say that the marrow contains cells with immune memory, but no statement can be made regarding their identity, origin, or circulating characteristics.

The above data raises the question of the marrow role in the induction of immunological tolerance. The in vitro proliferative response of rabbit marrow cells to a variety of antigens was eliminated when the cells were exposed to high antigen concentrations. The response to other, noncross-reacting antigens, was unaffected.[165] In the rabbit, studies have confirmed these data.[166] Kaplan and Cinader,[167] in mice, showed that immunological unresponsiveness resided in the differentiated, i.e., SIg-bearing B-cell population of the marrow but that their precursors generate a progeny which is no longer unresponsive. Thus, the duration of immunologic tolerance in the marrow is determined by the life span of tolerant B cells and their length of residence within the marrow. The unresponsiveness state is of shorter duration in the marrow than in the thymus.

Human and other primate marrow contain immunocompetent cells in sufficiently high concentrations to limit the therapeutic uses of bone marrow transplantation, due to the acute and chronic lethal reactions mounted by the transplanted cells against the tissues of a genetically incompatible host. This graft-vs.-host reaction is considered a cell mediated immune response. Presumably, only a fraction of marrow lymphocytes react against histocompatibility antigens (HLA). In vitro treatment of marrow cells with antithymocyte serum eliminates the graft-vs.-host reaction.[168] There are several reports supporting the T lymphocyte as the HLA-reactive cells in the marrow. Chronic thoracic duct drainage depletes rat marrow of HLA reactive cells[169] and eliminates cells which react with antithymocyte serum.[170] Following hydrocortisone lysis of mouse T cells further suggests that histocompatibility antigen-reactive lymphocytes of the marrow are likely to be part of the circulating pool of T cells.[171]

In spite of these findings, the possibility exists that the GVH reaction is, in part, truly mediated by marrow B cells. This caution is based on the fact that marrow-derived B lymphocytes were required together with thymocytes for the cell mediated killing of allogeneic cells[172] and that GVH reactive lymphocytes are generated in the bone marrow of thymectomized, bone marrow-reconstituted mice.[173] It must be remembered, however, that prethymic T cells are found in marrow, and that in these experiments the design has not ruled out the possibility of contaminating T cells from blood and/or lymph.[62]

The precursors of histocompatibility antigen-reactive lymphocytes that reside in the marrow are nonmigrating.[169,174] In the mouse these precursor cells sediment on a density gradient in different fractions than the immunocompetent lymphocytes.[175–177] Only the fraction containing the precursors were capable of repopulating the thymus; the fractions that contained the immunocompetent cells were not.[178] The precursors were also shown to acquire histocompatibility antigen reactivity if they were circulated in a perfusate through the thymus.[175] These nonmigrating population cells have characteristics of prethymocytes so that these data also must be viewed cautiously.

V. BONE MARROW MANIFESTATIONS OF LYMPHOPROLIFERATIVE DISORDERS AND HODGKIN'S DISEASE

The distinction between lymphoproliferative disease in the marrow and benign lymphoid lesions is of critical clinical importance. Although most lymphoproliferative disease involving the marrow are detected as part of a clinical staging procedure. Bone marrow involvement by lymphoid malignancies is frequently encountered as part of a diagnostic evaluation for an abnormal peripheral blood picture, fever of unknown causes, or unexplained lymphadenopathy and organomegaly. Because the demonstration of marrow involvement is *a priori* evidence of systemic disease its detection is of therapeutic significance. Bone marrow involvement is also important for diagnosing recurrent disease and in monitoring the efficacy of chemotherapy.

A. Anatomical Distribution of Normal Marrow Lymphocytes

The bone marrow contains small and large lymphoid cells. Together, these cells total one quarter of all nucleated marrow cells in adult mice (5×10^5 lymphocytes per mm^3 of marrow); in younger animals the total lymphoid population is even greater. It has been estimated that the whole marrow organ contains a population of lymphocytes considerably larger than that seen in the spleen.

The many lymphocytes found in human marrow are either dispersed or are found as aggregates or nodules. By definition, these nodular structures of lymphoid tissue are composed of lymphoid cells, devoid of myeloid and adipose tissue, and most importantly, devoid of venous sinuses. Benign lymphoid aggregates vary in size from less than 50 to greater than 1000 mm^3 in diameter. The number per biopsy specimen varies from a solitary nodule to numerous scattered nodules. They are randomly distributed with no predilection for a paratrabecular distribution. They are well circumscribed and clearly demarcated from the surrounding marrow. When nodules are particularly large and numerous it may be difficult to distinguish benign lymphoid hyperplasis from well-differentiated lymphocytic (small cell) lymphoma. Lymphoid nodules are invariably supplied by arterial vessels. Careful sectioning of lymphocyte aggregates show that each aggregate has one or several branches of an artery. Entwining along with the arterial vessels one can see argyrophilic fibers formed into a fibrillar net extending from the center of the nodule toward its periphery and some forming into a concentric retial sac at the margin of the nodule.[179] Another type of concentric, fibrillar pattern is seen in the layers of lymphocyte around germinal centers in the rare nodules that contain centers. The presence of fibers serves as a criterion in distinguishing between a true lymphocyte aggregate and a lymphomatous infiltration. Most aggregates lack germinal centers or mitotic figures. When germinal centers contain cells in mitosis a marked inflammatory response is occurring in the host.[180]

The frequency of occurrence of lymphocyte aggregates has varied, ranging from 60% in Fischer's[181] work to 3% in the reports of Rohr.[182] In Hashimoto's series[183] aggregates were seen in 26% of cases. These later investigators obtained specimens somewhat indiscriminately from different bones, and therefore suggested that lymphoid aggregates are more numerous than their data indicates. In large autopsy series the incidence is from 25 to 30%. Nodule detectability is directly related to the hematopoietic activity of the marrow sample; they are rarely detected in fatty marrow. The earliest period of life in which lymphocyte aggregates occur is 10 months after birth.[184] In general, detectability of aggregates in human marrow varies with age—lower in infancy and greater in later life. In people greater than 60 years of age the percentage of cases with detectable aggregates is 40%.

Occasionally bone marrow specimens with nonmalignant and nonhematologic disorders contain increased numbers of lymphoid appearing cells that are characterized by sparse cytoplasm and hyperchromatic nuclei that are frequently indented or have irregular outlines. These are referred to as hematogones. These cells vary in size but range between 10 to 20 μm. They are present in low numbers of very young children and probably represent marrow precursor cells, e.g., transitional cells. They are most commonly found in increased numbers in the marrow of children with diverse disorders as iron-deficiency anemia, neuroblastoma, and ITP. Because they are hyperchromatic with indented nuclei they may be misinterpreted as lymphoma cells. Unlike lymphoma cells hematogones do not manifest prominent nucleoli. The chromatin is very clumped and homogeneous in appearance. In bone marrow sections hematogones do not form dense accumulations, as lymphoma cells usually do.

B. Hodgkin's Disease (HD)

Marrow involvement by HD is usually found by marrow biopsies or sections of marrow particle preparations. Because of the invariable fibrosis found in marrow involved with HD an aspiration smear is of limited value although occasionally a Reed-Sternberg cell may be identified.

The incidence of marrow involvement in HD ranges from 5 to 23% in studies analyzing treated and untreated patients.[185] The marrow at the time may be the only diagnostic tissue obtainable. Because the histopathology of the marrow lesions in HD may not be identical to that obtained by lymph node biopsy classification of HD is difficult by marrow analysis alone.

A histologic diagnosis of HD in the marrow requires the demonstration of Reed-Sternberg (RS) cells. The classic type of RS cell is a large cell with abundant acidophilic cytoplasm which is often pyroninophilic. It may contain two or more nuclei or a lobated nucleus with prominent, large, acidophilic nucleoli that have perinucleolar halo (Figure 2). Three RS variants have been described:

1. The lacunar-type, seen predominating in the nodular sclerosis type
2. A polypoid type, seen predominating in lymphocyte-predominant histology
3. A pleomorphic, sarcomatous variant seen in lymphocyte-depleted type

The histopathologic criteria for the diagnosis of HD in marrow has been defined by the Committee on Histopathological Criteria Contributing to Staging of HD. HD in marrow can be diagnosed when Reed-Sternberg (RS) cells are found in the cellular environment containing swirls of fibrous tissue together with lymphocytes, plasma cells, eosinophils, histiocytes, and fibroblasts. The presence of the mononuclear cell

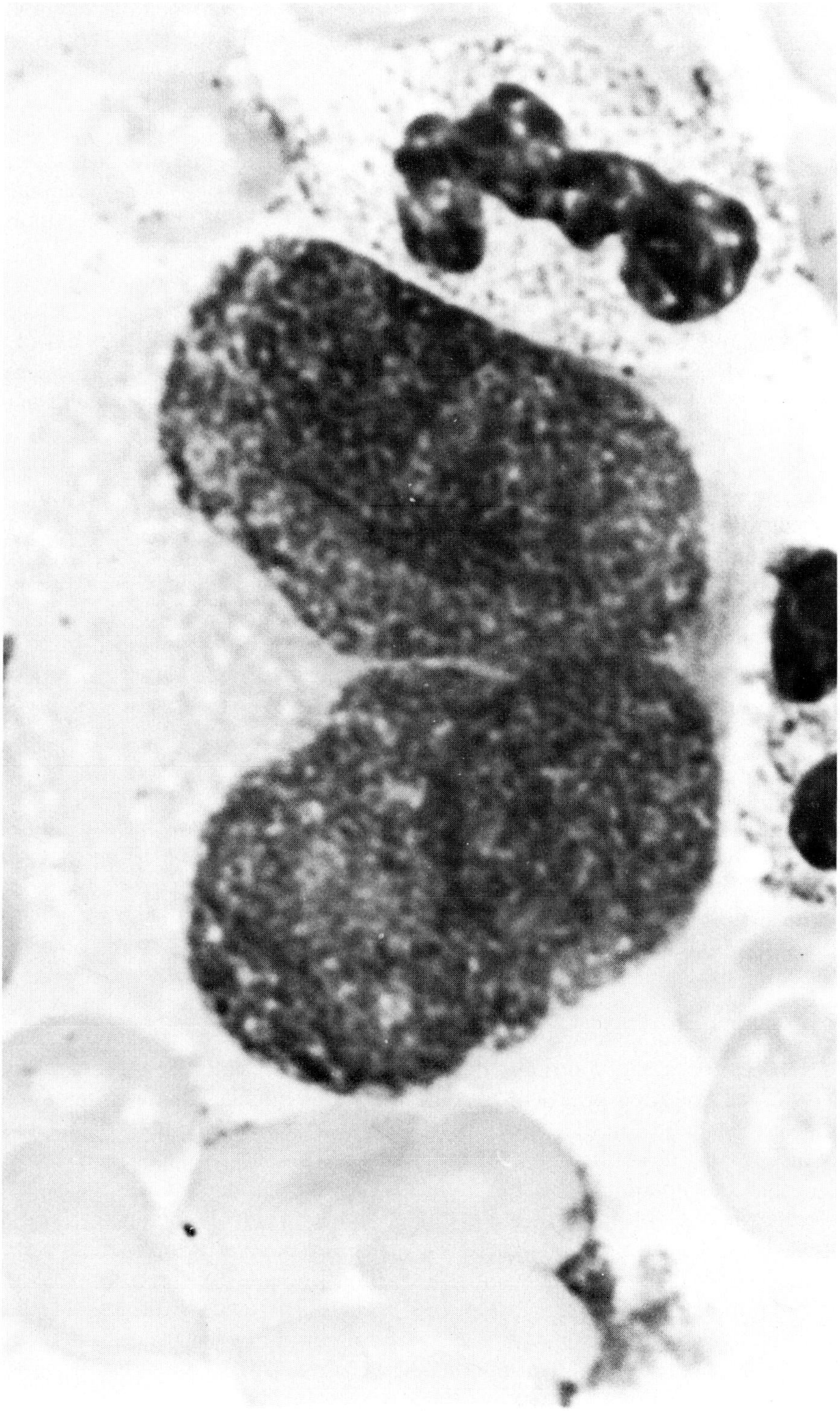

FIGURE 2. A Reed-Sternberg cell in the marrow. Approximately ×2000.

environment described should be regarded as indicative of marrow involvement. The presence of histiocytes, not characteristic of RS cells, in the polycellular environment or focal or diffuse area of fibrosis is highly suggestive of marrow HD. The finding of marrow fibrosis alone should be considered suspicious for HD; however, the diagnosis must be proven by lymph node biopsy.[185,186]

The pattern of marrow HD is highly variable. The most common pattern (80%) is diffuse involvement. In this situation HD tissue occupies the entire area between the bony trabeculae. A focal pattern is characterized by isolated lesions that are completely surrounded by normal marrow cells or are paratrabecular in location. Reticulum and collagen fibrosis is characteristic of all HD involving the marrow.

The cellular infiltrate in HD marrow is subject to considerable variation. The lesions may consist of polycellular infiltrate, and may in some cases lack some of the specific cell types or rarely be composed solely of lymphocytic proliferation. The areas of marrow uninvolved with disease may be normal or demonstrate nonspecific changes such as myeloid hyperplasia. In cases of lymphocyte-depleted HD the surrounding marrow may be hypoplastic. In an analysis of marrow from HD patients by te Velde et al.,[196] the unaffected marrow was characterized by specific damage, inflammatory infiltrates, disturbed hematopoiesis and intramedullary phagocytosis. The disturbed erythropoiesis was correlated to the stage of the disease.

A certain amount of caution must be exercised in interpreting marrow sections even if characteristic RS cells are identified, since RS-like cells have been reported in myeloproliferative disease, myeloma, and chronic lymphocytic leukemia.[185] Lesions of the marrow most commonly causing difficulty in the diagnosis of HD include noncaseating granulomas and benign lymphoid nodules. It has been reported that 12% of patients with HD with no marrow involvement at the time of diagnosis exhibit granulomas or lymphoid aggregates.

C. Lymphoma and Leukemia

The topic of marrow involvement in malignant lymphoma has been the subject of several recent reports. Since 80% of all lymphoma present with marrow invasion, marrow interpretation is critical in patient care.

Well-differentiated (small cell) lymphocytic lymphoma (WDL) is a tumor which is considered the tissue counterpart of chronic lymphocytic leukemia. At the present time no definite morphologic criteria differentiate CLL from WDL. CLL is defined as an absolute lymphocytosis ($>5000/\mu\ell$) in the blood; WDL is defined as marrow infiltration with small lymphocytes but with no peripheral lymphocytosis. The lymphocytes from WDL are considered a proliferation of B cells, whereas, CLL appears to involve an abnormal proliferation of T and B cells.[187] Cell membrane immunoglobulin is detected in sparse amounts in CLL lymphocytes and in ''normal'' amounts on WDL cells. CLL lymphocytes in addition, have high frequency avidity for mouse erythrocytes, whereas, B-cell lymphomas in leukemic phase lack these receptors.

In the marrow the lymphocytes are extremely uniform in cell and nuclear size, configuration, and chromatin pattern. There is a sparse rim of clear cytoplasm. The nucleus is round without evidence of indentation or clefting. The nuclear chromatin shows considerable clumping. Nucleoli are absent. In WDL the marrow is infiltrated diffusely or in a focal pattern. The focal pattern has poorly circumscribed margins without a predilection for a paratrabecular distribution. Approximately 70% of WDL present in a nonparatrabecular pattern.[188]

Poorly differentiated lymphocytic lymphoma (PDL) in the Rappaport classification exists as a nodular or diffuse type. Both are diseases of the follicular center cell. Approximately 40% of cases of diffuse PDL present with marrow involvement. The diffuse

PDL have diverse morphologic patterns. The cells are large but vary in size. Cytoplasm is sparse to moderate and slightly basophilic. Cytoplasm vacuoles may be present. The vacuoles usually stain positively with PAS. The chromatin is hyperchromatic. Clefting and nuclei folding is common and nucleoli are variable in number.[185,189]

Marrow sections may show minimal or focal tumor, or the entire marrow may be infiltrated. Large areas of lymphomatous involvement may be in direct apposition to normal hemopoietic tissue. Bone trabeculae commonly form a demarcation line. Occasionally, the lymphomatous lesion is composed of histiocytes or epitheloid cells.

In nodular PDL, Rosenberg[190] reported marrow involvement at initial presentation to be 85%. Brunning's series reported a 54% incidence. Marrow involvement in the majority of cases is characterized by focal infiltrates frequently in a paratrabecular distribution. Occasionally, focal lesions simulate germinal centers and proteinaceous material may be observed within the lymphomatous nodule in a fashion similar to that seen in lymph nodes. If we analyze marrow biopsies according to the Lukes-Collins classification small cleaved follicular center cell (FCC) lymphomas have the highest incidence of marrow involvement and noncleaved the least frequent. Small cleaved FCC have the greater tendency for a paratrabecular distribution, i.e., 65%.[188]

Cytologically, nodular PDL lymphoma in the marrow may reveal large transformed lymphocytes, i.e., immunoblasts. Brunning et al.[185] have described a "small nodular lymphoma" cell in patients with marrow involvement. The cell measures 7 to 10 μ with a uniformly staining, frequently indented nucleus. These investigators feel that this cell when seen is highly suggestive of nodular PDL lymphoma (FCC). In a minority of nodular PDL patients the marrow contains large numbers of histocytes with abundant eosinophilic cytoplasm and nucleoli. These lesions must be distinguished from HD and Lennert's lymphoma.

Barcos and Lukes[191] described a lymphocytic lymphoma which is distinguishable from PDL by a high mitotic index and its morphologic similarity with acute lymphoblastic leukemia cells. Clinically, these tumors present with a mediastinal mass early and blood-marrow involvement as the disease progresses. In some patients marrow involvement is present at the time of diagnosis.

Two major morphologic subtypes can be distinguished, one with a convoluted nucleus, and another with a nonconvoluted nucleus. The convoluted type contains a somewhat small cell and manifests a high incidence of cells exhibiting prolymphocytic differentiation. This lymphoma may be distinguished from the lymphoblastic type in that the former has extreme nuclear contortion. The lymphoma cells stain strongly with acid phosphatase, usually in a focal paranuclear distribution. Involvement of the marrow is generally diffuse. The origin of lymphoblastic lymphoma cells is believed to be the T cell.[191]

The three categories of acute lymphoblastic leukemia (ALL) as designated by the French-American-British group are the common childhood type (L_1), the adult, morphologically heterogeneous group (L_2), and the very rare Burkitt-like group (L_3). Immunologic studies using antisera against common ALL antigen (cALL), human T cell antigen (HuTLA), the ability to form E-rosettes (ER), and to fluoresce membrane Ig are used to classify ALL (in adults and children) into common ALL (cALLA +; 40% of children, 30% of adults), common T cell ALL (cALLA +, HuTLA +; 31% of children, 15% of adults), pre-T-ALL (cALLA−, HuTLA +, ER−; 13% of children, 17% of adults), and T-ALL (HuTLA +, ER+; 13% children 17% adults). The remaining few percent are B cell (sIg + only). Cytochemically, coarse granular PAS positivity is seen in all forms except pre-T-ALL; similarly, acid phosphatase (granular and/or paranuclear pattern) staining and acid esterase staining are present in all groups (excluding B-ALL). Definite survival advantage following therapy is seen in the cALL group when compared to other subtypes.[192] There appears to be a clear correlation between immunologic subtype and clinical response when both children and adults are analyzed independently.[193,194] The immunologic subtypes of ALL have been expanded greatly by the use of monoclonal antibodies, but at the present time, add no further insight into the therapy of ALL.

Undifferentiated lymphoma, Burkitt's type (small noncleaved), patients are generally young adults, who tend to present initially with abdominal disease. The lymphoma is FCC in origin. Approximately 50% of patients present initially with marrow involvement. The FAB classification places this lymphoma when in leukemia phase into the L3 group. Cytologically, the cells are large with intensely basophilic cytoplasm. Nucleoli are multiple. The cytoplasm tends to contain multiple oil-O staining vacuoles; the cytoplasm itself stains intensely with methyl green pyronine.[186] Nuclear chromatin in finely distributed and marrow involvement in this lymphoma is usually extensive.[185,186] Although nodal tissue characteristically show numerous macrophages, i.e., ''starry sky'' appearance, this finding is absent from marrow sections. Mitotic figures are abundant and the cells are relatively uniform in size. The cell membrane Ig staining pattern is ''dot-like'' rather than the ring pattern of the other lymphomata.

Marrow involvement in histiocytic (large cell) lymphoma (HL) as classified in the Rappaport scheme occurs infrequently (approximately 5 to 25% of cases).[186–190] The pattern of marrow involvement may be focal or diffuse without a paratrabecular predilection. Cell size is extremely variable as is nuclear size. In the Lukes-Collins scheme large FCC lymphomas have a 30% incidence of bone marrow involvement.[188]

Cytologically HL included a spectrum of cells including immunoblasts to histiocytes with large nuclei and abundant cytoplasm. The histiocytes may approach the size of megakaryocytes. The cells may contain azurophilic granules; the cell outline is generally irregular with pseudopod formation common.

The cell of origin of HL is a point of controversy but true ''histiocytic lymphoma'' is rare. Cell membrane marker studies suggest that 60% of the malignant cells B cells origin and 60% have no detectable markers but morphologically resemble B-cell lymphomata. In a minority of cases the HL are truly derived from the monocyte-macrophage line which originates exclusively in marrow. Straus et al.[195] used agar culture techniques to demonstrate leukemic cluster formation in 11 of 15 cases of true HL. Morphologically these cells could be classified as acute monocytic leukemia (M5a, M5b) using the FAB scheme. The patients responded to leukemic therapy.[195]

Cytologically, the cells in hairy cell leukemia(LR) show a moderate rim of cytoplasm and a delicate nuclear chromatin structure intermediate between coarse and evenly distributed. The nuclear outline is contorted and may be clefted or monocytoid in configuration. Nucleoli tend to be prominent. The most frequent misdiagnosis applied to LR cases is PDL. The LR cell can be characterized histochemically by the presence of tartrate resistant acid phosphatase activity. A variable percent of cells stain with PAS and α-naphthyl acetate esterase. The cytoplasm contains numerous vacuoles and the cytoplasmic outline is irregular with delicate cytoplasmic projections. It is perhaps best appreciated under phase contrast microscopy. The surface Ig staining is bright but cIg is absent. No mouse erythrocyte or complement receptors are detectable.

The marrow is difficult to aspirate in LR and ''dry taps'' are common; LR, like other lymphomas, may present as a focal or diffuse pattern. In LR, however, the cellular infiltrate is loosely structured in a random distribution. In PDL, the cells are in close opposition and the tumor infiltrate is usually compact.

REFERENCES

1. **Yoffey, J. M.,** Stem cell role: lymphocyte-transition cell in LT compartment, in *Haemopoietic Stem Cells,* Ciba Found. Symp., Elsevier, North-Holland, 1973, 5.

1a. **McCulloch, E.,** Cellular communication early in hemopoietic differention, *Haemopoietic Stem Cells,* Ciba Found. Symp., Elsevier, North-Holland, 1973, 183.

2. **Yoshida, Y. and Osmond, D. G.,** Identification and proliferation of small lymphocyte precursors in culture of lymphocyte-rich fractions of guinea pig bone marrow, *Blood,* 37, 73, 1971.
3. **Miller, S. C. and Osmond, D. G.,** The proliferation of lymphoid cells in guinea pig bone marrow, *Cell Tissue Kinet.,* 6, 259, 1973.
4. **Yoffey, J. M., Thomas, D. B., Moffat, D. J., Sutherland, I. H., and Rosse, C.,** Biological Activity of the Leucocyte, *Ciba Found. Study Group,* 10, 45, 1961.
5. **Rosse, C.,** Small lymphocyte and transitional cell populations of bone marrow: their role in the mediation of immune and hemopoietic progenitor cell functions, *Int. Rev. Cytol.,* 45, 155, 1976.
6. **Rosse, C. and Yoffey, J. M.,** The morphology of the transitional lymphocyte in guinea pig bone marrow, *J. Anat.,* 102, 113, 1967.
7. **Yoffey, J. M., Hudson, G., and Osmond, D. G.,** The lymphocyte in guinea pig bone marrow, *J. Anat.,* 99, 841, 1965.
8. **Simar, L. J., Hact, J., and Betz, E. H.,** Etude Ultrastructurale de la Moelle Hematopoietique au Cours de la Regeneration apres Irradiation, *Eur. J. Cancer,* 4, 529, 1968.
9. **Yoffey, J. M. and Courtice, F. C.,** *Lymphatics, Lymph and the Lymphomyeloid Complex,* Academic Press, New York, 1970.
10. **Rosse, C. and Trotter, J. A.,** Cytochemical and radioautographic identification of cells induced to synthesize hemoglobin, *Blood,* 43, 885, 1974.
11. **Garcia, A. M. and Sullivan, S. A. N.,** The ribonucleic acid and deoxyribonucleic acid content of mononuclear leukocytes of different sizes studied by ultraviolet cytophotometry, *J. Histochem. Cytochem.,* 21, 628, 1973.
12. **Frenster, J. H., Allfrey, V. G., and Mirsky, A. E.,** Repressed and active chromatin isolated from interphase lymphocytes, *Proc. Natl. Acad. Sci., U.S.A.,* 50, 1026, 1963.
13. **Littau, V. C., Allfrey, V. G., Frenster, J. H., and Mirsky, A. E.,** Active and inactive regions of nuclear chromatin as revealed by electron microscopic autoradiography, *Proc. Nat. Acad. Sci., U.S.A.,* 52, 93, 1964.
14. **To-Kuyasu, K., Madden, S. C., and Zeldis, L. J.,** Fine structural alterations of interphase nuclei of lymphocyte stimulated to growth actively *in vitro, J. Cell. Biol.,* 39, 630, 1968.
15. **Moffat, D. J., Rosse, C., and Yoffey, J. M.,** Identity of the hemopoietic stem cell, *Lancet,* 2, 547, 1967.
16. **Osmond, D. G., Miller, S. C., and Yoshida, Y.,** in Kinetics and hemopoietic properties of lymphoid cells, *Haemopoietic Stem Cells,* Ciba Found. Symp., North-Holland, 1973.
17. **Pathak, V. B., Reinhardt, W. D., and Yoffey, J. M.,** Lymphocytes in thoracic duct lymph and bone marrow of the guinea pig, *J. Reticuloendothel. Soc.,* 7, 197, 1968.
18. **Ackerman, G. A.,** in *Regulation of Hematopoiesis,* Vol. II, Gordon, A. S., Eds., Appleton, New York, 1971, 1297.
19. **Ambs, E. and Granemeyer, R.,** Die Mukleden-morphologue van lymphozyten des peripheren blutes, *Acta Haematol.,* 68, 104, 1972.
20. **Rosse, C. and Trotter, J. A.,** A cytochemical and radioautographic analysis of erythropoiesis at the ultrastructural level, *Am. J. Anat.,* 141, 41, 1974.
21. **Ben-Ishay, Z. and Yoffey, J. M.,** Ultrastructural studies of erythroblastic islands of rat bone marrow, II. The resumption of erythropoiesis in erythropoietically depressed rebound marrow, *Lab. Invest.,* 26, 637, 1972.
22. **Yoffey, J. M.,** *Bone Marrow in Hypoxia and Rebound,* Charles C. Thomas, Springfield, Ill., 1974.
23. **Safier, S., Cottier, H., Cronkite, E. P., Jansen, C. R., Kanti, R., and Wagner, H. P.,** Studies on lymphocytes. VI. Evidence showing different generation times for cytologically different lymphoid cell lines in the thoracic duct of the calf, *Blood,* 30, 301, 1967.
24. **Beathard, G. A., Fish, J. C., Folse, D. S., Sarles, H. E., Remmers, A. R., and Ritzmann, S. E.,** Characterization of lymphocytes in calf thoracic duct lymph, *J. Reticuloendothel. Soc.,* 10, 293, 1971.
25. **Tanaka, Y. and Goodman, G. R.,** *Electron Microscopy of Human Blood Cells,* Harper, New York, 1972.
26. **Glick, B., Perkins, W. D., Rosse, C., and Schwartz, M. R.,** Comparison of lymphocyte population bearing surface immunoglobulins in avian bone marrow, bursa and spleen, *Int. Arch. Allergy. Appl. Immunol.,* 49, 332, 1975.

27. **Clawson, C. C., Cooper, M. D. and Good, R. A.,** Lymphocyte fine structure in the bursa of Fabricius, the thymus and the germinal center, *Lab. Invest.,* 16, 407, 1967.
28. **Leene, W., Duyzings, M. J. M., and van Steeg, J.,** Lymphoid stem cell identification in the developing thymus and bursa of Fabricius in the chick, *Zelforsds. Mikrask. Anat.,* 136, 521, 1973.
29. **Thomas, D. B., Russel, P. M., and Yoffey, J. M.,** Pattern of haematopoiesis in the fetal liver, *Nature,* 187, 876, 1960.
30. **Thomas, D. B.,** Radiation chimaeras as an experimental model for stem cells, in *Haemopoietic Stem Cells,* Ciba Found. Symp., Elsevier, North-Holland, 1973.
31. **Thomas, D. B. and Yoffey, J. M.,** Human fetal haemopoiesis in the cellular composition of fetal blood, *Br. J. Haematol.,* 8, 290, 1962.
32. **Yoffey, J. M.,** The stem cell problem in the fetus, *Gen. Med. Sci.,* 7, 825, 1971.
33. **Winter, G. C. B., Byles, A. B., and Yoffey, J. M.,** Blood lymphocytes in newborn and adult, *Lancet,* 2, 932, 1965.
34. **Blackfan, K. D. and Diamond, L. K.,** *Atlas of Blood in Children,* Oxford University Press, London, 1944.
35. **Yoffey, J. M., Winter, G. C. B., Osmond, D. G., and Meek, E. S.,** Morphological studies in the culture of human leukocytes with phytohaemagglutinin, *Br. J. Haematol.,* 11, 688, 1965.
36. **Rosse, C.,** In *Haematopoietic Stem Cells,* Ciba Found. Symp., Elsevier, North-Holland, 1973.
37. **Zucker-Franklin, D.,** The ultrastructure of the lymphocytes, *Semin. Haematol.,* 6, 4, 1969.
38. **Douglas, S. D.,** Electron microscopic and functional aspects of human lymphocyte responses to mitogens, *Transplant. Rev.,* 11, 39, 1972.
39. **Douglas, S. D.,** Human lymphocyte growth *in vitro:* morphologic, biochemical and immunologic significance, *Int. Rev. Exp. Pathol.,* 10, 41, 1971.
40. **Curry, J. L. and Trentin, J. J.,** Hemopoietic spleen colony studies. I. Growth and differentiation, *Dev. Biol.,* 15, 395, 1967.
41. **Abramson, S., Miller, R. G., and Philips, R. A.,** The identification in adult bone marrow of pluripotent and restricted stem cells of the myeloid and lymphoid systems, *J. Exp. Med.,* 145, 1567, 1977.
42. **Rosse, C., Griffith, D. A., Edwards, A. E., Gadres, C. G. C., Long, A. L. H., Wright, J. L. W., and Yoffey, J. M.,** Identity of erythroblast precursors in bone marrow, *Acta Haematol.,* 63, 80, 1970.
43. **Orlic, D.,** In *Regulation of Hematopoiesis,* Gordon, A. S., Ed., Vol. 1, Appleton, New York, 1970.
44. **Moore, M. A. S., Williams, N., and Metcalf, D.,** Purification and characterization of the *in vitro* colony forming cell in monkey hemopoietic tissue, *J. Cell. Physiol.,* 79, 283, 1972.
45. **Zucali, J. R., Rakowitz, F., Van Zaut, G., and Gordon, A. S.,** Separation of agar colony forming cells from rat bone marrow, *Proc. Soc. Exp. Med.,* 145, 519, 1974.
46. **Daniels, E.,** *In vitro* colony formation by lymphocyte fractions of guinea pig bone marrow, *Anat. Rec.,* 178, 339, 1974.
47. **Lucas, A. M. and Jonnroz, C.,** in *Atlas of Avian Hematology, U.S. Dep. Agr., Agr. Mono. No. 25,* 1961.
48. **Lukic, M. L., Vujanovic, N. L., and Jankovic, B. D.,** Lymphocyte differentiation in the chicken embryo-relationship to the microenvironment, *Adv. Exp. Med. Biol.,* 29, 27, 1973.
49. **Burkart, P. T. and Meuwisien, H. J.,** Immunocompetent lymphocyte in human and primate marrow, *Transplantation,* 16, 372, 1973.
50. **Borella, L. and Sen, L.,** The distribution of lymphocytes with T and B cell surface markers in human bone marrow, *J. Immunol.,* 112, 836, 1974.
51. **Everett, N. B. and Tyler, R. W.,** Lymphopoiesis in the thymus and other tissues; functional implications, *Int. Rev. Cytol.,* 22, 205, 1967.
52. **Everett, N. B. and Tyler, R. W.,** In *Blood Cells as a Tissue,* Holmes, W. L., Ed., Plenum Press, New York, 1970.
53. **Everett, N. B. and Tyler, R. W.,** In *Formation and Destruction of Blood Cells,* Greenwalt, T. J. and Jameson, G. A., Eds., Lippincott, Philadelphia, 1970, 264.
54. **Osmond, D. G.,** In Proc. Leucocyte Bult. Cong. 6th, Rosario, Washington, 1971.
55. **Yoffey, J. M.,** In *Regulation of Hematopoiesis,* Gordon, A. S., Ed., Vol. 1, Appleton, New York, 1970.
56. **Osmond, D. G. and Everett, N. B.,** Radioautographic studies of bone marrow lymphocytes *in vivo* and in diffusions chambers, *Blood,* 23, 1, 1964.
57. **Osmond, D. B.,** In *The Lymphocyte in Immunology and Haemopoiesis,* Yoffey, J. M., Ed., Arnold, London, 1967.
58. **Rosse, C.,** Lymphocyte production and life-span in the bone marrow of the guinea pig, *Blood,* 38, 372, 1971.

59. **Ropke, C. and Everett, N. B.,** Small lymphocyte populations in the mouse bone marrow, *Cell Tissue Kinet.,* 6, 499, 1973.
60. **Miller, S. C. and Osmond, D. G.,** Quantitative changes with age in bone marrow cell population of C3H mice, *Exp. Hematol.,* 2, 227, 1974.
61. **Rosse, C.,** Migration of long-lived lymphocytes to the bone marrow and to other lymphomyeloid tissues in normal parabiotic guinea pigs, *Blood,* 40, 90, 1972.
62. **Ropke, C. and Everett, N. B.,** Migration of small lymphocytes in adult mice demonstrated by parabiosis, *Cell Tissue Kinet.,* 7, 137, 1974.
63. **Howard, J. G.,** Cellular events in the induction and loss of tolerance of pneumonococcal polysaccharides, *Transplant. Rev.,* 8, 50, 1972.
64. **Sprent, J. and Basten, A.,** Circulating T and B lymphocyte of the mouse. II. Lifespan, *Cell Immunol.,* 7, 40, 1973.
65. **Ropke, C. and Haugen, H. P.,** In *Proc. Int. Workshop Nude Mice,* Denmark, 1974, 62.
66. **Linna, T. J. and Liden, S.,** Cell migration from the bone marrow to the spleen in young guinea pigs, *Int. Arch. Allergy Appl. Immunol.,* 35, 35, 1969.
67. **Brahim, F. and Osmond, D. G.,** Migration of bone marrow lymphocytes demonstrated by selective bone marrow labeling with thymidine-H3, *Anat. Rec.,* 168, 139, 1970.
68. **Parrot, D. M. V. and DeSousa M.,** Thymus dependent and thymus independent populations: origin, migrations patterns and life span, *Clin. Exp. Immunol.,* 8, 663, 1971.
69. **Howard, J. C. and Scott, D. W.,** H3-uridine incorporation as a T lymphocyte indicator in the rat, *Cell Immunol.,* 8, 270, 1973.
70. **Goldscheider, I. and McGregory, D. D.,** Anatomical distribution of T and B lymphocytes in the rat, development of lymphocyte specific anti-sera, *J. Exp. Med.,* 138, 1441, 1973.
71. **Back, D., Back, R., Hemmingson, E. J., Linden, S., and Linna, T.,** Migration of bone marrow cells to the bursa of Fabricius and the spleen in the chicken, *Scand. J. Immunol.,* 2, 357, 1973.
72. **Nossal, G. J. V.,** Studies on the rate of seeding of lymphocytes from the intact guinea pig thymus, *Ann. N.Y. Acad. Sci.,* 120, 171, 1964.
73. **Linna, J. J.,** Cell migration from the thymus to other lymphoid organs in hamsters of different ages, *Blood,* 31, 727, 1968.
74. **Iorio, R. J., Chanana, A. D., Cronkite, E. P., and Joel, D. D.,** Studies on lymphocytes. XVI. Distribution of bovine thymic lymphocytes in the spleen and lymph nodes, *Cell. Tissue Kinet.,* 3, 161, 1970.
75. **Weissman, I. L.,** Thymus cell migration, *J. Exp. Med.,* 126, 291, 1967.
76. **Joel, D. D., Hess, M. W., and Cottier, H.,** Magnitude and pattern of thymic lymphocyte migration in neonatal mice, *J. Exp. Med.,* 135, 907, 1972.
77. **Hemmingson, E. J.,** Ontogenetic studies on lymphoid cell traffic in the chicken: cell traffic from the thymus, *Int. Arch. Allergy Appl. Immunol.,* 43, 481, 1972.
78. **Tyler, R. W. and Everett, N. V.,** Radioautographic study of cellular migration using parabiotic rats, *Blood,* 39, 249, 1972.
79. **Hemmingson, E. J. and Linna, T. J.,** Ontogenetic studies on lymphoid cell traffic in the chicken. I. Cell migration from the bursa of fabricius, *Int. Arch. Allergy Appl. Immunol.,* 42, 693, 1972.
80. **Metcalf, D. and Moore, M. A. S.,** in *Haemopoietic Cells,* Elsevier, North-Holland, Amsterdam, 1971.
81. **Bierring, F.,** The lymphocyte count of the bone marrow in thymectomized lymphade nectomized rats, *Acta Anat.,* 55, 9, 1963.
82. **Rieke, W. O. and Schwartz, M. R.,** In *The Lymphocyte in Immunology and Haematopoiesis,* Yoffey, J. M., Ed., Arnold, London, 1967.
83. **Carrsa, J.,** Action of purified thymus hormone in the thymectomized guinea pig, *Am. J. Med. Sci.,* 250, 79, 1965.
84. **Hays, E. F.,** The effects of allografts of thymic epithelial reticular cells on the lymphoid tissues of neonatal thymectomized mice, *Blood,* 29, 29, 1967.
85. **Claesson, M. H., Ropke, C., and Hargen, H. P.,** Distribution of short lived and long lived small lymphocytes in the lymphomyeloid tissue of germ free mice, *Scand. J. Immunol.,* 11, 345, 1971.
86. **Osmond, D. G. and Nossal, G. J. V.,** Differentiation of lymphocytes in mouse bone marrow: quantitative radioautographic studies of antiglobulin binding by lymphocytes in bone marrow and lymphoid tissue, *Cell Immunol.,* 13, 117, 1974.
87. **Vaughan, W. P. and McGregor, D. D.,** Lymphopoiesis in the rat. I. The effect of pool size on lymphocyte production, *J. Cell. Physiol.,* 80, 1, 1972.
88. **Esteban, J. N.,** The differential effect of hydrocortisone on the short-lived small lymphocyte, *Anat. Rec.,* 162, 349, 1968.

89. **North, R. J.,** The action of cortisone acetate on cell mediated immunity to infection: histogenesis of the lymphoid cell response and selective elimination of committed lymphocytes, *Cell Immunol.*, 3, 501, 1972.
90. **Claman, H. N., Moorhead, J. W., and Bermer, W. H.,** Corticosteroids on lymphoid cells *in vitro.* I. Hydrocortisone lysis of human guinea pig and mouse thymus cells, *J. Lab. Clin. Med.*, 78, 499, 1971.
91. **Harris, P. F., Menkins, V., and Yoffey, J. M.,** The action of leukocytosis promoting factor on the blood and bone marrow of the guinea pig, *Blood,* 11, 243, 1956.
92. **Griffiths, D. A.,** Radioautographic studies of the lymphocytic bone marrow, *Blood,* 34, 696, 1969.
93. **Wicklein, H. S., Ford, C. E., Evans, E. P., and Gray, J. G.,** Interrelationships of myeloid and lymphoid cells: studies with chromosome marked cells transfused into lethally irradiated mice, *Proc. Royal. Soc. London,* 165, 78, 1966.
94. **El-Arini, M. O. and Osoba, D.,** Differentiation of thymus derived cells from mouse bone marrow, *J. Exp. Med.*, 137, 821, 1973.
95. **Basch, R. S. and Kadish, J. L.,** Hematopoietic thymocyte precursors. II. Properties of the precursors, *J. Exp. Med.*, 145, 405, 1977.
96. **Roelants, G. E., Mayor, K. S., Hagg, L. B., and Loor, F.,** Immature T lineage lymphocytes in athymic mice, presence of TL, lifespan and homeostatic regulation, *Eur. J. Immunol.*, 6, 75, 1976.
97. **Pantelauris, E. M.,** Absence of thymus in a mouse mutant, *Nature (London),* 217, 370, 1968.
98. **Wortis, H., Nehlsen, S., and Alveir, J.,** Abnormal development of the thymus in ''nude'' mice, *J. Exp. Med.*, 134, 681, 1971.
99. **Scheid, M. P., Goldstein, G., Hammerling, V., and Bajse, E. A.,** Lymphocyte differentiation from precursor cells *in vitro, Ann. N.Y. Acad. Sci.*, 249, 521, 1975.
100. **Kamiro, K., Goldstein, G., and Boyse, E. A.,** Thymus-repopulating capacity of cells that can be induced to differentiate to T cells *in vitro, J. Immunol.*, 115, 196, 1975.
101. **Bollum, F. J.,** Terminal deoxynucleotidyl transferase as a hematopoietic cell marker, *Blood,* 54, 1203, 1979.
102. **Baltimore, D.,** Is terminal deoxynucleotidyl transferase a somatic mitogen in lymphocytes? *Nature,* 248, 409, 1974.
103. **Goldschneider, I.,** Early stages of lymphocyte development, in *Current Topics in Development Biology,* Vol. 12, Friedlander, M., Monroy, A., and Moscona, A. A., Eds.: Academic Press, New York, 1979.
104. **Bollum, F. J.,** Terminal transferase: Biological studies, in *Advanced Enzymology,* Vol. 47, Meister, A., Ed., John Wiley & Sons, 1978.
105. **Vines, R. L., Coleman, M. S., and Hutton, J. J.,** Reappearance of terminal deoxynucleotidyl transferase containing cells in rat bone marrow following corticosteroid administration, *Blood,* 56, 501, 1980.
106. **Gregoire, K. E., Goldschneider, I., and Barton, R. W.,** Ontogeny of terminal deoxynucleotidyl transferase positive cells in lymphohemopoietic tissues, *J. Immunol.*, 123, 1347, 1979.
107. **Unanaue, E. R., Grey, H. M., and Rabellino, E.,** Immunoglobulins on the surface of lymphocytes: the bone marrow as the main source of lymphocytes with detectable surface-bound immunoglobulins, *J. Exp. Med.*, 133, 1188, 1971.
108. **Dukor, P., Bianco, C., and Nussenzweig, V.,** Bone marrow origin of complement receptor lymphocytes, *Eur. J. Immunol.*, 1, 491, 1971.
109. **Nossal, G. J. V. and Pike, B. L.,** Studies of the differentiation of B lymphocytes in the mouse, *Immunology,* 25, 33, 1973.
110. **Trentin, J., Wolf, N., Cheng, V., Bahlberg, W., Weiss, D., and Bonhag, G. R.,** Antibody production by mice repopulated with limited numbers of clones of lymphoid cell precursors, *J. Immunol.*, 98, 1326, 1967.
111. **Yung, L. L. L., Wyne-Evans, T. C., and Diener, E.,** Ontogeny of the immune murine system: development of antigen recognition and immune responsiveness, *Eur. J. Immunol.*, 3, 224, 1973.
112. **Warner, N. L., Szenberg, A., and Burnet, F. M.,** The immunological role of different lymphoid organs in the chickens. I. Dissociation of immunologic responsiveness, *Aust. J. Exp. Biol. Med. Sci.*, 40, 373, 1962.
113. **Cooper, M. D., Peterson, R. D. A., South, M. A., and Good, R. A.,** The functions of the thymus system and the bursa system in the chicken, *J. Exp. Med.*, 123, 75, 1966.
114. **Kincade, P. W., Lawton, R. D. A., South, M. A., and Good, R. A.,** The functions of the thymus system and the bursa system in the chicken, *J. Exp. Med.*, 123, 75, 1966.
115. **Toivanen, P. and Toivanen, A.,** Bursal and post-bursal stem cells in chicken: functional charactersitics, *Eur. J. Immunol.*, 3, 585, 1973.

116. **Toivanen, P., Toivanen, A., and Good, R. A.,** Ontogeny of bursal function in chicken. I. Embryonic stem cell for humoral immunity, *J. Immunol.,* 109, 1058, 1972.
117. **Toivanen, P., Toivanen, A., and Good, R. A.,** Ontogeny of bursal function in chicken. III. Immunocompetent cell for humoral immunity, *J. Exp. Med.,* 136, 816, 1972.
118. **Toivanen, P., Toivanen, A., and Good, R. A.,** Ontogeny of bursal function in chicken. II. Postembryonic stem cell for humoral immunity, *J. Immunol.,* 109, 1071, 1972.
119. **Lafleur, L., Miller, R. G., and Phillips, R. A.,** A quantitative assay for the progenitors of bone marrow associated lymphocytes, *J. Exp. Med.,* 135, 1363, 1972.
120. **Lafleur, L., Underwood, B. J., Miller, R. G., and Phillips, R. A.,** Differentiation of lymphocytes. Characterization of early precursors of B lymphocytes, *Sem. Haematol.,* 52, 5c, 1972.
121. **Lafleur, L., Miller, R. G., and Phillips, R. A.,** Restriction of specificity in the precursors of bone marrow associated lymphocytes, *J. Exp. Med.,* 137, 954, 1973.
122. **Hayes, L. L. and Claman, H. N.,** Recovery of immunocompetence of bone marrow and spleen following sublethal irradiation, *Proc. Soc. Exp. Biol. Med.,* 133, 57, 1970.
123. **Osmond, D. G. and Nossal, G. J. V.,** Differentiation of lymphocytes in mouse bone marrow. II. Kinetics of maturation and renewal of antiglobulin binding cells studied by double labeling, *Cell Immunol.,* 13, 132, 1974.
124. **Stocker, J. W., Osmond, D. G., and Nossal, G. J.,** Differentiation of lymphocytes in the mouse bone marrow. The adoptive response of bone marrow cells to a thymus cell independent antigen, *Immunology,* 27, 795, 1974.
125. **Ryser, J. E. and Vassalli, P.,** Mouse bone marrow lymphocytes and their differentiation, *J. Immunol.,* 113, 719, 1974.
126. **Gathings, W. E., Lawton, A. R., and Cooper, M. D.,** Immunofluorescent studies of the development of pre-B cell, B lymphocyte and immunoglobulin isotype diversity in humans, *Eur. J. Immunol.,* 7, 804, 1977.
127. **Raff, M. C., Megson, M., Owen, J. J., and Cooper, M. D.,** Early production of intracellular IgM by B lymphocyte precursors in mouse, *Nature,* 259, 224, 1976.
128. **Lawton, A. R. and Cooper, M. D.,** Two new stages of antigen independent B cell development in mice and humans, in *Development of Immune Defenses,* Cooper, M. D. and Dayton, D. H., Eds, Raven Press, New York, 1977.
129. **Kagen, W. A., Siegal, F. P., Gupta, S., Goldstein, G., and Good, R. A.,** Early stages of human marrow lymphocyte differentiation induction *in vitro* by thymopoietin and ubiquitin, *J. Immunol.,* 122, 686, 1979.
130. **Nossal, G. J. V. and Pike, B.,** Studies on the differentiation of B lymphocytes in the mouse, *Immunology,* 25, 33, 1973.
131. **Owen, J. J. T., Raff, M., and Cooper, M. D.,** Generation of B lymphocytes in the mouse embryo, *Eur. J. Immunol.,* 5, 468, 1975.
132. **Raff, M. C., Megson, M., Owen, J. J., and Cooper, M. D.,** Early production of intracellular IgM by B lymphocytes in fetal liver and bone marrow, *J. Immunol.,* 118, 2067, 1977.
133. **Owen, J. J., Wright, D. E., Haber, S., Raff, M. C., and Cooper, M. D.,** Studies on the generation of B lymphocytes in fetal liver and bone marrow, *J. Immunol.,* 118, 2067, 1977.
134. **Gupta, S. R., Pahwa, R., O'Reilly, R., Good, R. A., and Siegal, F. P.,** Ontogeny of lymphocyte subpopulations in humans fetal liver, *Proc. Natl. Acad. Sci. U.S.A.,* 73, 919, 1976.
135. **Kearney, J. F., Cooper, M. D., Klein, J., Abney, E. R., Parkhouse, R. M. E., and Lawton, A. R.,** Ontogeny of Ia and IgD or IgM bearing B lymphocytes in mice, *J. Exp. Med.,* 146, 297, 1977.
136. **Abney, E. R., Cooper, M. D., Kearney, J. F., Lawton, A. R., and Parkhouse, R. M. E.,** Sequential expression of immunoglobulin in developing mouse B lymphocytes: a systematic survey that suggests a model for the generation of immunoglobulin isotype diversity, *J. Immunol.,* 120, 2041, 1978.
137. **Vitetta, E. S. and Uhr, J. W.,** IgD and B cell differentiation, *Immunol. Rev.,* 37, 50, 1977.
138. **Rosenberg, Y. J. and Parish, C. R.,** Ontogeny of the antibody forming cell line in mice. IV. Appearance of cells bearing Fc receptors, complement receptors, and surface immunoglobulins, *J. Immunol.,* 118, 612, 1977.
139. **Hammerling, U., Chin, A. F., and Abbott, J.,** Ontogeny of murine B lymphocytes: sequence of B cell differentiation from surface immunoglobulin negative precursors to plasma cells, *Proc. Nat. Acad. Sci. U.S.A.,* 73, 2008, 1976.
140. **Melchers, F.,** B lymphocyte development in fetal liver. II. Frequency of precursors B cells during gestation, *Eur. J. Immunol.,* 7, 482, 1977.
141. **Golde, E. A. and Siskind, G. W.,** Ontogeny of B lymphocyte function. I. Restricted heterogeneity of the antibody response of B lymphocytes from newborn and fetal mice, *J. Exp. Med.,* 140, 1285, 1974.

142. **Sherr, D., Szewczuk, M. R., and Siskind, G. W.,** Ontogeny of B lymphocyte function. IV. Kinetics of maturation of B lymphocytes from fetal and newborn mice when transferred into adult irradiated hosts, *J. Immunol.,* 119, 1674, 1977.
143. **Szewczuk, M. R., Sherr, D. H., and Siskind, G. W.,** Ontogeny of B lymphocyte function. V. Ontogeny of thymus cells capacity to facilitate the functional maturation of B lymphocytes, *Eur. J. Immunol.,* 8, 370, 1978.
144. **Askonas, B. A. and Rhodes, J. M.,** Immunogenicity of antigen containing ribonucleic acid from macrophages, *Nature,* 205, 470, 1965.
145. **Fishman, M.,** Antibody formation *in vitro, J. Exp. Med.,* 114, 837, 1965.
146. **Thiery, J. P.,** Microcinematographic contribution to the study of plasma cells, in *Ciba Found. Symp. on Cellular Aspects of Immunity,* Wolstenholme, G. E. W. and O'Connor, M., Eds., Little Brown, Boston, 1959.
147. **Sharp, J. A. and Burwell, R. G.,** Interaction ''peripolesis'' of macrophages and lymphocytes after skin homografting of challenges with soluble antigen, *Nature,* 188, 474, 1960.
148. **Shoenberg, M. D., Murrow, V., Moore, R. D., et al.,** Cytoplasmic interaction between macrophages and lymphocytic cells in antibody synthesis, *Science,* 143, 964, 1964.
149. **Azar, H. A., Pham, T. C., and Kurban, A. K.,** An electron microscopic study of a syphilitic chancre: engulfment of *Treponema pallidum* by plasma cells, *Arch. Pathol.,* 90, 143, 1970.
150. **Aronson, M.,** Bridge formation and cytoplasmic flow between phagocytic cells, *J. Exp. Med.,* 118, 1083, 1963.
151. **Gordon, S. and Cohn, Z. A.,** The macrophage, *Int. Rev. Cytol.,* 36, 171, 1973.
152. **Farrar, J. J. and Koopman, W. J.,** Characterization of monocytogenic factors and their effect on the antibody response *in vitro,* in *Biology of the Lymphokines,* Cohen, S., Pick, E., and Oppenheim, J. J., Eds., Academic Press, New York, 1979.
153. **Opitz, H. G., Niethammer, D., and Jackson, R. C.,** Biochemical characterization of a factor released by macrophages, *Cell Immunol.,* 18, 70, 1975.
154. **Lutz, C. T. and Fitch, F. W.,** Accessory cell requirements in the generation of cytolytic T lymphocytes, *J. Immunol.,* 122, 2188, 1979.
155. **Rosenstreich, D. L. and Oppenheim, J. J.,** The role of macrophages in the activation of T and B lymphocytes, in *Immunobiology of the Macrophage,* Nathan, D. S., Ed., Academic Press, London, 1976.
156. **Aarden, L. A., Brunner, T. K., and Cerottini, J. C.,** Revised nomenclature for antigen-nonspecific T cell proliferation and helper factors, *Cell Immunol.,* 48, 433, 1979.
157. **Unanaue, E. R.,** Antigen binding cells. II. Effect of highly radioactive antigen on the immunoglobulin function of the bone marrow cells, *J. Immunol.,* 107, 1063, 1971.
158. **Green, A. A. and Borella, L.,** Immunologic rebound after cessation of long term chemotherapy in acute leukemia. *In vitro* response to phytohemagglutinin and antigens by peripheral blood and bone marrow lymphocytes, *Blood,* 42, 99, 1973.
159. **Thorbecke, G. J. and Kenning, F. J.,** Antibody formation *in vitro* by haemopoietic organs after subcutaneous and intravenous immunization, *J. Immunol.,* 70, 129, 1952.
160. **Hay, J. B., Murphy, M. J., Morris, B., and Bessis, M. C.,** Quantitative studies on the proliferation and differentiation of antibody forming cells in lymph, *Am. J. Pathol.,* 66, 1, 1972.
161. **Gudat, F. G., Harris, T. N., Harris, S., and Hummeler, K.,** Studies of antibody-producing cells. 1. Ultrastructure of 19S and 7S antibody producing cells, *J. Exp. Med.,* 132, 448, 1970.
162. **Storb, V., Bauer, W., Storb, R., Fliedner, T. M., and Weiser, R. S.,** Ultrastructure of rosette forming cells in the mouse during the antibody response, *J. Immunol.,* 102, 1474, 1969.
163. **Miller, H. C. and Cudkowicz, I.,** Immunologic memory cells of bone marrow origin. Increased burst size of specific immunocyte precursors, *J. Exp. Med.,* 135, 1028, 1972.
164. **McGregor, D. D. and Gowans, J. L.,** The antibody response of rats depleted of lympocytes by chronic drainage from the thoracic duct, *J. Exp. Med.,* 117, 303, 1963.
165. **Singhal, S. K. and Wigzell, H.,** *in vitro* induction of specific unresponsiveness of immunologically reactive normal marrow cells, *J. Exp. Med.,* 131, 149, 1970.
166. **Abdou, N. I. and Richter, M.,** Cells involved in the immune response. XI. Identification of the antigen reactive cell as the tolerant cell in the immunologically tolerant rabbit, *J. Exp. Med.,* 130, 164, 1970.
167. **Kaplan, A. M. and Cinader, B.,** Cellular aspects of tolerance. Unresponsiveness of B cells, *Cell Immunol.,* 6, 442, 1973.
168. **Lydyard, P. and Ivanyi, J.,** Suppression of graft versus host reactive lymphocyte by heterologous antithymus serum *in vitro, Transplantation,* 12, 493, 1971.
169. **McGregor, D. D.,** Bone marrow origin of immunologically competent lymphocytes in the rat, *J. Exp. Med.,* 127, 953, 1968.

170. **Goldschneider, I. and McGregor, D. D.**, Anatomical distribution of T and B lymphocytes in the rat, *J. Exp. Med.*, 138, 1443, 1973.
171. **Cohen, J. J. and Claman, H. N.**, Thymus and marrow immunocompetance. Hydrocortisone resistant cells and processes in the hemolytic antibody response of mice, *J. Exp. Med.*, 133, 1026, 1971.
172. **Lonai, P. and Feldman, J.**, Cooperation of lymphoid cells in an *in vitro* graft reaction system, *Transplantation,* 11, 446, 1971.
173. **Osmond, D. G. and Nakatsu, T.**, Graft versus host activity of lymphoid tissue and bone marrow cells following x-irradiation and bone marrow transfusion in normal and thymectomized rats, *Anat. Rec.*, 172, 377, 1972.
174. **Goldschneider, I. and McGregor, D. D.**, Development of immunologically competent cells in the rat, *Nature (London),* 212, 1433, 1966.
175. **Burleson, R. and Levey, R. H.**, Demonstration of thymic function *in vitro, Transplant. Proc.*, 3, 918, 1971.
176. **Burleson, R. and Levey, R. H.**, Studies on the isolation of lymphocytes active in cell mediated immune response. Demonstration of an active population of thymus derived cells in mouse bone marrow, *Cell Immunol.*, 4, 305, 1972.
177. **El-Arini, M. O. and Osoba, D.**, Differentiation of thymus derived cells from precursors in mouse bone marrow, *J. Exp. Med.*, 137, 821, 1973.
178. **Levey, R. H. and Burleson, R.**, Studies on the isolation of lymphocytes active in cell mediated immune response. Identification and recovery of an immunocompetent subpopulation of mouse thymocytes, *Cell Immunol.*, 4, 316, 1972.
179. **Orsos, F.**, Das Bindegewebesgerust des Knochenmarks in normalen und pathologischen, Zustand, *Zieglers Beitr. z. Path. Anat.*, 76, 36, 1927.
180. **Sundberg, R. D.**, Lymphocytes and plasma cells, Ann. N.Y. Acad. Sci., 57, 671, 1957.
181. **Fischer, O.**, Uber die Lymphknotchen im menschlechen Humerus-Wirbel und Rippermark, *Frankf. Z. Path.*, 20, 347, 1917.
182. **Rohr, K.**, *Das Menschliche Knochenmark,* Georg Thiem Verlag, Leipzig, 1927.
183. **Hashimoto, M., Higuchi, M., and Saito, T.**, Lymph nodules in human bone marrow, *Acta Pathol. Japonica.*, 7, 33, 1957.
184. **Askanazy, M.**, Uber die Lymphfollikel in menschlichen Knockenmark, *Virchows. Arch.*, 220, 257, 1915.
185. **Brunning, R. D., Bloomfield, C. D., and McKenna, R. W.**, Bilateral trephine bone marrow biopsies in lymphoma and other neoplastic disease, *Ann. Intern. Med.*, 82, 365, 1975.
186. **Rappaport, H.**, *Tumors of the Hematopoietic System,* Armed Forces Institute of Pathology, Washington, D.C., 1966.
187. **Rambotti, P. and Davis, S.**, Lactic dehydrogenase in normal and leukemic lymphocyte subpopulation: evidence for abnormal T and B cells in CLL, *Blood,* 57, 325, 1981.
188. **Foucar, K., McKenna, R. W., Frizzera, G., and Brunning, R. D.**, Incidence and patterns of bone marrow and blood involvement by lymphoma in relations to the Lukes-Collins classification, *Blood,* 54, 1417, 1979.
189. **Jones, S. E., Rosenberg, S. A., and Kaplan, H. S.**, Non-Hodgkin's lymphoma. I. Bone marrow involvement, *Cancer,* 29, 954, 1972.
190. **Rosenberg, S. A.**, Bone marrow involvement in non-Hodgkin's lymphomata, *Br. J. Cancer,* 32, 261, 1975.
191. **Barcos, M. F. and Lukes, R. J.**, Malignant lymphoma of convoluted lymphocytes: a new entity of possible T cell type. In *Conflicts in Childhood Cancer,* Sink, L. F. and Godden, J. O., Eds., Alan R. Liss, New York, 1975.
192. **Thiel, E., Rodt, H., Huhn, D., et al.**, Multimarkers classification of acute lymphoblastic leukemia. Evidence for further T subgroups and evaluation of their clinical significance, *Blood,* 56, 759, 1980.
193. **Greaves, M. F. and Lister, T. A.**, Prognostic importance of immunologic markers in adult acute lymphoblastic leukemia, *N. Engl. J. Med.*, 304, 119, 1981.
194. **Foon, K. A., Billing, R. J., Teraski, P. I., and Cline, M. J.**, Immunologic classification of acute lymphoblastic leukemia. Implications for normal lymphoid differentiation, *Blood,* 56, 1120, 1980.
195. **Straus, D. J., Koziner, B., Broxmeyer, et al.**, True histiocytic lymphoma is an extramedullary manifestation of acute monocytic leukemia, *Proc. Am. Assoc. Cancer Res.*, 21, 136, 1980.
196. **te Velde J., Den Ottolander, G. J., Spaander, P. J., Van den Berg, C., and Hartgrink-Groveneveld, C. A.**, The bone marrow in Hodgkin's disease: the non-involved marrow, *Histopathology,* 2, 31, 1978.

Chapter 14

PLASMA CELL IN THE BONE MARROW

Young K. Park, Sidney Trubowitz, and Stephen Davis

TABLE OF CONTENTS

I. INTRODUCTION

Plasma cells are normal constituents of many organs, but are particularly abundant in lymph nodes, spleen, skin, intestine, and bone marrow. The total plasma cell mass may be remarkably increased in certain disease states. In the normal bone marrow, however, the plasma cells constitute a small percentage of the nucleated cells.[1] Plasma cells are readily identifiable but display considerable morphologic variability both in reactive plasmacytosis and malignant proliferation.

II. MORPHOLOGY OF PLASMA CELLS

A. The Typical Plasma Cell (the Plasma Cell of Marschalko)

Plasma cells have a characteristic appearance consisting of a basophilic cytoplasm with eccentrically located nucleus. The typical plasma cell has an average diameter of 14 μm. The mean diameter of the nucleus is 8.5 μm.[2] The eccentricity of the nuclear location is attributed to a large perinuclear zone occupied by the Golgi complex. The nucleus is round or oval in shape. Overall the nuclear morphology is similar to that of mature lymphocytes, i.e., the nuclear chromatin is coarse and clumped. The clumped chromatin is often distributed along the periphery of the nucleus with a clear interchromatin space, which in histological section sometimes gives the appearance of "the spokes of a wheel."[3] Nuceloli are usually not visualized with the light microscope. The cytoplasm is deeply basophilic due to its abundant ribonucleoprotein content. The large, pale perinuclear halo or "hof" is quite characteristic of the plasma cell and is the site of the Golgi complex. Often, various intracytoplasmic inclusions, vacuoles or hyaline sphericles may be observed in the cytoplasm.

On electron microscopy,[4–7] the nuclear heterochromatin aggregates into clumps, characteristically distributed around the nuclear membrane. Nucleoli may be observed in a minority of cells, but are frequently small and inconspicuous. The most prominent feature of the cytoplasm is the abundant rough-surfaced endoplasmic reticulum. The rough-surfaced endoplasmic reticulum does not differ structurally from that seen in other secretory cells, such as pancreatic acinar cells, gastric peptic cells, or follicular cells of the thyroid.[8] The endoplasmic reticulum helps to distinguish the plasma cell from the lymphocytes and reticulum cells. The ribosomes of the rough-surfaced membranes are responsible for the deep blue staining of the cytoplasm with basic dyes. The cisternae are frequently flattened giving rise to a parallel lamellar configuration. Accumulation of synthesized protein within the cisternae of the plasma cell may dilate these canalicular structures in varying degrees. As a consequence the cisternae are filled with electron-dense, amorphous material which is the presecretory immunoglobulin. These spherical inclusions vary in size, and are the Russell bodies seen in stained histological preparations.

The Golgi apparatus is usually moderately developed but varies considerably in size and structure. Vesicles, vacuoles, and granules are frequently observed. Mitochondria also vary considerably in size, shape and number. The cytoplasmic membrane is thin and frequently closely apposed to the bone marrow macrophage.[1,9–11] The cell surfaces possess microvilli with a varying number of pseudopods, containing endoplasmic reticulum and cisternae. The pseudopods appear to be budding and on careful examination, invagination of cytoplasmic membrane or micropinocytosis may be observed.[6,12] Recently, the scanning electron microscope has demonstrated the presence of microvilli, pseudopods and budding of the cytoplasmic membrane.[13–15]

B. Morphologic Variation

Departure from the well-defined characteristics of the typical plasma cell of Marschalko is common: the plasma cell displays an extreme degree of variation in its morphology. Its size ranges from a small lymphoid plasmacyte (4 μm) to a large blast form (up to 30 μm). Variability may be expressed in the form of cytoplasmic inclusions, such as Russell bodies or vacuoles as seen in Mott cells and thesaurocytes, or as divergent histochemical staining properties as in the flaming cells. The significance of the inclusions and their relationship to plasma cell activity have not been clarified.

1. Immature Plasma Cell (Plasmablast, Proplasmacyte)

The immature plasma cell is rarely seen in the normal bone marrow, but is increased in conditions associated with plasmacytosis either reactive or ''malignant.'' The plasmablast or proplasmacyte is a large cell (14 to 24 μm) which has a centrally located or slightly eccentric nucleus. The nuclear cytoplasmic ratio is increased between 1:1 to 1:2. The nucleus of the plasmablast has a fine and delicate chromatin, which may contain one to four large nucleoli. The cytoplasm stains a light blue and tends to stain rather unevenly. The cytoplasmic margin tends to be irregular and indistinct (Figure 1). On electron microscopy, the rough-surfaced endoplasmic reticulum is scanty and frequently occurs in irregular shapes,[4–7] and free ribosomes are scattered throughout the cytoplasm. As maturation proceeds from proplasmacyte to plasma cell, the nuclear chromatin becomes clumped and polarizes toward the periphery of the nucleus. Nucleoli become less distinct on light microscopy, but their inconspicuous persistance may be seen in electron microscopy. With further maturation the cytoplasm is packed with endoplasmic reticulum as the Golgi apparatus progressively develops to its full size. This immature plasma cell may be confused with some ''myeloma'' cells, in which nucleocytoplasmic maturation is said to be asynchronous.[7,10,16,17]

The so-called Türk cell is believed to be a variant of the immature plasma cell. This cell, described by Türk,[18,19] refers to as a large cell which has a lymphoid nucleus with deeply basophilic cytoplasm. Türk cells have been described in certain viral infections, particularly rubella and measles, as well as during recovery from severe pyogenic infections and in hypersensitivity reactions. Pappenheim[20] considered this cell to be a plasma cell of lymphoid derivation and called it Türk's irritation cell (''Reizungsformen''). His concept was recently resurrected when immature plasma cells were demonstrated in lymphocyte cultures stimulated by various antigens. Türk cells, observed by electron microscopy,[21,22] resemble immature plasma cells as well as large lymphocytes. Circulating Türk cells have been shown to contain detectable amounts of immunoglobulin.[23] Türk cells may best be defined as transitional cells that follow lymphocyte stimulation.

2. Nuclear Variation

a. Nuclear Multiplicity, Lobulation, and Indentation

Binucleated and even tetranucleated plasma cells are seen in reactive plasmacytosis. The more highly multinucleated cells (hexa- or even octaploid) are more likely allied to a neoplastic plasma cell proliferative marrow. Sometimes these multiple nuclei are connected by a fine thread.

Nuclear indentation, irregular contour, or lobulation is observed in both myeloma and in the immature plasma cells found in benign plasmacytosis. The nuclear indentation is usually associated with cytoplasmic invagination.[10,24,25] Whether the irregularity indicates immaturity or degenerating changes as seen in Sezary cells is not clear.[24]

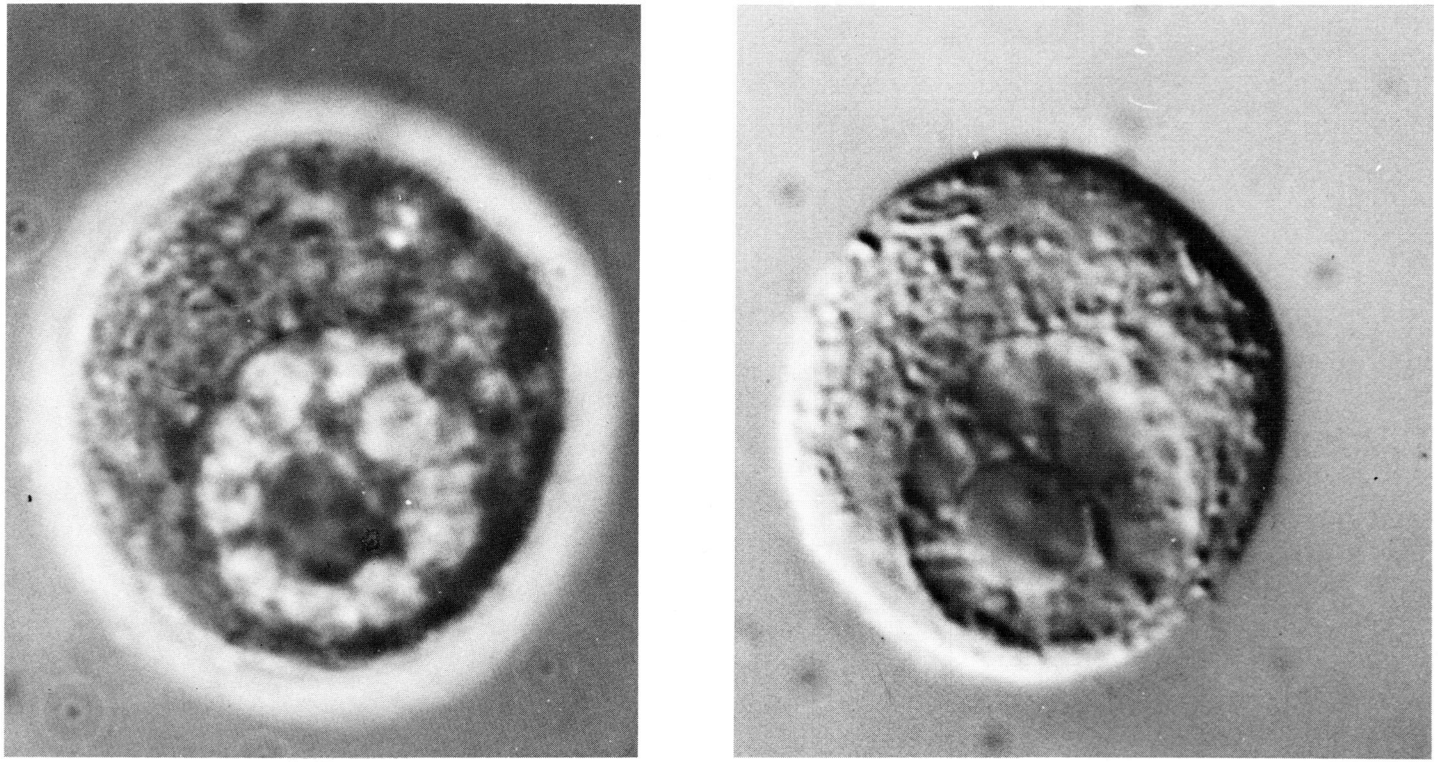

A B

FIGURE 1. A plasma cell from a patient with myeloma as seen by phase-contrast (A) and interference (B) microscopy. Note the large central nucleolus. Approximately 2500 ×.

b. Nucleolar Variation

The presence of a large nucleolus in the plasma cell has been interpreted by some as nuclear-cytoplasmic asynchrony, a morphologic characteristic of malignancy, by others, as the normal morphologic expression of very active protein synthesis in secretory cells.[26,27]

The measured nucleolar size and nucleolar/nuclear ratio of bone marrow plasma cells appear to correlate roughly with the percentage of plasma cells in the bone marrow and with the concentration of M globulin in the serum.[28] The large, compact nucleoli of the proplasmacyte gradually decrease in size and granularity resulting in small and frequently, ring-shaped structures of the plasmacyte.[16,29] This sequence of maturation from proplasmacyte to plasmacyte is accompanied by a decreasing production of RNA. The persistent RNA synthesis seen in a high proportion of "myeloma" cells[30,31] may then represent the normal requirement for very active protein-synthesis by the immature plasma cells, rather than asynchronism. Smetana,[16] however, reported relatively immature nucleoli in the otherwise mature nucleus and cytoplasm of "myeloma" cells, which he interpreted as maturation asynchrony of the nucleolus.

c. Intranuclear Inclusions

Several types of nuclear inclusions have been observed in plasma cells; the most frequent are round or oval shaped. Inclusions vary from extremely small, identifiable only by electron microscopy, to inclusions occupying almost the entire nucleus. In the later case, the inclusion can be seen on light microscopy as hyaline spheres on staining with acid dyes. These inclusions are often dissolved by the May-Grunwald-Giemsa stain resulting in nuclear vacuoles. PAS staining is variously positive or negative.[32,33] On electron microscopy, these inclusions show a homogeneous material with varying degrees of electron density, but more commonly, high electron density.[33–40] Intranuclear inclusions in plasma cells, when studied by immunofluorescence techniques, are shown to contain immunoglobulins secreted by the plasma cells themselves.[35,37,39] The round shaped intranuclear inclusions are observed in all immunoglobulin subgroups associated with disease, including IgG, IgA myeloma, pure Bence-Jones protein variant myeloma, and Waldenstrom's macroglobulinemia. Its occurrence in reactive plasmacytosis has not been observed.

According to Brunning[33] the low density intranuclear inclusions seen by electron microscopy are PAS positive. He postulated that the electron-light inclusions have a higher carbohydrate content than the osmiophilic electron-dense inclusion. The histochemical and electron density differences seem to be related more to differences in the terminal sequence of immunoglobulin synthesis than to the nature of the specific immunoglobulin subtypes or chains.[41–43] Whether the intranuclear inclusions originate from the nucleus[36,37,39] or from perinuclear cisternae[25,35,40,44] has been debated, but a perinuclear cisternal origin is supported by the following data:

1. The inclusion is an immunoglobulin which is identical to the cytoplasmic Russell body (evidence for nuclear synthesis of immunoglobulin is lacking).
2. Immunoglobulin production is understood to begin in the perinuclear cisterna.[45,46]
3. In numerous instances the nuclear inclusions are smooth-membrane bound, and surrounded by clumped chromatin. Therefore it is likely that immunoglobulin in the perinuclear cisterna is invaginated into the nucleus with eventual loss of its connection to the perinuclear cisterna.[33]

Nuclear body and nucleoloid body are other nuclear inclusions found in plasma cells. The electron microscopic feature of these inclusions is, basically, composed of fine filaments with or without dense granules. This filamentous structure appears to be RNA and seems to be increased in active plasma cells.[47,48] These inclusions have been observed in myeloma cells[10,25] and in nonmyeloma cells as well.[48,49] The significance of these nuclear RNA fragments is not known.

3. Cytoplasmic Variation

Perhaps the most striking variation in the morphology of the plasma cell is due to the variable degrees of dilatation or collapse of the cisternae of the endoplasmic reticulum, a property of its function as a secretory cell. Maldonado[36] described six different variations in the cytoplasm of plasma cells based on endoplasmic reticulum shapes: a lamellar type, moderately dilated type, markedly dilated type, globular dilatation, flaming cells, and cells with dense bodies (Russell bodies). This classification is basically similar to the seven types described by Tanaka.[5]

The regular array of parallel, flattened cisternae is common in the mature normal plasma cell and in the plasma cell of myeloma.[10] Globular or vesicular dilatation of RER are also seen frequently in myeloma. Russell bodies and flaming cells are discussed below. Other cytoplasmic inclusions include crystals,[44,50] fibrillar formation,[25,51–53] and dense body.[6,44,51] These probably represent protein fragments.

Russell bodies were originally described by Russell in 1890 as "fuchin bodies,"[54] which he regarded as the "characteristic organisms of cancer." On light microscopy Russell bodies are seen as hyaline spheres of varying size, sometimes reaching 2 to 3 μm in diameter. They stain with acid dyes, but more often are dissolved by May-Grunwald-Giemsa stain. In such cases, the plasmacyte seem to be more or less filled with colorless vacuoles. The PAS reaction of the Russell body is variable.[55]

On electron microscopy the bodies are round and of homogeneous material of high electron density within the cisternae of RER. Morphologically the bodies are similar to the intranuclear round shaped inclusions. By immunofluorescence techniques these vacuoles contain immunoglobulins.[56,57] It is postulated that these bodies are condensations of synthesized immunoglobulin in the RER or excess light chains.[58]

Russell bodies are usually seen in conditions of intense and sustained immunologic stimulation. They are often present along the gastrointestinal (GI) tract, particularly in chronic gastritis and chronic enteritis. In myeloma the Russell bodies are, in fact, not commonly observed.[59,60] Oikawa could find Russell bodies only in 3 of 35 patients with myeloma and Waldenström macroglobulinemia.[44]

The term "Mott cell" refers to a cell with multiple Russell bodies. Under the light microscope Mott cells have a grape-like appearance. With Giemsa staining it may be confused with fat-containing histiocytes. The Mott cell is not regarded as pathognomic of any particular disease. The Mott cell appears under similar clinical conditions to that of Russell bodies. Interestingly, Mott originally described these cells in 1906[61] in the cerebrospinal fluid of the patient with trypanosomiasis. Later Stefanopoulo[62] produced the same cell experimentally in rats infected with *Trypanosoma gambiense*. It appears that the Mott cell occurs primarily in situations of chronic antigenemia, notably typhus, malaria, and kala-azar.[63] The occurrence of the Mott cell in myeloma is regarded as an unusual event.[59,60]

The "flaming cell" was first described by Undritz.[64] This cell has a characteristically distinct reddish tinge or bright red cytoplasm with an eccentrically located nucleus. On electron microscopy, the cisternae are moderately dilated and are filled with electron dense granular or flocculant material.[65]

Thesaurocyte, named by Paraskevas and Waldenström,[66] is defined as a plasma cell variant in which the cytoplasm is filled with several thin-walled sacs resulting from the extremely dilated cisterna. The nucleus is frequently small, pycnotic, and eccentrically located. The cytoplasm is characteristically pale staining. The electron microscope findings suggest that the flaming cell and thesaurocyte are similar and probably represent different stages of the same cell. Flaming cells and thesaurocytes have been observed in both myeloma and reactive plasmacytosis. Although the flaming cell is not specific for any particular immunoglobulin subgroup, the occurrence of these cells has been more frequently reported in IgA myeloma.[59,65]

Recently, Hayhoe[60] studied the incidence of flaming cells in the various immunoglobulin groups of myeloma. Of 195 patients, flaming cells were observed in approximately 60% of patients with IgA myeloma, compared with approximately 30% of patients with IgG myeloma. However, the percentage of flaming cells per patient were not different within the IgA and IgG myeloma groups. Jacobs et al.[67] reported that flaming cells were not more common in IgA myeloma. The higher content of carbohydrate in the IgA and IgM molecule than in the IgG molecule is thought to lend these proteins a higher affinity for the basic dyes and PAS, and thus account for the supposed frequent association of flaming cells with IgA myeloma. Waldenström[59] postulated that the flaming cell probably stores immunoglobulin within the dilated cisternae which eventually burst discharging their contents into the cytoplasm (clasmatosis). The clinical significance of the flaming cell is not known.

Phagocytic activity is a characteristic feature of monocytes, macrophages, and polymorphonuclear cells. Although phagocytic capacity has been reported occasionally in lymphocytes in certain conditions,[68–71] the occurrence of phagocytosis by normal plasma cells appears to be a rare phenomenon. However, clear demonstration of the phagocytic activity of plasma cells in myeloma has been reported.[44,58,72–75]

These reports show an incidence of phagocytic plasma cells from less than 1% to 21% of bone marrow plasma cells. In one of the reported cases, plasma cells were shown to phagocytose latex particles in vitro.[75] Phagocytosis of other cells by the plasma cell is indeed rare, however, phagocytosis of foreign materials ranging from iron particles to *Treponema pallida*[76–85] has been reported more frequently. Speculation of possible transfer of iron from macrophage to the plasma cell has been raised.[78] Recently, Ottosen et al.[12] demonstrated that ferritin bound to plasma cell surfaces was taken up in endocytic vesicles by invagination of the surface membrane. Within 30 to 60 min, the ferritin was concentrated within lysosomes and in several secretory compartments. This endocytotic activity appears to be much lower in myeloma cells than in benign plasma cells.

III. MATURATION AND FUNCTION OF PLASMA CELL

A. Origin of Plasma Cell

The origin of the plasma cell has been debated since Cajal,[86] Unna,[87] and Marschalko[88] described the cell in the last decade of the 19th century. The origin of the plasma cell has been linked to an independent precursor system, and to the lymphocyte. Studies on the origin of the plasma cell have been aided by the introduction of modern immunobiologic techniques.

McMaster and Hudack[89] found that antibody appeared in the lymphatic tissue draining the site of injected antigen. Fagraeus[90] observed a large "transitional cell" in splenic tissue during an antibody response that preceded the appearance of the plasma cell. Nossal[91,92] confirmed this finding in murine lymph nodes by autoradiography. The earliest cells taking up the labeled thymidine were large immunoblastic cells; eventually the label passed to the smaller plasma cell. The subsequent delination of the lymphoid system, i.e., T and B lymphocytes, helped to clarify the situation.

It is now well established that plasma cells are derived from B lymphocytes in the process of a normal immune response. The B-lymphocyte transformation into a plasma cell can be initiated by B-lymphocyte-dependent mitogens, e.g., bacterial lipopolysaccharide in the mouse,[93,94] *Nocardia opaca* in man,[95,96] or by T-lymphocyte-dependent mitogens, e.g., pokeweed in both mouse and man. In the latter, the helper factor produced from stimulated T lymphocyte causes differentiation of the B lymphocyte into a plasma cell.[97] Alternatively it is also known that B-lymphocyte activation is suppressed by T cells after interaction with antigen.[98] Although mitogens or antigens for the most part induce polyclonal immunoglobulin, recent studies with antiidiotypic antibodies suggest that a plasma cell secreting immunoglobulin of a given specificity is derived from a precursor B lymphocyte with surface-bound immunoglobulin of identical specificity.[99–101]

B. Maturation Sequence

Small lymphocytes are immunologically competent cells which can undergo a complex sequence of immunological differentiation and morphological transformation when stimulated. The mature-looking small lymphocytes, in fact, always contain nucleoli when carefully examined on electron microscopy.

The morphologic and cytokinetic features of lymphocyte transformation have been studied in man. Douglas et al.[103–106] studied human peripheral lymphocytes following stimulation with pokeweed mitogen. They observed within the first 24 hr of culture that the nucleoli became enlarged, frequently were multiple, and were composed of a granular component with compact form. By 48 hr this event was followed by the appearance of large cells, apparently T and B immunoblasts. The immunoblasts developed into two distinctly different morphologic types by 60 to 72 hr of culture. One type, about 20 to 30% of all cultured cells, was compatible with plasmablast-proplasmacyte on electron microscopic examination. The other cells were immature lymphoid cells which resembled the phytohemagglutinin-induced T immunoblast. On extended cultures, up to 7 to 10 days, 10 to 20% of the cells showed development of abundant rough-surfaced endoplasmic reticulum. The T-immunoblastic cell line failed to show any plasma cell differentiation.[105]

The cytokinetic sequence[94,98,102] during the maturation largely reflected the morphologic changes. The RNA synthetic activity as measured by uridine-H^3 incorporation of peripheral lymphocytes displayed significant labeling after 2 hr of exposure to pokeweed stimulation. The RNA synthetic activity increased rapidly during the first 12 to 30 hr of incubation and reached a plateau by 48 to 64 hr. The DNA synthesis, measured by [^{3}H]thymidine incorporation increased slowly during the first 3 days, then reached a plateau in 3 to 5 days. The thymidine incorporation began to decrease at 7 days of incubation independent of culture modification, but the number of plasma cells seemed to increase continuously through 7 days of incubation. Immunoglobulin could be detected on day 3, and reached a maximum by day 7 in cultures of human peripheral or tonsilar lymphocytes stimulated with pokeweed or *Nocardia opaca* mitogen, both polyclonal mitogens. The characteristic B-cell markers including surface immunoglobulins and C_3 receptors appeared to be lost progressively during the B-cell transformation into a plasma cell.[107]

C. Function

The plasma cell is an immunoglobulin-secreting cell. Its function is to synthesize and release antibody. The secretory function of the plasma cell is very active. In normal adult man, about 2.2 g of immunoglobulin G (IgG) is synthesized each day.[108] Expressed differently, about 10^{13}IgG molecules are synthesized per second.

The structure of the immunoglobulin molecule is determined by the genetic information encoded in the DNA. Chromosome abnormalities have been described in myeloma, but little is known about their specificity.[109] The nuclear DNA is transcribed into mRNA, which is transported from nucleus to the ribosomes in the cytoplasm. The sequence of immunoglobulin synthesis, intracellular transportation, and secretion has been determined using techniques including pulse-chase biosynthetic labeling, subcellular fractionation, electron microscopic autoradiography, various inhibitors of glycosylations, etc. The membrane-bound ribosomes are the sites of light and heavy chain synthesis.[110]

During the formation of the polypeptides on the membrane of the endoplasmic reticulum, carbohydrate is added starting with monosaccharides and concluding when the polysaccharide chain reaches its full length. The light chains are then freed from the membrane structure of the endoplasmic reticulum and released into an intracellular pool within the cytoplasm or the cisternae of the endoplasmic reticulum. The free light chains then combine with the ribosome-bound heavy chains, forming half of an immunoglobulin molecule, i.e., a heavy-light chain dimer. The two halves are then linked by disulfide bonds to form the four polypeptide chain immunoglobulin, i.e., IgG. Assembly of immunoglobulin monomer is a very rapid process and is followed within a few minutes by polymerization to make 19S pentamers, i.e., IgM. It appears that almost all IgM is assembled intracellularly before secretion.[111] The completed immunoglobulin enters the cisternae of the Golgi complex and carbohydrates, like glucosamine galactose and sialic acid, are attached.

The secretion of the immunoglobulin molecule is probably facilitated by the presence of carbohydrate but there is no clear evidence that carbohydrate incorporation is obligatory to the normal secretory process.[112] In actively secreting plasma cells, the free light chains are secreted within 20 min of synthesis and fully assembled IgG from 30 to 40 min after synthesis. Recent studies demonstrate that immunoglobulin secretion is mediated by a constant traffic of smooth vesicles to the cell surface where immunoglobulin is discharged by exocytosis.[111,113] The plasma cell stores little, if any, intracellular immunoglobulin. Unlike other glandular, secretory cells the immunoglobulins are not concentrated intracellularly.

The regulatory mechanisms of immunoglobulin secretion are not known. Plasma cell secretion is insensitive to a variety of hormones, mediators, cyclic nucleotide derivatives, extracellular calcium depletion, and agents acting on microtubules or microfilaments which regulate secretion in other glandular cells.[111] In the nonsecretory "myeloma" cells found in about 1% of all cases of myeloma, the cells do not secrete immunoglobulin, although intracellular immunoglobulin synthesis is demonstrated. Electron microscopic and histochemical analysis are not able to differentiate secretory from nonsecretory cells. Recently, a possible block related to glycosylation at the level of Golgi apparatus was postulated as the cause of the failure of secretion by the nonsecretory myeloma cells.[114]

IV. REACTIVE PLASMACYTOSIS

The occurrence of increased plasma cells at any given anatomical site is the result of antigenic stimulation. In fact, plasmacytosis or plasmacytomas never develop in germ-free mice and plasma cells are rarely found in the tissues of the fetus or in the newborn.

In the normal adult, plasma cells are distributed strategically at the site of entry of antigens. The tonsils, mucosal surfaces of GI tract, upper respiratory tract, and squamocolumnar junction of the cervix are the favorite sites of local reactive plasmacytosis. Their reaction is accompanied by local inflammatory changes. In certain infections or inflammatory disease and other intense immunologic reactions diffuse plasmacytosis may be observed in the lymph nodes, spleen, and bone marrow. Transient plasma cell circulation in peripheral blood is not uncommon in these circumstances especially when looked for by immunofluorescence techniques.[115] In general, the total body plasma cell mass correlates well with the quantity of circulating immunoglobulin and percentage of bone marrow plasma cell.[116–119] The criteria for the diagnosis of reactive plasmacytosis are

1. An increase of the plasma cell population in the bone marrow above the normal range (>3%)
2. Presence of a clinical disease which is known to be associated with an acute or chronic immune reaction
3. No clinical evidence of malignant plasma cell dyscrascia

The percentage of plasma cells estimated from Giemsa-stained smears in the bone marrow of a normal adult ranges from 0 to 3%.[1] In a recent study of 1000 bone marrow examinations from a general community hospital approximately one fourth had 2% or more plasma cells in the bone marrow; 3.8% of the cases, excluding myeloma, had more than 5% of plasma cells.[120] More than 10% plasma cell infiltration of the bone marrow appears to be uncommon in reactive plasmacytosis,[117,120] although bone marrow evaluation is usually not performed in cases of polyclonal gammopathy.

The most common diseases associated with reactive plasmacytosis include viral, bacterial, protozoal or parasitic infections, especially pneumonia, lung abscess, pulmonary tuberculosis and pyelonephritis, cirrhosis of liver, collagen disease, carcinomas, diabetes mellitus, and granulomatous disease.[115,120]

The bone marrow findings in reactive plasmacytosis may demonstrate, in addition to the plasma cells, any structural or cellular alteration characteristic of the underlying diseases for which the bone marrow examination was initially performed. Plasma cells are frequently observed in perivascular and perisinusoid sites in histologic section of the bone marrow (Figure 2). Hyun et al.[120,122] recently reported on the bone marrow findings of 276 specimens with reactive plasmacytosis. They found macrophages frequently surrounded by numerous plasma cells, the plasmacytosis islet[121] or plasmacytic satellitosis which is believed to be a morphologic expression of the immune reaction in the process of immunoglobulin production. They observed plasmacytic satellitosis, defined as three or more plasma cells surrounding a macrophage, in 46% of the reactive specimens compared to 10% of the specimens with normal percentage of plasma cells. Interestingly, plasmacyte satellitosis was not found in any of their cases of myeloma.[122] In addition, they also observed lymphoid follicles more frequently in the marrow of reactive plasmacytosis than in the normal. In contrast with above observations Blom et al. reported macrophage-apposed plasma cells in all myeloma cases on the electron microscope.[10]

Significant variation of the plasma cell from the typical Marschako cells is often observed in reactive plasmacytosis. In fact, Russell bodies and Mott cells appear more frequently in the marrow of patients with reactive plasmacytosis than in patients with myeloma. Multinucleated cells (even four nuclei), thesaurocytes, and various intracellular crystals have been observed in reactive states.[120]

V. PATHOLOGIC PLASMACYTOSIS

A. Multiple Myeloma

Myelomatosis represents a disease of plasma cells in which the axial skeleton is the predominate site of proliferation and accumulation. The disease occurs after the age of

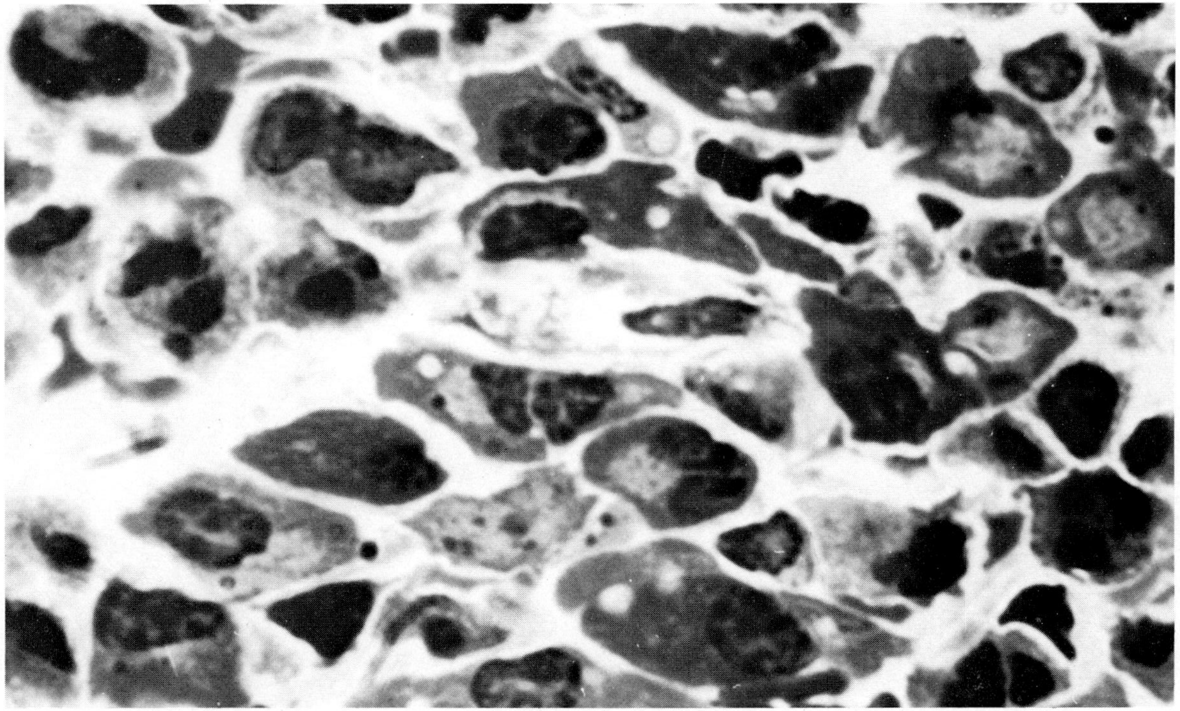

FIGURE 2. Perisinusoidal accumulation of plasma cells in benign reactive plasmocytosis. Histologic section of marrow particles. Approximately 1500 ×.

40. Bone pain, anemia, renal insufficiency, hypercalcemia, infection, and hyperviscosity syndrome comprise the major symptom complexes. About 5% of patients present with extraosseous involvement. Approximately half of the patients have an IgG paraprotein, 22% IgA, 20% Bence-Jones protein only; the remainder have IgM, IgD, and IgE monoclonal spikes. About 1% have no serum and urine paraprotein.

1. General Pathology of the Skeletal System

The pattern of skeletal lesions in multiple myeloma varies from case to case. The myeloma lesions can infiltrate almost the entire red marrow and to a great extent, the yellow marrow. The ''myeloma'' lesions may be observed in any bone of the human skeletal system, even for example the laryngeal bones. On gross examination, myeloma is characterized by diffuse confluent, gelatinous tumor nodules of up to 1.0 cm in size. Less commonly, myeloma is seen as discrete multiple plasmacytomas with normal looking surrounding marrow. These two types, diffuse nodular and discrete tumoral lesions, are not distinctly separate entities. There is considerable overlap and truly discrete lesions without microscopic infiltration of intervening marrow is a rare finding.

Myeloma lesions frequently invade paraskeletal areas by direct extension from the bone, resulting in subdural, epidural, or paracostal lesions. The extent of these lesions vary from small periosteal infiltrations to large plasmacytomas with destruction of the underlying bony structure. The myeloma lesions, roentgenographically, can be seen as osteolytic lesions. Rarely, osteosclerotic lesions have been reported in an atypical form of myeloma, usually associated with a polyneuropathy, hypertrichosis or diabetes.[123] The presence of monoclonal paraprotein in this variant is uncommon. X-ray examination of the skeleton of myeloma reveals descrete round or oval lytic lesions and/or diffuse mottled osteoporosis.

2. Microscopic Bone Marrow Findings

The distribution of plasma cells in the biopsy specimen most often shows a diffuse infiltration throughout the sections with preference for the endosteal region and the vascular sinusoids. In Burkhardt's[124] study, 5% of his cases of multiple myeloma showed a focal circumscribed arrangement of plasma cells. The plasma cell population, as a percentage of all nucleated cells in the bone marrow, ranges from normal (below 3%) to 98%.[125–127] Schneider and Mazabrand[128] reported that 20% of patients with multiple myeoloma had a plasma cell count below 10%. The presence of more than 10% of plasma cells in a given specimen is suggestive and more than 40% is indicative of multiple myeloma. The presence of a plasma cell infiltration on marrow analysis does not, in itself, confirm the diagnosis of myeloma.

Bone marrow aspirate and clot examination should be performed if possible in an area of pain or demonstrable lesion on the X-ray. Bone marrow biopsy may give more information about the true population and distribution of the plasma cells. It may also be possible to observe the osseous remodeling. Osteolysis may be characterized by a markedly decreased trabecular volume and by increased osteoid volume.[124]

The hematopoietic compartment in myeloma is replaced by the plasma cells. According to Hansen and Burkhardt,[124,129] there is no inverse correlation between fat cell area and the plasma cell area. There is also no correlation found between the fat cell area and the degree of anemia. These findings, however, should be carefully interpreted: a random biopsy specimen may not be a reliably representative sample of the whole marrow.

The pathogenesis of anemia in multiple myeloma is not completely understood and appears to be multifactorial. The degree of anemia seems to be roughly correlated with the measured total myeloma cell mass.[130] Of 22 patients evaluated by Hansen,[129] the serum creatinine level correlated best with the degree of anemia. There are numerous reports and discussions about the relationship of the anemia of myeloma and megaloblastic changes in bone marrow cells,[131] low serum folate values,[132] depletion of bone marrow iron store,[133] normal iron saturation of serum transferrin,[134] and myelopoiesis depressing factor from kidney.

3. *Myeloma Cell*

The cytology of the myeloma cell has been extensively studied. Since Braunsteiner described the characteristic electron microscopic features of plasma cells in 1953, numerous morphologic changes have been advanced as pathognomic markers of myeloma cells.

a. Size

Many textbooks of hematology state that myeloma cells are generally larger than the plasma cells of benign plasmacotysis but this finding is not pathognomic. Recently, Hayhoe and Neuman measured the size of plasma cells from 100 cases of multiple myeloma.[60] The major diameter of IgG, IgA, and Bence-Jones myeloma cells was 13 to 15 μm and the minor diameter, 11 to 12 μm without statistical difference between subgroup. The diameter of mature plasmacytes is 12 to 15 μm with an average of 14.4 μm.

b. Nucleus

An immature nucleus is frequently observed in myeloma plasma cells and in reactive plasmacytosis. Nuclear cytoplasmic maturation asynchrony is said to be a significantly more common finding in multiple myeloma. Graham and Bernier[7] described asynchrony in the bone marrow cells of 33 of 34 patients with multiple myeloma or macroglobulinemia. Definite asynchromy was not found in any of the patients with reactive plasmacytosis. Although the degree of asynchrony was not always uniform in all the plasma cells observed in a particular marrow specimen, moderate to marked asynchrony was observed in all of the clinically advanced multiple myeloma cases. Mild degrees of asynchrony were observed in about one third of patients with myeloma and one half of patients with benign gammopathy. Thus, it is not clear whether the described asynchrony is a transient phenomenon reflecting an active secretory function or a characteristic feature associated with neoplasia. The same authors subsequently compared light and electron microscopy for the identification and quantification of the asynchrony of plasma cells in myeloma.[135] They demonstrated relatively good correlation between the degree of asynchrony and clinical extent of disease, but the correlation between light and electron microscopy was poor.

Review of cytogenetic literature reveals that the plasma cells in patients with myeloma have a high degree (40%) of hypodiploid karyocytes suggesting that DNA content may be a useful marker for the disease.[136]

c. Nucleolus

Large, prominent, and conspicious nucleoli with poor perinucleolar chromatin condensation represent a typical finding of immature plasma cells. Immature nucleoli are found in either reactive plasmacytosis or myeloma. Smetana,[16] however, observed immature nucleoli in the mature nuclei of the myeloma cells (nucleolar nuclear asynchrony).

d. Other Nuclear Variations

The binucleated cell or multinucleate plasma cell is most often observed in multiple myeloma or related neoplastic diseases. It is postulated that this may represent nuclear/ cytoplasmic maturation asynchrony; however, binucleated cells are also seen in reactive plasmacytosis.

An irregular contour of the nucleus is a common feature of myeloma cells but also of plasma cells of reactive plasmacytosis or during mitogen-induced lymphocyte transformation. The significance of these morphologic changes is not known, but is thought to be either a normal variation of immaturity or degenerative changes.[24]

The other intranuclear inclusions are thought of as dysplastic changes and not considered pathognomic for malignancy.

e. Cytoplasmic Variation

The various configurations of the endoplasmic reticulum and cytoplasmic inclusions are considered nonspecific. The exact metabolic role of these variations is not known. The Russell bodies, grape-like cell, or Mott cell are rarely observed in myeloma, whereas the flaming cell is more often observed. Variation of cell shape and changes in the number of mitochondria are not considered specific for multiple myeloma.

Cytoplasmic membrane, pseudopods, microvilli, budding, and endocytosis have been observed in the myeloma cell; however, this is believed to represent normal cellular activities not neoplastic change.

4. Cytokinetics

The usual course for myeloma patients consists of an initial reduction in ''tumor'' load after chemotherapy followed by a variable interval of disease stabilization, and then relapse with increasing ''tumor'' burden. Drewinko and Alexanian[137] have postulated the existence of a chemotherapy sensitive and resistant cell fraction. These clinical findings can be amplified into a working model for the pathogenesis of myeloma.

Plasma cells in the bone marrow contain the same distribution of immunoglobulin classes that are seen in the serum.[138–141] These data have led to the hypothesis that the marrow is the major site of immunoglobulin production. Bone marrow lymphocytes in myeloma patients have been shown to be monoclonal as determined by antiidiotypic sera suggesting that the myelomatous process begins at the level of the marrow B lymphocyte.[142] The appearance of monoclonal lymphocytes in the peripheral blood and lymph nodes of myeloma patients appears to be the result of a leukemia-like dissemination. It is known that plasma cell leukemia is predominantly seen, but rarely so, during the terminal phase of myeloma.[143] The bone lesions of myeloma consist of an indolent cell population whose capacity for cell division and turnover is limited. This is true even though bone destruction and the rise in M-component may occur at extremely rapid rates. Most plasma cells in myeloma are probably terminally differentiated and do not undergo cell division; plasma cells in myeloma label at a very low rate (1%) following exposure to ^{3}H-thymidine, but can synthesize immunoglobulin and osteoclast-promoting factors at prolific rates.

Since the plasma cells in myeloma do not actively divide, the progression of disease can only be explained by the continuing contribution of a precursor cell. The idiotypic specificity of the marrow B lymphocytes and the fact that the marrow B lymphocytes in myeloma patients show a higher labeling index than plasma cells (15% vs. 1%) suggest that the marrow lymphocytes may be the precursor tumor cell.[141] This hypothesis would explain the rapid fall of the M-component following chemotherapy since therapy in our opinion, would be more likely to effect immunoglobulin-producing B lymphocytes. The kinetic data formulated by Sullivan and Salmon[143] using the M component as the index of tumor mass may be valid if we include lymphocytes in the calculation of tumor burden. Support of this hypothesis comes from Drewinko et al.[137] who found that the myeloma tumor arises from a proliferating population of marrow cells. Alternatively, the absence of significant numbers of lymphocytes in the marrow of advanced cases of myeloma suggest that the abnormal clone of B lymphocytes do not differentiate within the marrow.

Plasma cell leukemia is considered to be a variety of plasma cell dyscrasia characterized by a high proliferative capacity and the production of a great variety of immunoglobulin products ranging from complete immunoglobulins to light chains or immunoglobulin fragments. It appears that asynchronous or incompleted synthesis of heavy and light chains is pronounced in plasma cell leukemia. This disease may represent a true plasma cell malignancy if we compare its cellular kinetics to that of other leukemias.

Durie and Salmon[145] have developed a clinical staging system for myeloma based upon the initial hemoglobin, calcium, extent of osteolytic lesions, and size of the M component. These investigators have extrapolated the size of the M protein into a concept of ''cell mass.'' Simply, the cell mass = total body M protein synthetic rate divided by the cellular M protein synthetic rate. The presence of a high cell mass and a high labeling index in marrow plasma cells (>3%) connotes a particularly bad prognosis.[146]

B. Waldenström's Macroglobulinemia

Waldenström's macroglobulinemia is a malignant disorder of differentiating B lymphocytes associated with the production of monoclonal macroglobulins. The common clinical manifestations, hyperviscosity, bleeding, renal failure, malabsorption, anemia, hepatospenomegaly, and lymphadenopathy are the direct or indirect effect of increased macroglobulin production and cellular infiltration. The serum concentration of monoclonal macroglobulin ranges between 1 to 12 g/dℓ; the monoclonal protein usually comprised 20 to 70% of the total serum proteins. Autopsy studies on patients with Waldenström's macroglobulinemia show involvement of bone marrow in 100%, liver 76%, spleen 70%, lymph nodes 76%, kidney 69%, and brain in 19% of cases.[147] Lymph nodes and bone marrow represent the most accesible sources for histologic examination although the diagnosis of Waldenström's macroglobulinemia is not solely dependent on histology. Bone marrow aspiration may result in a ''dry tap'' or may show decreased cellularity because of the hypercellularity of the bone marrow and the high viscosity of marrow blood.

The bone marrow biopsy specimen is hypercellular and characteristically reveals a pleomorphic cellular infiltration which is composed, in varying degrees, of small lymphocytes, intermediate size lymphocytes, lymphocytoid plasma cells, and plasma cells. Increased mast cells and reticulum cells are also noted. Although the degree of pleomorphism is variable, the predominant cells are usually the lymphocytoid plasma cells. This cell usually shows a very basophilic cytoplasm. The periodic-acid-Schiff (PAS) stain is frequently positive. A significant proportion of plasma cells or lymphocytoid plasma cells contain intranuclear PAS-positive inclusions or show a diffuse positive PAS reaction in the cytoplasm most likely due to the high carbohydrate concentration of IgM.[152] On electron microscopy, these lymphocytoid plasma cells resemble immature plasmacytes or plasmacytes containing developed rough endoplasmic reticulum.

The pattern of cellular infiltration in the marrow can be differentiated into two types, nodular and diffuse. The nodular type consists of well-circumscribed lymphoid aggregates with relatively well-preserved bone marrow tissue; the diffuse type shows cells infiltrating the marrow with replacement of hematopoietic and fat compartments. Re-

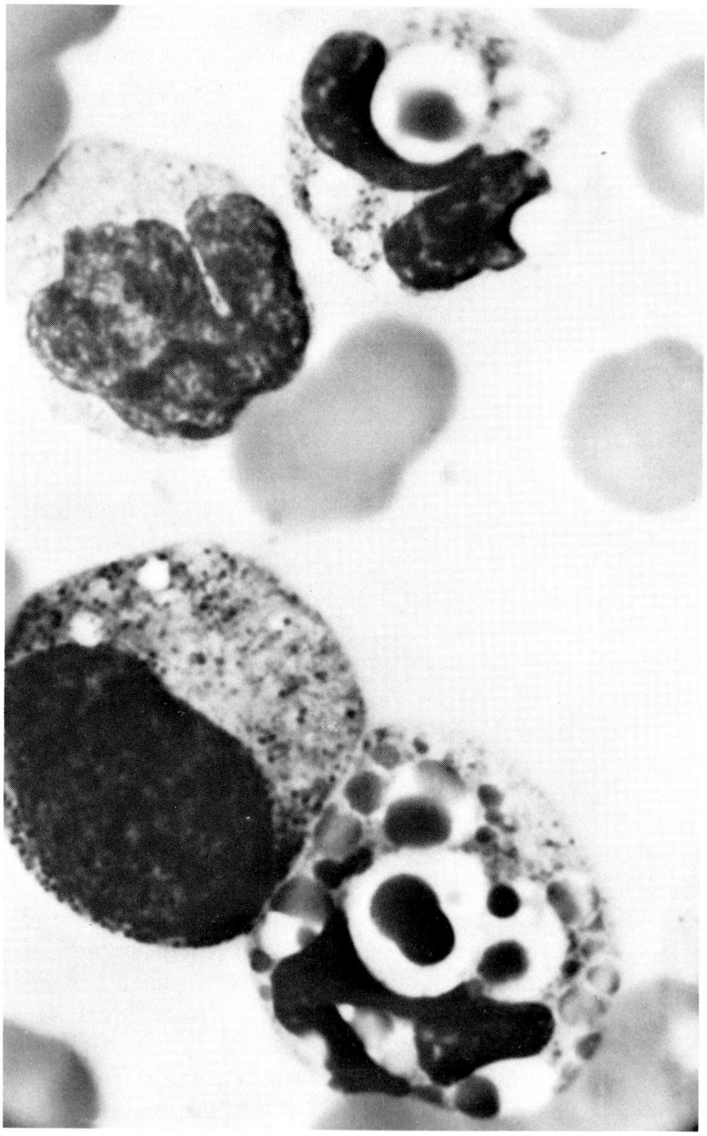

FIGURE 3. Marrow amyloid. Bone marrow granulocytes with engulfed amyloid material. Approximately 2500 ×.

cently, Duhamel[148] compared the bone marrow histology and the clinical course of patients with Waldenström's macroglobulinemia. The nodular type was found in 29% of patients and the diffuse type in 66% of patients. The patients with diffuse type presented with more advanced clinical manifestations and had a poorer prognosis than the nodular type. Chelazzi[149] also reported a poorer prognosis in patients with diffuse pattern on bone marrow histology. The histologic pattern in the bone marrow reflects the pattern that is seen in other organs like lymph nodes and spleen.[150] Although the cells infiltrating the bone marrow are pleomorphic, it is known that the pleomorphic cells are, in fact, differentiating B lymphocytes.

With antiidiotypic antibodies it can be demonstrated that most of the infiltrating cells in the bone marrow are monoclonal in origin, and that the immunoglobulin idiotype pattern is the same in bone marrow and peripheral blood lymphocytes.[138,150,151] Although Waldenström's macroglobulinemia is frequently characterized by a unique clinical syndrome, the histopathologic patterns and general clinical course more often resemble the classic lymphocytic lymphomas. In this respect, Waldenström's macroglobulinemia is considered as one type of lymphoplasmacytic malignant lymphoma.[153]

C. Amyloidosis

Amyloidosis is a disease characterized by the deposition of a homogeneous, eosinophilic material in various tissues throughout the body. The clinical presentation is attributed to the extent of organ or tissue dysfunction caused by the infiltration of "amyloid material."

Under the electron microscope, amyloid is seen to consist of rigid, nonbranching fibrils. Biochemically, amyloid fibrils are either light chains, or light chain fragments of immunoglobulin or various nonimmunoglobulin proteins. The pathogenesis of amyloid formation in multiple myeloma and related disease has been extensively studied, but the other types of amyloidosis are poorly understood. Amyloid may deposit in almost any organ including kidney, heart, lung, GI tract, liver, spleen, and nervous system. A biopsy can be performed from any organ depending on clinical presentation, although, when systemic amyloidosis is suspected, rectal biopsy is preferable. The incidence of positive rectal biopsies in systemic amyloidosis is about 80% with rare complication. Bone involvement may not be apparent on clinical presentation in patients with systemic amyloidosis without myeloma. The bone roentogenograms are normal in 95% of cases.[154] Despite this, amyloid deposition can be identified frequently from bone marrow specimen either by special stain or Wright-Giemsa stain.

Amyloid appears as a structureless, homogeneous material which stains as pale pink to colorless with hematoxylin and eosin, purple-red with crystal violet, dark blue-purple with methyl violet stain. Amyloid stained with congo red displays a green birefringence in polarized light. Kyle[155] reported a 42% positivity in antemortem bone marrow biopsies in patients with systemic amyloidosis. Interestingly, amyloid was also identified by Wright stain from the bone marrow aspirate.[155,157]

Bone marrow biopsy examination reveals amyloid deposition within the walls of small blood vessels close to the basement membrane usually associated with marked thickening of the wall itself and occluded lumina. The amyloid can be seen as discrete isolated masses or diffusely dispersed throughout the marrow with replacement or normal hemopoietic tissue. The amyloid may be surrounded by histocytes and giant cells and can occasionally be phagocytized by marrow granulocytes (Figure 3). Plasma cells are increased to as much as 15% of nucleated cells.[154]

REFERENCES

1. **Hyun, B. H., Kwa, D., Gabaldon, H., and Ashton, J. K.,** Reactive plasmacytic lesions of the bone marrow, *Am. J. Clin. Pathol.,* 65, 921, 1976.
2. **Sacchetti, D.,** Le plasmacellule nel midollo osseo dell'uomo nella norma e nella pathologica: richerche quantitative citometriche et auxologiche, *Hematologica (Pavia),* 35, 13, 1951.
3. **von Marschalko, T.,** Ueber die sogenannten Plasmazellen: Ein Beitrag zur Kenntnis der Herkunft der entzündlichen Infiltrationzellen, *Arch. Dermat. Syph.,* 30, 3, 1895.
4. **Cawley, J. C. and Hayhoe, F. G.,** Ultrastructure of haemic cells, *A Cytological Atlas of Normal and Leukemic Blood and Bone Marrow,* W. B. Saunders, London, 1973.
5. **Tanaka, Y. and Goodman, J. R.,** *Electron Microscopy of Human Blood Cells,* Harper and Row, New York, 1972, 273.
6. **Maldonado, J. E., Brown, A. L., Bayrd, E. D., and Pease, G. L.,** Ultrastructure of the myeloma cell, *Cancer,* 19, 1613, 1966.
7. **Graham, R. C. and Bernier, G. M.,** The bone marrow in multiple myeloma: correlation of plasma cell ultrastructure and clinical state, *Medicine (Baltimore),* 54, 225, 1975.
8. **Fawcett, D. W.,** *An Atlas of Fine Structure. The Cell, its Organelles and Inclusions,* W. B. Saunders, Philadelphia, 1966, 135.
9. **Blom, J.,** The ultrastructure of contact zones between plasma cells and macrophages in the bone marrow of patients with multiple myeloma, *Acta Patho. Microbiol. Scand., Sect. A,* 85, 345, 1977.
10. **Blom, J., Hansen, O. P., and Mansa, B.,** The ultrastructure of bone marrow plasma cells obtained from patients with multiple myeloma during the clinical course of the disease, *Acta Pathol. Microbiol. Scan. Sect. A,* 88, 25, 1980.
11. **Blom, J.,** The ultrastructure of macrophages found in contact with plasma cells in the bone marrow of patients with multiple myeloma, *Acta Pathol. Microbiol. Scand. Sect. A,* 85, 335, 1977.
12. **Ottosen, P. D., Courtoy, P. J., and Farquhar, M. G.,** Pathway followed by membrane recovered from the surface of plasma cells and myeloma cells, *J. Exp. Med.,* 152, 1, 1980.
13. **Polliack, A., Gamliel, H., Froimovici, M., and Laskov, R.,** Myeloma cells: surface morphology as seen by scanning and transmission electron microscopy, *Isr. J. Med. S.C.,* 14, 1252, 1978.
14. **Polliack, A., Nilsson, K., Laskow, R., and Biberfeld, P.,** Characteristic surface morphology of human and murine myeloma cells: a scanning and transmission electron microscopic study, *Br. J. Haematol.,* 39, 25, 1978.
15. **Djaldetti, M. and Fishman, P.,** Scanning and transmission electron microscopy study on the plasma cells of patients with multiple myeloma, *Acta Haematol.,* 58, 173, 1977.
16. **Smetana, K., Gyorkey, F., Gyorkey, P., and Bush, H.,** Ultrastructural studies on human myeloma plasmacytes, *Cancer Res.,* 33, 2300, 1973.
17. **Bernier, G. M. and Graham, R. C., Jr.,** Plasma cell asynchrony in myeloma: correlation of light and electron microscopy, *Semin. Hematol.,* 13, 239, 1976.
18. **Türk, W.,** *Untersuchungen über den Verhalten des Blutes bei akuten Infektionskrankheiten,* Braumüller, Vienna, 1898.
19. **Türk, W.,** *Vorlesungen über Klinische Haëmatologie,* Pt. I. Braumüler, Vienna, 1904.
20. **Pappenheim, A.,** Wie verhalten sich die Unnaschen plasmazellen zu lymphocyten? *Arch. Pathol. Anat.,* 165, 365, 1901.
21. **Bessis, M. and Thiery, J. P.,** Electron microscopy of human white blood cells and their stem cells, *Int. Rev. Cytol.,* 12, 199, 1961.
22. **Spriggs, A. I. and Jerrome, D. W.,** Electron microscopy of Türk cells, *Br. J. Haematol.,* 13, 764, 1967.
23. **Herbeuval, R. and Herbeuval, H.,** *Cellules Cancéreuses et Insolites du Sang Circulant,* Masson, Paris, 1965.
24. **Zucker-Franklin, D.,** Cellular structure and neoplastic in normal and function lymphoid cells, *Arch. Intern. Med.,* 135, 55, 1975.
25. **Smetana, K., Hermansky, F., Koblizkova, H., and Pospisil, V.,** A further note on the ultrastructure of myeloma plasmacytes, *Neoplasma,* 18, 3, 1971.
26. **Bush, H. and Smetana, K.,** *The Nucleolus,* Academic Press, New York, 1970.
27. **Bernhard, W. and Granboulan, N.,** Electronmicroscopy of the nucleolus in vertebrate cells, in *The Nucleus,* Dalton, A. J. and Haguenau, F., Eds., Academic Press, New York, 1968, 81.
28. **Turesson, I.,** Nucleolar size in benign and malignant plasma cell proliferation, *Acta Med. Scand.,* 197, 7, 1975.
29. **Smetana, K., Lane, M., and Busch, H.,** Studies of nucleoli of leucemic agranulocytes and plasmacytes in multiple myeloma, *Exp. Molec. Pathol.,* 5, 236, 1966.

30. **Quaglino, D., Torelli, U., Sauli, S., and Mauri, C.**, Cytochemical and autoradiographic investigations on normal and myelomatous plasma cells, *Acta Haematol.*, 38, 79, 1967.
31. **Schmid, J., Kiely, J. et al.**, *In vitro* DNA and RNA synthesis in human bone marrow cells: a study of 12 normal subjects and 12 patients with lymphoplasmacytic disorders, *Blood*, 27, 310, 1966.
32. **Dutcher, T. F. and Fahey, J. L.**, The histopathology of the macroglobulinemia of Waldenström, *J. Natl. Cancer Inst.*, 22, 887, 1959.
33. **Brunning, R. D. and Parkin, J.**, Intranuclear inclusions in plasma cells and lymphocytes from patients with monoclonal gammopathies, *Am. J. Clin. Pathol.*, 66, 10, 1976.
34. **Bessis, M. C.**, Ultrastructure of lymphoid and plasma cells in relation to globulin and antibody formation, *Lab. Invest.*, 10, 1040, 1961.
35. **Brittin, G. M., Tanaka, Y., and Blecher, G.**, Intranuclear inclusions in multiple myeloma and macroglobinemia, *Blood*, 21, 334, 1963.
36. **Maldonado, J. E., Brown, A. L., Bayrd, E. D., and Pease, G. L.**, Cytoplasmic and intranuclear electron dense bodies in the myeloma cells, *Arch. Pathol.*, 81, 484, 1966.
37. **Stavem, P., Hovig, T., Frpland, S., and Skrede, S.**, Immunoglobulin containing intranuclear inclusions in plasma cells in a case of IgG myeloma, *Scand. J. Haematol.*, 13, 266, 1974.
38. **Ito, K., Ito, N., and Katsunuma, H.**, A case of myeloma demonstrating an interesting nuclear structure; review on nuclear inclusions body in myeloma, *Acta Hematol. Jpn.*, 27, 87, 1964.
39. **Cohen, H. J. and Lefer, L. G.**, Intranuclear inclusions in Bence-Jones Lambda plasma cell myeloma, *Blood*, 45, 131, 1975.
40. **Kuhn, C.**, Nuclear bodies and intranuclear globulin inclusions in Waldenström's macroglobulinemia, *Lab. Invest.*, 17, 404, 1967.
41. **Uhr, J. W. and Schenkein, I.**, Immunoglobulin synthesis and secretion. IV. Studies of incorporation of sugars as determined by subcellular fractionation, *Proc. Natl. Acad. Sci. U.S.A.*, 66, 952, 1970.
42. **Buxbaum, J. N.**, The biosynthesis assembly, and secretion of immunoglobulins, *Semin. Hematol.*, 10, 33, 1973.
43. **Tartakoff, V. and Vassali, P.**, Plasma cell immunoglobulin M molecules, *J. Cell. Biol.*, 83, 284, 1979.
44. **Oikawa, K.**, Electron microscopic observation of inclusion bodies in plasma cells of multiple myeloma and Waldenström's macroglobulinemia, *Tohoku J. Exp. Med.*, 117, 257, 1975.
45. **Leduc, E. H., Aurameas, S., and Bouteille, M.**, Ultrastructural localization of antibody in differentiating plasma cells, *J. Exp. Med.*, 127, 109, 1968.
46. **Aurameas, S. and Ledus, E. H.**, Detection of simultaneous antibody synthesis in plasma cells and specialized lymphocytes in rabbit lymph nodes, *J. Exp. Med.*, 131, 1137, 1970.
47. **Simar, L. J.**, Ultrastructure et constitution des corps nucleáires dan les plasmocytes, *Z. Zellforsch.*, 99, 235, 1969.
48. **Ishii, Y., Mori, M., and Onoe, T.**, Electron microscopic study of nuclear bodies in plasma cells of mouse lymph nodes during the primary immune response, *J. Electron. Microsc.*, 20, 182, 1971.
49. **Krishan, A., Uzman, B. G., and Hedley Whyte, E. T.**, Nuclear bodies: a component of cell nuclei in hamster tissue and human tumors, *J. Ultrastruct. Res.*, 19, 563, 1967.
50. **Suzuki, I., Takahashi, M., and Itoh, S.**, Ultrastructural study of human myeloma cells in relation to its function, *J. Clin. Pathol.*, 23, 339, 1970.
51. **Sorenson, G. D.**, Electron microscopic observations of bone marrow from patients with multiple myeloma, *Lab. Invest.*, 13, 196, 1964.
52. **Ogawa, M., Preston, R. A., Carson, M. D., Komiyama, A., and Spicer, S. S.**, Cytoplasmic fibrils in plasma cell leukemia, *Acta Haematol.*, 56, 123, 1976.
53. **Zucker-Franklin, D., and Franklin, E. C.**, Intracellular localization of human amyloid by fluorescence and electron microscopy, *Am. J. Pathol.*, 59, 23, 1970.
54. **Russell, W.**, An address on a characteristic organism of cancer, *Br. Med. J.*, 2, 1356, 1890.
55. **Welsh, R. A.**, Light and electron microscopic correlation of the periodic acid-Schiff reaction in the human plasma cell, *Am. J. Pathol.*, 40, 285, 1962.
56. **Ortega, L. G. and Mellors, R. C.**, Cellular sites of formation of gammaglobulin, *J. Exp. Med.*, 106, 627, 1957.
57. **White, R. G.**, Observation on the formation and nature of Russell bodies, *Br. J. Exp. Pathol.*, 35, 365, 1954.
58. **Fisher, E. R. and Zawadzki, Z. A.**, Ultrastructural features of plasma cells in patients with paraproteinemias, *Am. J. Clin. Pathol.*, 54, 779, 1970.
59. **Waldenström, J.**, *Diagnosis and Treatment of Multiple Myeloma*, Grune and Stratton, New York, 1970, 15.
60. **Hayhoe, F. G. J. and Neuman, Z.**, Cytology of myeloma cells, *J. Clin. Pathol.*, 29, 916, 1976.
61. **Mott, F. W.**, Report of the sleeping sickness, *Commission of the Royal Society*, 7, 15, 1906.

62. **Stefanopoulo, G., Graubet, P., and Davolan, S.**, Presence de cellules mariformes de Mott chez les rats inféctés de *Trypanosoma Gambiense, Bull. Soc. Pathol. Exot.*, 37, 296, 1944.
63. **Jude, A. and Frabiani, G.**, Presence de cellules mariformes dan la moelle osseuse au Cours du typhus, du paludisme, du kala-azar, *C. R. Soc. Biol.*, 139, 706, 1945.
64. **Undritz, E.**, *Sandoz Atlas of Hematology*, Basel, Sandoz, 1952, 91.
65. **Maldonado, J. E., Bayrd, E. D., and Brown, A. L., Jr.**, The flaming cell in multiple myeloma. A light and electron microscopy study, *Am. J. Clin. Pathol.*, 44, 605, 1965.
66. **Paraskevas, F., Heremans, J., and Waldenström, J.**, Cytology and electrophoretic pattern in 1A (B2A) myeloma, *Acta Med. Scand.*, 170, 575, 1961.
67. **Jacobs, P., Kinnear, B., and Richards, J. D.**, Diagnostic significance of ''flaming'' plasma cells in multiple myeloma, *Lancet*, 2, 363, 1980.
68. **Utsinger, P., Yount, W. J., Fuller, C. R., Logue, M. J., and Orringer, E. P.**, Hairy cell leukemia: B lymphocyte and phagocytic properties, *Blood*, 49, 19, 1977.
69. **Catowsky, D., Sperandio, P., O'Brien, M., et al.**, Phagocytic potential of leukemic B lymphocytes, *Scand. J. Haematol.*, 19, 211, 1977.
70. **Fioadi, M. D., Slater, A. G., and Pegrum, G. D.**, Erythrophagocytosis by acute lymphoblastic leukemia cells, *Scand. J. Haematol.*, 20, 85, 1978.
71. **Hughes, N. R.**, Erythrocyte phagocytosis by human lymphocytes, *Nature*, 212, 1575, 1966.
72. **Ludwig, H. and Pavelka, M.**, Phagocytic plasma cells in a patient with multiple myeloma, *Blood*, 56, 173, 1980.
73. **Butterworth, C. E., Frommeyer, W. B., and Riser, W. H.**, Erythrophagocytosis in a case of plasma cell leukemia, *Blood*, 8, 519, 1953.
74. **Abramson, N., Von Kapff, B. S., and Ginsburg, A. D.**, The phagocytic plasma cells, *N. Engl. J. Med.*, 283, 248, 1970.
75. **Fitchen, J. H. and Lee, S.**, Phagocytic myeloma cells, *Am. J. Clin. Pathol.*, 71, 722, 1979.
76. **Jaffe, R. H.**, The Reticuloendothelial System, in *Handbook of Hematology*, Vol. 2, Downey, H., Ed., Harper, New York, 1938.
77. **Koszweski, B. J.**, Megaloblastic erythropoiesis with hemochromatosis, *Blood*, 7, 1182, 1952.
78. **Shanmugathasa, M., Sobel, H. J., Marquet, E., and Trubowitz, S.**, Plasma cells with inclusions containing iron, *Arch. Pathol. Lab. Med.*, 103, 577, 1979.
79. **Izarn, P. and Enbarger, J.**, Plasmocytes avec inclusion d' hémosiderine, *Sang*, 29, 701, 1958.
80. **Lerner, R. G. and Parker, J. W.**, Dysglobulinemia and iron in plasma cells, *Arch. Int. Med.*, 121, 284, 1968.
81. **Goodman, J. R. and Hall, S. G.**, Plasma cells containing iron, *Blood*, 28, 83, 1966.
82. **Karcioglu, G. L. and Hardison, J. E.**, Iron containing plasma cells, *Arch. Int. Med.*, 138, 97, 1978.
83. **Cardinale, G. and Carrescia, P. M.**, Phagocytose plasmocytaire dans un cas de B-plasmocytome, *Sang*, 27, 682, 1956.
84. **De Lellis, R.**, Iron containing plasma cells in a healed spider bite, *Arch. Pathol.*, 92, 254, 1971.
85. **Azar, H. A., Pham, T. C., and Kurban, A. K.**, An electron microscopic study of a syphilitic chancre: engulfment of treponemia pallidum by plasma cells, *Arch. Pathol.*, 90, 143, 1970.
86. **Cajal, S. R.**, Quelques antecedents historiques ignores sur les plasmazellen, *Anat. Anzeiger*, 29, 666, 1906.
87. **Unna, P. G.**, Uber plasmazellen insbesondere beim lupus, *Monatsschr. Prakt. Dermat.*, 12, 296, 1891.
88. **Marschalko, T.**, Zur plasmazellenfrage, *Centralbl. Allg. Path. Path. Anat.*, 10, 851, 1899.
89. **McMaster, P. D. and Hudack, S. S.**, The formation of agglutinins within lymph nodes, *J. Exp. Med.*, 61, 783, 1935.
90. **Fagraeus, A.**, Antibody production in relation to the development of plasma cells, *Acta Med. Scand.*, 130 (suppl. 204), 3, 1948.
91. **Nossal, G. J. V.**, Antibody production by single cells, *Br. J. Exp. Path.*, 41, 89, 1960.
92. **Nossal, G. J. V. and Makelao, O.**, Autoradiographic studies of the immune response. I. The kinetics of plasma cell proliferation, *J. Exp. Med.*, 115, 209, 1962.
93. **Gery, I., Kruger, J., and Spiesel, S. Z.**, Stimulation of B lymphocytes by endotoxin in reactions of thymus deprived mice and karyotypic analysis of dividing cells in mice bearing T6T6 thymus grafts, *J. Immunol.*, 108, 1088, 1972.
94. **Shands, J. W., Peavy, D. L., and Smith, R. T.**, Differential morphology of mouse spleen cells stimulated *in vitro* by endotoxin, phytohemagglutinin, pokeweed mitogen and staphylococcal enterotoxin B., *Am. J. Pathol.*, 70, 1, 1973.
95. **Brochier, J., Bona, C., Ciorbaru, R., Revillard, J. P., and Chedid, L.**, A human T independent B lymphocyte mitogen extracted from Nocardia opacak, *J. Immunol.*, 117, 1434, 1976.

96. **LethiBich-Thuy, R., Ciorbaru, R., and Brochier, J.,** Human B cell differentiation. I. Immunoglobulin synthesis induced by Nocardia mitogen, *Eur. J. Immunol.*, 8, 119, 1978.
97. **Insen, R. A. and Merler, E.,** The necessity for T cell help for human tonsil B cell responses to pokeweed mitogen: induction of DNA synthesis, immunoglobulin, and specific antibody production with a T cell helper factor produced with pokeweed mitogen, *J. Immunol.*, 118, 1009, 1977.
98. **LethiBich-Thuy, Brochier, J.,** Human B cell differentiation. II. Suppression by T cell of B dependent and T independent plasma cell maturation, *J. Immunol.*, 122, 1842, 1979.
99. **Hall, J. C., Wang, A. L., Pawlak, L. L., et al.,** Suppression of idiotypic specificities in adult mice by administration of anti-idiotypic antibody, *J. Exp. Med.*, 135, 1293, 1972.
100. **Abdou, N. I. and Abdou, N. L.,** The monoclonal nature of lymphocytes in multiple myeloma. Effects of therapy, *Ann. Intern. Med.*, 83, 42, 1975.
101. **van Camp, B., Reynaert, Ph, and Broodtaerts, L.,** Studies on the origin of the precursor cells in multiple myeloma, Waldenstrom's macroglobulinemia and benign monoclonal gammopathy, *Clin. Exp. Immunol.*, 44, 82, 1981.
102. **Borjeson, J., Reisfeld, R., Chessin, L. N., Welsh, P., and Douglas, S. D.,** Studies on human peripheral blood lymphocytes *in vitro*. I. Biological and physiochemical properties of the pokeweed mitogen, *J. Exp. Med.*, 124, 859, 1966.
103. **Chessin, L. N., Borjeson, J., Welsh, P., Douglas, S. D., and Cooper, H. L.,** Studies on human peripheral blood lymphocytes *in vitro*. II. Morphological and biochemical studies on the transformation of lymphocytes by pokeweed mitogen, *J. Exp. Med.*, 124, 873, 1966.
104. **Douglas, S. D., Hoffman, P. T., Borjeson, J., and Chessin, L. N.,** Studies on peripheral blood lymphocytes *in vitro*. III. Fine structural features of lymphocytes transformation by pokeweed mitogen, *J. Immunol.*, 98, 1730, 1967.
105. **Douglas, S. D. and Fudenberg, H. H.,** *in vitro* development of plasma cells from lymphocytes following pokeweed mitogen stimulation: a fine structural study, *Exp. Cell. Res.*, 54, 277, 1969.
106. **Douglas, S. D.,** Human lymphocyte growth *in vitro:* morphologic, biochemical and immunologic significance, *Int. Rev. Exp. Pathol.*, 10, 42, 1971.
107. **Ramasamy, R. and Munro, A. J.,** Surface B and T cell markers on murine lymphomas and plasmacytoma, *Immunology,* 26, 563, 1974.
108. **Solomon, A., Waldman, T. A., and Fahey, J. L.,** Metabolism of normal globulin in normal subjects and in patients with macroglobulinemia and multiple myeloma, *J. Lab. Clin. Med.*, 62, 1, 1963.
109. **Liang, W. and Rowley, J. D.,** 149 + marker chromosomes in multiple myeloma and plasma cell leukemia, *Lancet,* 1, 96, 1978.
110. **Cioli, D. and Lennox, E.,** Ig nascent chains on membrane bound ribosomes of myeloma cells, *Biochemistry,* 12, 3211, 1973.
111. **Tartakoff, A. M., Vassalli, P., and Detraz, M.,** Plasma cell immunoglobulin secretion, arrest is accompanied by alteration of the Golgi complex, *J. Exp. Med.*, 146, 1332, 1977.
112. **Tartakoff, A., Vassalli, P., and Detraz, M.,** Plasma cell immunoglobulin M molecules: their biosynthesis, assembly and intracellular transport, *J. Cell. Biol.*, 83, 284, 1979.
113. **Ottosen, P. D., Courtoy, P. J., and Farquhar, M. G.,** Pathways followed by membrane recovered from the surface of plasma cells and myeloma cells, *J. Exp. Med.*, 152, 1, 1980.
114. **Mabry, R. J., Shelburne, J., and Cohen, H. J.,** *In vitro* kinetics of immunoglobulin synthesis and secretion by nonsecretory human myeloma cells, *Blood,* 50, 1031, 1977.
115. **Moake, J. L., Landry, R. P., Oren, M. E., Sayer, B. L., and Heffner, T.,** Transient peripheral plasmacytosis, *Am. J. Clin. Pathol.*, 62, 8, 1974.
116. **Klein, H. and Block, M.,** Bone marrow plasmacytosis: a review of 60 cases, *Blood,* 8, 1034, 1953.
117. **Callaway, M. W., Braud, E. L., McDonald, C. R., et al.,** Clinical correlates of bone marrow plasmacytosis, *South. Med. J.*, 70, 138, 1977.
118. **Hijmans, W., Schuit, H. R. E., and Hulsing-Hesselink, E.,** An immunofluorescence study in human bone marrow cells, *Ann. N.Y. Acad. Sci.*, 177, 290, 1971.
119. **van Furth, R.,** The formation of immunoglobulins by circulating lymphocytes, *Semin. Hematol.*, 6, 84, 1969.
120. **Hyun, B. H., Kwa, D., Gabaldon, H., and Ashton, J. K.,** Reactive plasmacytic lesions of the bone marrow, *Am. J. Clin. Pathol.*, 65, 921, 1976.
121. **Undritz, E.,** Die regionaren Monocyten der Blutkorperchennester, *Folia Haematol.*, 70, 32, 1950.
122. **Hyun, B. H.,** Plasmacytic lesions of the bone marrow: a critical review, in *Topics in Hematology,* Seno, S. and Takaku, F., Eds., Excerpta Medica, Amsterdam, 1977, 28.
123. **Waldenström, J. C., Adner, A., Gydell, K., and Zettervall, O.,** Osteosclerotic plasmocytoma with polyneuropathy, hypertichosis and diabetes, *Acta Medica. Scand.*, 203, 297, 1978.
124. **Bartl, R., Burkhardt, R., Gierster, P., Sandel, P., and Frateh-Moghadam, A.,** Significance of bone marrow biopsy in the multiple myeloma, *Rec. Prog. Cell. Biol.*, 45, 81, 1978.

125. **Bayrd, E. D.**, The bone marrow on sternal aspiration in multiple myeloma, *Blood*, 3, 987, 1948.
126. **Snapper, I., Turner, L. B., and Moscovitz, H. L.**, *Multiple Myeloma*, Grune, New York, 1953, 168.
127. **Morell, A., Maurer, W., Skvaril, F., and Barandun, S.**, Differentiation between benign and malignant monoclonal gammopathies by discriminant analysis on serum and bone marrow parameter, *Acta Haematol.*, 60, 129, 1978.
128. **Schneider, M. and Mazabraud, M.**, les signes revelateurs du myelome et leur frequence relative, *Rev. Rhum.*, 27, 660, 1959.
129. **Hansen, O. P.**, Bone marrow studies in myelomatosis, *Scand. J. Hematol.*, 21, 265, 1978.
130. **Durie, B. G. M. and Salmon, S. E.**, A clinical staging system for multiple myeloma, *Cancer*, 36, 842, 1975.
131. **Hoffbrand, A. V., Hobbs, J. R., Kremenshuzky, S., and Mollin, D. L.**, Incidence and pathogenesis of megaloblastic erythropoiesis in multiple myeloma, *J. Clin. Pathol.*, 20, 699, 1967.
132. **Magnus, E. M.**, Folate studies, folate and vitamin B_{12} values in relation to bone marrow pattern, *Scand. J. Haematol.*, 24 (suppl.), 1975.
133. **Cline, M. J. and Berlin, N. I.**, Studies of the anemia of multiple myeloma, *Am. J. Med.*, 33, 510, 1962.
134. **Bainton, D. F. and Finch, C. A.**, The diagnosis of iron deficiency anemia, *Am. J. Med.*, 37, 62, 1970.
135. **Bernier, G. and Graham, R., Jr.**, Plasma cell asynchrony in myeloma: correlation of light and electron microscopy, *Semin. Hematol.*, 13, 239, 1976.
136. **Latreille, J., Barlogie, B., Dosik, G., Johnston, D. A., Drewinko, B., and Alexanian, R.**, Cellular DNA content as a marker of human multiple myeloma, *Blood*, 55, 403, 1980.
137. **Drewinko, B. and Alexanian, R.**, Growth kinetics in multiple myeloma, *Proc. Am. Soc. Cancer Res.*, 15, 194, 1974.
138. **Skvaril, A. M., Huser, M. J., Spengler, G., and Barandun, S.**, Cytoplasmic immunoglobulins in bone marrow cells of polyclonal and monoclonal origin, *Acta Haematol.*, 60, 137, 1978.
139. **Husz, S., Krizsa, F., Dobozy, A., Munyadi, J., and Simon, N.**, B and T cell markers of bone marrow and peripheral blood lymphoid cells in patients with paraproteinaemia, *Acta Haematol.*, 57, 321, 1977.
140. **Morell, A., Skvavil, F., Huser, H. J., Spengler, G., and Barandun, S.**, Cytoplasmic immunoglobulins in bone marrow cells of polyclonal and monoclonal origin, *Acta Haematol.*, 60, 137, 1978.
141. **Mellstedt, H., Killander, P., and Pettersson, D.**, Bone marrow kinetic studies on three patients with myelomatosis, *Acta Med. Scand.*, 202, 413, 1977.
142. **van Camp, Reynaert, Ph., and Broodtaerts, L.**, Studies on the origin of the precursor cells in multiple myeloma, Waldenström's macroglobulinaemia and benign monoclonal gammopathy, *Clin. Exp. Immunol.*, 44, 82, 1981.
143. **Sullivan, P. W. and Salmon, S. E.**, Kinetics of tumor growth and regression in IgG multiple myeloma, *J. Clin. Invest.*, 51, 1697, 1972.
144. **Parker, D. and Malpas, J. S.**, Multiple myeloma, *J. Roy. Coll. Phy. London*, 13, 146, 1979.
145. **Durie, B. G. M. and Salmon, S. E.**, A clinical staging system for multiple myeloma, *Cancer*, 36, 842, 1975.
146. **Durie, B. G. M., Salmon, S., and Moon, T. E.**, Pretreatment tumor mass cell kinetics and prognosis in multiple myeloma, *Blood*, 55, 364, 1980.
147. **Yamaguchi, K.**, Pathology of macroglobulinemia: a review of Japanese cases, *Acta Pathol. Jpn.*, 23, 917, 1973.
148. **Duhamel, J. S., Govin, A. N., and Duhamel, de Mme, E.**, Étude histologique de la moelle osseuse dans 96 cas de maladie de Waldenstrom, *Sem. Hop. Paris*, 1596, 1979.
149. **Chelazzi, G., Bettini, R., and Pinotti, G.**, Bone marrow patterns and survival in Waldenstrom's macroglobulinemia, *Lancet*, 8149, 965, 1979.
150. **Aozasa, K. and Uda, H.**, Lymph node involvement in Waldenstrom's macroglobulinemia, *Acta Pathol. Jpn.*, 30, 437, 1980.
151. **Mellstedt, D. P. and Holm, G.**, Characterization of the monoclonal blood and bone marrow B lymphocytes in Waldenstrom's macroglobulinemia, *Scan. J. Immunol.*, 11, 593, 1980.
152. **Kim, H., Heller, P., and Rappaport, H.**, Monoclonal gammopathies associated with lymphoproliferative disorder, a morphologic study, *Am. J. Clin. Pathol.*, 59, 282, 1973.
153. **Lennert, K.**, *Malignant Lymphomas*, Springer-Verlag, New York, 1978, 209.
154. **Kyle, R. and Bayrd, E. D.**, *The Monoclonal Gammopathies*, Charles C Thomas, Springfield, Ill., 1976, 229.
155. **Kyle, R. A., Pease, G. L., Richmond, H., and Sullivan, L.**, Bone marrow aspiration in the antemortem diagnosis of primary systemic amyloidosis, *Am. J. Clin. Pathol.*, 45, 252, 1966.

156. **Conn, R. B. and Sunderg, R. D.,** Amyloid disease of the bone marrow, *Am. J. Pathol.*, 38, 61, 1961.
157. **Stavem, P., Larsen, I. F., Ly, B., and Rorvik, T. O.,** Amyloid deposits in bone marrow aspirates in primary amyloidosis, *Acta Med. Scand.*, 208, 111, 1980.

Chapter 15

MARROW APLASIA

Stephen Davis and Sidney Trubowitz

TABLE OF CONTENTS

I. INTRODUCTION

Hematopoietic failure is clinically defined as peripheral blood pancytopenia associated with marrow hypocellularity not associated with an infiltrative process. The diagnosis encompasses a heterogeneous group of conditions with multiple etiologies and diverse natural histories. Aplasia can be congenital, inherited, but most often is acquired. Deficiencies may occur in single cell lines, i.e., isolated anemia, granulocytopenia, thrombocytopenia, or manifest as complete marrow failure, i.e., aplastic anemia. The single cell aplasias have been discussed briefly in previous chapters. In this monograph we will develop the concept of aplastic anemia. The principles described in this section must equally apply to single cell deficiencies as they do to total aplasia, as well as to mild or severe cytopenias.

II. PATHOGENESIS OF APLASTIC ANEMIA

In previous chapters of this volume we have developed the concept that pluripotent stem cells (CFU-S)* and committed stem cells (CFU-C, BFU-E, CFU-M) are capable of selfrenewal. Differentiation occurs under circumstances that are, in part, regulated by specific factors. In vivo differentiation depends upon interaction between different cell types, soluble factors, and the microenvironment. Stohlman[1] and Trentin[2] showed that the microenvironment influenced hematopoiesis and that a damaged microenvironment prevented normal hematopoiesis. Ershler[3] demonstrated "exuberant" in vitro growth of erythroid colonies from marrow aspirates from an anemic patient with reduced morphologically recognizable erythroid precursors. When whole bone fragments were similarly cultured no appreciable hemoglobin synthesis was observed. The data suggest that an unfavorable microenvironment resulted in the anemia.

Aplasia theoretically can result from aberrations at several steps during normal hematopoiesis. The pluripotential stem cell (CFU-S) may be decreased in absolute number or in its selfrenewal potential.[4] CFU-S may be unable to differentiate into committed stem cells because of an instrinsic abnormality or inability to respond to normal stimuli. Similarly, the committed stem cells may be decreased in number, defective in amplification, or unable to respond to differentiation factors, despite the fact these factors might be elevated in concentration. Lack of colony stimulating factor or of erythropoietin or thrombopoietin might explain an isolated single cell aplasia, but all stimulators would be necessarily missing to produce the pancytopenia of aplastic anemia. Soluble cofactors derived from lymphocytes could be absent if the cells producing them are deficient. There may be humoral inhibitors such as antibodies, or inhibitors such as suppressor T lymphocytes.

Aplastic anemia may occur as a result of damage to all the cell lines in the maturation compartment and/or damage to the pluripotent stem cells (CFU-S). If the former occurred it would imply a continuously acting toxin since normally the regenerative capacity of the CFU-S compartment would readily replenish the differentiating compartments of each cell line.

Successful hematopoietic reconstitution by syngeneic marrow infusion from identical or HLA matched donors add further support to the hypothesis that aplastic anemia, is, in most cases, due to a disorder of CFU-S.[5] Ragab et al.[6] reported on committed stem cell (CFU-C) numbers in 10 cases of aplastic anemia. All cases had extremely decreased numbers of CFU-C. Singer and Brown[7] measured CFU-C concentrations in 22 patients

*This term has been used to designate the pluripotent stem cell in mice. The human equivalent has recently been described and termed CFU-GEMM.

with severe aplastic anemia; only two had colony formation. Similar results have been reported by Kern et al.[8] The absence of extramedullary hematopoiesis in aplasia may indicate an immediate inability of CFU-S in the marrow to migrate and repopulate the liver and spleen as sites for new hematopoiesis, as well as their total absence.

Using broad categories there are two basic mechanisms for marrow aplasia: aplasia induced by toxins that kill marrow cells in a dose-related fashion; and aplasia developing in an unpredictable and perhaps unidentifiable fashion, affecting both the marrow cells and the micro-environment.

A. Nonimmune Marrow Failure

Benzene, chemotherapeutic agents, and irradiation clearly cause a dose-related toxicity to marrow cells resulting in aplasia. If the dose is high enough or given with rapidity the microenvironment may be additionally and irreversibly damaged. This type of dose-related, and usually reversible aplasia, is distinguishable from the aplasia due to exposure to toxins that are believed to be noninjurious to marrow (idiosyncratic). Idiosyncratic reactions are unpredictable and not dose related; neither the microenvironmental nor the stem cell compartments appear to be irrepairably damaged. Idiosyncratic aplasia would seem to involve mechanisms that would imply that either the stem cells or drug metabolism is abnormal and that such a defect is likely to be based on a genetic predisposition. Morley et al.[9] suggested that idiosyncratic aplasia resulting from toxins that are only mildly myelotoxic might be explicable if the CFU-S compartment had already sustained damage from an earlier, unrecognized insult.

1. Drugs

Drugs, like chloramphenicol, can produce aplasia by simultaneously damaging the stem cell and transit compartment probably secondary to its ability to inhibit protein synthesis.[10] Dilantin appears to be able to cause aplasia by a similar mechanism.[11]

Gold salts produce marrow damage by a different mechanism. In most patients treated with gold, aplasia appears dose related; in a minority, however, small doses cause marrow aplasia.[12] In these latter cases aplasia results from damage to the transit compartment. Since gold salts persist for long periods in the body the marrow damage may remain long after gold administration has ceased.[13]

Benzene causes dose-dependent aplasia and disordered maturation. In experimental animals, CFU-S are unaffected by benzene exposure. Radioautograph labeling indices with thymidine and cytidine for the proerythroblast compartment are normal, whereas, in the basophilic normoblast, promyelocyte, and myelocyte compartments it is 40% of normal. This suggests a direct effect on DNA and RNA synthesis in the recognizable transit compartment.[14]

2. Radiation

Boggs and Boggs[15] have studied the effects of whole body irradiation (WBI) on the CFU-E compartment. These investigators found that interruption of CFU-E differentiation began at a dose of 200 r and that the delay in resumption of erythropoiesis was directly proportion to the increase in WBI. Furthermore, if WBI reduced the CFU-E compartment to 10% of normal no CFU-E differentiation occurred; however CFU-E regrowth continued. If a stimulus to erythropoiesis, i.e., bleeding, was performed immediately after irradiation a transient wave of erythropoiesis was induced. If bleeding was delayed for 2 days this effect was lost. The data suggested that the recognition phenomenon for the depletion of the CFU-E compartment was delayed but that once the phenomenon was recognized CFU-E differentiation could not be forced or increased.

3. Paroxysmal Nocturnal Hemoglobinuria

Paroxysmal nocturnal hemoglobinuria (PNH) is an acquired disorder in which erythrocytes and platelets show increased sensitivity to the lytic action of complement. PNH marrow erythroid, platelet and myeloid precursors have also an increased sensitivity to complement-mediated lysis. Despite the increased sensitivity of marrow erythroid and myeloid precursor cells during hemolytic episodes, the marrow aspirate invariably shows a compensating hyperplasia which, if one measures the reticulocyte index, is ineffectual. This trilineal complement-lysis along with the association of PNH with aplastic anemia, myelosclerosis, and acute luekemia suggested a clonal marrow defect at the level of the CFU-S. CFU-C growth in PNH is decreased in patients with PNH thereby implicating a proliferative abnormality.[16] In two cases reported by Applebaum[17] twin marrow infusion restored marrow function in both cases without concomitant cyclophosphamide therapy. The fact that immunosuppression was unnecessary reinforces the stem cell defect hypothesis in PNH.

4. Fanconi's Anemia

Fanconi's anemia is the best-defined aplastic syndrome included in the category of constitutional aplasia. Bone marrow failure appears to be only one manifestation of a generalized cellular defect. It has been suggested that these patients have a defect in DNA repair mechanisms. Ragab et al.[6] studied two patients with Fanconi-type aplastic anemia and found decreased colony formation in both marrow CFU-C and CFU-E. Singer et al.[7] reported similar findings in the sibling of a patient with Fanconi anemia although the sibling was hematologically normal. The CFU studies suggested that, although hematologically unimpaired, an intrinsic defect in committed stem cell function was apparent and that intrinsic abnormalities in stem cell function were not as yet expressed clinically. It is possible that those patients represent marrow aplasia of congenital or genetic type in which nonhematologic features are absent, i.e., formes frustes. This subgroup might also be those patients who have the propensity to develop aplasia following nonmyelosuppressive toxin exposure, i.e., idiosyncratic reactions.

5. Viral Hepatitis

Virus-induced aplasia appears to be a common but transient occurrence; however, there is little doubt that irreversible aplasia may occur. In a series of 193 patients with aplasia following infectious hepatitis Hagler et al.[18] reported that 19% had received chloramphenicol, it was suggested that chloramphenicol predisposed this group of patients to marrow damage. The marrow suppressant effects of drugs and toxins may be addictive or synergistic. Williams et al.[19] suggest that viral infection may cause direct marrow damage, damage to the microenvironment, failure of a diseased liver to clear toxins, and/or an immunologically mediated toxicity (see below).

6. Pregnancy

The first reported case of aplastic anemia reported by Ehrlich[21] was in a pregnant woman with no associated disease. Eight cases occurring during and remitting following pregnancy were reviewed by Fleming;[22] in three this cycle of aplasia and remission recurred in a second pregnancy suggesting a cause and effect relationship. The pathogenesis remains speculative but might be related to the hyperestrogenemia of pregnancy in a genetically susceptible individual.

7. Thymoma

Twelve cases of marrow aplasia associated with thymoma have been reported.[23] Except for a single case all the patients were adults above the age of 50 and four were being treated simultaneously with drugs or radiotherapy. Therefore, toxins might have contributed to the development of the pancytopenia. Immunologic mechanisms have been implicated in the syndrome of thymoma and red cell aplasia.[24]

B. Immune Basis of Marrow Failure

Immune mechanisms have been identified as the basis for a variety of human hematological disorders. We will deal here only with disorders in which immune mechanisms have been implicated in the intramedullary destruction of hematopoietic cells and/or in the inhibition of normal hematopoietic differentiation as related to aplastic anemia.

1. Antibody-Mediated Aplasia

Systemic lupus erythematosus (SLE) is an immune disorder in which autoantibodies to denatured DNA and nucleoproteins can be detected. It represents the prototype for antibody-mediated marrow failures. The majority of patients with SLE have a normochromic microcytic anemia due to marrow depression, possibly mediated by antibodies to developing erythroid elements. There may also be production of antibodies to circulating platelets producing immune thrombocytopenia. In a minority of patients, pancytopenia is found.[20] Marrow aspirates show a marked decrease of all normal hematopoietic marrow elements with replacement by lymphoid and other mononuclear cells. The marrow failure may be caused by the destruction of the committed stem cells by antibodies against their differentiation antigens, but this is speculative.

Freedman et al.[25] reported a case of aplastic anemia in which the patient's serum inhibited CFU-E and CFU-C growth in normal marrow. The patient's B lymphocytes similarly decreased CFU-C's when cocultured with normal marrow. The authors suggested antibody-mediated marrow failure. Herron et al.[26] described a patient suffering from aplastic anemia who had an anti-Vel autoantibody. No in vitro colony forming studies were performed so that the pathophysiology of this association is speculative.

Yoda et al.[27] studied five cases of aplastic anemia (AA) with antisplenic tissue antibody. This antibody was an IgG and was directed to a component of the marginal sinus or capillaries of the spleen. A possible correlation between this antibody and microenvironment failure as a cause of AA was suggested.

2. Cell-Mediated Aplasia

The identification of naturally occurring cytotoxic cells[28] and specific cytotoxic lymphocytes in various autoimmune disorders[29] has raised the possibility that aplastic anemia may be produced by lymphocytes cytotoxic to the differentiation antigens of the pluripotential or committed stem cells. Patients with aplastic anemia have been described whose bone marrow had a markedly reduced number of CFU-C, but in whom the number of CFU-C increased after the treatment of bone marrow cells with antithymocyte globulin and complement.[30]

In a series of aplastic anemia patients, Hoffman et al.[31] demonstrated that peripheral blood lymphocytes from five of seven produced a 79 to 94% reduction in the number of CFU-E when their peripheral lymphocytes were cocultured with normal bone marrow cells. There was no inhibition of normal CFU-E growth by the serum of the aplastic anemia patients; therefore, the inhibition of erythroid growth was not due to an antibody against erythropoietin or the erythroblasts. Individuals who had been multiply transfused for other hematological disorders were controls in these studies. No inhibition of CFU-E growth was observed when the control peripheral lymphocytes were cocultured with normal bone marrow cells, suggesting that the inhibition was not due to reactivity to histocompatibility antigens.

The presence of cytotoxic lymphocytes in the peripheral blood of 117 patients with aplastic anemia has been studied by Warren et al.[32] Lymphocytes from 29% of patients exhibited cytotoxicity against their own lymphocytes. Lymphocytes from 50% of patients showed cytotoxicity against lymphocytes from their HLA-identical siblings.

Recently, Applebaum et al.[17] studied mononuclear cells for the presence of suppressor activity prior to transplant in identical twins. Cells from the two patients who ultimately required cyclophosphamide appeared to inhibit CFU-C or BFU-E by donor marrow, whereas cells from one patient who responded to marrow infusion alone did not. These data in identical twins permit the clearest test of coculture suppression assays. The data by these investigators suggest that aplastic anemia is correctable by simple marrow infusion or in some cases due to active marrow suppression and require immunosuppression prior to transplant. The differences might reflect variable etiologies for AA or, alternatively, different stages of a common mechanism. In contrast, Sullivan et al.[33] studied 18 untreated patients and found an absolute deficiency of stem cells that is not effected or sustained by lymphocytes.

A subset of aplastic anemia that has a particularly poor prognosis is posthepatitis aplastic anemia.[34] Several lines of evidence support an immunologic basis for the marrow injury. In aplastic anemia patients an increase in the reactivity of recipient peripheral blood lymphocytes to autologous PHA-stimulated lymphoblasts has been noted when compared to the reactivity of HLA identical sibling lymphocytes. Individuals with posthepatitis aplastic anemia may destroy their stem cells because of the presence of lymphocytes cytotoxic to hepatitis antigens expressed on stem cells, or to shared antigens of liver and marrow elements. The cytotoxicity of virally infected cells may be HLA restricted, i.e., the target and effector cell have to be HLA compatible.[35] The Royal Marsden Hospital Bone Marrow Transplant Team reported on a case of posthepatitic AA treated by twin marrow infusion in which hematopoiesis was not restored until cyclophosphamide pretreatment preceded marrow infusion.[36] Applebaum et al.[17] reported a similar case in which prompt marrow function resulted without immunosuppression. Hepatitis-associated aplastic anemia, similar to idiopathic AA, may have more than one pathogenesis or present at different states of a spectrum.[37]

Some aplastic anemia patients who have received immunosuppression and allogeneic bone marrow transplants, either HLA identical or parental, have had a spontaneous return of their own normal hematopoietic function.[38] Such patients are believed to have some residual pluripotent stem cells that were capable, under appropriate conditions, of repopulating the marrow. It is not clear whether the immunosuppression destroyed lymphocytes cytotoxic to the host stem cells or suppressor cells that interfered with normal hematopoietic differentiation. Another possibility is that the graft-vs.-host or the host-vs.-graft reaction induced by the transplanted marrow produced factors which stimulated stem cell differentiation as has been described in murine graft-vs.-host disease.[39] A few patients with aplastic anemia for whom no donor was available have received immunosuppression alone with return of normal hematopoiesis.[14] However, these cases must still be reviewed with caution since there was a significant hiatus between the discontinuance of the immunosuppression and the return of hematopoietic function; these may represent spontaneous recovery. Parkman reported on six patients with aplastic anemia treated with antithymocyte serum alone. In no case has there been any improvement in hematopoietic function.[40]

Because of the danger of immunosuppression in patients with reduced numbers of granulocytes and monocytes, it would be preferable to have a reliable in vitro test to detect those individuals in whom an immune mechanism is probable. Immunosuppression could then be used only in those individuals in whom there was a high possibility of success. Recently, Bagby et al.[41] cultured marrow cells from 54 patients with pancytopenia (preleukemia) for the presence of CFU-C. Cultures were performed with or without cortisol. Cortisol failed to enhance colony growth in 29 of 34 cases tested; none of these 29 patients responded in vivo to steroids. Cortisol enhanced CFU-C in five patients, three of whom responded clinically.

III. BONE MARROW PHYSIOLOGY IN APLASIA

Intuitively, the marrow biopsy should provide a reliable estimate of functional hypoplasia of the marrow, but several studies have failed to show a correlation of cellularity with prognosis.[42,43] This may be the result of sampling error[44] or that "functional hot spots," i.e., cellularity,[45] frequently occur. By contrast, an increase in the numbers of lymphocytes and/or plasma cells has been associated with a poorer prognosis.[43] This observation might simply reflect a greater depletion of erythroid and myeloid elements; however, teVelde and Haak[43] showed that the presence of diffuse lymphoid infiltrates are associated with increased mortality.

Patients with aplastic anemia have an impaired ability to incorporate iron into marrow erythroid precursors.[46] Scott et al.[47] showed that ferrokinetic data correlated well with hypoplastic appearance of the marrow. In patients with aplastic anemia, plasma iron is increased, disappearance of iron is prolonged, plasma iron turnover is reduced, and iron incorporation into erythrocytes diminished. In the study of Najean[46] iron utilization in patients who died within 6 months was 11%, whereas, in patients living more than 1 year iron utilization was 14%. Unfortunately, ferrokinetic studies in aplastic patients are difficult to perform. Therefore, indium chloride scintigraphy has been advocated as a measure of severity of aplastic anemia.[48] In 22 patients a diminished indium uptake correlated well with clinical severity and survival.

Patients with severe aplastic anemia have slight lymphopenia and hypogammaglobulinemia. However, it appears that despite reduced or undetectable CFU-S, CFU-C and CFU-E, lymphoid colony formation is normal.[49] Elfenbein et al.[50] found that aplastic patients have modest lymphopenia (70% of normal levels); T and B cells were equally depressed. Cytotoxic effector cells mediating natural killing, i.e., lymphocytes bearing Fc receptors only, are decreased as is antibody-dependent cytotoxicity. Hypogammaglobulinemia is common but in vitro responses to mitogens are normal. Elfenbein[50] suggested that these findings are secondary to previous glucocorticoid therapy and not disease related. Since these studies were performed on treated patients, more data on this subject will be needed.

IV. BONE MARROW MORPHOLOGY BEFORE AND FOLLOWING MARROW RECOVERY

Hypoplastic marrow of less cellularity than normal is obviously the constant feature of aplastic anemia. Characteristically there is a marked decrease to total absence of hemopoietic islands. Isolated groups of two to four cells with varying maturity are seen but the orderly arrangement of proliferating and maturing cells in islands connected by vascular channels is completely lacking. All normal types of cells are present including granulocytes and increases in early erythroid cells and cells essembling transitional cells. At the same time percentages of myelocytes and normoblasts are increased. Hence, morphologically the changes observed in the marrow is that of a deficiency of all blood cells plus a suppression of maturation resulting in a greater percentage of primitive cells.

Umehara[52] classified the morphologic appearance of the marrow in aplastic anemia patients into three main types, A, B, and C. The type A (65% of cases) was further subdivided into a completely aplastic type, hypoplastic type, exudative type, and fibroid type. The exudative subtype was seen in 10% of cases and was characterized watery, thick, granular, fine fibrous, hyalin-like with a torn spiderweb-like appearance. The cases with extensive fibrin-like exudation were classified as fibroid. The B type (31% of cases) was the proliferative type. This consisted of a normoplastic and diffuse proliferative type. The C group (6% of cases) was considered to be the red cell accumulation type.[52]

The fat cell in aplastic marrow biopsies appears to irregular with loss of membrane elasticity. In occasional cases infusion of exudate into fat cells (''Gallert Mark'') is seen. Fat cell degeneration is almost uniformly seen in type A marrows. The sinusoidal wall can be thickened with ribbon-like dilatation by which the spaces between the fat cells appear unusually wide.

Ultrastructurally, the sinusoidal lining cells are atrophic with amorphous tangling, hyperdigitation and ''weed like'' changes; or hypertrophic with thickening, lumps and frosted glass-like sclerosis.

Allogeneic marrow transplantation has allowed analysis of marrow cell proliferation following destruction of the pluripotent stem cells since the nature of the transplant conditioning leaves the microenvironment intact.

Postconditioning (day 0 transplantation) marrow is devoid of hematopoietic precursors. Only stromal cells, adipocytes, histiocytes, and scattered lymphocytes are recognizable. By 1 week following transplant small clusters of early hemapoietic precursors are seen usually located within the adipocytes and far from bone trabeculae. Scattered blast cells and early erythroid and myeloid forms are found in small groups. In marrow samples obtained 3 weeks after transplantation small clusters were seen as erythoid or myeloid cells. Committed progenitor cells, i.e., CFU-C, CFU-E, are more common in marrow than pluripotent stem cells. This may explain the high frequency of single cell line clusters. In a study by Naeim et al.[51] 60% of early transplant cell clusters were composed of one line, 25% contained clusters with mixed elements, and 15% of clusters were unclassifiable. In 3-week marrow samples the myeloid: erythroid ratio was 1:1 or less. Dysplasia was prominent as was megaloblastosis. Eight-week marrow specimens had greater cellularity with large clusters of cells. These were most often composed of mixed cellular elements, including megakaryocytes. Mast cells are usually found in great numbers in the areas where clusters of fatty tissue and stromal cells are found in posttransplant patients in which rejection occurred, whereas successful marrow engraftment biopsies failed to show mast cells. An inverse correlation between marrow ''takes'' and mast cells is suggested.[51]

REFERENCES

1. **Stohlman, F., Jr.,** Aplastic anemia, *Blood,* 40, 282, 1972.
2. **Trentin, J. J.,** Influence of hemapoietic organ stroma (hematopoietic inductive microenvironments) on stem cell differentiation, in *Regulation of Hematopoiesis,* Vol. 1, Gordon, A. S., Ed., Appleton-Century-Crofts, New York, 1971.
3. **Ershler, W. B., Ross, J., Finlay, J. L., and Shahidi, N. T.,** Bone marrow microenvironment defect in congenital hypoplastic anemia, *N. Engl. J. Med.,* 302, 1321, 1980.
4. **Lajtha, L. G. and Schofeld, R.,** Regulation of stem cell renewal and differentiation: possible significance in aging, *Adv. Gerontol. Res.,* 3, 131, 1971.
5. **Boggs, D. R. and Boggs, S. S.,** The pathogenesis of aplastic anemia: a defective pluripotent hematopoietic stem cell with inappropriate balance of differentiation and selfreplication, *Blood,* 48, 71, 1976.
6. **Ragab, A. H., Gilkerson, E., Crist, W. M., and Phelan, E.,** Granulopoiesis in childhood aplastic anemia, *J. Pediatr.,* 88, 790, 1976.

7. **Singer, J. W., Brown, J. E., Storb, R., and Thomas, E. D.,** The effect of peripheral blood lymphocytes from patients with aplastic anemia on granulocytic colony growth from HLA-matched and mismatched marrows: effect of transfusion sensitization, *Blood,* 52, 37, 1978.
8. **Kern, P., Heit, W., Kubanek, B., and Heimpe, I. H.,** Granulocytic colony forming cells *in vitro.* II. Patients with aplastic anemia, *Blut,* 34, 406, 1977.
9. **Morley, A., Trainor, K., and Reines, J.,** Residual marrow damage, possible explanation for idiosyncrasy to chloramphenicol, *Br. J. Haematol.,* 32, 525, 1976.
10. **Yunis, A. A.,** Chloramphenicol-induced bone marrow suppression, *Semin. Hematol.,* 10, 225, 1973.
11. **Yunis, A. A.,** Drug-induced bone marrow injury, *Adv. Intern. Med.,* 15, 357, 1969.
12. **Kay, A.,** Depression of bone marrow associated with crysotherapy, *Ann. Rheum. Dis.,* 33, 277, 1973.
13. **Reid, G. and Patterson, A. C.,** *Br. Med. J.,* ii, 1457, 1977.
14. **Speck, B., Cornu, P., Sartorius, J., Nissen, C., Groff, P., Burri, H. P., and Jeannet, M.,** Immunologic aspects of aplasia, *Transpl. Proc.,* 10, 131, 1978.
15. **Boggs, D. R. and Boggs, S. S.,** Possible pathogenic mechanisms in aplastic anemia, *Transpl. Proc.,* 10, 125, 1978.
16. **Tumen, J., Kline, L. B., Fay, J. W., Schllin, D. C., Reisner, E. G., Rosse, W. F., and Huang, A. T.,** Complement sensitivity of paroxysmal nocturnal hemoglobinuria bone marrow cells, *Blood,* 55, 1040, 1980.
17. **Applebaum, F. R., Fefer, A., Cheever, M. A., Sanders, J. E., Singer, J. W., Adamson, J. W., Mickelson, E. M., Hansen, J. A., Greenberg, P. D., and Thomas, E. D.,** Treatment of aplastic anemia by bone marrow transplantation in identical twins, *Blood,* 55, 1033, 1980.
18. **Hagler, L., Pastore, R. A., and Bergin, J. J.,** Aplastic anemia following viral hepatitis, *Medicine (Baltimore),* 54, 139, 1975.
19. **Williams, D. M., Lynch, R. E., and Cartwright, G. E.,** Drug-induced aplastic anemia, *Semin. Hematol.,* 10, 195, 1973.
20. **Estes, D. and Christian, C. L.,** The natural history of systemic lupus erythematosus by prospective analysis, *Medicine, (Baltimore),* 50, 85, 1971.
21. **Ehrlich, P.,** Ueber einen Fall von Anamie mit Bemerkungen uber regenerative Veranderundgen des Inochenmarks, *Charite-Annalen,* 13, 300, 1888.
22. **Fleming, A. F.,** Hypoplastic anemia of pregnancy, *Clin. Haematol.,* 2, 477, 1973.
23. **Alter, B. P., Potter, N. U., and Li, F. P.,** Classification and etiology of the aplastic anemias, *Clin. Haematol.,* 7, 431, 1980.
24. **Karntz, S. B. and Zaentz, S. D.,** Pure red cell aplasia, in *A Year of Hematology,* Silber, R., Gordon, A. S., and Lo Bue, J., Eds., Plenum Press, New York, 1977.
25. **Freedman, M. H., Gelfand, E. W., and Saunders, E. F.,** Acquired aplastic anemia, antibody-mediated hematopoietic failure, *Am. J. Hematol.,* 6, 135, 1979.
26. **Herron, R., Hyde, R. D., and Hillier, S. J.,** The second example of an Anti-Vel autoantibody, *Vox Sang,* 36, 179, 1979.
27. **Yoda, Y., Abe, T., and Komiya, M.,** Antisplenic tissue antibody in aplastic anemia, *Acta Haem. Jpn.,* 38, 315, 1975.
28. **Parkman, R. and Rosen, F. S.,** Identification of a subpopulation of lymphocytes in human peripheral blood cytotoxic to autologous fibroblasts, *J. Exp. Med.,* 144, 1520, 1976.
29. **Currie, S., Saunders, M., Knowles, M., and Brown, A. E.,** Immunological aspects of polymyositis, *Q. J. Med.,* 40, 63, 1970.
30. **Ascensao, J., Pahwa, R., Kajar, W., Hansen, J., Moore, M. A., and Good, R. A.,** Aplastic anemia, evidence for an immunologic mechanism, *Lancet,* 1, 669, 1976.
31. **Hoffman, R., Zanjani, E. D., Lutton, J. D., Zalusky, R., and Wasserman, L. R.,** Suppression of erythroid-colony formation by lympohcytes from patients with aplastic anemia, *N. Engl. J. Med.,* 292, 10, 1977.
32. **Warren, R. P., Storb, R., Thomas, E. D., et al.,** Autoimmune and alloimmune phenomena in patients with aplastic anemia, *Blood,* 56, 583, 1980.
33. **Sullivan, R., Quesenberry, P. J., Parkman, R., Zuckerman, K. S., Levey, R. H., Rappeport, J., and Ryan, M.,** Aplastic anemia, lack of inhibitory effect of bone marrow lymphocytes on *in vitro* granulopoiesis, *Blood,* 56, 625, 1980.
34. **Calmitta, B., Nathan, D. G., Forman, E. N., Parkman, R., Rappeport, J. M., and Orillana, T.,** Posthepatitic severe aplastic anemia—an indication for early bone marrow transplantation, *Blood,* 43, 572, 1974.
35. **Doherty, P. C., Blanden, R. V., and Zinkernagel, R. M.,** Specificity of virus-immune effector T cells for H-2K or H-2D compatible interaction, implications for H-antigen diversity, *Transpl. Rev.,* 29, 89, 1976.
36. **Royal Marsden Hospital Bone Marrow Transplantation Team,** Failure of syngeneic bone marrow graft without preconditioning in post-hepatitis marrow aplasia, *Lancet,* 2, 742, 1977.

37. **Wilson, H. A., McLarsen, G. D., Dworken, H. J., and Tebbi, K.,** Transient pure red cell aplasia, cell mediated suppression of erythropoiesis associated with hepatitis, *Ann. Intern. Med.*, 92, 196, 1980.
38. **Jeannet, M., Rubinstein, A., Pelet, B., and Kummer, H.,** Prolonged remission of severe aplastic anemia after ALG pretreatment and HLA-semi-incompatible bone marrow cell transfusion, *Transpl. Proc.*, 6, 359, 1974.
39. **Parker, J. W. and Metcalf, D.,** Production of colony stimulating factor in mixed leukocyte cultures, *Immunology*, 26, 1039, 1974.
40. **Parkman, R.,** The immunopathology of marrow failure, *Clon. Haematol.*, 7, 475, 1978.
41. **Bagby, G. C., Gabourel, J. D., and Linman, J. W.,** Glucocorticoid therapy in the pre leukemic syndrome, *Ann. Intern. Med.*, 92, 55, 1980.
42. **Frisch, B. and Lewis, S. M.,** The bone marrow in aplastic anemia, diagnostic and prognostic features, *J. Clin. Pathol.*, 27, 231, 1974.
43. **teVelde, J. and Haak, H. L.,** Aplastic anemia. Histological investigation of methacrylate embedded bone marrow biopsy specimens, correlation with survival after conventional treatment in 15 adult patients, *Br. J. Haematol.*, 38, 119, 1977.
44. **Lewis, S. M.,** Course and prognosis in aplastic anemia, *Br. Med. J.*, 1, 1027, 1965.
45. **Kansu, E. and Erslev, A. S.,** Aplastic anemia with hot pockets, *Scand. J. Haematol.*, 17, 326, 1976.
46. **Najean, Y. and Seligmann, M.,** Evolution et prognostic des pancytopenies idiopathiques, *Nouv. Fr. Hematol.*, 5, 639, 1965.
47. **Scott, J. L., Cartwrigth, G. E., and Wintrobe, M. M.,** Acquired aplastic anemia, an analysis of 39 cases and review of the pertinent literature, *Medicine*, 38, 119, 1959.
48. **McNeil, B. J., Rappeport, J. M., and Nathan, D. G.,** Indium chloride scintography, an index of severity in patients with aplastic anemia, *Br. J. Haematol.*, 34, 599, 1976.
49. **Gorski, A., Rowinska, D., Skopinska, E., and Orlowski, T.,** Circulating suppressor cells in aplastic anemia, *Vox Sang*, 36, 356, 1979.
50. **Elfenbein, G. J., Kallman, C. H., Tutschka, P. J., Adkinson, N. F., Jr., Bias, W. B., Braine, H. G., Humphrey, R. L., Saral, R., Mellits, E. D., and Santos, G. W.,** The immune system in 40 aplastic anemia patients receiving conventional therapy, *Blood*, 53, 652, 1979.
51. **Naeim, F., Smith, G. S., and Gale, R. P.,** Morphologic aspects of bone marrow transplantation in patients with aplastic anemia, *Human Pathol.*, 9, 295, 1978.
52. **Umehara, S.,** Bone marrow stroma in aplastic anemia, in *Aplastic Anemia*, Hibino, S., Takaku, F., and Shahidi, N. T., Eds., University Park Press, Baltimore, 1978.

Chapter 16

BONE MARROW MAST CELLS

Stephen Davis and Sidney Trubowitz

TABLE OF CONTENTS

I. INTRODUCTION

Since the concept of mast cells was first elucidated by Ehrlich some 100 years ago mast cells still remain enigmatic elements. Little is known about the fate, regulation, or function of marrow mast cells; and only recently have data on their origin been accumulated. The purpose of this section is to report qualitative and quantitative observations on marrow mast cells with the goal of presenting reasonable current insight into these peculiar cells.

II. MORPHOLOGY

The mammalian mast cell is generally elliptical in shape when viewed in tissue sections. Their average diameter is approximately 12 μm depending on the stage of maturation.[1,2] Some mast cells show pseudopodia-like extensions which are spindled-shaped and elongated, while others have a blunted head containing the nucleus with the remainder of the cytoplasm drawn into a long filamentous process, at times bifid. The nucleus is usually obscured by densely packed granules which in H and E sections resembles a plasma cell nucleus in its dispersed chromatin pattern, unsegmentation, and eccentric location. This represents a source of confusion since H and E staining does not allow identification of the cytoplasmic granules.[3] Basophil nuclei have a segmented appearance with a chromatin pattern similar to other granulocytes.

As originally observed by Erhlich the cytoplasmic granules stain metachromatically. The size of these granules range between 0.5 and 2.0 μm in diameter and are evenly distributed in the cytoplasm.[4] In contrast to basophil granules, mast cell granules are almost always spherical in shape. Electron microscopically the granules may be amorphous or display crystals, cyclindrical lamellae, "scrolls," or whorls."[5] The granules of marrow mast cells are not water soluble and are therefore easily differentiated from basophils in alcoholic fixed tissue specimens. For their ultrastructural description, therefore, basophil granules require aldehyde fixative and epoxy embedding media.

Lison[6] first attributed the metachromasia of mast cell granules to polysulfated polymers. Evidence that heparin accounted for the metachromasia soon followed.[7] Histamine and histamine decarboxylase have been clearly demonstrated in mast cells.[8] Mast cells contain hydrolytic proteases. On the basis of histochemical studies and analysis of purified granules the proteases appear to be active *in situ*. The presence of proteolytic enzymes clearly distinguishes marrow mast cells from basophils.[9] Bone marrow mast cells granules contain no peroxidase products, whereas the mature basophil clearly demonstrate peroxidase-positive granules.

Staining of the mast cell granules in the rat with Alcian blue and safranin has enabled the distinction, respectively, between the content of weakly and strongly sulfated mucopolysaccharides. Based on staining with these stains as well as morphology, Coombs[10] delineated four stages of development of the mature mast cell. Pretlow and Cassidy[11] subsequently observed that Stage 1 cells were separable by rate-zonal sedimentation into two distinct subtypes, 1a and 1b. Briefly, Stage 1 cells have a mean diameter of 8.3 μm. The cytoplasm contains a variable number of granules which stain only with Alcian blue. Stage 2 cells have a mean diameter of 11.0 μm with more than half the granules stained by Alcian blue, the rest being safranin-positive. Stage 3 mast cells have a 12.7 μm mean diameter with more than half the granules stained by safranin. In Stage 4 the mast cells are very large (16.0 μm) with large safranin staining granules only.

Toluidine blue staining can identify true mast cells in marrow by the demonstration of metachromatic granules. If overdecalcification occurs diminished staining of the granules by toluidine blue results. This can be prevented by treatment of the marrow sections with potassium permanganate followed by oxalic acid prior to staining. Giemsa staining results in a purple-blue coloration of mast cells.

III. ANATOMICAL DISTRIBUTION

Examining tissue sections, Johnstone[12] enumerated mast cells in human marrow and divided his findings into three categories:

1. No mast cells seen
2. One to five cells/hpf
3. More than five cells/hpf

No mast cells were seen in 30% of patients, one to five cells/hpf in 60% cases, and more than five cells/hpf in 10% of cases. Peart and Ellis[13] found mast cells in all but 5% of iliac bone marrow sections. They ranged from 0 to 33 cells per mm^2 with a median count of $1.95/mm^2$. The majority had less than five mast cells per mm^2 marrow with 38% having less than one cell per mm^2 marrow.

Bone marrow mast cells, like all tissue mast cells, occur in relation to the adventitia of small blood vessels but are not confined to this anatomical situation (Figure 1). They occur irregularly within the hemopoietic elements, in the reticular framework, and stretched around marrow fat cells. They are most numerous in and about the endosteum and scanty toward the center of the medullary cavity of bone.[12] Mast cells appear consistently in the periphery of marrow lymphoid aggregates (nodules), but never in the center. The number of mast cells varies in the aggregate from occasional to abundant. This distribution limits the precise value of mast cell counts and makes interpretation of serial biopsies difficult.

IV. ONTOGENY OF MAST CELLS

At birth and in the initial month of life rat mast cells are numerous in the liver and spleen and lie free in the sinusoids of the hemopoietic foci. The red marrow of the rat is scanty until 3 days of age; therefore the bone marrow has few mast cells until the third week of life but the number subsequently increases rapidly. The increase in marrow mast cells is matched by a corresponding decrease in extramedullary hematopoietic foci. These kinetics are similar to the findings of Metcalf and Moore[14] for granulopoiesis. In 4-day-old rats 63% of mast cells belong to Stage 1 maturation, 24% to Stage 2, 12% to Stage 3, and 1% to Stage 4. The percentage of Stage 1 cells falls over the next two weeks but then rises to a steady state by four weeks.[15]

Recently, Kitamura et al.[16–20] used various experimental systems to investigate the origin of precursor cells which differentiate into mast cells. The number of mast cells was examined in various tissues of genetically mast cell-depleted mice (WBB6F, WB × 57BL/6-W/W^v) after injection of hemopoietic and lymphoid tissue from cogenic +/+ mice. Similarly, the number of mast cells with giant granules (Chediak-Higashi, beige, C 57BL/6-bg^J/bg^J) was studied in irradiated congenic +/+ mice after the injection of lymphoid cells. Their results indicated that mast cell precursors are derived from hematopoietic tissue rather than lymphoid tissue. Similar findings were obtained when mouse embryonic liver was used in reconstitution experiments.

Following bone marrow transplantation with a beige-type mouse donor discrete clusters of mast cells are seen in mesentery located mainly in fat tissue near blood vessels. These clusters are derived from a single precursor cell which migrates through the

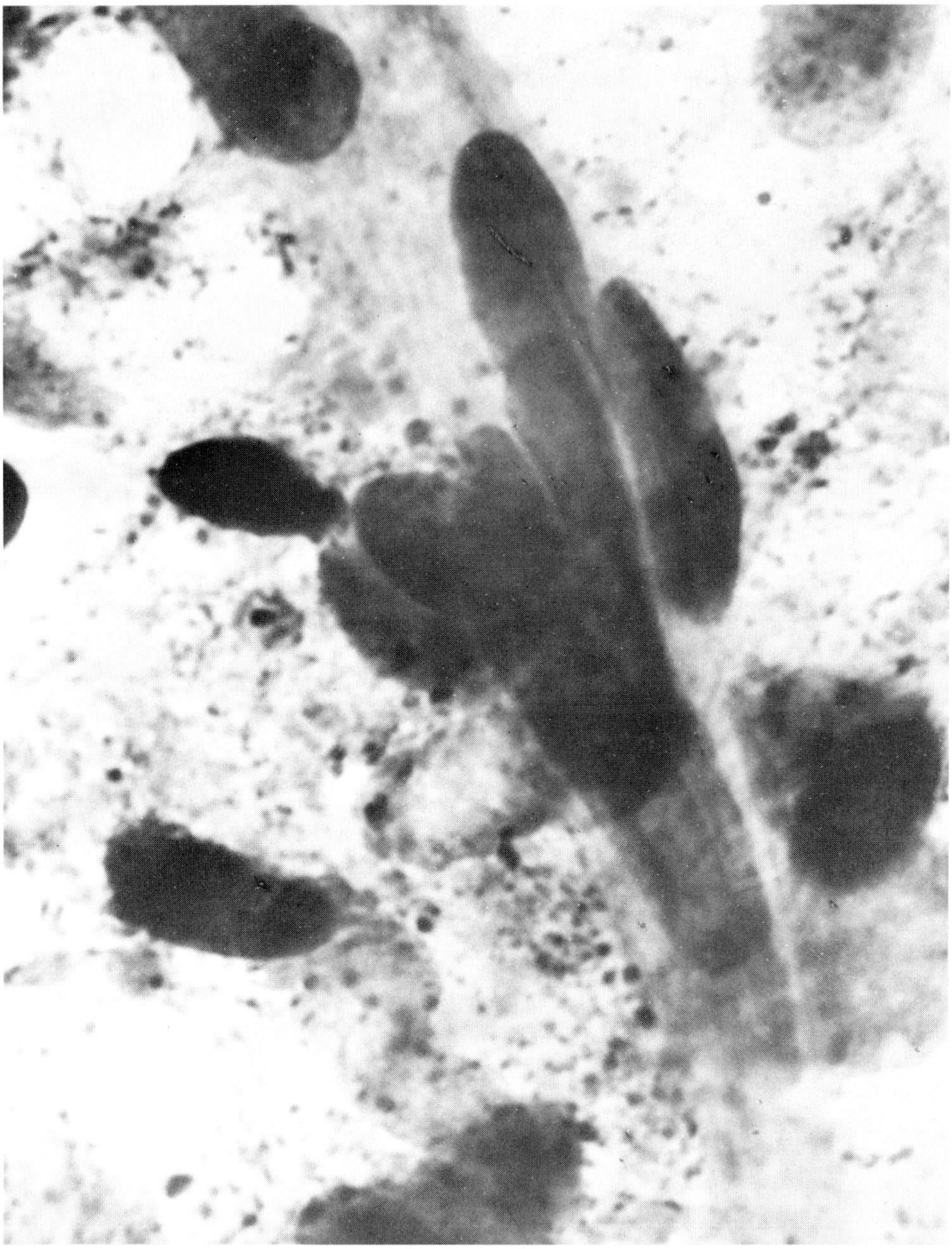

FIGURE 1. Highly magnified light microscopic photograph of mast cells lining the adventitia of a blood vessel. Magnification approximately ×1875.

bloodstream and proliferates at the site of differentiation. Kitamura and his associates have found that Sl/Sl^d mice like W/W^v mice have markedly decreased numbers of skin and mesenteric mast cells. This latter strain of mouse is unique in that following bone marrow transplantation with congenic +/+ mouse cells the number of mast cells do not increase in mesenteric sites. Alternatively, transplantation of Sl/Sl^d marrow cells to W/W^v mice increased the number of tissue mast cells. This suggests that Sl/Sl^d mouse marrow contains mast cell precursors and that the failure of Sl/Sl^d mice to develop tissue mast cells is due to a defect in the microenvironment of skin and mesentery.[17,19,20]

The possibility the mast cells originate from lymphoid cells has gained some experimental support. Burnet[21] reported that in the thymus of NZB mice large numbers of mast cells appear in the cortical regions bordering the medullary germinal centers. Burnet presented an hypothesis suggesting that mast cells are transformed thymocytes, the transformation being brought on by various stimuli analogous to the transformation of lymphocytes to plasma cells. Yong et al.[15] presented data supporting this observation in that the thymus in neonatal rats contains about 5000 mast cells/mm^3 of tissue. The distribution of mast cells in rat thymus does not change with increasing age. Tissue culture studies also support the lymphoid origin of mast cells.[21] The development of mast cell colonies in soft agar from rat peripheral blood "lymphocyte" fractions has been described by Zucker-Franklin,[22] but the presence of CFU-S cells in this fraction obviously can not be excluded. However, Keller et al.[23] showed that congenitally athymic (nude) mice have a normal density and connective tissue distribution of mast cells. In addition, thymectomy or the treatment of bone marrow cells with antithymocyte (Thy1.2) serum does not alter the distribution or quantity of mast cells generated following marrow transplantation of mast cell depleted W/W^v mice. Mast cell precursors are detected in the thymus in amounts less than 0.1% of that found in marrow.[18]

Recent observations in nude mice and adult thymectomized, irradiated, bone marrow-reconstituted rats show that the mucosal mast cell proliferation that follows infestation with nematode parasites is T-cell dependent.[24,25] This hyperplasia is independent of the thymus but dependent on circulating T cells. It has been suggested the mucosal mast cells form from the granular intraepithelial lymphocytes (GIEL) of the intestinal tract.[26] These cells contain small numbers of granules with staining properties similar to mucosal mast cells. Granular intraepithelial lymphocytes do not have lymphocyte membrane markers, their proliferation is thymus-independent, and may represent a nonlymphoid leukocyte of bone marrow origin, data compatible with that of Kitamura.

It has been suggested that although marrow mast cells and basophils are different in morphology and enzyme content it is possible both cells are derived from a common marrow precursor cell. Support of this hypothesis comes from Zucker-Franklin who found cells with overlapping morphology in patients with myeloproliferative disorders.[22]

V. FUNCTION OF MARROW MAST CELLS

The function of bone marrow mast cells is unknown. That mast cells are intimately associated with blood vessels is well known. Such a relationship has led to the speculation that mast cells must necessarily play an important role in circulatory dynamics, perhaps by the secretion of histamine, heparin, or other substances. Direct evidence to this effect is lacking although partial amelioration of symptoms in patients with systemic mastocytosis has occurred with histamine antagonists. Similarly, mast cells are numerous in connective tissues. It has been postulated that the development and integrity of collagen and bone, especially endochondral trabeculae, are dependent on marrow mast cells.[27] Riley[28] postulated that mast cells provide heparin necessary for mucopolysaccharide synthesis by fibroblasts. However, Benditt and Lagunoff[3] argue that this hypothesis is unlikely because not enough heparin is produced by mast cells for the relatively large need.

It is important to note that the mast cells found in mucosal linings of the bronchus and stomach may differ from marrow-derived mast cells. Mucosal mast cells (MMC) appear allied to the APUD (Amine Precursor Uptake Decarboxylation) system because of the pharmacologic properties of their granules and therefore, are derived from neural crest tissue.[29] Distinction of mast cells from "mucosal mast cells" can be made by the inability of the latter to demonstrate metachromasia when fixed in buffered 10% formalin.[29] Mayrhofer[26] suggests that MMC were bone-marrow derived.

Austen and his co-workers[30] have shown that prostaglandin D_2 is the major arachidonic acid metabolite synthesized by rat serosal mast cells and human lung-parenchymal mast cells. In two cases of systemic mastocytosis manifesting severe hypotensive episodes Roberts et al.[31] found marked overproduction of prostaglandin D_2 and modest increases in histamine production. The hypotension could not be reversed by therapeutic doses of cimetidine. These data suggest that prostaglandin D_2 and histamine are mast cell-derived mediators of mast cell function. The role of these mediators in normal patients is lacking.

VI. MAST CELLS IN PATHOLOGIC CONDITIONS

In patients with chronic renal failure marrow mast cells are increased. Peart and Ellis[13] found the arithmetic mean to be 13.75 and the median to be 9.55 cells/mm^2. Following renal transplantation marrow mast cell numbers return to normal range (mean, 3.9; median, 1.95 cells/mm^2). In chronic renal failure mast cells were most significant within zones of osteitis fibrosa. Similarly, marrow mast cells accumulate in areas of fracture callus; areas where there is connective tissue proliferation.[32] That marrow mast cells are increased in fatty marrow and hematopoietically active marrow suggests that other factors present in renal failure contribute to the fibrous tissue formation. It appears that resorption and remodeling of bone, whatever the cause, is associated with increased marrow mast cells.[27] The precise relationship between marrow mast cells and bone resorption and remodeling is unclear. Local effects of heparin may be responsible since it is known that heparin administration is associated with osteoporosis.[33] Others have suggested that the bone resorptive effect of heparin is an indirect one mediated through hyperparathyroidism resulting from the hypocalcemia following binding of serum calcium to heparin.[34] This hypothesis is not supported by data showing that parathyroidectomy does not prevent heparin osteopathy.[33] In systemic mastocytosis, a condition where bone marrow and other tissue is infiltrated by mast cells, bone marrow sections show resorption of trabeculae at collections of mast cells, deposition of fibrillary lamelar bone, and trabecular thickening.[35] Despite these data there does not appear to be a direct relationship to marrow mast cell numbers and the presence or severity of bone mineralization defects.[36]

Rywlin[37] described a distinct bone marrow finding showing agglomerates of eosinophils, lymphocytes, and elongated "fibrohistiocytes." The author suggested that the lesion is associated with a drug hypersensitivity reaction. The lesion was called the "eosinophilic fibrohistiocyte lesion" of marrow. Te Velde et al.[38] have recently shown that these "fibrohistiocytes" are mast cells. All of these later patients had severe osteoporosis. These infiltrates vary from 0.1 to 2 mm in diameter, and were present centrally in the marrow, or around arterioles, or in a crescentic form along sinuses. This lesion is distinctly different from the diffuse increase of mast cells seen in metabolic bone disease, e.g., osteitis fibrosa, but also from the monomorphic infiltrate with osteosclerosis and eosinophilia in the surrounding hyperplastic marrow seen in systemic mastocytosis.

In lymphoproliferative disorders involving the marrow benign or malignant appearing mast cells may be present in increased numbers. Nixon[39] noted increased mast cells in chronic lymphocytic leukemia, well-differentiated lymphoma, and Waldenström's macroglobulinemia (Figure 2). Using a semiquantitative method, Yoo et al.[40] showed a

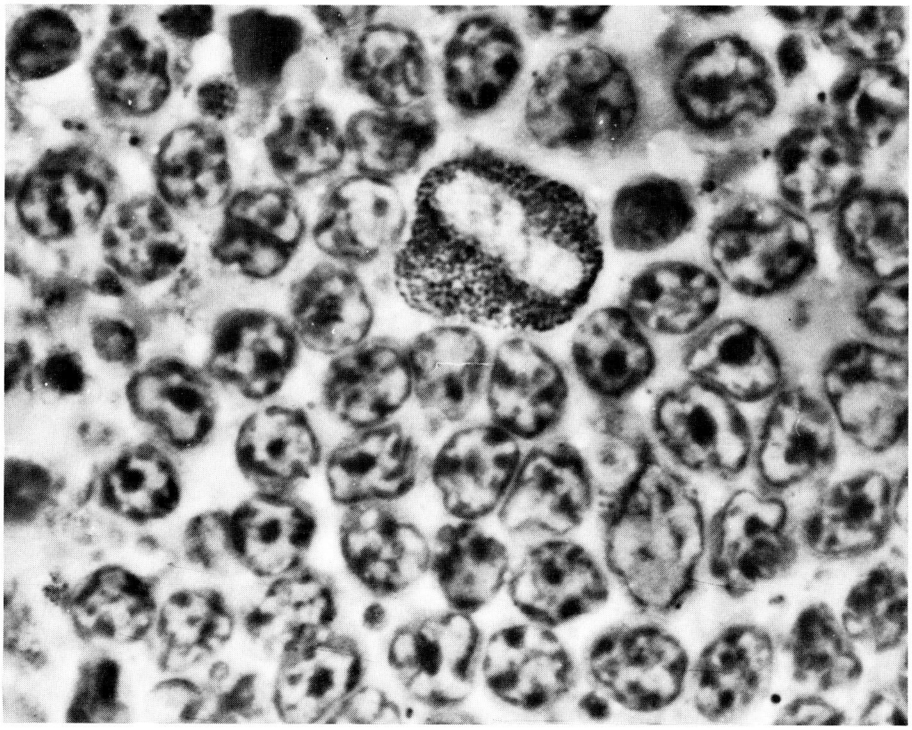

FIGURE 2. Bone marrow mast cell among the mature appearing lymphocytes of chronic lymphocytic leukemia. Magnification ×1100.

direct relation between the percentage of marrow lymphocytes and marrow mast cells in lymphoproliferative diseases and reactive lymphocytosis. These investigators believe that mast cell density may be related to the degree of lymphoid proliferation. Patients with myeloma had decreased mast cell content. Increase marrow mast cell content may support the diagnosis of lymphoproliferative disorders. The reason for the mast cell increase is unknown.

Systemic mastocytosis is a rare disorder characterized by infiltration of mast cells in various organs. The most commonly involved organ is the skin, usually in the form of urticaria pigmentosa. At times, systemic mastocytosis can occur in the absence of urticaria pigmentosa; in such situations a bone marrow biopsy may be diagnostic. Usually a marrow specimen is obtained because of abnormal blood counts or radiographic bone changes.

In systemic mastocytosis the marrow lesions may be local with slight increases in mast cells, or diffuse with replacement of normal marrow elements. The mast cells may be found in granuloma-like masses, occur in clusters, or be distributed throughout the section. Perivascular arrangement of the infiltrates are common. Both normal and abnormal-appearing mast cells are identifiable, occasionally with giant forms. Numerous inflammatory cells may be scattered throughout the lesions. Lymphocytes are frequently abundant and may surround or be surrounded by mast cells. Eosinophils can be seen within and about the periphery of a lesion. Reticulin fibers are abundant and arterioles show prominent medial and advential hypertrophy.

The bone may show increased osteoblastic activity with deposition of osteoid at the periphery of the bone trabeculae associated with a decrease in bone mass. Both osteoclerosis and osteoporosis may be seen in the same section.

Aspirated bone marrow may show increased mast cells, but because of the frequency of fibrosis in mastocytosis aspirated specimens may not truly reflect a mast cell proliferation. A marrow particle preparation is more useful than smear preparations.

Most frequently the marrow lesions in systemic mastocytosis are confused with nonspecific inflammatory disease, Hodgkin's disease, myelofibrosis, lymphoma, and eosinophilic granuloma.

REFERENCES

1. **Faden, R. S.,** Tissue mast cells in human bone marrow, *Blood,* 6, 614, 1951.
2. **Benditt, E. P.,** Morphology, chemistry and function of mast cells, *Ann. N.Y. Acad. Sci.,* 73, 204, 1957.
3. **Benditt, E. P. and Lagunoff, D.,** The mast cell: its structure and function, *Prog. Allerg.,* 8, 195, 1964.
4. **Keller, R. and Mühlethaler, K.,** Cytologishe Untersuchungen zum Verhalten isolierter Mastzellen bei deranaphytaktisohen Reakton, *Path. Microbiol.,* 25, 115, 1962.
5. **Fedorko, M. E. and Hirsch, J. G.,** Crystalloid structure in granules of guinea pig basophils and human mast cells, *J. Cell. Biol.,* 26, 973, 1965.
6. **Lison, L.,** Etudes sur la metachromasie, colorants metachromatiques et substances chromotropes, *Arch. Biol. (Paris),* 46, 599, 1935.
7. **Parekh, A. C. and Glick, D.,** Studies in histochemistry. LXV. Heparin and hexosamine in isolated mast cells: determination, intracellular distribution, and effects of biological state, *J. Biol. Chem.,* 237, 280, 1962.
8. **Schayer, R. W.,** Formation and binding of histamine by free mast cells of rat peritoneal fluid, *Am. J. Physiol.,* 186, 199, 1956.
9. **Lagunoff, D. and Benditt, E. P.,** Proteolytic enzymes of mast cells, *Ann. N.Y. Acad. Sci.,* 103, 185, 1963.
10. **Coombs, J. W., Lagunoff, D., and Benditt, E. P.,** Differentiation and proliferation of embryonic mast cells of the rat, *J. Cell. Biol.,* 25, 277, 1965.
11. **Pretlow, T. G. and Cassidy, I. M.,** Separation of mast cells in successive stages of differentiation using programmed gradient sedimentation, *Am. J. Pathol.,* 61, 323, 1970.
12. **Johnstone, J. M.,** The appearance and significance of tissue mast cells in human bone marrow, *J. Clin. Pathol.,* 7, 275, 1954.
13. **Peart, K. M. and Ellis, H. A.,** Quantitative observations on iliac bone marrow mast cells in chronic renal failure, *J. Clin. Pathol.,* 28, 947, 1975.
14. **Metcalf, D. and Moore, M. A. S.,** In *Hemopoietic Cells,* North-Holland, Amsterdam, 1971.
15. **Yong, L. C., Watkins, S. G., and Boland, J. E.,** The mast cell. III. Distribution and maturation in various organs of the young rat, *Pathology,* 11, 427, 1979.
16. **Kitamura, Y., Shimada, Y., Hatanaka, K., and Miyano, Y.,** Development of mast cells from grafted bone marrow cells in irradiated mice, *Nature,* 268, 442, 1977.
17. **Kitamura, Y., Shunada, M., Go, S., Matsuda, H., Hatanaka, K., and Seki, M.,** Distribution of mast cell precursors in hematopoietic and lymphopoietic tissues of mice, *J. Exp. Med.,* 150, 482, 1979.
18. **Kitamura, Y., Matsuda, H., and Hatauaka, K.,** Clonal nature of mast cell cultures formed in W/W^v mice after bone marrow transplantation, *Nature,* 281, 154, 1979.
19. **Kitamura, Y. and Go, S.,** Decreased production of mast cells in $S1/S1^d$ anemic mice, *Blood,* 53, 492, 1979.
20. **Hatanaka, K., Kitamura, Y., and Nishimune, Y.,** Local development of mast cells from bone marrow derived precursors, *Blood,* 53, 142, 1979.
21. **Burnet, F. M.,** The probable relationship of some or all mast cells to T cell system, *Cell Immunol.,* 30, 258, 1977.
22. **Zucker-Franklin, D.,** Ultrastructural evidence for the common origin of human mast cells and basophils, *Blood,* 56, 534, 1980.
23. **Keller, R., Hess, M. W., and Riley, J. F.,** Mast cells in the skin of normal, hairless and athymic mice, *Experimentia,* 32, 171, 1976.

24. **Ruitenberg, E. J. and Elgersma, A.,** Absence of intestinal mast cell response in athymic mice during Trichinella spiralis infection, *Nature,* 264, 258, 1976.
25. **Mayrhofer, G. and Fisher, R.,** Mast cells in severely T cell depleted rats and the response to infestation with *Nippostrongylos brasiliensis, Immunology,* 37, 145, 1979.
26. **Mayrhofer, G.,** Thymus-dependent and thymus-independent subpopulations of intestinal intraepithelial lymphocytes: a granular subpopulations of probable bone marrow origin and relationship to mucosal mast cells, *Blood,* 55, 532, 1980.
27. **Severson, A. R.,** Mast cells in areas of experimental bone resorption and remodelling, *Br. J. Exp. Pathol.,* 50, 17, 1969.
28. **Riley, J. F.,** *The Mast Cells,* Livingston, Edinburgh, 1959.
29. **Enerback, L.,** Mucosal mast cells in humans, *Acta Path. Micro. Biol. Scand.,* 66, 289, 1966.
30. **Roberts, L. J., Lewis, R. A., Oates, J. A., and Austen, K. F.,** Prostaglandin, Thromboxane, and 12-hydroxy-5,8,10,14-eicosatetranoic acid production by ionophore-stimulated rat serosal mast cells, *Biochim. Biophys. Acta,* 575, 185, 1979.
31. **Roberts, L. J., Sweetman, B. J., Lewis, R. A., Austen, K. F., and Oates, J. A.,** Increased production of prostaglandin D_2 in patients with systemic mastocytosis, *N. Engl. J. Med.,* 303, 1400, 1980.
32. **Selye, H.,** *The Mast Cells,* Butterworths, Washington, D.C., 1965.
33. **Ellis, H. A. and Peart, K. M.,** The effects of heparin and dextran sulfate on cultured mouse limb bones, *Br. J. Exp. Pathol.,* 51, 43, 1970.
34. **Hahnemann, S.,** Heparin and osteoporosis, *Lancet,* 2, 855, 1965.
35. **Jensen, W. H. and Lasser, E. C.,** Uriticaria pigmentosa associated with widespread sclerosis of the spongiosa of bone, *Radiology,* 71, 826, 1958.
36. **Ellis, H. A. and Peart, K. M.,** Azotemic renal osteodystrophy: a quantitative study on iliac bone, *J. Clin. Path.,* 26, 83, 1973.
37. **Rywlin, A. M., Hoffman, E. P., and Ortega, R. S.,** Eosinophilic fibrohistiocytic lesion of bone marrow: a new morphologic finding, probably related to drug hypersensitivity, *Blood,* 40, 464, 1972.
38. **te Velde, J., Vismans, F. J. F. E., Leenheers-Binnendijk, L., et al.,** The eosinophilic fibrohistiocytic lesion of the bone marrow, *Virchows Arch. Path. Anat. Histol.,* 377, 277, 1978.
39. **Nixon, R. K.,** The relationship of mastocytosis and lymphomatous disease, *Ann. Intern. Med.,* 59, 856, 1956.
40. **Yoo, D. and Lessin, L. S.,** Bone marrow mast cells in lymphoproliferative disease, *Ann. Intern. Med.,* 88, 753, 1978.

Chapter 17

BONE CELLS AND MULTINUCLEATED GIANT CELLS OF THE MARROW

Stephen Davis and Sidney Trubowitz

TABLE OF CONTENTS

I. INTRODUCTION

The specialized functions of bone cells determine calcium homeostasis and the quantity and quality of the skeleton. However, the process of bone cell specialization is not well understood. This situation is not surprising in light of the inherent complexity of bone and the difficulty in studying the tissue. The forthcoming discussions will attempt to emphasize the evolving concepts of marrow bone cells.

The "classical" model of bone cell differentiation reflects the work of many investigators. According to this model, the lineage of all bone cells begins with the mesenchymal cell. Mesenchymal cells are morphologically identified as spindle cells with small elongated, hyperchromatic nuclei. They contain large glycogen stores and little endoplasmic reticulum. These cells constitute 95% of the total lining of normal bone surfaces.[1] They line the external endosteal surfaces of both cortical and trabecular bone and the internal endosteal surfaces of haversian bone. It is believed that these cells are the osteoprogenitor cells which are the source of cells active in bone remodeling (Figure 1). The classical theory of bone cell differentiation holds that both osteoblasts and osteoclasts are derived from osteoprogenitor cells but that the two cell lines diverge at an early stage of differentiation.

Two major modifications of this classic model were subsequently proposed. The first, originated by Frost[2] and Rassmusen and Bordier,[1] holds that the osteoclast fragments nonmitotically into osteoblasts. This theory provides a cellular basis for the precedence of bone resorption over bone formation. However, the evidence was indirect and has remained unconvincing. The second modification pointed to the origin of osteoclasts and all normal multinucleate cells from the fusion of circulating monocytes. This later theory is supported by a large body of experimental data, and forms the basis of our current understanding of bone cell physiology.

II. OSTEOPROGENITOR CELLS

These cells were first defined as the population of cells enveloping bone surfaces that are labeled shortly after ^{3}H-thymidine injection into animals. The location of these cells is the main criterion defining them since their morphological appearance is indistinguishable from cells previously termed marrow mesenchymal cells, fibroblasts, reticulum cells, and marrow vascular endothelial cells. Young believed, using ^{3}H-thymidine kinetics studies, that they are the immediate precursors of bone cells and so termed them osteoprogenitor cells. His method was to determine the labeling of osteoprogenitor cells and then to follow the rate of appearance of labeled nuclei in both osteoclasts and osteoblasts at various times thereafter. In 1 hr about 20% of osteoprogenitor cells, 0% of osteoclasts and less than 5% of osteoblasts were labeled. With increasing time the percentage of labeled osteoclasts and osteoblasts equaled that of osteoprogenitor cells. Young concluded that osteoclasts and osteoblasts were derived from osteoprogenitor cells.[3,4]

Further information on the origin of osteogenic cells was obtained from studies on bone marrow. The data obtained suggested that marrow contains two main cellular systems, the stroma and the hematopoietic system, each derived from histogenetically distinct cell lines in the postnatal organism. The stroma of marrow consists mainly of a network of reticular cells and fibrils together with the endothelial cells lining the walls of the sinusoidal vessels. The cytoplasm of reticular and endothelial cells is rich in filaments and rough endoplasmic reticulum and there are fine fibrous structures associated with the cell surfaces. These cells appear to be members of the fibroblast family in that they are capable of producing connective tissue. The hematopoietic cells are

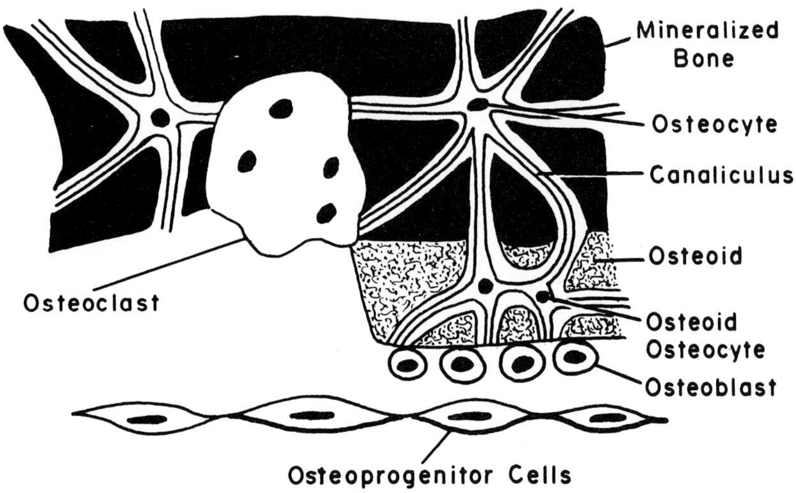

FIGURE 1. Schematic representation of the bone cells to the boney trabeculae.

supported by the stromal network. An exception is the macrophage whose long processes appears to interwine with and entrap the stromal cells.

Morphologically the osteogenic connective tissue of periostial and endosteal surfaces and that of haversian canals is continuous with the marrow stromal elements. Stromal cells merge into preosteoblasts and osteoblasts near bone surfaces. Osteoclasts and their precursors are found both near bone surfaces and within bone cavities.

The potential for differentiation of marrow stroma and osteogenic connective tissue has been evaluated in experimental systems. Following localized removal of marrow from the midshaft of long bones a blood clot fills the depleted region in the marrow within 2 days. Then, active proliferation of connective tissue budding from the endothelial surfaces and from the haversian spaces within the bone is noted, and, as the marrow blood clot contracts, this connective tissue advances into the cavity. Differentiation of this tissue occurs to form bone trabeculae and the sinusoidal capillaries. Hematopoietic cells arrive last and hematopoiesis is established. The trabecular bone is then resorbed.[5] At the present time experimental data suggest that in the postnatal mammal stromal tissue is derived from a cell line separate from that of hematopoietic tissue, i.e., no common stem cell gives rise to both.

III. OSTEOCLASTS

Osteoclasts are multinucleate giant cells appearing at the surface of bone undergoing resorption typically located in Howship's lacunae (Figure 1). At the light microscopic level these cells contain from 1 to 100 nuclei. A characteristic feature of the osteoclast is the ruffled border which seems to consist of a complex system of cytoplasmic folds and projections at the point of the osteoclasts with bone. These processes interdigitate between collagen fibers which are free of mineral in the resorptive process.[6] Adjacent to the ruffled border, the osteoclast cytoplasm shows many vacuoles which appear to be pinocytic vesicles, some containing apatite crystals or collagen fibers.[7] In addition, osteoclasts contain many mitochondria and lysosomes.[8]

On Romanowsky staining of the marrow, osteoclasts show a fine reticular chromatin with an occasionally observed nucleolus. The cytoplasmic is red violet and finely granular. Each nucleus is discrete not multilobulated as that of the megakaryocyte.

Another unique feature of osteoclasts is their high content of acid phosphatase.[8] Walker[9] found that bone marrow cells contain 2.03 moles of acid phosphatase per kg of dry tissue, whereas osteoclasts contain 29.23 moles per kg of dry tissue. He also found that osteoclasts contain four times the amount of citrate as that found in marrow cells. In undecalcified bone marrow sections, osteoclasts contain a mean number of four nuclei. In people over 70 years of age the mean number of nuclei per osteoclast decreases to 2.25, which is similar to the number found in patients with postmenopausal osteoporosis (2.6). In contrast, in primary hyperparathyroidism the mean number of nuclei is 4.8. Conversely, in Paget's disease the mean number increases to 22 per cell, with many large forms seen.[1]

A. Origin

It is now quite clear from experiments with parabiotic rats that osteoclasts are derived from circulating cells. Gothlin and Ericsson[10] joined a pair of inbred rats by skin flaps, thus establishing a cross-circulation. One animal was irradiated with a dose sufficient to destroy all hematopoietic cells, while the other animal was shielded. A fracture of the femur of each animal was produced. The cross-circulation was arrested, and tritiated-labeled thymidine was injected into the shielded rats. After 20 min cross-circulation was reestablished. Animals were then sacrificed and the healing fractures evaluated by electron microscopy. In the shielded animals both osteoblasts and osteoclasts were labeled, while in the irradiated animal only osteoclasts showed uptake. Those data were verified by Buring,[11] and van Furth et al.,[12] who provided further evidence that the circulating cells are fused monocytes.

Skeletal changes in mice subjected to continuous external whole body irradiation support the fact that osteoclast precursors occur in the hemopoietic compartment.[13] Irradiation causes marrow aplasia. Histologic and morphometric studies on such irradiated bones provided no evidence of osteoblast dysfunction since linear bone growth continues unimpaired. However, bone remodeling, i.e., osteoclast function, is deficient. Osteoclast counts decline progressively following irradiation which can not be reversed by parathormone or infusions with circulating mononuclear cells. When bone marrow cellularity recovered bone remodeling resumed.

It is generally believed that osteoclasts (and all multinucleate giant cells) represent an end stage in cell differentiation, and that after serving their particular function they die. Recent data argue against this theory.[14,15] The most important observation deals with the effect of calcitonin upon osteoclast structure. When animals are given calcitonin there is a dramatic fall (greater than 70%) in the number of osteoclasts. These cells withdraw almost immediately from their characteristic position on the bone surface, they become smaller, and within 15 min their ruffled border becomes flattened and the cells begin to appear as mononucleated cells.[16] If cell death had occurred one would expect to see cellular debris, but no such evidence is seen. These observations suggest that osteoclasts are not irreversibly differentiated cells.

B. Osteoclast Function

In 1873 Kölliker[17] suggested that the osteoclast is responsible for bone resorption. Many laboratories have shown that osteoclasts resorb bone and that the ruffled border is the site of resorption. The reaction products of several lysosomal enzymes are found at the bone-osteoclast interface.[18] The osteoclast cytoplasm contain phagosomes and vacuoles which make them ideally suited for removing dead bone both by endocytosis and secretion of extracellular enzymes.

The exact mechanism by which osteoclasts induce bone resorption is uncertain. Parathormone increases the number of osteoclasts after about 18 hr in vivo.[19] Calcitonin causes osteoclasts to leave the bone surface and lose their ruffled border.[16] Although hormones control osteoclastic activity they do not account for the localized nature of bone remodeling which occurs in the skeleton. Since osteoclasts are formed from macrophages their involvement in bone removal implies a phagocytic recognition of outworn bone. This presumes that there is a recognition phenomenon. Areas of bone compression are electronegative and areas of tension are electropositive. Since in long bone fractures osteoclast activity occurs in area of bone tension the associated electropositivity may be responsible for phagocytic recognition by osteoclasts.[20]

Osteopetrosis is a disease of mammals, including man, associated with a defect of bone resorption. Osteoclasts may be increased, decreased, or normal in numbers in this disease, but they are always qualitatively abnormal.[21] Animal models of this disease have yielded new insight into the function of osteoclasts.

In mice osteopetrosis is determined by the presence of homozygous recessive mutant genes at one or another of four loci.[21] These loci are termed *mi mi, gl gl, oc oc, op op*. In rats this condition is due to recessive mutant genes termed, *ia ia, op op,* and *tl tl*. Affected *ia ia* rats have osteopetrosis from birth but recover spontaneously soon after birth. *op op* rats are normal at birth but osteopetrosis develops in infancy and is associated with progressive depletion of T lymphocytes and thymic atrophy. It has been shown that thymus grafting from a normal sibling cures the osteopetrosis and thymic atrophy in *op op* rats.[22] *tl tl* rat osteopetrosis is resistant to all attempts at transplantation.

Apparently, *gl gl* and *mi mi* mice have similar degrees of osteopetrosis. The petrosis in such mice is curable by lethal irradiation and bone marrow transplantation,[23] but in contrast to *op op* rats, *mi mi* mice are not subject to thymic atrophy nor cured by thymic grafting or by infusion of circulating T and B lymphocytes. Loutit and Nisbet[24] suggest that the irradiation is unnecessary and the cure occurs with syngenic marrow cells. In addition, *mi mi* mice possess defects in T and B lymphocytes, at least in regard to mitogen responses. The association of osteoclast dysfunction and lymphocyte dysfunction, therefore, appear to be linked.

Milhead and Labat[22] feel that the thymus is crucial to osteoclast function. They suggested that a thymic hormone acts directly to activate osteoclasts or that such a hormone promotes differentiation of thymocytes to osteoclast formation. Neither hypothesis seems likely since thymectomized or nude mice do not develop osteopetrosis.

As previously stated, the macrophage is the most likely candidate for the osteoclast precursor. Loutit[24] has shown that the macrophages of *mi mi* mice release less calcium from bone powder than do macrophages of normal mice. They suggest that *mi mi* mice osteoclasts have defects in recognition phenomenon. Thus, in *mi mi* mice phagocyte and lymphocyte defects occur in osteopetrosis which is cured by bone marrow transplant but not lymphocyte infusions. Therefore, the defect of lymphocytes may be incidental, not causative, in *mi mi* mouse osteopetrosis.

In *op op* rats the repair of the osteopetrosis seems to be dependent on thymic lymphocytes, i.e., a thymus graft restores adequate osteoclast function. Since it is well known that T lymphocytes "activate" macrophages in inflammatory states independent of antigen it appears reasonable to suggest that a thymic cell acts in a helper function to macrophages in the removal of outworn mineral bone. From studies in these rodent models it appears the degree of T lymphocyte contribution to osteoclast function is genetically determined and thus variable. These animal models will provide useful tools in studying human osteopetrosis. Bone marrow transplantation has been successfully applied to a case of human osteopetrosis.

IV. BONE CELL FUNCTION IN AGING

It is generally believed that skeletal mass decreases with age, a phenomenon which is independent of differences in physical activity, diet, and expectations of aging. It has been suggested that the age-related bone loss simply reflects the product of age-dependent changes in vascular, renal, neural, and hormonal activities.[26]

Studies by Flanagan and Nichols[27] using human bone samples ranging in age from newborn to 67 years, showed that bone cellularity decreased with age. Despite the wide age range of the subjects, oxygen utilization rates were fairly constant at 0.47 μmoles/mg DNA/hr. Similarly, the rates of bone aerobic lactate production were constant in this varied aged group at 0.79 μmoles/mg DNA/hr. These authors suggested that despite the decrease in the number of bone cells with senescence, metabolic activity of bone remains relatively constant and is not a factor in bone loss.

Schulz and Delling[28] have shown that osteoblastic activity is reduced with advancing age, a process which is accompanied by an antagonistic increase in the inactive osteoid surface with osteoclasts. These findings became most significant in the sixth decade of life. This age-related decrease in osteoblastic activity, coupled with age-related increases in osteoclastic activity, could readily account for the steady and progressive bone loss with senescence.

The percentage of small osteocytes decreases after the age of 40 while large osteocytes increase in number after the age of 40. Whereas the small osteocyte is considered to play an active role in transport of bone substances, large osteocytes function primarily to resorb bone.[29,30] Since activation of osteocytes is an indicator of parathormone function, the age-related increment mentioned may represent the response to progress with increases of parathormone with age.

Changes in endocrine functions with age include an increase in circulating parathormone, and a decrease in tri-iodothyronine, estrogens, testosterone, calcitonin, somatomedin, and 1,25-dihyroxycholecalciferol.[31,32] Bone cell metabolism may be altered in diabetics with premature osteopenia since insulin stimulates bone uptake of amino-acids and exerts a stimulatory effect on collagen synthesis.[33] Thus, relative degrees of insulin, calcitonin, and estrogen deficiency may result in age-related bone changes—calcitonin, due to its effect on osteoclasts, as previously described. The effect, of estrogen on bone cells is unknown. These data must be interpreted with caution until purified bone cells can be examined in the proper clinical situation.

V. OSTEOBLASTS AND OSTEOCYTES

Of all bone cells osteoblasts are the most uniform in size and appearance. Their most striking aspects are their extensive rough endoplasmic reticulum and associated cytoplasmic basophilia which are measurements of active protein synthesis.[34,35] Within the cytoplasm are a number of mitochondria and many vesicles 200 to 400 Å in diameter. These vesicles contain a dense amorphous material which probably represents mucopolysaccharide. The osteoblasts are characteristically lined up along the bone surface in a fairly regular and ordered array, but the contiguous cells do not form tight junctions (Figure 1). Osteoblasts viewed in the marrow aspirate appear elongated with their greatest diameter being approximately 30 μm^3. The nucleus is somewhat eccentric with a coarse trabeculated chromatin and several deep blue nucleoli. The cytoplasm is dark blue and at a certain distance from the nucleus reveals a lighter zone called the archoplasm. Because of eccentric location of the nucleus, it is important to avoid confusion with plasma cells; since osteoblasts tend also to occur in clusters, as in Paget's disease, they must be clearly delineated from tumor cells.

All active osteoblasts are in intimate contact with the underlying osteoid. At sites of bone formation the cell layer overlying these sites may be several cell layers thick. The cells not in opposition to the osteoid are considered preosteoblasts. These later cells are normally basophilic with minimal endoplasmic reticulum and large amounts of glycogen. They are clearly distinguishable from osteoprogenitor cells by their larger size, more extensive cytoplasm, larger paler nuclei, and increased glycogen content.

Osteoblasts exhibit polarity in that they secrete collagen into the matrix space adjacent to the osteoid surface, at that time they send out cellular processes only into the underlying osteoid not into the preosteoblast cell layer. Within these cellular extensions are electron-dense material which may be bone mineral needed for collagen calcification.[36] After secreting collagen for a time, the osteoblast is converted into an osteoid osteoblast, and the layer of preosteoblasts is converted into osteoblasts which begin to secrete collagen and encase the former osteoblast, now an osteocyte (Figure 1). The distinguishing feature of the osteoid osteocyte is that it has lost considerable cytoplasm but retains most of its endoplasmic reticulum. The osteocyte is the most numerous of bone cells lining bone surfaces. Baud estimated approximately 25,000 osteocytes per cubic millimeter of bone.[37] It is important to note that as preosteoblasts become osteoblasts they send out cellular processes which form junctions with the underlying osteocytes, thus establishing the cellular extensions responsible for the canalicular system of cell to cell communication within bone.

Osteopenia simplistically can be defined as a decrease in the amount of bone, i.e., too little bone. Pathophysiologically this may be due to decreased matrix, decreased mineralization or too much resorption. Deficient osteoblastic function can result in a quantitative decrease in trabecular bone resulting in osteoporosis. Defects in mineralization result in osteomalacia of rickets, whereas, osteoclast dysfunction occurs in multiple myeloma, malignancies, and hyperparathyroidism. Osteopenia can be reliably diagnosed roentgenographically, but X-rays can not differentiate the multitude of etiologies.

The assessment of osteopenia requires evaluation of thin-cut, undecalcified bone biopsies from the iliac crest. Decalcified bone is not suitable for the identification of osteoid (unmineralized matrix). Undecalcified sections permits distinction of mineralized and nonmineralized matrix.

With the aid of the fluorescent properties of tetracycline the kinetics of human bone formation can be evaluated by a single biopsy specimen. Tetracycline stoichiometrically binds to divalent cations in newly deposited bone mineral. If one administers two time-spaced doses of the drug the rates of bone mineralization can be determined by studying the two resulting parallel fluorescent bands. The more superficial fluorescent band forms at the interface of osteoid and mineralized bone, whereas, the deeper band reflects the first tetracycline dose. The mean distance between these two bands divided by the interdose time reflects the quantity of bone mineralized per time. These techniques add insight into the heterogeneity of osteopenia.

VI. BONE MARROW MULTINUCLEATED GIANT CELLS

Mammalian tissues normally contain a single nucleus. This biologic "rule" is broken in skeletal muscle, placenta, and bone marrow where cells with several nuclei can be seen to share the same cytoplasm. Otherwise, the recognition of polykaryons in tissue should be considered abnormal.

A. Mechanisms of Fusion

The current concept of the cell membrane is that it consists of a lipid bilayer in which proteins move with varying degrees of lateral mobility.[38] The lipid bilayer is an inherently stable structure and needs to be altered by some destabilizing force before it will fuse with other lipid membranes.[39] The mechanism by which these cell surface alterations lead to fusion is essentially unknown. The plasma membranes of mammalian cells are normally separated by a 15-nm gap; since the membrane lipid bilayer is inherently stable the close approach of cell surfaces beyond the normally observed separation distance must be accompanied by changes which render the bilayer unstable. All mammalian cells carry a net negative charge on their surface. Poste and Allison[40] suggest that the close approach of negatively charged membranes, which is allowed by the reduced surface coat thickness seen preceeding fusion, leads to electrostatic displacement of intramembranes calcium. Calcium is known to be vital to membrane stability and the destabilization of membranes which follows its removal may be the common denominator allowing membrane fusion.[41] Papahadjopoulos et al.[42] have shown that cells fuse with negatively charged but not neutral lipid vesicles.

B. Inflammatory Giant Cells

Inflammatory multinucleate cells are commonly seen in many pathologic conditions in response to a variety of foreign or insoluble substances. Because of this association and because they often contain ingested material these cells are assumed to represent a mechanism for improved phagocytosis. They have, however, been shown to have poor phagocytic function.

The multinucleate cell described by Langhans is characterized by a circular peripheral arrangement of nuclei around a central granular mass. In the foreign body giant cell the nuclei are scattered in an irregular fashion throughout the cell. These two types of inflammatory giant cells may be found in infective and sterile granulomas. The nomenclature of these two types of granuloma is arbitrary and nondiagnostic.

Borrel[43] was the first to suggest that inflammatory multinucleate giant cells were fused mononuclear leukocytes. Lambert[44] and Lewis[45] confirmed these data. Spector and Lykke[46] reported that circulating monocytes fuse to form multinucleate cells appearing in inflammatory granulomas. It can thus be concluded that the mononuclear phagocyte is the precursor of inflammatory multinucleate giant cells as they are for osteoclasts.

It is generally believed that mononuclear phagocyte form giant cells by fusion rather than nuclear division. Using two macrophage populations, one with radioactive label, the other unlabeled, Mariano and Spector[47] showed that the nuclei of both populations appeared in giant cells in vivo. They also showed electron microscopically macrophages active in the fusion process. Sutton and Weiss[48] demonstrated fusion of chicken macrophages in vitro in the absence of mitosis.

In common with other cell types macrophages can be fused, either with other macrophages or other cell types, by viruses.[49] At this time no evidence exists that links viruses to macrophage fusion in vivo except, perhaps, in viral infections known to be associated with granuloma. Macrophage polykaryons are commonly found in areas containing poorly removable foreign material. Frequently the material is antigenic, e.g., tuberculosis, although it need not necessarily be so. Parks and Weiser[50] have suggested that the immune system is intimately linked to macrophage fusion. These investigators found pulmonary lavage fluid from animals mounting a secondary response to intravenous BCG caused fusion of normal alveolar macrophages in vitro. Galindo[51] reported fusion of BCG-sensitized rabbit alveolar macrophages on in vitro challenge with BCG. The same investigators showed identical results with lymph node cells.[52] To assess the role of the immune system in macrophage giant cell formation Papadimitrious[53] implanted glass coverslips into normal and nude (athymic) mice. He found no difference in the rate or extent of giant cell formation. This data suggested that the cellular immune system is not responsible for macrophage fusion. Weir[54] performed a series of experiments suggesting that lymphocyte derived fluids (lymphokines) lack the ability to induced macrophage fusion. Parks[50] data would lead us to a different interpretation. When he incubated rabbit alveolar macrophages with immune pulmonary lavage fluids, together with particulate matter, he found giant cells contained the particles. If giant cells were formed prior to the addition of particles only the remaining mononuclear cells took up the particles. These findings suggest that it is phagocytosing macrophages which fuse under the influence of lymphokines. Park believed that under the influence of lymphokines membrane changes associated with phagocytosis facilitate the adherence and fusion of macrophages. These interpretations are reminiscent of the role of lymphokines in animal models of osteopetrosis.

Attachment of many substances to macrophage surfaces is followed by the formation of endosome margins which eventually approach each other and fuse to complete endosome formation. Chambers[55,56] suggested that in material attached to the surface of two macrophages each macrophage would form endosome margins. The margins of one macrophage would then meet the phagosome margins of the other and fusion might result between the two cells.

It can be seen from our discussion that all proposed mechanisms for cell fusion involve close membrane opposition, made possible by membrane alterations or differentiation, followed by membrane fusion. There is no loss of membrane from the cell surface. Accordingly, Gordon and Cohn[49] found no reduction of cell membrane in cells subjected to virally induced fusion. During fusion membrane receptors are interiorized, and this should lead to the formation of polykaryons with reduced capacity for further ingestion of the same material requiring membrane receptors but normal capacity for substances ingested by different receptors.[57]

From the available experimental data the Langhans and foreign body cell inflammatory granulomas can be seen as a dynamic structure with constant recruitment of new macrophages among the already fused macrophages.[58] The fusion process described above is selflimiting, since following fusion the multinucleate cell has less surface receptors and is therefore progressively less likely to undergo further phenomena of simultaneous attachment. The degree of fusion seen with different granuloma-inducing agents varies. Chambers believes this variability is due to the different amounts of energy needed during phagosome closure to overcome the forces responsible for membrane separation. If the forces of attachment of the phagosome margin are low in relation to the forces opposing the phagosome margin fusion does not occur. Similarly, following attachment of endocytic material to two macrophages in vivo, a strongly attached substrate may lead to fusion, while a more weakly adherent substrate will be removed from one or the other macrophage. This model of fusion following simultaneous endocytosis resolves the paradox of the presence of ingested material in giant cells which have poor phagocytic activity.[59]

C. Tumor Giant Cells

It has been known for many years that benign and malignant epithelial and mesenchymal neoplasm contain multinucleated giant cells.[60] They are usually associated with undifferentiated tumors and the nuclei of the giant cells resemble those of the mononuclear tumor population. The nuclei are pleomorphic, often hyperdiploid, and show abnormal mitosis. Unlike inflammatory giant cells, their mode of formation is unknown but all of the previous discussed mechanisms appear likely. Harris[61] suggests that it is unlikely that repeated nuclear division without cell separation could account for tumor giant cell formation since tumor giant cells contain a single mitotic spindle. Nuclei sharing cytoplasm normally form a single mitotic spindle leading to the formation of a single hyperdiploid nucleus. The formation of a shared spindle following tumor cell fusion may account for the bizarre hyperdiploid cells.

A second group of giant cells in tumors in which mitosis is almost never seen among the giant cell nuclei; the nuclei are uniform in size and shape. They resemble inflammatory multinucleate giant cells. These cells are now believed to be secondarily formed from macrophages and not by fusion of neoplastic cells.

REFERENCES

1. **Rassmusen, H. and Bordier, P.,** *The Physiological and Cellular Basis of Metabolic Bone Disease,* Williams and Wilkins, Baltimore, 1974.
2. **Frost, H. M.,** *The Bone Dynamics of Osteoporosis and Osteomalacia,* Charles C Thomas, Springfield, Ill., 1966.
3. **Young, R. W.,** In *Bone Biodynamics,* Frost, H. M., Ed., Little, Brown, Boston, 1964.
4. **Young, R. W.,** In *Biology of Hard Tissue,* Proc. 2nd Conf., Budy, A. M., Ed., National Aeronautics and Space Administration, Washington, D.C., 1968.
5. **Owen, M.,** Histogenesis of bone cells, *Calcif. Tissue Res.,* 25, 205, 1977.
6. **Ham, A. W.,** *Histology,* 7th ed., Lippincott, Philadelphia, 1974.
7. **Gothlin, G. and Ericsson, J. L. E.,** The osteoclast, *Clin. Orthop. Rel. Res.,* 120, 201, 1976.
8. **Lucht, U.,** Acid phosphatase of osteoclasts demonstrated by electron microscopic histochemistry, *Histochemie,* 28, 103, 1971.
9. **Walker, D. G.,** Enzymatic and electron microscopic analysis of isolated osteoclast, *Calcif. Tissue Res.,* 9, 296, 1972.
10. **Gothlin, G. and Ericsson, J. L. E.,** On the histogenesis of the cells in fracture callus. Electron, microscopic autoradiographic observations in parabiotic rats and studies on labelled monocytes, *Virchows Arch. Zell. Pathol.,* 12, 318, 1973.
11. **Buring, K.,** On the origin of cells in heterotopic bone formation, *Clin. Orthop. Rel. Res.,* 110, 293, 1975.
12. **van Furth, R., Cohn, Z. A., Hirsch, J. G., Humphrey, J. H., Spector, W. G., and Langevoort, H. L.,** The mononuclear phoagocyte system, a new classification of macrophages, monocytes, and their precursor cells, *Bull. WHO* 46, 845, 1972.
13. **Anderson, N. D., Colyer, R. A., and Riley, L. H., Jr.,** Skeletal changes during prolonged external irradiation, alterations in marrow, growth plate and osteoclast populations, *John Hopkins Med. J.,* 145, 73, 1979.
14. **Gaillard, P. J.,** Parathyroid gland and bone *in vivo, Schweiz. Med. Wochenschr.,* 14, 447, 1957.
15. **Mills, B. G., Harontinian, A. M., Holst, P., Bordier, P., and Tun-Chot, S.,**Ultrastructural and cellular changes at the costochondral junction following *in vivo* treatment with calcitonin or calcium chloride in the rabbit, in *Endocrinology,* Heinemann Books, London, 1972.
16. **Kallio, D. M., Garant, P. R., and Minkin, C.,** Evidence of coated membranes in the ruffled border of the osteoclast, *J. Ultrastruct. Res.,* 37, 169, 1971.
17. **Kölliker, A.,** *Die Normale Resportion der Knochengewebe,* Leipzig, Vogel, 1873.
18. **Schofield, B. H., Levin, L. S., and Doty, S. B.,** Ultrastructure and lysosomal histochemistry of 1α rat osteoclasts, *Calcif. Tissue Res.,* 14, 153, 1974.
19. **Bingham, P. J., Brazell, I. A., and Owen, M.,** The effect of parathyroid extract on cellular activity and plasma calcium levels *in vivo, J. Endocrinol.,* 45, 387, 1969.
20. **Rabinovitch, M. P.,** Phagocytic recognition, in *Mononuclear Phagocytes,* van Furth, R., Ed., Blackwell, Oxford, 1970.
21. **Marks, S. C. and Walker, D. G.,** Mammalian osteopetrosis a model for studying cellular and humoral factors in bone resorption, in *The Biochemistry and Physiology* of Bone, Bourne, IV, G. H., Ed., New York, Academic Press, 1976.
22. **Milhead, G. and Labat, M. L.,** Thymus and osteopetrosis, *Clin. Orthoped.,* 135, 260, 1978.

23. **Walker, D. G.,** Bone resorption restored in osteopetrotic mice by transplants of normal bone marrow and spleen cells, *Science,* 190, 784, 1972.
24. **Loutit, J. F. and Nisbet, N. W.,** Resorption of bone, *Lancet,* 2, 27, 1979.
25. **Loutit, J. F. and Samsom, J. M.,** Osteopetrosis of microphthalmic mice, a defect of the hematopoietic stem cell, *Calcif. Tissue Res.,* 20, 251, 1976.
26. **Garn, S. M.,** Bone loss and aging, in *The Physiology and Pathology of Human Aging,* Goldman, R. and Rockstein, M., Eds., Academic Press, New York, 1975.
27. **Flanagan, B. and Nichols, G., Jr.,** Metabolic studies of human bone *in vitro* I. Normal bone, *J. Clin. Invest.,* 44, 1788, 1965.
28. **Schulz, A. and Delling, G.,** Age-related changes of bone resorption parameters in iliac crest trabecular bone, *Proc. 1st Workshop on Bone Morphometry,* University of Ottawa Press, Ottawa, 1976.
29. **Baud, C. A.,** Histophysiology of the osteocyte, an introduction to the morphometry of periosteocytic lacunae, *Proc. 1st Workshop on Bone Morphometry,* University of Ottawa Press, Ottawa, 1976.
30. **Belanger, L. F., Robichon, J., Migicovsky, B. B., Copp, D. G., and Vincent, J.,** Resorption without osteoclasts, in *Mechanisms of Hard Tissue Destruction,* Sognnaes, R. F., Ed., American Association for the Advancement of Science, Washington, D.C., 1963.
31. **Berlyne, G. M., Ben-Ari, J., Kusheloevsky, A., and Idelman, A.,** The etiology of senile osteoporisis, secondary hyperparathyroidism due to renal failure, *Q. J. Med.,* 44, 505, 1975.
32. **Bartizal, F. J., Coulain, C. B., and Gaffey, T. A.,** Impaired binding of estradiol to vaginal mucosal cells in post menopausal osteoporosis, *Calcif. Tissue,Proc. 11th Eur. Symp.,* PorsNielsen, S., Hjorting-Hauen, E., Ed., 1975.
33. **Davis, P. J.,** Endocrine and aging, *Hosp. Prac.,* 1977, 133.
34. **Gaillard, P. J.,** The physiology and biochemistry of parathyroid function, in *Parathyroid Hormone and Thyrocalcitonin,* Talmage, R. V., Belanger, L. F., and Clark, S., Eds., Excerpta Medica Foundation, Amsterdam, 1968.
35. **Cameron, D. A.,** The fine structure of osteoblasts in the metaphysis of the tibia of the young rat, *J. Biophys. Biochem. Cytol.,* 9, 583, 1961.
36. **Pautard, F. G. E.,** Anatomolecular survey of calcification, in *Calcified Tissues,* Fleish, H., Blackwood, J., and Owen, M., Eds., Springer-Verlag, New York, 1966.
37. **Baud, C. A. and Amil, E.,** Osteocyte differential count in normal human alveolar bone, *Acta Anat.,* 78, 321, 1971.
38. **Nicolson, G. L.,**Transmembrane control of the receptors on normal and tumor cells, *Biochim. Biophys. Acta,* 457, 57, 1976.
39. **Lucy, J. A.,** Aspects of the fusion of cells *in vitro* without viruses, *J. Reprod. Fertil.,* 44, 193, 1975.
40. **Poste, G. and Allison, A. C.,** Membrane fusion reaction, a therapy, *J. Theoret. Biol.,* 32, 165, 1971.
41. **Weiss, L.,** The Cell Periphery, Metastasis and Other Contact Phenomena, North-Holland, Amsterdam, 1967.
42. **Papahadjopoulos, D., Poste, G., and Schaeffer, B. D.,** Fusion of mammalian cells by unilamellar lipid vesicles, influence of lipid surface charge, fluidity, and cholesterol, *Biochim. Biophys. Acta.,* 323, 23, 1973.
43. **Borrel, A.,** Tuberculose pulmonaire experimentale, *Ann. Inst. Pasteur.,* 7, 593, 1893.
44. **Lambert, R. A.,** The production of foreign body giant cells *in vitro, J. Exp. Med.,* 15, 510, 1912.
45. **Lewis, W. H.,** The formation of giant cells in tissue cultures and their similarity to those in tuberculous lesions, *Am. Rev. Tuberc.,* 15, 616, 1927.
46. **Spector, W. G. and Lykke, A. W. J.,** The cellular evolution of inflammatory granuloma, *J. Pathol. Bact.,* 92, 163, 1966.
47. **Mariano, M. and Spector, W. G.,** The formation and properties of macrophage polykaryons, *J. Pathol.,* 113, 1, 1974.
48. **Sutton, J. S. and Weiss, L.,** Transformation of monocytes in tissue culture into macrophages, epitheloid cells, and multinucleate giant cells, *J. Cell Biol.,* 28, 303, 2966.
49. **Gordon, S. and Cohn, Z. A.,** Macrophage-melanocyte heterokaryons, *J. Exp. Med.,* 131, 981, 1970.
50. **Parks, D. E. and Weiser, R.,** The role of phagocytosis and natural lymphokines in the fusion of alveolar macrophages to form Langhans giant cells, *J. Reticuloendothel. Soc.,* 17, 218, 1975.
51. **Galindo, B.,** Antigen-mediated fusion of specifically sensitized rabbit alveolar macrophages, *Infect. Immun.,* 9, 212, 1974.
52. **Galindo, B., Myrvik, Q. N., and Love, S. H.,** A macrophage agglutinating factor produced during a pulmonary delayed hypersensitivity reaction, *J. Reticuloendothel. Soc.,* 18, 295, 1975.
53. **Papadimitrious, J. M.,** The influence of the thymus on multinucleate foreign body giant cells, *J. Pathol.,* 118, 153, 1976.
54. **Weir, D. M.,** A Handbook of Experimental Immunology, Blackwell, Oxford, 1973.

55. **Chambers, T. J.,** Fusion of macrophages following simultaneous attempted phagocytosis of glutaraldehyde-fixed red cells, *J. Pathol.,* 122, 71, 1977.
56. **Chambers, T. J.,** The mechanisms of fusion of hamster macrophages induced by antimacrophage serum, *J. Pathol.,* 122, 163, 1977.
57. **Chambers, T. J.,** Failure of altered macrophage surfaces to lead to the formation of polykaryons, *J. Pathol.,* 122, 185, 1977.
58. **Spector, W. G.,** The macrophage, its origin and role in pathology, *Pathobiol. Annu.,* 4, 33, 1974.
59. **Chambers, T. J.,** Multinucleate giant cells, *J. Pathol.,* 126, 1, 1978.
60. **Roizman, B.,** Polykaryocytosis, Cold Spring Harbor Symp. Quant. Biol., 27, 327, 1962.
61. **Harris, H.,** In *Nucleus and Cytoplasm,* Clarendon Press, Oxford, 1968.

Chapter 18

PATHOLOGIC REACTIONS INVOLVING THE BONE MARROW

Stephen Davis and Sidney Trubowitz

TABLE OF CONTENTS

I. GROSS AND MICROSCOPIC APPEARANCE

Hidden from view and secluded within the confines of the skeleton, the size and scope of the human marrow has been poorly appreciated and difficult to assess. At birth, active hemopoietic marrow exists in all of the osseous cavities, but by 4 years of age the red hemopoietic marrow in the more distal portions of the skeleton is replaced by fat. The fatty, yellow marrow progressively replaces the red hemopoietic marrow in a centripetal direction, so that by age 20 the red marrow is confined to the skull, clavicles, scapulae, sternum, ribs, pelvis, and the most proximal ends of the long bones. The total amount of marrow in an average 70-kilogram individual measures about 3000 g half of which is active, red hemopoietic marrow, and half inactive, fatty yellow marrow. Thus, the hemopoietic marrow is an organ comparable in size to that of the liver and represents about 2% of the individual's total body weight.

In the mature adult about 40% of the red marrow is housed in the pelvis, 29% in the vertebrae, 13% in the ribs and the remainder in the humeri, scapulae, clavicles, and skull.[1] The gross examination of the human marrow is obviously impossible in life and traditionally, pathologists have limited their examination of the marrow at post-mortem to the inspection of frontal section through the bodies of the lower vertebrae. The normal human marrow is bright red in color and firm in consistency. In polycythemia the marrow is dark red and soft; in the leukemias, muddy-brown or grey-white. Metastatic disease manifests as grey to white localized nodules, varying in size and in consistency from soft friable, gumous material to hard, dense structures. The myelomatous marrow is often dark red, soft, almost liquid, accompanied by marked osteopenia and fractures. In semistarvation and in cachexia marrow fat is lost and the marrow presents grossly as a collapsed gelatinous mass. For the most part gross pathologic changes bespeak advanced disease; the more subtle changes of marrow architecture and function escape recognition on gross examination.

In an attempt at developing an assay for hemopoietic function and mineral content of the marrow by gross inspection Brandt[2] introduced a semiquantitative histometric method for analysis of the human marrow. Brandt examined the upper end of the femur obtained at autopsy. He selected the upper end of the femur for study because he found the pelvis unsuitable for histometric analysis. Brandt[2] transected the upper end of the femur in its frontal plane and scored the intensity of the red marrow as follows:

1. For a totally fatty marrow.
2. For marrow, containing about 25% red marrow.
3. Containing about 50% red marrow.
4. Seventy-five percent red marrow.
5. A totally red marrow.

The mean "intensity index" of 195 femurs so analyzed was 2.08 + 0.6. A value below 1.4 was felt to represent deficient hemopoietic activity and above 2.6, increased activity. There was no correlation between the intensity score and age or the underlying illness. The nuclear or cellular content of the marrows scored at 50, 75, and 100% was constant. The scores reflected a decrease in fat content and an increase in the number of red blood cells and sinusoids. The level of hemopoietic activity did not correlate with the color index of the marrow. An increase in marrow iron was found with increasing intensity scores. Copper and zinc concentrations were also higher in the intensely red marrow.

It is clear that the information obtained from the gross examination of the marrow is limited and reliance must be placed on the microscopic study of the material obtained by needle biopsy during life or of the sections prepared from the marrow removed at autopsy. Bone marrow cells, however, undergo rapid disintegration after death: the more mature cells (granulocytes and normoblasts) degenerate earlier than the more immature cells, the lymphocytes, and the plasma cells. The human pluripotent hematopoietic stem cells can apparently survive as long as 19 post-mortem hours.[3] The recognizable marrow cells usually degenerate beyond recognition after 15 post-mortem hours and thus impose an important time limit on the post-mortem examination of the marrow. The needle core biopsy of the bone marrow is safe, free of morbidity, repeatable, and provides adequate and well-preserved material for study.

The histologic preparation of the marrow consists of fat, a matrix of reticulum cells and macrophages, a sinusoidal system, the hemopoietic cells, lymphocytes, and plasma cells, and the bony spicules. About 50% of the surface of a normal bone marrow section is occupied by fat. The fat and the hemopoietic cells bear an inverse relationship to each other in the aplastic and hyperplastic states. The bone marrow, like all other organs, can be heir to developmental anomalies, metabolic disturbances, inflammatory reactions, circulatory compromise, infarction and necrosis, and to tumor and malignant proliferation.

II. DEVELOPMENTAL ABNORMALITIES

A. Constitutional

The constitutional aplastic anemias constitute a group of congenital, genetic, or familial diseases which feature an inherent propensity for bone marrow failure.

1. Fanconi's Anemia

Fanconi's anemia is an inherited disorder of autosomal recessive transmission. The afflicted homozygote has bone marrow failure which first becomes clinically manifest at 5 to 10 years of age.[4] The patients are generally short and present with one or more characteristic physical abnormalities, such as hyperpigmentation, absent or hypoplastic thumbs, radial aplasia, structural renal anomalies, microopthalmia, strabismus, microcephaly, mental retardation, and deafness.[5] Similar physical anomalies, and/or leukemia,[6] tumors,[7,8] and diabetes mellitus[9] may exist in other members of afflicted families without marrow failure and may represent either an incomplete expression of the homozygous state or heterozygosity.

The bone marrow of Fanconi's anemia is aplastic; the defect is probably at the level of the stem cells, both CFU-E and BFU-E.[10–12] A most striking and characteristic feature of the Fanconi anemia is the random chromosome breaks and rearrangements in the peripheral blood lymphocytes and the bone marrow cells.[13] Evidence has been presented to suggest a defect in the DNA repair mechanisms.[14,15]

2. Familial Aplastic Anemia

Familial aplastic anemia probably represents an ill-defined group of familial constitutional anemias similar to Fanconi's anemia in hematologic expression, but without the associated physical abnormalities.[16] Whether familial aplasia represents incomplete expression of the genes for Fanconi's anemia or other defective alleles at the same locus for Fanconi's anemia is not clear.[17] As more cases are analyzed it may become necessary to broaden the diagnostic criteria of Fanconi's anemia and yet separate this syndrome from other familial aplastic anemias and leukemia which resemble Fanconi's anemia but are probably different in origin.[18]

3. Amegakaryocytic Thrombocytopenic Purpura

Amegakaryocytic thrombocytopenia is a rare disorder of uncertain identity in which thrombocytopenia appears at birth or shortly thereafter to be followed by complete aplasia within months or years. At onset, the marrow is normally cellular with absent megakaryocytes or populated by small megakaryocytes.[16,19]

4. Dyskeratosis Congenita

Dyskeratosis cogenita is thought to be a sex-linked, male predominant disorder which involves skin and mucous membranes to produce dyskeratosis (reticular hyperpigmentation, dystrophic nails) and leukoplakia, and subsequently involves the bone marrow as well, leading to marrow aplasia and total marrow failure.[20]

5. Schwachman-Diamond Syndrome

This syndrome combines two essential features—pancreatic insufficiency and neutropenia. The disorder is probably autosomal recessive with a one to one male:female ratio. Elevated fetal hemoglobin and metaphysial dysostosis may be present. In some cases marrow failure may proceed to involve all of the hemopoietic elements with a resultant peripheral blood pancytopenia. These children are highly susceptible to infections to which they frequently succumb.[21]

6. Congenital Hypoplastic Anemia

The Blackfan-Diamond syndrome is a pure red cell anemia characterized by mild macrocytosis, reticulocytopenia, and a marked diminution of the erythroid precursors in the bone marrow. Hemoglobin levels at birth are normal, but the majority of the patients become anemic by the fourth month of age. Minor physical abnormalities, particularly abnormal thumbs, either triphalangeal or duplicated, may be present. The inheritance pattern of the disease has not been determined but an autosomal dominant pattern has been suggested in some families.[22]

The pathogenesis of the disorder has not been elucidated but it does not seem to be related to soluble inhibitors of erythropoietin or of the erythroid precursor cells.[23,24] Some evidence has been elicited which suggests that the defect is intrinsic to the stem cell population[25] or presents a cellular inhibitor of erythropoiesis.[26] An abnormality of the bone marrow microenvironment as the major pathogenetic mechanism in congenital hypoplastic anemia has been found in some subjects.[27] The red cells of this disorder tend to show the characteristics of fetal red blood cells, namely, elevated F hemoglobin, presence of i antigen and fetal enzyme patterns.

7. Congenital Neutropenia

Congenital neutropenia may exist as a benign disorder or a severe autosomal recessive disease characterized by great susceptibility to infection.[28] For details on the marrow changes see the chapter on the pathophysiology of granulopoiesis. Congenital neutropenia is also seen in association with thymic alymphoplasia.

8. Congenital Thrombocytopenia

This disease may be encountered as a distinct entity in association with absent radii, the thrombocytopenia-absent radii syndrome (TAR). The disorder is thought to be due to an autosomal recessive gene which affects both hemopoiesis and forearm development, both of which occur at 4 to 8 weeks of embryonic life, suggesting a common prenatal factor.

B. Environmental

The fetus is subject to a host of environmental influences mediated via its intimate interconnection with the mother. These influences include the transmission of drugs, antibodies and infectious agents.

1. Transplacental Passage of Drugs

Many drugs and chemicals are known to be teratogenic and the administration of such agents to a pregnant woman may prove to be disastrous to the infant. A highly publicized and dramatic example of such an interaction was the unfortunate limb deformities of children born to mothers who had taken thalidomide for sedation. Hematologic abnormalities have been observed in the newborn following the induction of labor with quinine. Hapten-antibody production induced by quinine can give rise to marked thrombocytopenia and purpura in both mother and child. Severe hemorrhagic disease of the fetus has followed the ingestion of naphthalene (moth balls) by the mother or the administration of large doses of vitamin K to the mother. Little information is available on the marrow changes in the newborn in these circumstances, but one might anticipate changes similar to the changes found in the adult similarly afflicted.

Drugs such as dicoumerol, salicylates, sulfonamides, chloramphenicol, and others can negotiate passage through the placental circulation and place the fetus in jeopardy by initiating a hemorrhagic syndrome or marrow aplasia and pancytopenia. Heinz-body anemia in the new born has followed thiazide ingestion by the mother.[30] The administration of chemotherapeutic agents particularly in the first trimester of pregnancy, may seriously damage the marrow of the infant.[30] Detailed interrogation of parents of children suffering from aplasia of the marrow revealed exposure to a variety of drugs, chemicals, or toxins, predominantly in the fathers of such infants. In many instances exposure to multiple myelotoxic agents was found. Although many potentially myelotoxic agents were uncovered by such interviews, the role of these agents in the pathogenesis of the aplasia of a specific patient was difficult to assess.[31]

2. Transplacental Transmission of Antibodies

a. Hemolytic Disease of the Newborn

Fetal red blood cells regularly enter the maternal circulation and arouse antibody production against those fetal antigens that are not inherited from the mother. The maternal antibodies can cross into the fetal circulation and destroy the fetal red cells. Fetal-maternal incompatibility is responsible for two thirds of cases of hemolytic diseases of the newborn. Rh incompatibility is responsible for the remaining one third of cases of hemolytic disease of the newborn but is generally more serious and severe. Anemia, jaundice, and hepatosplenomegaly are invariably present and reflect in their magnitude the severity of the illness. Macrocytosis, polychromasia, and an elevated reticulocyte count accompany an intense outpouring of nucleated red cell precursors—hence the name, erythroblastosis fetalis. The circulating red cell precursors represent all levels of erythroid maturation but are not megaloblastic. Marked leucocytosis is usually present, but the platelet counts are generally normal. The bone marrow reflects these changes, being markedly hyperplastic and normoblastic. Extramedullary hematopoiesis is present in both liver and spleen.

b. Thrombocytopenic Purpura of the Newborn

Thrombocytopenia of the newborn may arise from the transplacental transfer of platelet antibodies. Similar to erythroblastosis fetalis, antibodies may be the product of active immunization of the mother by the isoantigens of the leaked fetal platelets, or autoantibodies passively transferred from the maternal circulation of a mother suffering from idiopathic thrombocytopenia purpura. The thrombocytopenia is usually quite severe and the bone marrow shows normal or increased numbers of megakaryocytes.

c. Transmission of the LE Factor

The LE factor, passively transmitted from the mother, has been identified in the newborn. This factor may persist in the infant for 7 to 8 weeks with no ill effects on the child. The baby remains healthy and displays none of the hematologic or other complications of lupus erythematosus.[32]

3. Transplacental Transmission of Virus

Congenital rubella is usually the result of maternal infection acquired during the first trimester of pregnancy. The syndrome embraces a broad constellation of manifestations consisting of heart malformations, eye lesions, microcephaly, deafness, mental retardation, and thrombocytopenic purpura.[33] Thrombocytopenia is found in more than half of newborn infants with congenital rubella. Bleeding may be severe and the child covered with the typical "blueberry muffin" lesions.[34] Bone marrow examination reveals a decrease and, rarely, a complete absence of the megakaryocytes, suggesting deficient platelet production.[35]

C. Miscellaneous

1. Cretinism

Mild anemia frequently accompanies thyroid lack, as in myxedema, as well as other endocrine deficiencies, and is due primarily to bone marrow failure. Cretinism, thyroid failure in the child, is rarely recognized at birth. The diagnosis of cretinism may be delayed for years, exemplified by a patient seen by us some years ago. The patient was a young man who was drafted into the armed forces apparently having no difficulty with the induction physical examination. However, it soon became apparent that he could not keep up with rigors of military training and he was discharged with a diagnosis of anemia, cause undetermined to a Veteran's Administration facility, where his bone marrow was normally cellular with no obvious abnormalities. His appearance was however highly suggestive of juvenile myxedema, a diagnosis supported by X-ray and laboratory evidence. Replacement therapy effected a metamorphosis and normal hematopoiesis.

The origin of the term, cretin, is obscure. The speculation has been made that the name may be derived from a Rhaeto-Romanic word meaning "clay", referring to the pale or clay color of the cretin,[36] though emphasis in most descriptions of the disease has been on the idiotic expression of the cretin. The presenting problems of the cretin, namely, anemia, constipation, and hyperostosis are often treated separately long before the true nature of the disorder is recognized.

2. Osteopetrosis

Marble-bone disease of Albers-Schonberg is a rare disorder throught to be due to a failure of the progenitor cells of the osteoclasts. The malignant form of this disease begins in utero, is autosomal recessive, and progresses rapidly. The more benign type is autosomal dominant, appears later and progresses more slowly. The bones appear dense and uniformly sclerotic on X-ray examination. Fractures are a frequent complication even with trivial trauma. Anemia is often present and attributed to the decrease in the size of the marrow cavity. Extramedullary foci of hematopoiesis are present in the liver, spleen, and lymph nodes and contribute to their enlargement.

Progressive diaphyseal dysplasia (Camarati-Engelmann Disease) is characterized by a symmetrical thickening and increased diameter of the long bones, particularly the femurs, tibias, fibulas, radii, and ulnas. The bones are hyperostotic and mild anemia may be present, presumably a result of marrow encroachment.

III. METABOLIC ABNORMALITIES

A. Nutritional

1. Semistarvation and Cachexia

The world is constantly confronted with famine despite the prodigious agrigultural output of the more advanced countries. Substandard nutrition and semistarvation remain among the most common of human afflictions which contribute to the valetudinarian conditions of millions of people. Semistarvation in the more affluent societies is more frequently associated with disease and some degree of cachexia is a common feature of chronic illness. The hematologic data obtained from studies of the semistarved in famine and war document the prevalence of anemia, normochromic and normocytic in type in prolonged starvation, and that the degree of anemia appears to be related to the degree of starvation. Reports on the leucocyte responses to starvation have been quite variable but the evidence does indicate that in uncomplicated starvation leucopenia is the rule.

Although considerable variability of the bone marrow changes in the semi-starved has been reported, most investigators describe depletion of the marrow cells with a mucoid degeneration of the fatty marrow, absorption of the fat cells, and hyperemia of the red marrow. The bone marrow of the cachectic patient dying of a chronic illness is grossly altered and presents as a gelatinous degeneration of the fatty marrow.[37,38]

The gelatinous or the "starved" marrow is characterized by the accumulation of a gelatinous, extra cellular material, fat atrophy, and associated focal marrow hypoplasia. The aspirate of a starved marrow contains no particles and consists of small globules of a gelatinous substance admixed with peripheral blood. The marrow biopsy contains foci of grey-pink gelatinous material which is made up predominantly of mucopolysaccharides, fat atrophy, and focal hypoplasia of the marrow. The lesions tend to be focal and the adjacent hemopoietic tissue is frequently hypercellular. The overall cellularity thus appears normal. The sinusoids are dilated and congested.[39] Identical histologic lesions have been produced in the rabbit by the drastic reduction of their food intake.[40] The relationship between the marrow findings and the peripheral blood alterations in semi-starvation is not completely clear.

2. *Alcoholism*

Alcohol in concert with dietary inadequacy, deficient vitamin intake, and abnormal liver function has been implicated as a causal factor in the development of the many hematologic abnormalities that occur commonly in the alcoholic patient. These abnormalities embrace a wide spectrum of manifestations ranging from the commonly occurring iron deficiency anemia due to alcohol-induced gastritis, megaloblastosis-secondary to folate deficiency, hemolytic anemia due to membrane alterations, vacuolization of marrow cells, sideroblastic anemia, granulocytopenia, thrombocytopenia, anemia due to chronic disease to hemochromatosis.[41]

Iron lack anemia is the obvious sequel to gastrointestinal (GI) blood loss and was seen in about a third of the patients admitted to the hospital for alcoholism.[42] Megaloblastosis due to folate deficiency is seen less frequently but its presence may be suspected by the presence of hypersegmented neutrophils in the peripheral blood.[43] Severe iron deficiency anemia can mask folate deficiency which may become manifest with the development of megaloblastosis following adequate iron therapy. Alcohol can induce vacuolization of the immature cells in the marrow, best seen in the proerythroblasts. No specific marrow changes are associated with the alcohol-induced vacuolization. Most often the marrow is normally cellular with an M/E ratio about one and in which all stages of red cell maturation are represented. Similar marrow findings of vacuolization of the proerythroblasts and red cell maturation are seen in phenylalanine deficiency, hyperosmolar coma, and pyrazinoic acid amide ingestion. Chloramphenicol can also cause vacuolization of the proerythroblasts, but is associated with marked depression of erythropoiesis and a marked reduction in the number of the more mature red cell precursors. Riboflavin and copper deficiency can be associated with vacuolization of the marrow cells with normoblastopenia. Ringed sideroblasts may also appear in the marrow of alcoholics. This phenomenon may be due to pyridoxine deficiency or an intracellular enzyme defect of the erythroid precursors. Frank sideroblastic anemia is seen more often in the alcoholic suffering from marked nutritional deficiency and megaloblastosis. Bone marrow iron is frequently increased, particularly in those alcoholics who consume large amounts of wine or other high iron containing beverages.

Production of granulocytes and of platelets may be depressed by alcohol; the bone marrow may be hypoplastic with a decrease in the precursor granulocytic cells and megakaryocytes.

3. *Iron, Folate, B_{12} Lack*

The bone marrow changes accompanying iron lack anemia and the megaloblastosis of folate and B_{12} deficiency are discussed in length in the chapter on pathophysiology of erythropoiesis.

B. Aging

The red blood cell count, white blood cell count, and the platelet count of the aged show no significant changes from those of young people. The mean red cell count and hemoglobin concentration of the aged is somewhat lower than the mean values of the young, but do not fall below the established lower limit. The aging process cannot be held responsible for anemia discovered in the elderly patient. The mean white cell and platelet counts remain relatively unaltered throughout life.[47]

Bone marrow cellularity is maximal in the first decade of life to be followed by a gradual reduction over the course of the subsequent two decades. The marrow cellularity remains fairly stable from 30 to 60 years of age when a second wave of diminishing marrow cellularity begins and proceeds to age 80 with a final decrease of about 24 percent of the cellular elements of the marrow.[48] The estimations of marrow cellularity rests on the appraisal of the relative concentrations of cells and fat, and hence a part of the apparent decrease of marrow cellularity of the aged may indeed be spurious and may be due to an absolute increase in the marrow fat, which occupies the space created by the bone loss of senile osteoporosis and not to an inherent and absolute decrease in the cellular component of the marrow. The cellular composition of the red marrow of the aged shows no significant change from the marrow of young subjects. No distinction can be made on morphologic grounds between the marrow samples obtained by biopsy or aspirate from the young or the old. The bone marrow reveals no morphologic evidence of aging.[49,50]

The concentration of hematopoietic stem cells does not decrease with aging in animals.[50] The immediate response of erythroid precursors to an erythropoietic stimulus, such as bleeding in the old animal is normal but the response is not sustained and falls off more rapidly than in young animals. This inability to sustain an erythroblastic response has been attributed to changes in the microenvironment of the marrow, not to the stem cells themselves.[52-54]

C. Bone Disease

Various metabolic bone diseases may cause alterations, principally as fibrosis in the neighboring marrow. In osteitis fibrosa cystica, the result of parathormone excess, whether due to primary hyperparathyroidism or to secondary hyperparathyroidism of chronic renal failure, bone pain and fracture may dominate the clinical picture. Parathormone activities the osteoclasts; the osteoblasts are also proliferative and are stimulated to an accelerated synthesis of collagen and the production of an enlarged osteoid seam.[55] The fibrotic component of osteitis fibrosa appears at first adjacent to the trabeculae, particularly in the areas undergoing active resorption. The fibrous component of the reaction is prominent more often in the secondary hyperparathyroidism of chronic renal failure and considerable compromise of the marrow may be encountered. How important these marrow changes are in the production of the anemia so commonly seen in such patients is difficult to evaluate, but improvement in the anemia has been reported following parathyroidectomy.

Somewhat similar changes in the marrow occur in hyperthyroidism. Thyroxin acts as a general stimulus of bone cell activity in which osteolysis predominates. Osteopenia and accelerated collagen synthesis follow and, as in hyperparathyroidism, marrow fibrosis may appear.[56,57]

In the active phase of Paget's disease the adjacent hematopoietic bone marrow is replaced by fibrous connective tissue. Paget's disease may exist in one or many bones and the reaction is generally focal. The fibrous replacement of marrow occurs in the areas of intense osteoblastic and osteoclastic activity. The marrow reaction is characterized by the appearance of many fibroblasts and undifferentiated mesenchymal cells. Many osteoclasts may be found interspersed in the fibrous matrix at a considerable distance from the bone surface. In addition, numerous large vascular channels are present, encircled by the fibrous tissue and adjacent hemosiderin laden macrophages. No arteriovenous shunts have been demonstrated.[58]

In the ''burned-out'' phase of Paget's disease the bone marrow reverts to a more normal state as the excessive vascularity and fibrosis disappear. Only the singular mosaic pattern of pagetoid bone remains. The contained bone marrow is generally hypocellular.[58]

Aspiration of the marrow of an active Paget lesion may yield many multinucleated osteoclasts as well as clusters of osteoblasts.[59] The former may be confused with megakaryocytes, Reed-Sternberg cells or other multinucleated giant cells, the latter with plasma cells or tumor cells.

The marrow changes of the skeletal reticuloses, the lipid and nonlipid histiocytoses are discussed elsewhere.

IV. TOXIC ALTERATIONS

The bone marrow is highly susceptible to injury by a host of drugs, chemical agents, and ionizing radiation. The ultimate expression of such injury is pancytopenia and marrow aplasia, and myelofibrosis and leukemia.

Drugs can produce an aplastic marrow by their direct myelosuppressive effects as typified by the commonly employed oncolytic agents. The action of these drugs is predictable and dose related. Dose-dependent suppression of the marrow is also encountered following the administration of various unrelated drugs such as chloramphenicol, diphenylhydantoin, chlorpromazine, thiouracil, methicillin, etc. The myelosuppression produced by these agents manifests as reticulocytopenia and granulocytopenia, rarely pancytopenia which rapidly revert to normal on withdrawal of the drug.[60-62]

The idiosyncratic drug reactions are not dose dependent and usually not reversible. Chloramphenicol, as well as other drugs, may be associated with either type of reaction. The idiosyncratic reaction is fortunately less common, but often fatal. The bone marrow is typically aplastic—a fatty marrow with a markedly decreased cellular component.

Drugs can induce a pure red cell aplasia characterized by anemia, reticulocytopenia and a normally cellular marrow with virtual absence of the red cell precursors. The reaction is dose related, but erythropoiesis may or may not regenerate on withdrawal of the drug.[63]

A host of widely employed chemicals, both in industry and at home, such as insecticides and organic solvents, notably benzene have been implicated in the pathogenesis of aplastic anemia, acute and possibly chronic myelocytic leukemia. The relationship of ionizing radiation to aplastic anemia and leukemia is well documented.

V. MALIGNANT DISEASE INVOLVING THE MARROW

Since Reich's report in 1935, it has been known that carcinoma cells can be identified in bone marrow aspirates. Tumor cells are easily differentiated from the loosely arranged cells of normal hemopoietic bone marrow. In general, malignant cells are large, measuring 15 to 25 μm with hyperchromatic nuclei which contain from one to three prominent nucleoli. The cytoplasm may be scanty or may occur in the form of a homogeneous matrix or a large cluster of nuclei. Mitotic figures may be numerous. The neoplastic cells usually occur in groups, nests, or sheets but occasionally occur singly. Phagocytosis of red cells is often observed around tumor foci.[64] Occasionally the general site of tumor origin can be suspected based on the size, the arrangement, and the staining properties of the cells. Where it is possible to obtain exudates or transudates for examination from areas approximating the primary tumor site, there appears to be a relatively high cytologic similarity between the cell types. Clusters of cells permit a reasonably reliable diagnosis, but individual cells are not always easily distinguished from primitive marrow cells, especially marrow reticulum cells. Single cells, however, are often recognized by their poorly defined outline and a susceptibility of the cell wall to fracture when it is imprinted or smeared.[65]

Immediately surrounding the tumor cluster in the marrow is the so-called marginal reaction, a dense lymphoplasmacytic infiltration with accompanying fibrosclerosis. The fibrosis secondary to intramedullary carcinomatous is never associated with immunoglobulin deposits as is the sclerosis of myeloproliferative disorders. Remote from the neoplastic tissue are nonspecific cytologic alterations, the most prominent being a reactive plasmacytosis. An increase of plasma cells in the marrow has been seen in a variety of other conditions (review by Fadem),[66] and cannot be considered specific for malignancy.

Some changes in the marrow do not appear to be the result of direct interference by the physical presence of tumor cells but instead may have been due to substances secreted by the tumors. While still in their early stages, various tumors are associated with an increased vascularity of the marrow.[67] In addition, generalized changes in the bony tissues, usually lysis but occasionally sclerosis, can be seen before dissemination of the malignancy. Further evidence for such humoral factors comes from Horton[68] who has shown osteoclast-stimulating substances in plasmacytomas and in monocytes.

Burkhardt[67] has looked at the generalized reaction of the bone marrow to tumor in 1876 cases which he divided into four groups, Hodgkin's lymphoma, non-Hodgkin's lymphoma, plasmacytoma, and carcinoma. Overall, he found the marrow showed a mixture of inflammatory changes and degenerative changes in the presence of tumor. The most important were an increased number of plasma cells, an abnormal accumulation of iron, a reduction of the marrow parenchyma, and a proliferation of megakaryocytes. These changes are generally most marked in Hodgkin's disease although they occurred with such regularity in all tumors examined, that Burkhardt proposed the term "tumor myelopathy" for the syndrome of nonspecific bone marrow reaction. When the generalized marrow reaction was related to the extent of neoplastic dissemination, all groups of tumor showed an increasing frequency of changes as the cancer became more widespread. The most common alteration in the peripheral blood of the tumor-bearing patient is the anemia of chronic disorder. Occasionally, neoplasia may induce hemolytic anemia, a leukemoid reaction, or leukoerythroblastosis (see Chapter 10). The most common form of hemolytic anemia is that of the microangiopathic form. The offending malignancy is generally a mucin-forming adenocarcinoma. Examination of the blood reveals aniso- and poikilocytosis with cellular fragmentation and reticulocytosis. The associated thrombocytopenia varies with the degree of fibrinogen turnover and fibrin split products and is reflected in the marrow by increased megakaryocytes. Additional erythrocyte destruction may be caused by the contact between red cells and tumor emboli within small vessels. An immune hemolytic anemia may also be associated with malignancy, most commonly with the lympho-proliferative disorders.

VI. INFECTIONS OF BONE MARROW

A. Bacterial

The most consistently observed peripheral blood changes in acute bacterial infections involve quantitative leukocyte alterations, the anemia of chronic disease, and the sequalae of disseminated intravascular coagulation.

Infections like staphylococcus, streptococcus, and E. coli are commonly associated with a neutrophilic leukocytosis in blood and bone marrow. Alternatively, typhoid and paratyphoid fever, brucellosis, and tularemia are characterized by leukopenia. Scarlet fever is often observed with an eosinophilia. Monocytosis may also be seen in typhoid fever and brucellosis.

Salmonellosis can present as a brief febrile illness or as an overwhelming massive toxemia. Organisms are usually initially localized to the Peyer's patches of the intestinal tract but in severe salmonellosis there is marked proliferation of marrow histiocytes with aggregations. The lymph node and marrow histiocytes often contain bacteria and cellular debris in their cytoplasm. The erythrophagocytosis by the histiocytes is virtually characteristic of a *Salmonella* infection. In addition, a scattered infiltrate of lymphocytes and plasma cells is seen about these phagocytic foci with the conspicuous absence of neutrophils. Bone marrow necrosis is common in systemic Salmonellosis.

Brucellosis is usually a chronic disease of a small Gram-negative coccobacillus. It is transmitted to humans by the ingestion of milk from infected farm animals. *Brucella* infection is characterized by invasion of the reticuloendothelial system with resultant histiocytic hyperplasia and the formation of small granuloma in liver, spleen nodes, and bone marrow. These disease foci consist principally of accumulations of macrophages surrounded by a collar of fibroblasts and inflammatory cells. Caseation does not occur but occasionally there is central accumulation of neutrophils and suppurative necrosis of the granuloma center.

Rickettsial infections result from a group of pleomorphic coccobacillary organisms that are obligate intracellular organisms. All rickettsia can be demonstrated by Giemsa staining. All systemic rickettsial infections are self-limited and accompanied by a prominent skin rash. Rickettsia display a vascular tropism by invading endothelial cells. Once inside the endothelial cell a characteristic acute vasculitis is produced manifested by swelling and proliferation of the cells. Invariably a perivascular leukocytic inflammatory infiltrate ensues. The vascular lesions may lead to focal necrosis, fibrin thrombi, and fibrinoid ring formation within or around a granuloma.

B. Mycobacterium Infection

The hematologic manifestations of tuberculosis are extremely variable. Characteristically, the anemia of chronic disorders is seen. In a small group of patients with hematogenous spread tuberculosis may present with aplastic anemia, myelosclerosis, leukemoid reaction, or a picture resembling chronic monocytic leukemia.

If the diagnosis of disseminated tuberculosis is suspected, a bone marrow should be performed both for culture and histology. Mice infected with *Mycobacterium* develop a disease that kills them in 6 months.[69] It has been found that bacterial division is particularly rapid in bone marrow (every 4 days). Because of the propensity of *Mycobacterium* to initially ''home'' to the marrow, cultures are of clinical value. Bacilli are probably taken up into the marrow either by way of the endothelial cells lining the marrow sinuses or directly into processes of the marrow macrophages protruding through the endothelial cells into the lumen of the sinuses. The notable exception to this clinical caveat on *Mycobacterium* infection is in leprosy were marrow cytology is normal and bacteria and granuloma are rarely seen. The most significant marrow finding in leprosy is a plasmacytosis with normal to moderate amounts of amyloid if the disease is longstanding.[70]

Following experimentally induced mycobacterial infection, bacteria are seen in the marrow singly or in groups in macrophage lysosomes, often surrounded by large amounts of electron-dense lysosomal material. Neutrophils rarely contain bacilli. Later in the infection, i.e., 4 to 6 weeks, bacilli are more numerous in the macrophages as demonstrated by Ziehl-Nelson staining. The marrow histiocytes are now enlarged and have elaborate folded margins interdigitating with neighboring cells. Thc rough endoplasmic reticulum which in uninfected histiocytes is sparse, becomes extensive and occurs in parallel arrays. Marrow sinusoidal architecture remains normal. Later in the mycobacterial infection the epitheloid cells appear; these cells contain large nuclei with closely adhering plasma membrane, polyribosomes, mitochondria, and vacuoles.[71]

Morphologically, the epitheloid cell is about 60 μm in size and has been subdivided into two types.[72] Type ''A'' cells appear heavily stained and ''B'' lightly stained. ''B'' type predominates in sarcoidosis and type ''A'' in tuberculosis. Neither show phagocytosized material nor significant evidence of pinocytosis. The type ''A'' cells ultrastructurally have an abundant lamellar RE system while ''B'' cells have prominant

Golgi apparatus and vesicles containing granular material. The function of epitheloid cells appear to be primarily biosynthetic rather than phagocytic.[72]

In tuberculous granulomata clusters of epitheloid cells, containing intact or fragmented bacilli, are surrounded by multinucleated Langhans giant cells. Characteristically, these giant cells contain numerous oval nuclei dispersed about the periphery of the cytoplasm to create a ring or horseshoe distribution. Giant multinucleated epitheloid cells (150 μm in size) are commonly seen in a tuberculous granuloma. A collar of fibroblasts and lymphocytes accompany the epitheloid and giant cells. With time, however, two changes occur which are characteristic of Mycobacterial granuloma. First, the central region of epitheloid cells undergoes granular caseous necrosis. Cellular detail is lost and the granuloma center changes into an amorphous pink region filled with lipid-rich debris. The second modification is the formation of a well-developed enclosing fibrocytic and fibroblast wall which creates a histologic barrier between the inflammatory focus and the surrounding marrow.[72]

Insight on the formation of noncaseating granuloma can be obtained in laboratory animals following injection of *Cryptococcus neoformans*.[73] Following injection in mice, all cryptococci are phagocytosed by neutrophils and monocytes. Larger yeast forms (30 μm) however, become surrounded by rings (rosettes) composed of neutrophils and monocytes. This rosetting phenomenon requires the formation of specific antisera. Low antibody concentrations do not result in granuloma formation. The resulting cellular response was ineffective and unorganized. High antibody titers resulted in the rapid formation of granuloma. In rabbits an identical process occurs. However, rabbits need no detectable antibody levels for granuloma formation to occur. Interestingly, heat inactivation of rabbit serum inhibits the rosette phenomena suggesting serum dependency for rabbit granuloma to form. It would appear that the rate of formation of granuloma is directly correlated with rate of antibody formation, or antibody-antigen complexes.[74]

The noncaseating granuloma can be the morphologic manifestation of many infectious, malignant, and inflammatory diseases, as well as sarcoidosis and berylliosis. Both the caseating and noncaseating granuloma are sharply circumscribed. In the noncaseating granuloma the central follicle is composed of tightly packed epitheloid cells. Surrounding the central follicle is a perimeter of lymphocytes, monocytes, and fibroblasts.[75] Epitheloid cells have secretory capabilities and all epitheloid cells have identical histochemical staining properties for the enzymes of the pentose monophosphate shunt. The epitheloid cells have intracytoplasmic granules (residual bodies) which stain weakly for phospholipid and mucopolysaccharides. Multinucleated giant cells (see Chapter 17) are found among the epitheloid cells within the follicle. Macrophages within the follicle are large and have numerous interdigitating processes. The nuclei are indented and contain finely dispersed chromatin. Like epitheloid cells the macrophages have small amounts of phagosomes suggesting that they are poorly are not actively phagocytosing.[76] Many of the lymphocytes of the follicle appeared to be "activated." They are larger than usual and contain an irregular nucleus. These "activated" lymphocytes probably have a role in monocyte recruitment into the area of inflammation.[77] The extracellular material within the follicle has been described as amorphous hyaline. Electron microscopically this material is "ground" substance with interspersed fibers of various diameters.

The fate of granulomata have been well-documented morphologically. Although they can appear active for years the granuloma ultimately resolves leaving few changes or undergoes progressive fibrosis.[78] The fibrosis begins as a rim of collagen around the granuloma and proceeds in a centripetal fashion. In older granulomas peripheral fibroblasts are extensive and the inflammatory and immune cells in the periphery of the granuloma disappear.[76]

Not all granulomas disappear so quietly. Following experimental beryllium exposure, irregular bone formation starts in the marrow cavity independent of the bone endosteum. The osteogenesis appears to be preceded by fibrosis resulting from residual granuloma. The abnormal osteogenesis results in the formation of osteogenic sarcoma.[79]

C. Malaria Infection

Malarial infection is man is caused by *Plasmodium falciparum, P. vivax, P. malariae,* and *P. ovale*. These parasites are transmitted by a bite from the Anopheline mosquito or from the injection of malarious blood. It is usually possible to identify plasmodium parasites on Giemsa-stained thin and thick smears of peripheral blood. Rarely the bone marrow aspirate can be helpful because of the concentration of parasitized erythrocytes in the marrow. An additional advantage to marrow aspirate examination may be the demonstration of malarial pigment.[80]

The mechanisms concerned in the anemia of malaria are poorly defined. Important factors are probably intravascular hemolysis and phagocytosis of erythrocytes. This increased erythrocyte removal results in normoblastic hyperplastic erythropoiesis in the marrow. There is also evidence the anemia may be aggravated by failure of the formation of reticulocytes during active parasitemia. On removal of erythrocytic parasites by treatment reticulocytosis results. Still additional data suggest a total marrow inhibition of the marrow during parasitemia which may explain the leukopenia commonly observed in acute infections.[81]

An analysis of bone marrow smears therefore generally results in panhypocellularity in acute infections and various degrees of normo- to hypercellularity in chronic disease. The erythroid series is reduced, with younger cells rarely seen during parasitemia except with *P. malariae*. During convalescence increased erythroid activity results. During active disease marrow eosinophilia, lymphocytosis, and plasmacytosis generally occur. Successful therapy results in a return toward normal. An increase of immature or mature megakaryocytes is seen before treatment.[82]

D. Leishmaniasis

This is a protean infection caused by *L. donovani* and is transmitted by the bite of sand flies. It occurs in various forms, the African, Mediterranean, and Indian type. The Mediterranean type occurs mainly in children up to 13 years of age and the Indian type has a peak incidence at 10 to 20 years. The African type is more common in adults with the mean age about 25 years.

Early in the course of the disease there may be marked granulocytopenia with a relative or absolute lymphocytosis and monocytosis. The bone marrow generally is hyperplastic with an increase in the erythroid compartment secondary to the invariable anemia. Parasitized marrow histiocytes become infiltrated with Leishman-Donovan bodies. Presumably because of extensive marrow involvement anemia and leukopenia become more severe with death due to secondary infection.

E. Trypanosomiasis

This is a protozoan disease caused by the hemoflagellates *Trypanosoma rhodiense* or *T. gambiense* and is transmitted by the *Glossina* species of fly. The African variety is characterized by fever, edema of the extremities, posterior cervical adenopathy, and splenomegaly. The leukocyte counts usually are normal but a monocytosis may be seen. Parasites are characteristically observed in peripheral blood, buffy coat preparations, and bone marrow. The American variety (Chagas' disease) is characterized by unilateral conjunctivities, edema of the eyelids, and swelling of the lacrymal glands, lymphadenopathy, and hepatosplenomegaly. The hematological changes, generally, are leukocytosis, anemia, and lymphocytosis. During the febrile phase parasites are identifiable in peripheral blood, buffy coat preparations, and bone marrow aspirates.

F. Histoplasmosis

A highly infectious disease caused by *H. capsulatum* with subsequent hepatosplenomegaly and lymphadenopathy. The organism is a round-to-oval, budding, yeast-like fungus that is 2 to 4 μm in diameter. The organisms are characteristically found packed within histiocytes. Within the histiocyte *H. capsulatum* may simulate *Leishmania donovani* but is differentiated from it by a clear halo. Histologically, this infection may cause collections of macrophages with development of multinucleated giant cells. The central necrosis of the histoplasma lesion is a bland, infarct-like necrosis that resembles caseation.

VII. CIRCULATORY DISTURBANCES OF BONE MARROW

The sinusoids, as previously discussed (see Volume I, Chapter 3), are composed of a thin layer of endothelial cells with an occasional tight junction and an interrupted basement membrane. Regardless of the antomical continuity of endothelium, the discontinuous portion of the sinusoidal endothelial cells functionally do not allow for the effective exchange of fluid and cells between the intra- and extravascular compartments.[83]

Following any circulatory injury to the marrow the sinusoidal lumina expand and become totally surrounded by endothelial cells. The endothelium now becomes visible under light microscopy and is functionally continuous. The sinusoidal lumen fills with plasma due to vascular stasis, and the adjacent hematopoietic areas are compressed by the sinusoidal expansion. Ultrastructurally there is extravascular thrombosis and a marked leukocytic reaction along the abluminal side of the continuous sinusoidal endothelium. At the venous end of the circulation the vascular lumen narrows due to compression by stagnated fluid which exudes across the venular wall into the nutrient canal. Leukocyte trapping from the blood stream by the sinusoidal endothelium is also marked. As a result of these changes in the marrow circulatory units, considerable leukocytic agglutination in hematopoietic areas occurs; this is the initial morphological manifestation of sterile microabscesses.

If the injury is purely circulatory, e.g., sickle cell disease, osteomyelitis may not occur but may result in marrow necrosis. These phenomena may be seen following bacterial infection due directly to the organism or to the formation of immune complexes with resultant vasculitis.[84]

A. Osteomyelitis

The principal pathologic changes in bone consist of new bone formation, bone resorption, and bone necrosis. The occurrence of all three reactions vary considerably resulting in a varied histologic presentation. New bone formation consisting of an inflammatory stimulation of the periosteal fibrous layer leading to osteoblast formation. This is most commonly seen in low grade infection. New bone formation morphologically is recognized by its mosaic pattern, acidophilic staining, and irregular bone margins. Bone resorption occurs in severe inflammatory processes from acute or chronic causes. The bone lamellae stain poorly, the nuclei of the osteocytes become pyknotic, and the bone is progressively resorbed predominantly by osteoclastic activity. Invasion of vascular tissue into bone may be seen which accelerates resorption by exposing new areas to the osteoclast. When bone becomes devitalized and loses its connections with the surrounding connective tissue its removal cannot occur, and a sequestrum is formed. A sequestrum may become demarcated from viable bone by osteoclasis and eventually become a loose fragment surrounded by granuloma, fibrosis, or pus.[85]

Inflammatory changes in the bone marrow in osteomyelitis start at the periphery of the marrow space and progress centrally. There is atrophy of fat cells and degeneration of hematopoietic elements to the point of forming a homogeneous, structureless mass which in turn is replaced by fibrous tissue or new bone. This reaction bears no histological resemblance to the nonspecific hyperplasia of marrow seen in systemic diseases. It is an inflammatory reaction in the marrow adjacent to infected bone. In severe osteomyelitis marrow necrosis without healing may ensue.

B. Bone Marrow Necrosis

Bone marrow necrosis is an unusual histologic finding antemortem. When diagnosed premortem the majority of patients had either carcinoma or leukemia. At autopsy, the conditions associated with this lesion include bacterial infection, sickle cell disease, chemo- and radiotherapy, neoplasia, and hypovolemic shock.

The only clinical symptom that can specifically be related to marrow necrosis is bone pain. It is usually very severe in intensity and localized in the lower back alone or together with extremities. Systemic symptoms of fever, weight loss, and malaise usually accompany the pain but may be a manifestation of the underlying disease rather than necrosis itself.[86]

The peripheral smear shows nucleated erythrocytes and schistocytes. This may be seen as part of a leukoerythroblastic picture. Depending on the underlying disease there are variable degrees of anemia, thrombocytopenia, and leukopenia. Leukocytosis is the obvious finding in some acute and chronic leukemias.

The bone marrow aspirate yields watery, yellowish to reddish-brown material with stringy consistency. The areas involved are hypocellular and contain indistinct marrow elements with smudged nuclei and scanty cytoplasm. There is a heavy proteinaceous basophilic material with degenerated neutrophils. Bone marrow biopsies reveal necrosis of all hemopoietic and bony tissue; the bony trabeculae lack osteocytes.[86,87] Variable degrees of fibrosis are present depending on the underlying disease. In patients with sickle cell disease the small intramedullary vascular channels are engorged with tangled, sickled erthrocytes. Large veins outside the bone cortex may be plugged with bone marrow emboli. In patients with leukemia, the periosteal blood vessels may be invaded by blasts. The prognosis for patients with bone marrow necrosis diagnosed antemortem is extremely poor. Patients with leukemia have less than 10% chance of obtaining a complete remission.[89] In patients with solid tumor, metastasis survival ranged from 5 days to 11 months with a median survival of 22 days.[86] The diagnosis of marrow necrosis in sickle cell diseases has been reported to be as high as one in six patients presenting with bone pain; autopsy series show a higher incidence of questionable significance. In Brown's autopsy review of 72 cases, 40 were associated with infection; *Salmonella* appears to have a particular predilection to cause this lesion.[87]

Therapeutic irradiation has been a contributing factor in patients with marrow necrosis. Typically, radiation does not cause necrosis but pyknosis and karyorrhexis of marrow cells followed by a fatty marrow.

As described earlier the pathophysiology of marrow necrosis is believed to involve vascular obstruction within the marrow. Widespread microvascular occlusion with resulting infarction of sickle cell disease is readily explained by obstruction of marrow sinusoids by sickled cells. In infectious diseases disseminated intravascular coagulopathy has been postulated but fibrin thrombi are rarely found in this lesion; a more likely mechanism involves immune complex formation or hypoperfusion. It is plausible that in neoplastic disease of the marrow masses of tumor cells or blast cells, which are essentially nondeformable, impede sinusoidal flow; tumor-associated fibrosis or a cell mass outgrowing its blood supply also are considerations.[89]

A major complication of marrow necrosis is bone marrow and fat embolization. The clinical features of this syndrome include tachycardia, tachypnea, shock, fever, obtundation, petechial hemorrhages, and funduscopic changes. Fat droplets are characteristically observed only 2 to 4 days after embolization occurs. The fat droplets are 7 to 12 μm in diameter.[88]

Bone marrow emboli are found almost exclusively in pulmonary vessels, probably because the fragments are usually too large to pass through the capillary bed of the lungs. Two cases of marrow embolism to the brain and a single case of multiorgan embolism have been reported.[90] Infarcted marrow fragments eventually dislodge and gain entry into venous channels within bone and into the systemic venous circulation. The hematopoietic marrow is separated by only a single endothelial cell layer from the intramedullary sinusoids which communicate freely with systemic circulation by way of the veins leaving through the nutrient canal. The nutrient veins do not collapse in the presence of surrounding injury since they tend to have areas firmly adherent to bone which augments expulsion of disrupted material.[88]

VIII. ENDOCRINE DISORDERS

Naegeli[91] was one of the first investigators to point out the importance of the endocrine system in the formation of blood. However, since that time there have been relatively few clinical reports delineating the effects of hormones on the bone marrow. The role of the endocrine system however, is in modifying the rate of erythropoiesis and its effects are, in general, relatively slight compared to the abnormalities which result from deficiencies of essential substances like iron, vitamin B_{12}, and folate.

A. Thyroid Hormone

The activity of the thyroid gland has been shown to exert an influence on hematopoiesis. The marrows of patients with hyperthyroidism have an M:E ratio of 5:1 to as high as 20:1. Hyperplasia of both myeloid and erythroid cell lines occur but the myeloid changes are much more striking, occasionally with a predominant neutrophilia and an increase in megakaryocytes. In patients who are overtly thyrotoxic, the hyperplasia may be so marked that the marrow closely resembled that found in CML.[92] Many patients with hyperthyroidism have a lymphocytosis of the marrow, comprising as much as 40% of nucleated cells. Plasma cells and histiocytes are not altered qualitatively and quantitatively. In hyperthyroidism the red or functioning marrow may extend into the shafts of the long bones with diminution or absence of fat. Tritiated thymidine uptake is increased in erythroblasts, as is plasma erythropoietin and iron kinetics. Anemia is therefore not an accompanying feature of thyrotoxicosis.[93]

In contrast to hyperthyroidism, anemia is a common finding in hypothyroidism. The typical anemia of uncomplicated hypothyroidism is a macrocytic hypochromic anemia of moderate severity. There is a decrease in total functioning marrow to roughly one third of the mean value in patients with hyperthyroidism. The marrow is, therefore, hypoplastic with M:E ratio of 1:1 to 3:1. The hypoplasia affects both the myeloid and erythroid series equally. There is no striking change in the differential distribution of the erythroblasts, although there may be a slight right shift with a relative increase of the polychromatophilic forms. No megaloblastic erythropoiesis is seen. The megakaryocytes may be reduced but this is not reflected in the peripheral platelet count. There are no significant changes in lymphocytes, plasma cells, or reticulum cells.[92, 93] Significant hemosiderosis of the marrow may be seen in advanced cases.[94] There are several isolated case reports of bone marrow changes observed in cretins at post-mortem. The marrow cells were all rich in fat with marked hyperplasia of the erythrocytic line.

Thyroid hormone affects erythropoiesis but may not be a fundamental factor in its control. In vitro thyroid hormone effects an increase in colony formation independent of its calorogenic properties. Tudhope[95] suggested that the hormone does not have a direct, selective action on the red cell precursors in the marrow. Experiments in which animals were exposed to reduced oxygen tension showed that removal of the thyroid did not interfere with the effect of hypoxia on red cell production.

It has been suggested that the uncomplicated anemia of hypothyroidism resulted from a reduced rate of erythropoiesis, consequent upon the diminished needs of the tissues for oxygen. This hypothesis was strengthened by showing that the regulation of total red cell volume depended directly on changes in the basal oxygen consumption and not the coincidental action of the thyroid hormone on the bone marrow.[96] Das[97] also proposed that the low basal metabolic rate in hypothyroidism leads to decreased oxygen consumption by the tissues and, as a consequence, the synthesis and release of erythropoietin is also reduced. He showed a significant reduction in the proliferative activity of the marrow using ^{3}H-thymidine labeling of erythroblasts. There was also a decrease in plasma iron clearance and a delayed peak absorption of ^{59}Fe by red cells. Plasma erythropoietin levels were reduced and often immeasurable.

B. Parathyroid Hormone

Unexplained anemia has been reported in patients with primary hyperparathyroidism. The anemia tends to be most pronounced in patients with the more advanced bone disease and higher levels of serum calcium, alkaline phosphatase, and parathyroid hormone. Bone marrow biopsies show variable degrees of patchy myelofibrosis,[98] although it has been reported that the bone marrows are normal in hyperparathyroid patients who are anemic.[99]

The pathogenesis of the anemia of primary hyperparathyroidism is obscure. Several authors have suggested that myelofibrosis is a factor and may be related to the elevated levels of parathyroid hormone.[98,100] Bone cysts contribute to the anemia by encroaching on the hemopoietic compartment. It is also possible that parathyroid hormone itself may have a suppressive effect on erythropoiesis. Levi[101] demonstrated inhibition of erythropoiesis in vitro by high levels of parathyroid hormone. Iron kinetic studies show the anemia of hyperthyroidism to be indistinguishable from the chronic disease anemias.

The anemia of primary hyperparathyroidism appears to be reversible in most patients after surgical removal of the gland.[98,99] Because of these observations, there has recently been interest in the role of secondary hyperparathyroidism in the anemia of chronic renal failure. Several investigators reported that the anemia of uremia improved significantly after parathyroidectomy.[102] However, more recent studies showed that only 44 to 50% of patients exhibited a postoperative rise in hematocrit. The responders appeared to have more severe bone disease, slightly more marrow fibrosis, and lower initial hematocrit than did nonresponders.[103]

C. Glucagon

In the recently described syndrome of excess glucagon accompanying tumors of the pancreatic alpha cells, patients had a normochromic, normocytic anemia accompanying the relapses of the rash.[104] Bone marrow aspirates in these patients showed normoblastic maturation with normal iron stores. In some there were changes suggesting dyserythropoiesis with an excess of sideroblasts. The anemia may return to normal after surgical removal of the pancreatic tumor.[105]

Virtually no work has been reported on the effect of glucagon on erythropoietin in man. All studies to date have been done in animals, most recently by Naet.[106] He injected glucagon into mice and rats and found that after 10 days there was a marked depression of erythropoiesis. The erythropoietic response to hypoxia was also found to be inhibited. The authors postulated that glucagon exerts its effect early in the stages of erythropoiesis because maximal inhibition seemed to occur if hypoxia was initiated 0 or 1 day after injection of the hormone. This would place the level of interference at the stem cell or erythropoietin-sensitive cell differentiation and not at the earlier level of heme synthesis. It is tempting to extrapolate from observations with glucagon in rodents to humans since other hormones such as estrogens and androgens have been found to have similar effects in both groups. There are other diseases in man beside pancreatic tumors where anemia and hyperglucagonemia occur, i.e., cirrhosis, chronic inflammatory syndrome, and renal failure.

D. Anterior Pituitary Hormones

Anemia is commonly present in patients suffering from hypopituitarism but there are only rare reports of its effect on the human bone marrow. The changes have been well described, however, in animals. Gordon[107] examined the marrows of hypophysectomized rats and found that an increasing degree of hypoplasia occurs postoperatively. The marrow atrophy was associated with the development of cavities within the marrow and the appearance of an increase in the numbers of fat vacuoles. The M:E ratio remained unchanged. There was a tendency for a slight shift toward more mature granulocytes and for a slight lymphocytosis but these changes were not significant.

The bone marrows in anemic prepubertal hypopituitary dwarfs while on maintenance thyroid hormone and adrenal steroids show normal cellularity with an M:E ratio of 3:1. Erythropoiesis is normoblastic and megakaryopoiesis is normal. Lymphocytes constitute 20 to 25% of the total marrow count. Hemosiderin deposition is normal. When these patients are treated with human growth hormone in doses sufficient to produce linear growth and weight gain, erythropoiesis appears normal to increased as evidenced by an increase in red cell mass and improved iron kinetic studies. The most striking changes are associated with an increase in the number of lymphocytes to 35 to 45% of the total marrow cells. These changes are associated with an increased concentration of erythropoietin-stimulating factor in the urine, increased transferrin levels, and expansion of plasma volume.[108]

There has been considerable controversy in the past as to whether the anemia of hypopituitarism resulted entirely from deficiency of the target organ hormones. From many animal experiments, it appears that the pituitary is not obligatory in the fundamental control of erythropoiesis but that it plays a conditioning role by means of the effects of thyroxine, cortisol, testosterone, and growth hormone. The anemia of hypophysectomized rats is only completely corrected by combined treatment with thyrotropin, corticotropin, and growth hormone.[109] (See Chapter 4, Volume I).

Anorexia nervosa involves a disorder of the hypothalamic-anterior pituitary-gonadal axis. Few investigators have examined the bone marrow of these patients because the hematologic abnormalities are usually clinically unimportant although intractable marrow aplasia occurs. Anemia occurs in only 30% of anorexia nervosa patients and is usually mild. The bone marrow consistently show hypocellularity with a notable accumulation of an amorphous homogeneous material that stains faintly positive with PAS; it occurs in fibrous streaks or in large islands in which cellular elements or vacuoles are dispersed. Differential cell counts reveal reduced erythroblasts to less than 20% of all marrow cells, with increases in lymphocytes, histiocytes, and reticulum cells. The M:E ratio is increased in the range of 4:1 to 8.5:1.[110] Mant[111] noted prominent blue-green granules by Romanowsky stains in many of the histiocytes. These cells represent the ''sea-blue'' histiocytes commonly associated with malnutrition. After clinical improvement manifested by restoration of body weight, the mucous material disappears and the differentials of the bone marrow return to almost normal. The PAS-positive background material can be present in normal marrow. It is thought that as marrow fat declines, acid mucopolysaccharide replaces it as the major structural support for marrow cells.[111,112] Cornbleet[113] did histochemical analysis of this material and found it was similar in staining characteristics to the changes seen in the fat atrophy that occasionally accompanies starvation marrows, suggesting that this lesion is part of a process secondary to longstanding malnutrition.

E. Androgens

Hematological changes are not prominent clinical features of diseases of the gonads but there is no doubt that the sex hormones exert an influence on erythropoiesis. Adult males have a significantly higher hemoglobin concentration, red cell count, and packed cell volume than adult females, but there is no sex difference in prepubertal children.

Androgens exert an effect on erythropoiesis by one or all of the following mechanisms:

1. Stimulating production of erythropoietin
2. Exerting direct effects on heme synthesis
3. Directly affecting erythroid colony forming cells
4. Affecting pluripotent stem cells[114,115]

Urabe[116] found that certain C_{19} and C_{20} steroid metabolites enhanced the in vitro growth of both early primitive erythroid progenitors (BFU-E) and later progenitors (CFU-E) of normal human marrow. He demonstrated that the 5 β metabolites were more potent than the 5 α epimers, a fact that may prove useful clinically since the 5 β derivatives lack androgenicity. Rosenblum[117] studied the effect of androgens on granulopoiesis and found that the addition of testosterone to in vitro cultures lead to an increase in granulocyte colony formation of 24 to 60% but that the mechanism is unclear.

McCullough and Jones[118] studied the effects of androgens in eunuchoid patients. They noted a rise in the erythrocyte count but no change in the leukocyte count following testosterone therapy. We have seen two patients with Klinefelter's syndrome in whom both red cell and white count increased following androgen replacement and an additional patient with primary hypogonadism and a normal hemogram which became polycythemic and leukocytemic following androgen therapy; the counts returned to normal upon cessation of therapy.[119]

F. Estrogen

There has been little evidence of the clinical importance of the influence of estrogens on the blood. Bone marrow changes are well described in animals.[120] The first change noted is a variable degree of hyperplasia of the myeloid elements. Marked vacuolization of the marrow erythroid precursors occurs with decreased cellularity compared to controls. Mirand,[121] using large doses of estrogen, found that it prevented the normal increase in erythropoiesis produced by hypoxia. He suggests that estrogens inhibit the activation of erythropoietin in the blood and do not influence the production of erythropoietin. Jepson[122] felt that estrogens in lower doses appeared to inhibit stem cell response to erythropoietin.

G. Adrenocortical Steroids

There is one brief case report in the literature on the bone marrow changes in Addison's disease. The marrow was very fatty with slight hypoplasia of the erythroid line.[123] Adrenalectomy in rats leads to a significant decrease in the nucleated erythroid cells, accompanied by hyperplasia of the granulocytes with an increase in the more immature precursors with a resultant increase in the M:E ratio. The marrow changes are maximum approximately 2 weeks postoperatively and tend to diminish in intensity thereafter. Extracts of the adrenal cortex bring the M:E ratio to normal. Cortisone alone causes fatty infiltration which are accompanied by increased percentages of nucleated erythrocytes and a decreased concentration of myeloid elements.[124]

The effect of cortisol on erythropoiesis is complex. The hormone may have a stimulatory or a suppressive effect on red-cell production depending on the endocrine status of the animal, the dose, and the duration of administration of the steroid. The granulopoietic stem cells (CFU-C) have been uniformly reported to be decreased by glucocorticoids in both in vitro and in vivo mouse bone marrow cultures. Because of the conflicting data in this area, Zalman[125] looked at the dose-response relationships of dexamethasone and cortisone on both the very early erythroid and granulopoietic progenitors. The results showed that the early erythropoietic progenitors (BFU-E) were considerably more sensitive to inhibition by physiologic concentrations of either steroid than the granulopoietic progenitors (CFU-C). The later erythroid cells (CFU-E) showed a statistically insignificant increase in numbers in the presence of dexamethasone. The reason for this difference in sensitivity is unclear but may be related to the fact that CFU-C includes a broad age distribution of cells whereas BFU-E includes only early progenitors making it a more homogeneous committed stem cell population. It has been proposed that the differential control of BFU-E and CFU-E in series would provide an efficient mechanism of dampening the effect of glucocorticoids.

IX. CHRONIC RENAL FAILURE

The successive development of anemia and renal osteodystrophy are regular clinical features associated with chronic renal failure. The bone marrow of azotemic patients are normo- or hypercellular with a normoblastic type of erythropoiesis. Generally, it is only after a BUN greater than 150 is reached that the bone marrow shows any quantitative evidence of hypoplasia. With progressive azotemia, several changes are apparent. Decreases in both myeloid and erythroid lines occurred but the reduction in the erythroid line is more prominent so that at a BUN of 40 the M:E ratio is approximately 2:1, while at a BUN of 200, the M:E ratio is 4:1. Nordenson[126] found a distinct hypoplasia of the erythroid line but reported an M:E ratio of 8:1. Progressive azotemia also leads to a progressive increase in the number of mature granulocytes (i.e., neutrophilic myelocytes, metamyelocytes, and eosinophils). Furthermore, there is a decrease in the number of basophilic normoblasts but the number of orthochromatic normoblasts remains about the same. The megakaryocytes are normal or increased and the histiocytes and plasma cells are increased.

Sjogren[127] examined the marrow of patients with uremia who were on maintenance hemodialysis twice weekly. There was a significant shift to the left in the granulocyte series compared to normals and to uremic patients who had not been dialyzed with a significant increase in the frequency of promyelocytes. Also, there were significantly more eosinophils and mast cells than the two control groups.

A mixture of pathologic abnormalities have been described in the bones of patients with renal osteodystrophy, including increased osteoclastic activity, marrow fibrosis, osteosclerosis, and osteomalacia. Interestingly, osteosclerosis has been experimentally induced by parathyroid hormone which is elevated in uremic patients.[126] Significant fibrosis and sclerosis have been documented in human bone marrow biopsy specimens by several authors and often these changes diminish after renal transplantation.[128] The bony changes of osteodystrophy impinging on the marrow cavity may result in hematologic decompensation. Systematic examination of a uremic population undergoing long-term dialysis show that the more severe bone disease was demonstrated in patients with leukopenia and thrombocytopenia than in a control group. Cytopenic patients had higher serum parathyroid hormone and alkaline phosphatase levels, greater amounts of sclerosis on bone survey, and a tendency to greater per cent fibrosis on bone marrow biopsy than control subjects.[51] Chromium red cell survival studies showed that the cytopenic patients who lacked marrow expansion on scan had extramedullary hematopoiesis, possibly as an attempt to compensate for the marrow fibrosis. Of the patients without cytopenia, only those with significant marrow fibrosis and sclerosis had peripheral marrow expansion on scan, again representing an alternate attempt at compensation.

Bone marrow histology and ferrokinetic data suggest that the anemia of chronic failure is primarily due to the underproduction of red cells.[126] Several authors report that this hypoproliferation is secondary to the inability of the diseased kidneys to produce adequate amounts of erythropoietin.[129] However, recent investigations using more sensitive techniques have demonstrated that serum erythropoietin levels may be greater than normal in patients with uremia, suggesting that a lack of marrow responsiveness is a major factor in the anemia.[130] Less significant factors include hemolysis initiated by the azotemia, iron and folate deficiencies, and blood loss secondary to the dialysis procedure. In addition, there is a large body of in vivo and in vitro data suggesting that the serum of patients with chronic renal failure contains a substance inhibitory to erythropoiesis.

Little is known of the nature or mode of action of the proposed uremic erythropoietic inhibitor. Possibilities include a direct antierythropoietic material or a substance that inhibits heme synthesis and/or erythroblast maturation. This material has been studied using different tissue culture systems employing techniques to assay the ability of bone marrow cells to form erythroid colonies and by evaluating the rate of heme synthesis in marrow cells. Bone marrow cells from uremic patients synthesis heme when not in uremic serum and responds to erythropoietin normally.

There is evidence that the uremic inhibitor acts at the level of heme and/or protein synthesis. Gonen[131] measured the incorporation of labeled nucleotides and amino acids into erythroblasts taken from uremic and normal subjects and found that is was reduced in cells taken from uremic patients. Wallner et al.[132] studied erythroid and granulocytic colony growth in a plasma clot system using normal mouse marrow cells as the target organ. Fewer colonies were found in the cultures containing uremic serum and the effect was greater as the concentration of serum was increased, but there was no change in the size or the morphology of the colonies. This indicated an effect on early erythroid cells because once the CFU-E formed colonies, they were normal. The inhibitory effect of uremic serum is not immediate but is noted after at least 24 hr of culture. Using a tissue culture system where ^{59}Fe heme synthesis was measured, evaluating iron transport into erythroblasts in the presence of normal serum and uremic serum and partially purified serum extracts there was no difference in the rate of iron binding to membranes or in iron transport into cells, indicating that adequate cellular iron was available for heme synthesis.[133] Ohno[134] demonstrated that sera from undialyzed anemic uremic patients inhibited the number of BFU-Es and CFU-Es in the normal rabbit bone marrow plasma clot cultures and that the inhibitor is partly removed by hemodialysis.

The identity of the uremic inhibitor remains speculative. The inhibitor appears to be of low molecular weight, approximately 2300 daltons, suggesting that it is not an antibody to erythropoietin. Serum extraction with organic solvents indicate that the erythropoietic inhibitory substance is most likely a polar lipid that is soluble in chloroform. There is speculation as to parathyroid hormone being the uremic toxin but it is a peptide hormone and not a polar lipid. Creatinine, guanidine hydrochloride, guanidinosuccinic acid, and guanidinobutyric, substances known to be elevated in the serum of patients with anemia of renal disease, do not affect the number of CFU-E normal rabbit bone marrow cultures.[134]

The increase in granulopoiesis occasionally observed in bone marrows of uremic patients may be related to the fact that during dialysis there is a loss of circulating granulocytes which adhere to or will be damaged by the dialyzing surfaces. The transient neutropenia may be compensated for by an influx of neutrophils from the bone marrow.[135]

REFERENCES

1. **Ellis, R. E.,** The distribution of the active bone marrow in the adult, *Phys. Med. Biol.,* 5, 255, 1961.
2. **Brandt, G.,** Mineralzanlytische und histometrische Untersuchungen an menschlichen Knochenmark, *Medizin Welt.,* 28, 1307, 1977.
3. **Liu, P. I., Ogawa, M., Crook, L. et al.,** Proliferative function of cadaveric bone marrow cells, *Am. J. Hematol.,* 5, 145, 1978.
4. **Schroeder, T. M., Tilgen, D., Kruger, J., and Vogel, F.,** Formal genetics of Fanconi's anemia, *Human Genet.,* 32, 257, 1976.
5. **Gmyrek, D. and Sylim-Rapoport, I.,** Zur Fanconi-Anaemia (FA). Analyse von 129 Beschriebene Fälle, *Z. Kinderheilkunde,* 91, 297, 1964.
6. **Garriga, S. and Crosby, W. H.,** The incidence of leukemia in families of patients with hypoplasia of the marrow, *Blood,* 14, 1008, 1959.
7. **Swift, M.,** Fanconi's anemia in the genetics of neoplasia, Nature, 230, 279, 1971.
8. **Swift, M.,** Fanconi's anemia: cellular abnormalities and clinical predisposition to malignant disease, in *Congenital Disorders of Erythropoiesis,* Ciba Found. Symp. 37, 115, 1976.
9. **Swift, M., Sholman, L., and Gilmour, D.,** Diabetes mellitus and the gene for Fanconi's anemia, *Science,* 178, 303, 1972.
10. **Saunders, E. F., Amato, D., and Freedman, M. H.,** Defective granulocyte colony formation in congenital aplastic anemia, *Blood,* 44(Abstr.), 913, 1974.
11. **Chu, J-Y., Ho, J., Monteleone, P., et al.,** Fanconi's aplastic anemia: Defect of both stem cell and microenvironment? *Pediatr. Res.,* 10(Abstr.), 375, 1976.
12. **Freedman, M. H., Amato, D., and Saunders, E. F.,** Erythroid colony growth in congenital hypoplastic anemia, *J. Clin. Invest.,* 57, 673, 1976.
13. **Bloom, G. E., Warner, S., Gerald, P. S., and Diamond, L. E.,** Chromosome abnormalities in constitutional aplastic anemia, *N. Engl. J. Med.,* 178, 104, 1966.
14. **Todaro, G. J., Green, H., and Swift, M. R.,** Susceptibility of human diploid fibroblast strains to transformation by SV 40 virus, *Science,* 153, 1252, 1966.
15. **Latt, S. A., Stetten, G., Juergens, L. A., et al.,** Induction by alkylating agents of sister chromatid exchanges and chromatid breaks in Fanconi's anemia, *Proc. Natl. Acad. Sci. U.S.A.,* 72, 4066, 1975.
16. **O'Gorman Hughes, D. W.,** Aplastic anemia in childhood. III. Constitutional aplastic anemia and related cytopenias, *Med. J. Aust.,* 1, 519, 1974.
17. **Beard, M. E. J., Young, D. E., Bateman, C. J. T. et al.,** Fanconi's anemia, *Q. J. Med.,* 42, 403, 1973.
18. **Gonzalez, C. H., Durkin-Stamm, M. V., Geimer, N. F. et al.,** The WT syndrome—a new autosomal dominant pleiotropic trait of radial-ulnar hypoplasia and high risk of bone marrow failure and/or leukemia, in *New Syndromes, Part B of Annual Reviews of Birth Defects, 1976, The National Foundation March of Dimes Birth Defects: Original Article Series,* Vol. 8, No. 10, Bergsma, D. and Lowry, R. B., Eds., Alan R. Liss, New York, 197, 11.
19. **Korn, D.,** Congenital hypoplastic thrombocytopenia. Report of a case and review of the literature, *Am. J. Clin. Pathol.,* 37, 405, 1962.
20. **Sirinavin, C. and Towbridge, A. A.,** Dyskeratosis congenita: clinical features and genetic aspects. Report of a family and review of the literature, *J. Med. Genet.,* 12, 139, 1975.

21. **Schwachman, H. and Holsclaw, D.,** Some clinical observations on the Schwachman syndrome (pancreatic insufficiency and bone marrow hypoplasia), *The National Foundation—March of Dimes Birth Defects: Original Article Series,* Vol. 8, No. 8, 1977, 46.
22. **Diamond, L. K., Wang, W. C., and Alter, B. P.,** Congenital hypoplastic anemia, *Adv. Pediatr.,* 22, 149, 1976.
23. **Geller, G., Krivet, W., Zalusky, R., and Zanjani, F. D.,** Lack of erythropoietic inhibitory activity of serum from patients with congenital pure red cell aplasia, *J. Pediatr.,* 86, 198, 1975.
24. **August, C. S., King, E., Githens, J. H., et al.,** Establishment of erythropoiesis following bone marrow transplantation in a patient with congenital hypoplastic anemia (Blackfan-Diamond syndrome), *Blood,* 48, 491, 1976.
25. **Nathan, D. G., Clarke, B. J., Hillman, D. G., et al.,** Erythroid precursors in congenital hypoplastic (Blackfan-Diamond) anemia, *J. Clin. Invest.,* 61, 489, 1978.
26. **Hoffman, R., Zanjani, E. D., Vila, J., et al.,** Diamond-Blackfan syndrome: lymphocyte-mediated suppression of erythropoiesis, *Science,* 193, 899, 1976.
27. **Ershler, W. B., Ross, J., Finlay, J. L., et al.,** Bone marrow microenvironment defect in congenital hypoplastic anemia, *N. Engl. J. Med.,* 302, 1321, 1980.
28. **Kostmann, R.,** Infantile genetic agranulocytosis. A review with presentation of two new cases, *Acta Paediatr. Scand.,* 64, 362, 1975.
29. **Masson, A., Cronmuller, G., Rousselot, P., et al.,** La thrombocytopenie hypoplastique congenitale avec aplasie radiale, *Ann. Pediatr.,* 18, 777, 1971.
30. **Cohlan, S. Q.,** Fetal and neonatal hazards from drugs administered during pregnancy, *N.Y. J. Med.,* 64, 493, 1964.
31. **Alter, B. P., Potter, N. U, and Li, F. P.,** Classification and aetiology of the aplastic anemias, *Clin. Haematol.,* 7, 431, 1978.
32. **Smith, C. H. and Miller, D. R.,** *Blood Diseases of Infancy and Childhood,* 3rd ed., C.V. Mosby. St. Louis, 1972, 23.
33. **Sever, J. L., Nelson, K. B., Gilkeson, M. E., et al.,** Rubella epidemic, 1964: effect on 6000 pregnancies, *Am. J. Dis. Child.,* 110, 395, 1965.
34. **Boyer, W. L., Sherman, F. E., Michaels, R. H., et al.,** Purpura in congenital and acquired rubella, *N. Engl. J. Med.,* 273, 1362, 1965.
35. **Berge, T., Brunnhage, F., and Nilssen, L. R.,** Congenital hyperplastic thrombocytopenia in rubella embryopathy, *Acta Paediatr.,* 52, 349, 1963.
36. **Gardner, L. E.,** *Endocrine and Genetic Diseases of Childhood and Adolescence,* W. B. Saunders, Philadelphia, 1975, 234.
37. **Keys, A., Brozek, J., Henschel, A. et al.,** *The Biology of Human Starvation,* Vol. 1, University of Minnesota Press, Minneapolis, 1950, 248.
38. **Szejnman, M.,** Changes in peripheral blood and bone marrow in hunger disease, *Curr. Concepts Nutr.,* 7, 161, 1979.
39. **Seaman, J. P., Kjeldsberg, C. R., and Linker, A.,** Gelatinous transformation of the bone marrow, *Human Pathol.,* 9, 685, 1978.
40. **Tavassoli, M., Eastlund, T. D., Yam, L. T. et al.,** Gelatinous transformation of bone marrow to prolonged self-induced starvation, *Scand. J. Haematol.,* 16, 311, 1976.
41. **Eichner, E. R.,** The hematologic disorders of alcoholism, *Am. J. Med.,* 54, 621, 1973.
42. **Trubowitz, S., Zamora, J., and Miller, W.,** Quantitative estimation of marrow nonheme iron in alcoholics, *Am. J. Clin. Pathol.,* 60, 912, 1973.
43. **Lindenbaum, J.,** Folate and vitamin B_{12} deficiencies in alcoholism, *Semin. Hematol.,* 17, 119, 1980.
44. **Das, K. C., Herbert, V., Colman, N., et al.,** Unmasking covert folate deficiency in iron-deficient subjects with neutrophils hypersegmentation. IV. Suppression tests of lymphocytes and bone marrow, *Br. J. Haematol.,* 39, 357, 1978.
45. **McCurdy, P. R. and Rath, C. E.,** Vacuolated nucleated bone marrow cells in alcoholism, *Semin. Hematol.,* 17, 100, 1980.
46. **Cowan, D. H.,** Effects of alcoholism on hemostasis, *Semin. Hematol.,* 17, 137, 1980.
47. **Brocklehurst, J. C.,** *Textbook of Geriatric Medicine and Gerontology,* Churchill Livingstone, Edinburgh, 1978, 560.
48. **Hartsock, R. J., Smith, E. B., and Petty, C. S.,** Normal variations with aging of the amount of hematopoietic tissue in bone marrow from the anterior iliac crest, *Am. J. Clin. Pathol.,* 43, 326, 1965.
49. **Reich, C., Swirsky, M., and Smith, D.,** Sternal bone marrow in the aged, *J. Lab. Clin. Med.,* 29, 508, 1944.
50. **Shapleigh, J. B., Mayer, S., and Moore, C. V.,** Hematologic values in the aged, *J. Gerontol.,* 7, 207, 1952.

51. **Chen, M. G.,** Age related changes in hematopoietic stem cell properties of long-lived hybrid mice, *J. Cell. Physiol.,* 78, 225, 1971.
52. **Coggle, J. R., Gordon, M. Y., Proukaxis, C., and Boggs, C. E.,** Age-related changes in the bone marrow and spleen of SAS/4 mice, *Gerontologie,* 21, 1, 1975.
53. **Reylance, P. J., Hanna, I. R. A., and Tarbutt, R. G.,** Changes with age in cell proliferation of the rat bone marrow, *J. Anat.,* 104, 191, 1969.
54. **Harris, D. E.,** Defective erythropoietic responses of aged mice not improved by young marrow, *J. Gerontol.,* 30, 286, 1975.
55. **Byers, P. D. and Smith, R. S.,** Quantitative histology of bone in hyperparathyroidism. Its relation to clinical features, X-ray and biochemistry, *Quant. J. Med.,* 40, 471, 1971.
56. **Meunier, P. J., Bianchi, G. S., Edouard, C. M., et al.,** Bony manifestations of thyrotoxicosis, *Orthop. Clin. N.A.,* 3, 745, 1972.
57. **Bordier, I., Miravet, R., Matrajt, H., et al.,** Bone change in adult patients with abnormal thyroid function (with special reference to ^{45}Ca kinetics and quantitative histology), *Proc. Roy. Soc. Med.,* 60, 1132, 1967.
58. **Singer, F. R.,** *Paget's Disease of Bone,* Plenum Press, New York, 1977, 44.
59. **Rubinstein, M. A., Smelin, A., and Freedman, A. L.,** Ostoblasts and osteoclasts in bone marrow aspiration, *Arch. Int. Med.,* 92, 964, 1953.
60. **Bithel, T. C. and Wintrobe, M. M.,** Drug-induced aplastic anemia, *Semin. Hematol.,* 4, 194, 1967.
61. **Pisciotta, A. V.,** Drug-induced leukopenia and aplastic anemia, *Clin. Pharmacol. Ther.,* 12, 13, 1971.
62. **Yunis, A. A.,** Chloramphemicol-induced bone marrow suppression, *Semin. Haemtol.,* 10, 225, 1973.
63. **Krantz, S. B. and Zaentz, S. D.,** Pure red cell aplasia, in *A Year of Hematology,* Silber, R., Golden, A. S., and LoBue, J., Eds., Plenum Press, New York, 1977, 153.
64. **Milch, R. A. and Changus, G. W.,** Response of bone to tumor invasion, *Cancer,* 9, 340, 1956.
65. **Agress, H.,** Comparative study of spreads and section of bone marrow, *Am. J. Clin. Pathol.,* 27, 282, 1957.
66. **Fadem, R. S. and McBirnie, J. E.,** Plasmacytosis in diseases other than the primary plasmacytic disease, *Blood,* 5, 191, 1950.
67. **Burkhardt, R., Bartl, B., Standel, P., and Binsack, T.,** Generalized reaction of bone marrow in neoplastic disorders, *Bibl. Haematol.,* 45, 55, 1978.
68. **Horton, J. E., Raisz, L. G., Simmons, H. A. et al.,** Bone resorbing activity in supernatant fluid from cultured human peripheral blood leukocytes, *Science,* 177, 793, 1972.
69. **Brown, I. N. and Draper, P.,** Growth of Mycobacterium lepraemurium in the mouse bone marrow: an ultrastructural study, *Infect. Immunity,* 13, 1199, 1976.
70. **Desikan, K. V. and Job, C. K.,** A review of postmortem findings in 37 cases of leprosy, *Int. J. Leprosy,* 36, 32, 1968.
71. **Papadimitriou, J. M. and Spector, W. G.,** The ultrastructure of high-and low turnover inflammatory granulomata, *J. Pathol.,* 106, 37, 1972.
72. **Jones-Williams, W., Erozmusk, D. A., Valerie-James, E. M., and Davies, T.,** The fine structure of sarcoid and tuberculous granulomas, *Postgrad. Med. J.,* 46, 496, 1970.
73. **Schneerson-Porat, S., Shahar, A., and Aronson, M.,** Formation of histiocyte rings in response to *Cryptococcus neoformans* infection, *J. Reticuloendothel. Soc.,* 2, 249, 1965.
74. **Shahar, A., Kletter, Y., and Aronson, M.,** Granuloma formation in Cryptococcus, *Isr. J. Med. Sci.,* 5, 1164, 1969.
75. **James, E. M. and Williams, W. J.,** Fine structure and histochemistry of epitheloid cells in sarcoidosis, *Thorax,* 29, 115, 1974.
76. **Soler, P. and Basset, F.,** Morphology and distribution of the cells of a sarcoid granuloma: ultrastructural study of serial sections, *Ann. N.Y. Acad. Sci.,* 278, 147, 1976.
77. **Hunninghake, G. W., Gadek, J. E., Young, R. C., Jr., et al.,** Mechanisms of granuloma formation in pulmonary sarcoidosis by T lympohocytes within the lung, *N. Engl. J. Med.,* 302, 594, 1979.
78. **Scadding, J. G.,** The late stages of pulmonary sarcoidosis, *Postgrad. Med. J.,* 46, 530, 1970.
79. **Fodor, I.,** Histogenesis of beryllium induced bone tumours, *Acta Morphol. Acad. Sci. Hung.,* 25, 99, 1977.
80. **Young, M. D.,** Malaria, in *A Manuel of Tropical Medicine,* 4th ed., Hunter, G. W. and Frye, W. W., Eds., W. B. Saunders, Philadelphia, 316.
81. **Frankenburg, S. and Greenblatt, C. L.,** Cellular changes in the bone marrow of *Plasmodium berghes* infected mice, *Isr. J. Med. Sci.,* 14, 582, 1978.
82. **Srichaikul, T., Panikbutr, N., and Jeumtrakul, P.,** Bone marrow changes in human malaria, *Am. J. Trop. Med.,* 15, 40, 1966.

83. **Weiss, L.**, An electron microscopic study of the vascular sinuses of the bone marrow of the rabbit, *Bull. Johns Hopkins Hosp.*, 108, 171, 1961.
84. **Yamaguchi, H., Takeuchi, H., Torikata, C., et al.**, Experimental osteomyelitis induced by repeated administration of soluble immune complexes: consideration of the fundamental pathogenesis of osteomyelitis, *Int. Arch. Allergy Appl. Immun.*, 49, 763, 1975.
85. **Allam, A. F. and Schuknedt, H. F.**, Pathology of petrositis, *Laryngoscope*, 78, 1813, 1968.
86. **Kiraly, J. F., III and Wheby, M. S.**, Bone marrow necrosis, *Am. J. Med.*, 60, 361, 1976.
87. **Brown, C. H.**, Bone marrow necrosis, a study of 70 cases, *Johns Hopkins Med. J.*, 131, 189, 1972.
88. **Shelley, W. M. and Curtis, E. M.**, Bone marrow and fat embolism in sickle cell anemia and sickle-cell hemoglobin C disease, *Bull. Johns Hopkins Hosp.*, 97, 8, 1959.
89. **Kundel, D. W., Brecher, G., Bodey, G. P., and Brittin, G. M.**, Reticular fibrosis and bone infarction in acute leukemia: implications for prognosis, *Blood*, 23, 526, 1964.
90. **Pynn, K. S. and Katzenstein, R. E.**, Widespread bone marrow embolism with myocardial involvement, *Arch. Pathol.*, 89, 378, 1970.
91. **Naegeli, O.**, *Blutkrankheiten and Blutdiagnostik*, J. Springer, Berlin, 1931.
92. **Jones, R. M.**, Human sternal marrow in hyperthyroid and myxedematous states, *Am. J. Med. Sci.*, 200, 211, 1940.
93. **Axelrod, A. R. and Berman, L.**, The bone marrow in hyperthyroidism and hypothyroidism, *Blood*, 6, 436, 1951.
94. **Douglass, R. C. and Jacobson, S. D.**, Pathologic changes in adult myxedema: survey of 10 necropsies, *J. Clin. Endo.*, 17, 1354, 1957.
95. **Tudhope, G. R.**, *The Thyroid and the Blood*, Heinemann Medical Books, London, 1969.
96. **Muldowney, F. D., Crooks, J., and Wayne, E. J.**, The total red cell mass in thyrotoxicosis and myexedema, *Clin. Sci.*, 16, 309, 1957.
97. **Das, K. C., Mukherjee, M., Sarkar, T. K., et al.**, Erythropoiesis and erythropoietin in hypo—and hyperthyroidism, *J. Clin. Endocrin. Metab.*, 40, 211, 1975.
98. **Boxer, M., Ellman, L., Geller, R., and Wang, C.**, Anemia in primary hyperparathyroidism, *Arch. Intern. Med.*, 137, 588, 1977.
99. **Mallette, L. E., Bilexikian, J. P., and Heath, D. A.**, Primary hyperparathyroidism. Clinical and biochemical features, *Medicine*, 53, 127, 1974.
100. **Hunter, D.**, Hyperparathyroidism: generalized osteoitis fibrosa, *Br. J. Surg.*, 19, 203, 1931.
101. **Levi, J., Bessler, H., Hirsch, I., and Djaldetti, M.**, Inhibition of erythropoiesis by parathyroid hormone, *Proc. 7th Int. Cong. Nephrol.*, 9(Abstr.), 1, 1976.
102. **Zingraff, J., Drueke, T., Marie, P., et al.**, Anemia and secondary hyperparathyroidism, *Arch. Intern. Med.*, 138, 1650, 1978.
103. **Podjarny, E., Rathaus, M., Korzets, A., et al.**, Is anemia of chronic renal failure related to secondary hyperparathyroidism? *Arch. Intern. Med.*, 141, 453, 1981.
104. **Mallinson, C. N., Bloom, S. R., Waren, A. P., et al.**, A glucagonoma syndrome, *Lancet*, 2, 1, 1974.
105. **Higgins, G. A., Recant, L., and Fischman, A. B.**, The glucagonoma syndrome: surgically curable diabetes, *Am. J. Surg.*, 137, 142, 1979.
106. **Naet, J. P. and Guns, M.**, Inhibitory effect of glucagon on erythropoiesis, *Blood*, 55, 997, 1980.
107. **Gordon, A. S.**, Endocrine influences upon the formed elements of blood and blood-forming organs, *Recent Prog. Hormone Res.*, 10, 339, 1952.
108. **Tudhope, G. R.**, Endocrine disease, *Clin. Haematol.*, 1, 475, 1972.
109. **Evans, E. S., van Dyke, D. C., Rosenberg, L. L.**, Interaction of the erythrocyte-stimulating factor with calorigenic hormones, *Endocrinology*, 75, 758, 1964.
110. **Amrein, P. C., Friedman, R., Kosinski, K., and Ellman, L.**, Hematologic changes in anorexia nervosa, *JAMA*, 241, 2190, 1979.
111. **Mant, M. and Faragher, B. S.**, The hematology of anorexia nervosa, *Br. J. Haematol.*, 27, 737, 1972.
112. **Lampert, J. and Lau, B.**, Bone marrow hypoplasia in anorexia nervosa, *Br. J. Haemat.*, 27, 737, 1972.
113. **Cornbleet, P. J., Moir, R. C., and Wolf, R. L.**, A histochemical study of bone marrow hypoplasia in anorexia nervosa, *Virchows Archiv.*, 374, 239, 1977.
114. **Paulo, L. G., Fink, G. D., Roh, B. L., and Fisher, J. W.**, Effects of several androgen and steroid metabolites on erythropoietin production in the isolated perfused dog kidney, *Blood*, 43, 39, 1974.
115. **Singer, J. W., Samuels, A. I., and Adamson, J. W.**, Steroids and hematopoiesis. I. Effect of steroids on in vitro erythroid colony growth, Structure/activity relationships, *J. Cell. Physiol.*, 88, 127, 1976.

116. **Urabe, A., Sassa, S., and Kappas, A.,** The influence of steroid hormone metabolites on the *in vitro* development of erythroid colonies derived from human bone marrow cells, *J. Exp. Med.*, 149, 1314, 1979.
117. **Rosenblum, A. L. and Carbone, P. P.,** Androgenic hormones and human granulopoiesis *in vitro, Blood,* 43, 351, 1974.
118. **McCullough, E. P. and Jones, R.,** Effect of androgens on the blood count of men, *J. Clin. Endocrinol.*, 2, 243, 1942.
119. **Reddy, G. N., Nager, S., and Trubowitz, S.,** Interaction of coexisting primary hypogonadism and polycythemia rubra vera, *J. Med. Soc. N.J.*, 77, 430, 1980.
120. **Piliero, S. J., Medici, P. T. and Haber, C.,** The interrelationships of the endocrine and erythropoietic systems in the rat with special reference to the mechanisms of action of estradiol and testosterone, *Ann. N.Y. Acad. Sci.*, 149, 336, 1968.
121. **Mirand, E. A. and Gordon, A. S.,** Mechanism of estrogen action in erythropoiesis, *Endocrinol.*, 78, 325, 1966.
122. **Jepson, J. and Lowenstein, L.,** Inhibition of the stem cell action of erythropoietin by estradiol, *Proc. Soc. Exp. Biol. Med.*, 123, 457, 1966.
123. **Leitner, S. J.,** Bone marrow biopsy. *Hematology in the Light of Sternal Puncture,* Grune & Stratton, 1949.
124. **Gordon, A. S.,** Endocrine influences upon the formed elements of blood and blood forming organs, *Recent Prog. Hormone Res.*, 10, 339, 1952.
125. **Zalman, F., Maloney, M. A., and Patt, H. M.,** Differentiation response of early erythropoietic and granulopoietic progenitors to dexamethasone and cortisone, *J. Exp. Med.*, 149, 67, 1979.
126. **Nordenson, N. S.,** The bone marrow in chronic nephritis, *Folia Haemat.*, 59, 1, 1968.
127. **Sjogren, U. and Thysell, H.,** Bone marrow morphology in patients on regular hemodialysis treatment, *Acta Haematol.*, 58, 332, 1977.
128. **Callen, I. R. and Limarz, L. R.,** Blood and bone marrow studies in renal disease, *Am. J. Pathol.*, 20, 3, 1950.
129. **Desforges, J. F.,** Anemia in uremia, *Arch. Intern. Med.*, 126, 808, 1970.
130. **Fisher, J. W., Foley, J. E., Moriyama, Y., et al.,** Studies on the mechanism of the anemia of renal insufficiency, *Proc. Clin. Dial. Transplant Forum,* 6, 42, 1976.
131. **Gonen, B., Levi, J., Van der Lyn E., and Aldelli, M.,** ^{3}H-thymidine, ^{3}H-uridine, and ^{3}H-leucine uptake in erythroblasts of patients with chronic renal failure, *Nephron,* 21, 95, 1978.
132. **Wallner, S. F., Vautrin, R., Kurnick, J. E., and Ward, H. P.,** The effect of serum from patients with chronic renal failure on erythroid colony growth *in vitro, J. Lab. Clin. Med.*, 92, 370, 1978.
133. **Wallner, S. F. and Vautrin, R. M.,** The anemia of chronic renal failure. Studies of iron transport *in vitro, J. Lab. Clin. Med.*, 96, 67, 1980.
134. **Ohno, Y., Rege, A. B., Fisher, J. W., and Barona, J.,** Inhibitors of erythroid colony-forming cells (CFU-E and BFU-E) in sera of azotemic patients with anemia of renal disease, *J. Lab. Clin. Med.*, 92, 916, 1978.
135. **Marshall, J. W., Ahearn, D. J., Nothum, R. J. et al.,** Adherence of blood component to dialyzer membranes. Morphological studies, *Nephron,* 12, 157, 1974.

INDEX

A

B

C

D

E

F

G

H

I

K

L

Lymphadenopathy, 61, 201, 256—257

M

N

O

P

R

S

T

U

V

W

X